AF352369

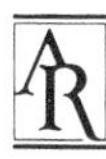

ANNUAL REVIEW OF MEDICINE: Selected Topics in the Clinical Sciences

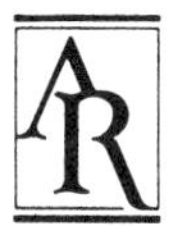

ANNUAL REVIEW OF MEDICINE: Selected Topics in the Clinical Sciences

VOLUME 53, 2002

C. THOMAS CASKEY, *Editor*
Cogentech, Inc.

CHRISTOPHER AUSTIN, *Associate Editor*
Merck Research Laboratories

JAMES HOXIE, *Associate Editor*
University of Pennsylvania

www.annualreviews.org   science@annualreviews.org   650-493-4400

ANNUAL REVIEWS
4139 El Camino Way • P.O. BOX 10139 • Palo Alto, California 94303-0139

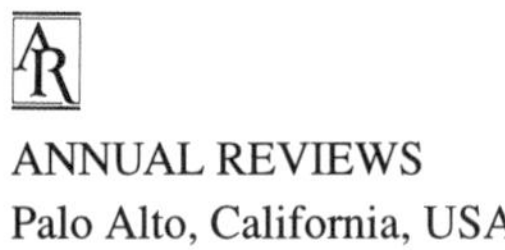

ANNUAL REVIEWS
Palo Alto, California, USA

International Standard Serial Number: 0066-4219
International Standard Book Number: 0-8243-0553-1
Library of Congress Catalog Card Number: A51-1659

Annual Review and publication titles are registered trademarks of Annual Reviews.
♾ The paper used in this publication meets the minimum requirements of American National Standards for Information Sciences—Permanence of Paper for Printed Library Materials, ANSI Z39.48-1992.

Annual Reviews and the Editors of its publications assume no responsibility for the statements expressed by the contributors to this *Annual Review*.

TYPESET BY TECHBOOKS, FAIRFAX, VA
PRINTED AND BOUND IN THE UNITED STATES OF AMERICA

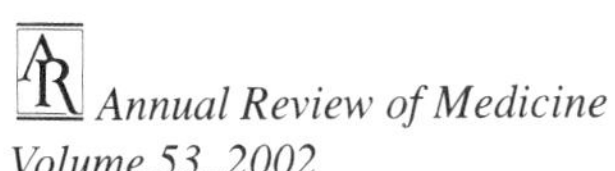

Annual Review of Medicine
Volume 53, 2002

CONTENTS

ERRATA
An online log of corrections to *Annual Review of Medicine*
chapters may be found at http://med.annualreviews.org/errata.shtml

Chapters by Category

From the ***Annual Review of Psychology***, Volume 53 (2002)

Insomnia: Conceptual Issues in the Development, Maintenance and Treatment of Sleep Disorder in Adults, Colin A. Espie

Depression: Perspectives from Affective Neuroscience, Richard J. Davidson, Diego Pizzagalli, Jack B. Nitschke, and Katherine Putnam

Emotions, Morbidity, and Mortality: New Perspectives from Psychoneuroimmunology, Janice K. Kiecolt-Glaser, Lynanne McGuire, Theodore F. Robles, and Ronald Glaser

Effects of Psychological and Social Factors on Organic Disease: A Critical Assessment of Research on Coronary Heart Disease, David S. Krantz, Melissa K. McCeney

From the ***Annual Review of Public Health***, Volume 23 (2002)

Tuberculosis, Parvathi Tiruviluamala and Lee B. Reichman

The Public Health Impact of Alzheimer's Disease, 2000–2050: Potential Implication of Treatment Advances, Phillip D. Sloane, Sheryl S. Zimmerman, Chirayath Suchindran, Peter Reed, Lily Wang, Malaz Boustani, and S. Sudha

Direct Marketing of Pharmaceuticals to Consumers, Alan Lyles

Morbidity and Mortality from Medical Errors: An Increasingly Serious Public Health Problem, David P. Phillips and Charlene C. Bredder

ERRATA

Erratum: *Annu. Rev. Med.* 2001. 52:371–400
Charis Eng, Heather Hampel, Albert de la Chapelle, GENETIC TESTING
FOR CANCER PREDISPOSITION

The copyright year was mistakenly printed as 2000. The correct year is 2001.

Erratum: *Annu. Rev. Med.* 2001. 52:147–60
Benjamin Samstein, Jean Emond, LIVER TRANSPLANTS FROM LIVING
RELATED DONORS

The copyright year was mistakenly printed as 2000. The correct year is 2001.

Erratum: *Annu. Rev. Med.* 2001. 52:125–45
Christine A. White, Robin L. Weaver, Antonio J. Grillo-López, ANTIBODY-
TARGETED IMMUNOTHERAPY FOR TREATMENT OF MALIGNANCY

The fourth paragraph on p. 138 should read as follows:

"Toxicity has been primarily hematologic with 27% Grade 4 neutropenia and
10% Grade 4 thrombocytopenia in the Phase I/II trial at the 0.4 mCi/kg dose.
A significant correlation was noted between percent bone marrow involvement
with NHL at baseline and hematologic toxicity. In that study, only 6% of patients
required hospitalization for infection (17)."

In Table 4 on p. 137, the results reported on "relapsed or refractory, LG/F, or
transformed" and "relapsed or refractory, LG/F, or transformed thrombocytopenic
patients" are from interim data. A footnote to that effect was omitted.

Erratum: *Annu. Rev. Med.* 2001. 52:259–74
Michael E. Ohl, Samuel I. Miller, SALMONELLA: A MODEL FOR
BACTERIAL PATHOGENESIS

Figure 3, p. 265: The image and caption have been revised as follows:

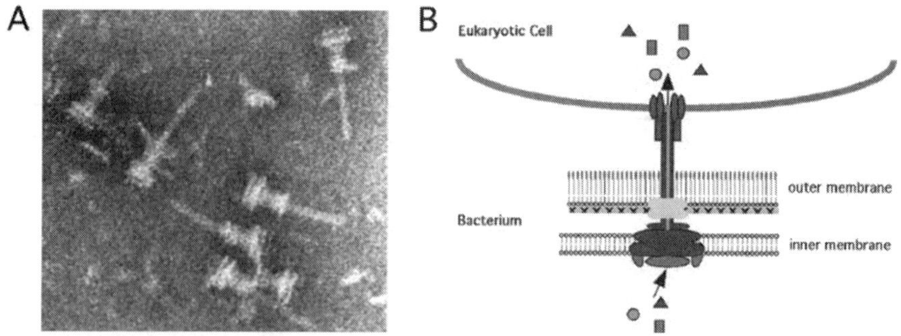

Figure 3   *Panel A:* Electron micrograph showing purified needle complexes. The two ring-shaped structures at the complex base associate with the bacterial inner and outer membranes and are homologous to the basal body of the flagellar export apparatus. The needle portion is unique to the type three secretion apparatus and is thought to bridge the bacterium and host cell during secretion of effector proteins. Micrograph courtesy of T. Kimbrough. *Panel B:* Diagram showing a needle complex spanning the bacterial and host cell membranes.

ANNUAL REVIEWS is a nonprofit scientific publisher established to promote the advancement of the sciences. Beginning in 1932 with the *Annual Review of Biochemistry*, the Company has pursued as its principal function the publication of high-quality, reasonably priced *Annual Review* volumes. The volumes are organized by Editors and Editorial Committees who invite qualified authors to contribute critical articles reviewing significant developments within each major discipline. The Editor-in-Chief invites those interested in serving as future Editorial Committee members to communicate directly with him. Annual Reviews is administered by a Board of Directors, whose members serve without compensation.

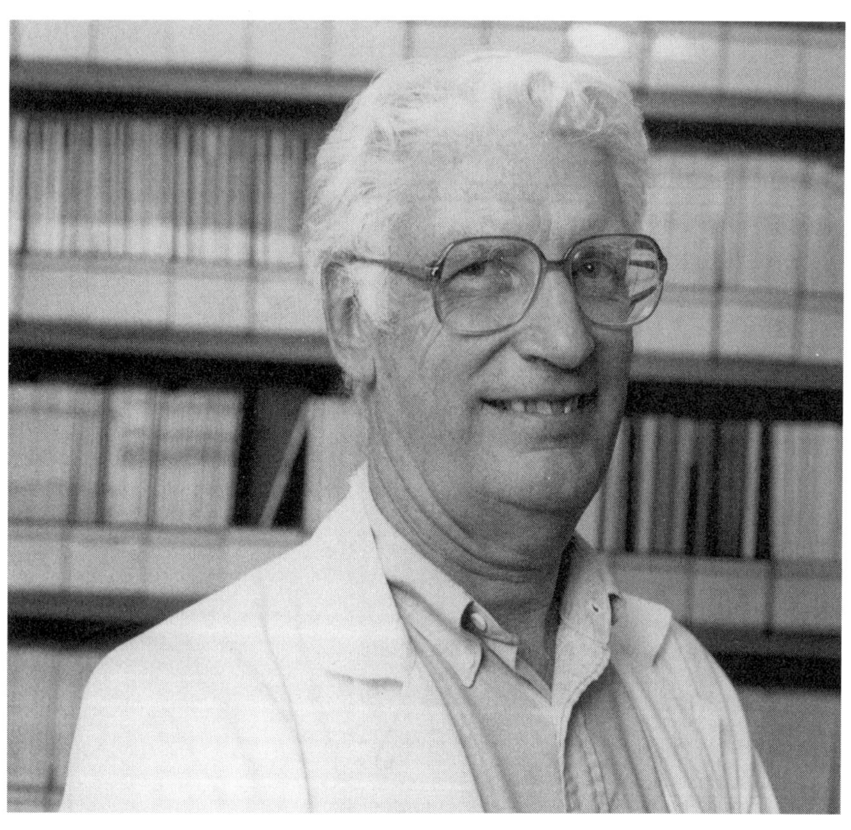

Peter C. Nowell

Annu. Rev. Med. 2002. 53:1–13

PROGRESS WITH CHRONIC MYELOGENOUS LEUKEMIA: A Personal Perspective over Four Decades

Peter C. Nowell

Department of Pathology and Laboratory Medicine, University of Pennsylvania School of Medicine, Philadelphia, Pennsylvania 19104; e-mail: nowell@mail.med.upenn.edu

Key Words BCR-ABL, CML, leukemia, Philadelphia chromosome, STI571

■ **Abstract** Our understanding and treatment of chronic myelogenous leukemia (CML) has progressed since 1960 in parallel with work on cancer in general. CML provided the first evidence of a specific genetic change associated with a human cancer (the Philadelphia chromosome) and the clonal nature of these disorders. With improved cytogenetic and molecular techniques over subsequent decades, the specific genetic rearrangements of CML and many other tumors were defined and the complex mechanisms of carcinogenesis gradually unraveled. During this period, improved treatments for CML (chemotherapy, interferon, bone marrow transplantation) were implemented, and therapy targeted to the specific genetic change in the leukemic cells has recently been brought to promising clinical trials. Similar efforts are under way for other human cancers, and although the problem is enormously complex, there is real hope for major improvements in controlling these disorders.

INTRODUCTION

In many respects, chronic myelogenous leukemia (CML) has been a model of our general progress over the past 40 years in discovering the fundamental nature of leukemias and lymphomas, as well as other human neoplasms, and in developing more sophisticated treatments. My personal involvement began with cytogenetic studies in the late 1950s. Although my subsequent research has focused primarily on other hematopoietic tumors, I have remained interested in CML and in the expansion of fundamental knowledge and the development of new therapies.

In this paper, I briefly review the history of these basic and clinical developments with respect to CML and the parallels with neoplasia in general. It has been a long, slow process. Today we have an enormous amount of new knowledge about neoplastic processes, with great potential for improvements in the control of cancer. However, we also face the frustrating recognition that different genetic alterations generate different tumors, and there is going to be no single, simple answer for the treatment of all cancers.

0066-4219/02/0218-0001$14.00

The story as presented here is a personal perspective, and in some areas, particularly the most recent molecular genetic developments, it lacks sophistication. A number of these newer aspects, both basic and clinical, are presented in other chapters in this volume.

CYTOGENETICS AND MOLECULAR GENETICS OF CML

The story has been told before (1) of how, as a junior faculty member in the pathology department of the University of Pennsylvania Medical School, I was growing leukemic cells in tissue culture, using a technique recently developed by Edwin Osgood (2), when I inadvertently rediscovered the value of hypotonic treatment in cytogenetics. I rinsed the slides with tap water before staining them with Giemsa for the morphological studies on cell differentiation that I was doing. I had had no intention of investigating the chromosomes of these cells and knew nothing about cytogenetics, but when I saw some metaphases with countable chromosomes on the slides, I felt that they might be worth examining. I had spent several previous years at the U.S. Naval Radiological Defense Laboratory in San Francisco, studying radiation effects and radiation carcinogenesis (3), and so the concept of a somatic genetic change contributing to carcinogenesis seemed reasonable.

Cancer cytogenetics was not a particularly active field (the correct number of human chromosomes, 46, had been determined only two years previously) (4), but after inquiring among local colleagues, I found a graduate student at the Fox Chase Institute for Cancer Research, David Hungerford, who was doing his doctoral thesis on human chromosomes and needed material to work with. This resulted in a collaboration in which I cultured leukemic cells from patients and Dave Hungerford used the slides to make the "squash" preparations that were then utilized for cytogenetic studies (Figure 1). We first examined several cases of acute myelogenous leukemia, found no obvious consistent chromosome change (5), and then moved on to CML. Here, David found an abnormally small chromosome in the metaphases of two cases (Figure 2). Because this first study involved only male patients, we originally thought that perhaps this was derived from the Y chromosome (6). As we expanded the study to women, however, it became clear that it was derived from one of the smallest autosomes (7). More importantly, because this abnormality was present in essentially every dividing cell and in every typical case of CML, it strongly suggested two major conclusions: first, that the leukemia in each patient had arisen from a single cell in which this somatic genetic change had occurred and given the progeny of that cell a selective growth advantage for clonal expansion, ultimately leading to systemic dispersion and clinical CML; and, second, that this specific genetic change, visible microscopically, was critical to the pathogenesis of this type of leukemia.

Our findings were quickly confirmed in several other laboratories (8), and at the First International Conference on Nomenclature in 1960, it was decided to name abnormal chromosomes in human tumors after the city of discovery, hence the name "Philadelphia chromosome" (9).

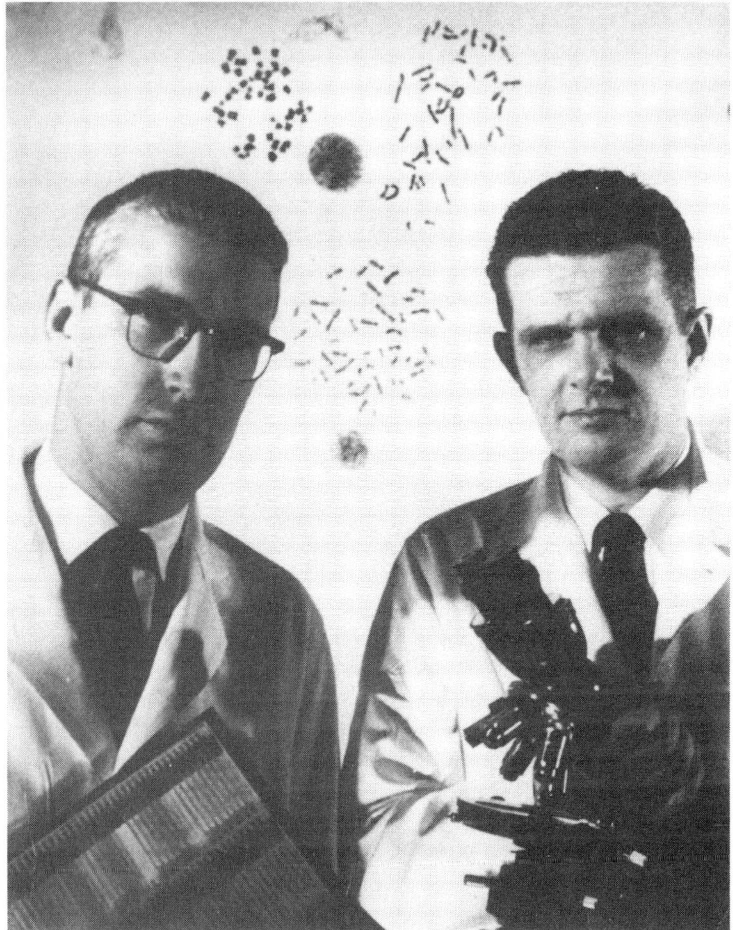

Figure 1   Peter Nowell and David Hungerford while collaborating on cytogenetic studies.

The 1960s and 1970s

The next decade was somewhat frustrating. Many cancer researchers preferred not to accept a genetic basis for neoplasia, since it implied irreversibility; and because of the relatively crude cytogenetic techniques of the 1960s, no other specific alterations were identified in human neoplasms. It was suggested that the Philadelphia chromosome was merely an epiphenomenon and was not directly involved in pathogenesis.

The climate changed in the 1970s with the development of "banding" techniques, which permitted identification of individual chromosomes and also abnormalities in small segments of each chromosome. Using these methods, Janet

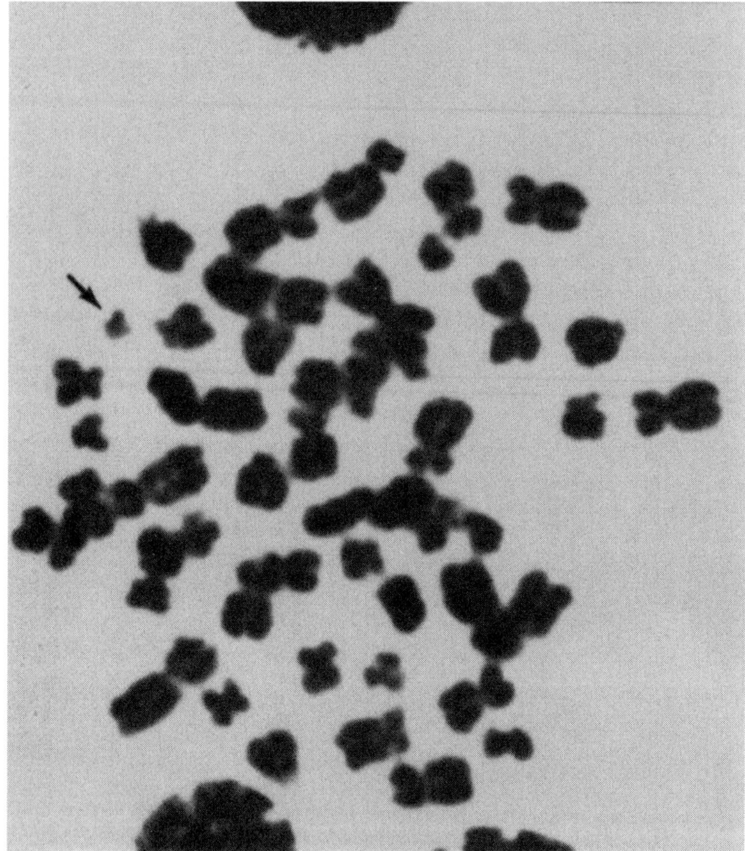

Figure 2 Metaphase from the first publication (6) describing the small abnormal chromosome (arrow) in CML cells.

Rowley (10) at the University of Chicago demonstrated that the Philadelphia chromosome resulted from an unequal translocation between terminal segments of the long arms of chromosomes 9 and 22 (Figure 3). More importantly, Rowley and many other laboratories were now able, with banding, to demonstrate other specific chromosomal translocations associated with nearly every other subtype of leukemia and lymphoma that was investigated (reviewed in 11). This clearly demonstrated that somatic genetic changes played a critical role in the pathogenesis of most, if not all, hematopoietic malignancies. This principle was rapidly extended to the more common epithelial cancers, although the cytogenetic changes were more variable and complex.

Also in the 1970s, more sophisticated cytogenetic findings in CML aided the development of the concept of clonal evolution as a basis for tumor progression, a concept that I had also found attractive during the previous decade (12). In CML,

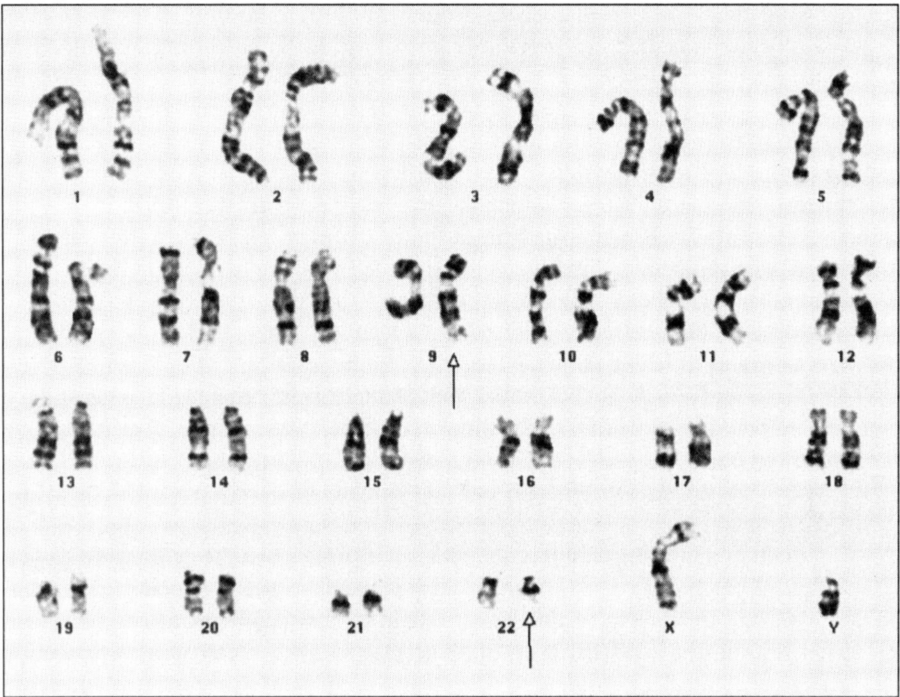

Figure 3   Banded karyotype illustrating the t(9;22) translocation that produces the Philadelphia chromosome (arrows).

it was shown that the characteristic clinical progression, resulting in the terminal blast crisis, was very commonly associated with the expansion of a subclone of the original neoplasm that had acquired one or more cytogenetic alterations in addition to the Philadelphia chromosome (e.g., a second Philadelphia chromosome, trisomy 8, isochromosome 17q) (13). This finding strongly supported the view, which had been suggested by animal studies in previous decades, that the tendency of tumors to become more malignant over time resulted from additional somatic genetic changes, which allowed a more aggressive subpopulation of the original clone to expand and to generate these additional biological and clinical characteristics (reviewed in 14). Like the original cytogenetic findings in CML, this clonal evolution concept was subsequently supported by additional cytogenetic, and ultimately molecular genetic, studies in many other leukemias and solid tumors, and it is now generally accepted as the basis for tumor progression.

The 1980s

In the 1980s, molecular genetic techniques became available, and the specific genes involved in the cytogenetic abnormalities in human neoplasia could be investigated. With respect to CML, Groffen et al. (15) found in 1984 that the t(9;22) translocation resulted in a previously known oncogene on chromosome 9, ABL, becoming fused with a previously unknown gene, named BCR, on chromosome 22. ABL encodes a tyrosine kinase, and the p210 kd chimeric protein (BCR-ABL) resulting from the translocation was presumed to have increased kinase activity, resulting in a proliferative advantage, particularly for cells differentiating along a myeloid lineage and so generating the expanded clone of CML cells.

Earlier studies had indicated that the initial cell carrying a Philadelphia chromosome was apparently a multipotential stem cell with the capacity to differentiate into all hematopoietic lineages (16). In vivo, however, the BCR-ABL product clearly provided the major proliferative advantage to the cells differentiating as granulocytes, although Ph-positive erythroid and megakaryocytic elements, as well as B cells and monocytes, were also demonstrable in the patient (17). Interestingly, this has not been true of T cells, which have typically remained Ph-negative. We followed one CML patient for 30 years without demonstrating Ph-positive T cells (18), which suggests that this lineage may actually be disadvantaged by the BCR-ABL protein.

Another interesting result of the molecular studies was the demonstration that patients presenting with Ph-positive *acute* leukemia (usually lymphocytic in phenotype) apparently had, in most cases, a slight structural difference in the translocation, resulting in a p190 BCR-ABL product (19, 20). This altered protein apparently had an even greater proliferative effect than the typical p210, resulting in the more aggressive clinical presentation. In a few cases these "acute leukemias" proved, on cytogenetic study, to be previously unrecognized CML that had progressed to blast crisis through additional karyotypic changes. These then showed the usual p210 product of CML.

Another result of the availability of molecular techniques in the 1980s was the identification of at least a few of the specific genes involved in progression of CML to the blast crisis. The gene or genes associated with the common additional change of trisomy 8 remain to be identified, but it has been shown that the also frequent isochromosome 17q, in this and several other neoplasms, involves loss of one p53 gene along with the short arm of the abnormal chromosome 17, and loss of function of the other p53 allele through various submicroscopic mechanisms (21, 22). It is now widely recognized that loss of p53's anticarcinogenic effects plays a major role in many different human malignancies, and it is not surprising that this is one of the most common contributors to tumor progression in CML.

Throughout the 1980s, the techniques used to identify BCR-ABL in CML also proved of great value in many other human tumors. In the leukemias and lymphomas particularly, chromosome translocations provided the clues for identifying a wide variety of genes involved in the pathogenesis of these disorders. Most of these were previously unknown genes, such as BCR. An exception was MYC, an oncogene previously identified in animal studies, which proved to be involved in a subset of both B-cell and T-cell neoplasms (reviewed in 23). The other genes, newly identified, were found to be generally lineage-specific, functioning only to generate a B-cell, T-cell, or myeloid neoplasm when deregulated by translocation. My own work during this period, with Carlo Croce, focused on lymphoid tumors and helped to identify a very interesting new gene, which he named BCL2, that turned out to be involved in regulating not proliferation but programmed cell death (apoptosis) (24, 25). This helped to initiate studies in altered apoptosis as a factor in tumorigenesis, which has proved important in a wide variety of human neoplasms.

By the end of the 1980s, it was apparent that essentially all human tumors resulted from specific genetic alterations, although it remains unclear why these are primarily translocations in hematopoietic neoplasms (with resultant increased activity of oncogenes) and deletions of genetic material (and associated "tumor suppressor genes") in solid tumors.

The 1990s

In the 1990s, with increasingly sophisticated molecular techniques, the extent of complexity, at both the gene and protein levels, continued to expand. Details of this progress are discussed elsewhere in this volume, so I limit my brief comments primarily to CML.

As numerous laboratories have explored the effects of the BCR-ABL p210 gene product, multiple functions have emerged. The protein has been shown to have constitutively activated tyrosine kinase activity, resulting in a major proliferative advantage, particularly for cells differentiating in the myeloid lineage (26). The p210 protein also appears to affect hematopoiesis through interactions with RAS-related pathways, SHIP proteins, and Stat5 (27–29). In addition, there is a anti-apoptotic effect, apparently primarily via BCL2 and related proteins, contributing to the expansion and survival of the Ph-positive clone (30). Finally, there is evidence that the BCR-ABL product influences adhesion molecules such as one beta 1 integrin (31), altering the interaction of Ph-positive cells with the local stroma. As has been demonstrated with these and other neoplastic cells, defects in adhesion can influence both proliferation and the ability of the cells to detach and move to other sites. Because leukemic cells metastasize "physiologically," a decrease in adhesion may not be as important in this respect as for the more common epithelial cancers, but it still may contribute to the easy escape of CML cells from the bone marrow and their spread throughout the body, generating the clinical and hematological characteristics of the leukemia.

Some recent data (32) suggest that the BCR-ABL product may also generate a degree of genetic instability in the Ph-positive cells, perhaps through interaction with the xeroderma pigmentosum group B (XPB) protein, which is important in DNA repair. This could be an important contributor to the almost invariable clinical progression of this disease, with the addition of further karyotypic changes that occur in the context of the blast crisis. This finding is of particular interest because the underlying basis for this instability in CML and its resultant clinical progression has been long debated. Hypotheses included some submicroscopic alteration in a "mutator" gene, unrelated to BCR-ABL, which occurred very early in the clonal expansion of CML cells, and even the possibility of other submicroscopic changes that led to such clonal expansion before the t(9;22) translocation occurred (33). It now seems likely that this mutator characteristic is one function of the p210 BCR-ABL product, and it may be possible for the CML clone to acquire all the characteristics of the chronic leukemic phenotype, including the high probability of further genetic changes, as the result of a single initial genetic alteration, the t(9;22) translocation producing the Philadelphia chromosome.

It is interesting that the other common chronic leukemia, chronic lymphocytic leukemia (CLL), which is characterized by a slowly expanding B-cell clone, does not show the same genetic instability as CML. Typically, CLL remains in the chronic stage for many years without clinical progression or the associated acquisition of additional genetic changes in the neoplastic cells. Unfortunately, the initiation of CLL—unlike nearly all other leukemias—has not been associated with a specific genetic alteration, so it has been difficult to clarify the basis for its unusual genetic stability (34).

In many respects, the increasingly complex molecular and functional findings in CML throughout the 1990s represent a prototype of the general results in other human cancers. It has become clear that not only growth-regulatory genes (involving proliferation, apoptosis, and differentiation) are important, but also genetic instability and, for the non-hematopoietic tumors, genetic changes that give the neoplastic cells the capacity for invasion and metastasis. As noted above, although a few genes such as p53 and MYC are associated with a variety of human cancers, in general most different types of tumors result from alterations in different genes.

With the increasing sophistication of molecular genetic techniques, such as microarray analysis, which permits the recognition of altered expression of numerous genes within a particular tumor, the levels of complexity have continued to expand. It is not certain how many steps are required for a fully developed neoplasm, although it is clear that for the common cancers these are multiple. CML may represent the other extreme, at which the single genetic change identified in the chronic phase may confer all the characteristics necessary for the primary low-grade leukemia, but other early alterations have not been ruled out (33).

Most important, the identification of both relatively simple levels of genetic change in the leukemias and more complex findings in the common carcinomas may eventually lead to specific targets for therapy and hence better control of these diseases. The evolving treatment of CML, as a prototype for this concept, is discussed in the next section.

TREATMENT OF CML

Changes in therapy for CML over the past four decades have in many respects paralleled the slow advances in knowledge of the basic biology of neoplasia and the gradually expanding applications of this knowledge to the control of cancer in general.

In the 1950s and 1960s, when various chemotherapies came into use for leukemia and other neoplasms, CML was included. Agents such as hydroxyurea and busulfan were utilized for most patients. Unfortunately, although many of these individuals achieved a significant degree of hematologic remission, the normal course of the disease, with progression to blast crisis, was very rarely altered significantly, and overall survival was generally not prolonged (35).

In the 1980s, our understanding of immune function increased and various immunological approaches to human cancer treatment were attempted. The cytokine interferon-α, either alone or in combination with conventional chemotherapy, was found to improve both the clinical course and overall survival of many CML patients (reviewed in 36, 37). Although individual responses vary considerably, hematologic and cytogenetic remissions are not uncommon, and this has represented a significant advance in the treatment of many CML patients. One limitation of interferon therapy has been its toxicity, and in some cases, interferon treatment must be discontinued despite a positive effect on the patient's leukemia.

In parallel with interferon, bone marrow transplantation has come into use for CML treatment. Although the possibility of successful allogeneic bone marrow transplantation was first demonstrated in the 1950s (38), it took several decades before graft-versus-host reactions (GVHR) were sufficiently controlled to make this a feasible therapeutic option for patients with CML and other leukemias (36, 37). In the 1990s, bone marrow transplantation for CML became significantly more sophisticated. Techniques were developed for generating populations of hematopoietic stem cells from the bone marrow and peripheral blood for allogeneic transplants, and also for isolating purified autologous stem cells, free of Ph-positive cells, from the patient's own hematopoietic system (39). In both circumstances, the patient is subjected to massive doses of chemotherapy, in an attempt to eliminate the leukemic cells before transplant, and this very aggressive approach limits, to some degree, the patients who are considered appropriate for such treatment.

There are positive and negative aspects to both allogeneic and autologous bone marrow transplantation. As indicated, allogeneic transplants generate GVHR, but a graft-versus-leukemia effect has also been recognized, which may in fact help to eliminate residual neoplastic cells in the patient. There are current efforts to enhance this graft-versus-leukemia effect (40). Similarly, although autologous transplants obviously lack GVHR risk, there is the issue of eliminating the patient's Ph-positive cells from the peripheral blood or bone marrow preparations transplanted. One recent approach to this issue has been the development of antisense oligonucleotides to specifically interfere with BCR-ABL RNA or to similarly block the MYB oncogene (41, 42). The former is a direct attack on the key genetic defect of CML; the latter is the result of the experimental observation that an anti-MYB construct had a greater inhibitory effect on leukemic cells than on normal cells. Both approaches are currently in clinical trials (43), and their ultimate value remains to be determined.

Bone marrow transplantation is one major current therapy for CML in which the identification of residual Ph-positive cells is critical, both in autologous cell preparations for infusion and in the patient after therapy. Again, the pluses and minuses of different approaches are currently under investigation. Cytogenetics is a relatively crude way of identifying residual leukemic cells, and fluorescence in situ hybridization (FISH) for the BCR-ABL translocation, in either proliferating or nondividing cells, is only somewhat more effective (44). The most sensitive technique is RT-PCR, either qualitative or quantitative, but if primitive Ph-positive cells are not transcribing the BCR-ABL RNA at the time of study, this approach may generate false negative results (45). Also, a very few cells with the BCR-ABL rearrangement have been identified in the blood of normal individuals (46), and although the significance of this finding is still unclear, this also could produce confusion if a very sensitive technique were being utilized to detect Ph-positive cells before or after bone marrow transplantation.

Until recently, although improved therapeutic techniques for CML had been developed, none of them, as a primary treatment, was directed specifically at the abnormal gene product in the Ph-positive cells. This has now changed with the introduction of a drug called STI571, which has a direct inhibitory effect on the tyrosine kinase activity of ABL. This drug appears to complex with the catalytic domain of ABL, keeping it in an inactive conformation, and having both antiproliferative and proapoptotic effects in Ph-positive cells (47). Although STI571, through this function, would be expected to interfere with normal ABL as well as with the BCR-ABL product in CML patients, its significant activity appears to be primarily related to the latter, and no major toxic effects involving other cells have yet been reported.

Results of clinical trials with STI571 are very encouraging (48). Most patients have shown a prolonged clinical and cytogenetic response, with little evidence of resistance to the drug, although there have been some indications of resistance in studies in vitro with Ph-positive cell lines (49). Obviously, these clinical results need to be extended, including the efficacy of STI571 in combination with other therapies, but to date it appears that CML may be one of the still very few human neoplasms in which we can specifically target the genetic alteration in the tumor cells, with minimal or no toxic effects on normal cells.

CONCLUSION

As is true of other human tumors, the past 40 years have brought a remarkable increase in what we know of the basic biology of CML, and now we are witnessing the beginnings of new, specific therapies based on that greater knowledge. It has been a long course, with literally decades being spent in moving from one stage to the next. Also, as our understanding has expanded, we have become increasingly aware of the complexity of the problem, recognizing that the specific approach to one neoplasm will probably not be useful in the treatment of another that involves a different genetic alteration.

It is encouraging that a specific attack (STI571) on the characteristic genetic change in CML has been developed, and that others, such as the antisense approach, are being actively explored. The hope is, of course, not only that this approach will be a major improvement for the treatment of CML but also that similar compounds, directed toward specific genetic changes in other tumors, will likewise attain clinical acceptance and provide specific treatments for many other human cancers. This may take several decades, but the long-term outlook is certainly a positive one.

Visit the Annual Reviews home page at www.AnnualReviews.org

LITERATURE CITED

1. Nowell PC. 1993. From chromosomes to oncogenes: a personal perspective. In *The Causes and Consequences of Chromosomal Aberrations*, ed. IR Kirsch, pp. 505–16. Boca Raton, FL: CRC

2. Osgood EE, Krippaehne ML. 1955. The gradient tissue culture method. *Exp. Cell Res.* 9:116–27

3. Nowell P, Cole L, Ellis M. 1956. Induction of intestinal carcinoma in the mouse by whole-body fast neutron irradiation. *Cancer Res.* 16:873–76

4. Tjio JM, Levan A. 1956. The chromosome number of man. *Hereditas* 42:1–6

5. Nowell P, Hungerford D, Brooks C. 1958. Chromosomal characteristics of normal and leukemic human leukocytes after short-term tissue culture. *Proc. Am. Assoc. Cancer Res.* 2:331 (Abstr.)

6. Nowell P, Hungerford D. 1960. Chromosomes of normal and leukemic human leukocytes. *J. Natl. Cancer Inst.* 25:85–109

7. Nowell P, Hungerford D. 1960. A minute chromosome in human chronic granulocytic leukemia. *Science* 132:1497 (Abstr.)

8. Tough IM, Court Brown WM, Baikie AG, et al. 1961. Cytogenetic studies in chronic myeloid leukaemia and acute leukaemia associated with mongolism. *Lancet* 1:411–17

9. Hsu TC. 1979. *Human and Mammalian Cytognetics*. New York: Springer-Verlag

10. Rowley JD. 1973. A new consistent chromosomal abnormality in chronic myelogenous leukaemia identified by quinacrine fluorescence and giemsa staining. *Nature* 243:290–93

11. Heim S, Mitelman F. 1987. *Cancer Cytogenetics*. New York: Liss

12. Cole L, Nowell P. 1965. Radiation carcinogenesis: the sequence of events. *Science* 150:1782–86

13. Rowley JD. 1980. Ph-positive leukaemia, including chronic myelogenous leukaemia. *Clin. Haematol.* 9:55–86

14. Nowell P. 1976. The clonal evolution of tumor cell populations. *Science* 194:23–28

15. Groffen J, Stephenson JR, Heisterkamp N, et al. 1984. Philadelphia chromosomal breakpoints are clustered within a limited region, bcr, on chromosome 22. *Cell* 36:93–99

16. Fialkow FJ, Denman AM, Jacobson RJ, et al. 1978. Chronic myelocytic leukemia: origin of some lymphocytes from leukemic stem cells. *J. Clin. Invest.* 62:815–20

17. Nitta M, Kato Y, Strife A, et al. 1985. Incidence of involvement of the B and T lymphocyte lineages in chronic myelogenous leukemia. *Blood* 66:1053–59

18. Nowell PC, Finan JB, Moore JS, et al. 1989. Ph-negative T cells in a patient with chronic myelogenous leukemia for twenty-eight years. *Leuk. Res.* 13:1019–23

19. Kurzrock R, Shtarid M, Romero P, et al. 1987. A novel c-Abl protein product in Philadelphia-positive acute lymphoblastic leukaemia. *Nature* 325:631–35

20. Chan LC, Karhi KK, Rayter SI, et al. 1987. A novel Abl protein expressed in Philadelphia chromosome positive acute lymphoblastic leukaemia. *Nature* 325:635–37

21. Feinstein E, Cimino G, Gale RP, et al. 1991. p53 in chronic myelogenous leukemia in acute phase. *Proc. Natl. Acad. Sci. USA* 88:6293–97

22. Nakai H, Misawa S. 1995. Chromosome 17 abnormalities and inactivation of the p53 gene in chronic myeloid leukemia and their prognostic significance. *Leuk. Lymphoma* 19:213–18

23. Nowell PC, Croce CM. 1990. Chromosome translocations and oncogenes in human lymphoid tumors. *Am. J. Clin. Pathol.* 94:229–37

24. Tsujimoto Y, Finger L, Yunis J, et al. 1984. Cloning of the chromosome breakpoint of neoplastic B-cells with the t(14;18) chromosome translocation. *Science* 226:1097–99

25. Hockenbury D, Nuñez G, Milliman C, et al. 1990. *Nature* 348:334–36

26. Lugo TG, Pendergast A-M, Muller AJ, et al. 1990. Tyrosine kinase activity and transformation potency of BCR-ABL oncogene products. *Science* 247:1079–82

27. Sawyers CL, McLaughlin J, Witte ON. 1995. Genetic requirement for Ras in the transformation of fibroblasts and hematopoietic cells by the BCR-ABL oncogene. *J. Exp. Med.* 181:307–13

28. Odai H, Sasaki K, Iwamatsu A, et al. 1997. Purification and molecular cloning of SH2- and SH3-containing inositol polyphosphate-5-phosphatase, which is involved in the signaling pathway of granulocyte-macrophage colony-stimulating factor, erythropoietin, and Bcr-Abl. *Blood* 89:2745–56

29. Shuai K, Halpern J, ten Hoeve J, et al. 1996. Constitutive activation of STATS by the BCR-ABL oncogene in chronic myelogenous leukemia. *Oncogene* 13:247–54

30. Sanchez-Garcia I, Grutz G. 1995. Tumorigenic activity of the BCR-ABL oncogene is mediated by BCL2. *Proc. Natl. Acad. Sci. USA* 92:5287–91

31. Verfaillie CM, Hurley R, Lundell BI, et al. 1997. Integrin-mediated regulation of hematopoiesis: Do Bcr/Abl-induced defects in integrin function underlie the abnormal circulation and proliferation of CML progenitors? *Acta Haematol.* 97:40–52

32. Takeda N, Shibuya M, Maru Y. 1999. The BCR-ABL oncoprotein potentially interacts with the xeroderma pigmentosum group B protein. *Proc. Natl. Acad. Sci. USA* 96:203–7

33. Fialkow PJ, Martin PJ, Najfeld V, et al. 1981. Evidence for a multistep pathogenesis of chronic myelogenous leukemia. *Blood* 58:158–63

34. Nowell PC, Moreau L, Growney P, et al. 1988. Karyotypic stability in chronic B cell leukemia. *Cancer Genet. Cytogenet.* 33:155–60

35. Cunningham I, Gee T, Dowling M, et al. 1979. Results of treatment of Ph-positive chronic myelogenous leukemia with an intensive treatment regimen (L-5 protocol). *Blood* 53:375–95

36. Faderl S, Talpaz M, Estrov Z, et al. 1999. Chronic myelogenous leukemia: biology and therapy. *Ann. Int. Med.* 131:207–19

37. Silver RT, Woolf SH, Hehlmann R, et al. 1999. An evidence-based analysis of the effect of busulfan, hydroxyurea, interferon, and allogeneic bone marrow transplantation in treating the chronic phase of chronic myeloid leukemia: developed for the American Society of Hematology. *Blood* 94:1517–36

38. Nowell P, Cole L, Habermeyer J, et al. 1956. Growth and continued function of rat marrow cells in X-irradiated mice. *Cancer Res.* 16:258–61

39. Apperly JF. 1998. Hematopoietic stem cell transplantation in chronic myeloid leukemia. *Curr. Opin. Hematol.* 5:445–53

40. Porter DL, Antin JH. 1999. The graft-versus-leukemia effects of allogeneic cell therapy. *Annu. Rev. Med.* 50:369–86

41. Kronenwett R, Haas R. 1998. Specific BCR-ABL-directed antisense nucleic acids and ribozymes: a tool for the treatment of chronic myelogenous leukemia? *Recent Results Cancer Res.* 144:127–38

42. Gewirtz AM, Sokol DL, Ratajczak MZ. 1998. Nucleic acid therapeutics: state of the art and future prospects. *Blood* 92:712–36

43. Luger S, O'Brien S, Ratajczak M, et al. 2000. Bone marrow purging with c-myb targeted oligodeoxynucleotides: results and long-term follow-up of a pilot study in CML patients. *Blood* 96:A609a (Abstr.)

44. Cuneo A, Bigoni R, Emmanuel B, et al. 1998. Fluorescence in situ hybridization for the detection and monitoring of the Ph-positive clone in chronic myelogenous leukemia: comparison with metaphase banding analysis. *Leukemia* 12:1718–23

45. Chomel J-C, Brizard F, Veinstein A, et al. 2000. Persistence of BCR-ABL genomic rearrangement in chronic myeloid leukemia patients in complete and sustained cytogenetic remission after interferon-α therapy or allogeneic bone marrow transplantation. *Blood* 95:404–9

46. Stryckmans P, Biernaux C, Sels A, et al. 1995. Very low levels of major BCR-ABL expression in blood of some healthy individuals. *Blood* 86:3118–22

47. Druker BJ, Tamura S, Buchdunger E, et al. 1996. Effects of a selective inhibitor of the Abl tyrosine kinase on the growth of Bcr-Abl positive cells. *Nat. Med.* 2:561–66

48. Druker BJ, Talpaz M, Resta D, et al. 1999. Clinical efficacy and safety of an Abl specific tyrosine kinase inhibitor as targeted therapy for chronic myelogenous leukemia. *Blood* 94(10):A1639 (Suppl. 1)

49. Weisberg E, Griffin JD. 2000. Mechanism of resistance to the ABL tyrosine kinase inhibitor STI571 in BCR/ABL-transformed hematopoietic cell lines. *Blood* 95:3498–3505

Annu. Rev. Med. 2002. 53:15–33

DIAGNOSIS AND TREATMENT OF VENOUS THROMBOEMBOLISM

Agnes Y. Y. Lee[1] and Jack Hirsh[2]

[1]Department of Medicine, McMaster University, Hamilton Health Sciences, Henderson Site, 711 Concession Street, Hamilton, Ontario, Canada L8V 1C3; e-mail: alee@thrombosis.hhscr.org; [2]Henderson Research Centre, McMaster University, 711 Concession Street, Hamilton, Ontario, Canada

Key Words   deep vein thrombosis, pulmonary embolism, D-dimer, low-molecular-weight heparin

■ **Abstract**   The diagnosis of deep vein thrombosis (DVT) and pulmonary embolism (PE) has been improved and simplified over the past decade thanks to advances in noninvasive and readily accessible technology. With high degrees of sensitivity and specificity, venous ultrasonography is favored as the initial investigation for DVT. To diagnose PE, most clinicians rely on diagnostic algorithms that combine clinical assessment, noninvasive lung studies, and, if necessary, venous ultrasonography of the legs and D-dimer testing. Substantial progress has also occurred in the treatment of acute venous thromboembolism with the introduction of low-molecular-weight heparins. This class of antithrombotic agents has changed initial therapy from an inpatient, intravenous regimen that required laborious monitoring to an outpatient practice using weight-adjusted doses of once-daily subcutaneous injections. In addition, several new anticoagulants with theoretical advantages over existing agents have entered phase III studies. Aspects of thrombosis treatment that remain controversial include vena caval interruption and the indications for thrombolysis and surgical thromboembolectomy.

INTRODUCTION

Venous thromboembolism (VTE) is a common condition in both outpatient and inpatient settings. The age- and sex-adjusted incidence of deep vein thrombosis (DVT) is 48 per 100,000 and that of pulmonary embolism (PE) is 69 per 100,000 (1). With increasing age, the risk of VTE almost doubles for every decade after age 60. This escalation in risk may reflect the higher prevalence of known risk factors for VTE in the older population, including malignancy, serious cardiac disease, hospitalization for surgery or trauma, and immobility. Since undiagnosed VTE can cause fatal PE, it is important to accurately diagnose VTE and effectively manage the acute and long-term sequelae of DVT and PE.

DIAGNOSIS OF DEEP VEIN THROMBOSIS

The use of objective investigations is essential for confirming a diagnosis of DVT because clinical diagnosis is insensitive and nonspecific. Patients with DVT may have minimal symptoms, and findings considered diagnostic of DVT can be found in nonthrombotic disorders. Only about 25% to 30% of patients with symptoms compatible with thrombosis are confirmed to have DVT on objective testing (2).

Clinical Assessment

The typical signs and symptoms of DVT are leg pain, tenderness, swelling, and occasionally discoloration. These clinical manifestations are nonspecific and can be found in patients with superficial thrombophlebitis, cellulitis, lymphedema, Baker's cyst, and other musculoskeletal conditions (2). The likelihood that these symptoms are caused by DVT is increased if the patient has any known risk factors associated with DVT. These risk factors include malignancy, major surgery or trauma, recent hospitalization or immobilization for medical illness, pregnancy and puerperium, use of hormonal agents (such as oral contraceptives and hormonal replacement therapy), and inherited thrombophilia. Outpatients with classical findings of DVT with at least one risk factor have an 85% probability of DVT, whereas those with atypical symptoms and no identifiable risk factors have only about a 5% probability (3). Hospitalized patients also can be reliably triaged using a clinical model and a bedside D-dimer assay (4).

Contrast Venography

Contrast venography remains the reference standard for diagnosing DVT. A thrombus is diagnosed by the presence of a constant intraluminal filling defect detected by radiography after injection of iodinated contrast dye into the leg veins. Because it can visualize the iliac vessels and the entire venous system in the legs, venography can detect pelvic thrombi and small, distal calf clots that are usually missed by noninvasive studies. However, venography is invasive and can be painful. It can be technically difficult to perform, which can lead to inadequate imaging and misinterpretation of results. Even when performed by experienced radiologists, 5% to 12% of venograms are inadequate (5). Other disadvantages include cost and limited accessibility. Rarely, the contrast medium can precipitate phlebitis, anaphylaxis, and renal failure.

Venous Ultrasonography

In contrast to venography, venous ultrasonography is painless, readily available, and has no adverse effects. In diagnosing DVT, compression B-mode or color duplex ultrasonography is highly accurate for symptomatic proximal thrombosis in the legs (6). With a positive predictive value of 97% and a negative predictive value of 98% for proximal DVT, venous ultrasonography has become the standard first-line screening test. Its major limitation is its poor sensitivity (about 60%) in detecting asymptomatic proximal or isolated symptomatic distal thrombosis (6).

By combining the results of venous ultrasound and clinical probability, DVT can be reliably diagnosed or excluded in almost all cases. When the results of these two tests are concordant, the accuracy and predictive values approach 100% (3). Therefore, when the clinical suspicion is high and the ultrasound is positive, DVT is confirmed; when the clinical suspicion is low and the ultrasound is negative, it is safe to exclude a diagnosis of clinically significant DVT and withhold treatment. In discordant cases, further testing is required, since the probability of DVT will range between 24% and 63%. Potential extension of a calf thrombus undetected at initial presentation can be identified by serial venous ultrasonography. Venography is indicated if a patient cannot return for repeated testing or has a high clinical probability (6). Figure 1 illustrates an algorithm for diagnosing DVT using clinical assessment and ultrasonography.

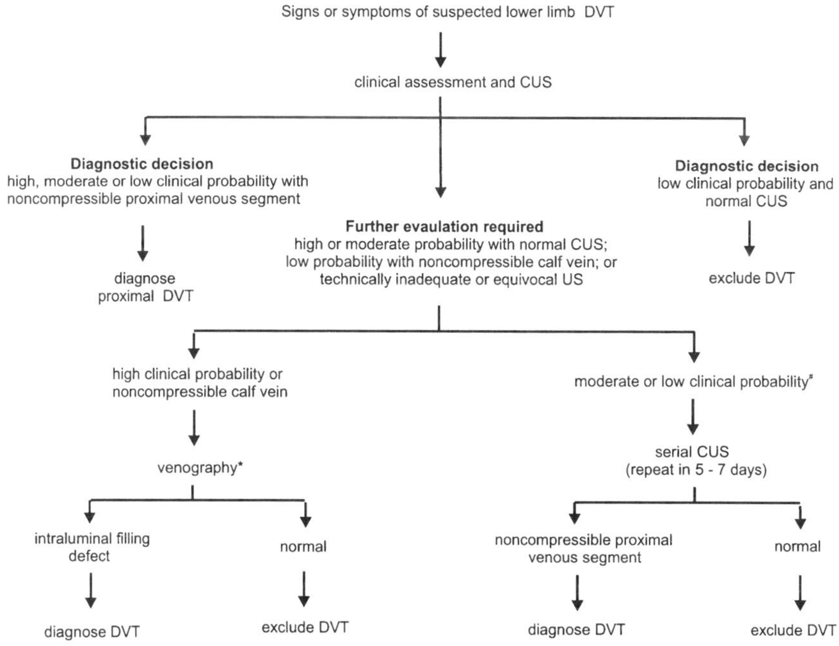

Figure 1   Diagnostic algorithm for diagnosing deep vein thrombosis.

Impedance Plethysmography

The use of impedance plethysmography (IPG) is becoming a matter of historical interest, as fewer instruments are available and as venous ultrasonography proves more reliable and much more accessible (7).

Despite its poor performance compared with ultrasonography, the IPG is useful for diagnosing DVT in combination with D-dimer testing. When a negative D-dimer result is combined with a normal IPG result, the probability of proximal thrombosis is less than 1% (8). This obviates further testing, and anticoagulant therapy can be withheld safely (9).

D-Dimer Assay

D-dimer testing has been validated as a useful adjunctive investigation for DVT. D-dimer is a plasmin-derived degradation product of crosslinked fibrin. Because D-dimer levels are elevated in other conditions besides acute thrombosis, such as pregnancy, acute inflammatory states, and malignancy, this test lacks specificity (10). Commercially available assays employ one of three basic techniques to measure D-dimer, including enzyme-linked immunosorbent assay (ELISA), latex agglutination, and whole blood red cell agglutination. These assays vary in their sensitivity, specificity, and clinical utility in detecting DVT (11, 12).

Using a D-dimer assay with high sensitivity, a negative result, in combination with a negative noninvasive leg study (IPG or ultrasound), can reliably rule out acute DVT (8). Several management studies have shown that outpatients who present with suspected acute DVT can be managed safely based on the combined results of D-dimer testing and either venous ultrasonography or standardized clinical assessment (9, 13, 14). A recent study demonstrated that D-dimer testing is also reliable in excluding acute DVT in hospitalized patients (4). However, in patients with a high risk for VTE (e.g., cancer patients), the negative predictive value of D-dimer assays is reduced and further testing is indicated (15, 16).

DIAGNOSIS OF PULMONARY EMBOLISM

Like DVT, the diagnosis of PE cannot be confirmed or excluded on clinical grounds. The clinical presentation is nonspecific, and objective investigations are essential. Only about 25% to 30% of patients with symptoms compatible with PE are confirmed to have thromboembolism on objective testing (17, 18). The remaining patients suffer from other more common disorders, such as viral or bacterial pneumonia, exacerbation of asthma or chronic obstructive lung disease, ischemic coronary events, and musculoskeletal conditions.

Clinical Assessment

Because a diagnosis of PE is often made or excluded on the basis of clinical manifestations and objective testing, a thorough history and physical examination are very important to establish the clinical likelihood of PE. Depending on the severity of the embolism, its manifestations may range from mild shortness of breath to circulatory collapse or sudden death. Physical findings range from an essentially normal exam to tachycardia, arrhythmia, pleural rub, loud second heart sound, elevated jugular venous pressure to right heart failure, hypotension, and shock. Because these findings are nonspecific, it is also important to examine the patient for signs of DVT and determine whether there are known risk factors for VTE. About 30% of patients with proven PE have clinical findings of DVT (19, 20). Although the absence of DVT features do not rule out PE, their presence makes the diagnosis of PE much more likely. Other potential but less common sources of embolism include the inferior vena cava, renal veins, upper limb veins, and right side of the heart. As for the diagnosis of DVT, a clinical model has been evaluated to standardize the clinical assessment of PE (21).

Pulmonary Angiography

Pulmonary angiography is the reference standard for diagnosing PE. It involves catheter-directed injection of iodinated contrast into the pulmonary arteries, which allows visualization of emboli to the subsegmental level on adequate angiograms. Persistent intraluminal filling defects or an abrupt cut-off in an artery with a diameter of >2 mm are diagnostic of PE. With modern techniques, pulmonary angiography is associated with a mortality rate of 0.1% and major nonfatal complication rate of 0.4% (22, 23). Approximately 4% of the results are nondiagnostic, and about 10% to 20% of patients are unable to undergo angiography (24, 25). The test requires considerable expertise and is not readily available. It is contraindicated if pulmonary artery pressures are high and if the patient has a history of anaphylactic reaction to contrast medium. Because of these limitations, pulmonary angiography is usually reserved for patients in whom an appropriate decision about management cannot be made using less invasive approaches.

Ventilation-Perfusion Lung Scintigraphy

To reduce the need for angiography, a diagnostic strategy using clinical assessment and an initial battery of investigations is commonly used. Figure 2 outlines two reasonable strategies for diagnosing PE, one using ventilation-perfusion (VQ) scanning, the other using spiral computed tomography (CT). The first routine screening test is VQ lung scintigraphy. By comparing the distribution of [99m]Technetium-labeled albumin in the pulmonary vasculature with the distribution of radioactive aerosol in the lung airspace, mismatches or differences in the perfusion and ventilation patterns can help diagnose PE. If the perfusion scan is normal, PE can almost always be ruled out and anticoagulant therapy withheld (17, 26, 27). If there are one or more perfusion defects of at least segmental size with normal matching ventilation, PE can usually be diagnosed, and treatment should be instituted (17, 28). All other lung scan imaging results, referred to as nondiagnostic scans, can be associated with PE in 15% to 65% of cases. Further diagnostic evaluation must be done in these cases, which make up about 50% to 60% of all patients presenting with suspected PE. In addition, even when the lung scan shows near normal perfusion or a high probability for PE, if the clinical assessment is discordant with the lung scan result, further tests should be performed using pulmonary angiography, bilateral venography, or venous ultrasonography (29, 30). Positive results on leg venography or venous ultrasound can be accepted as diagnostic for DVT, and anticoagulant therapy can be initiated. If the leg ultrasound is normal but the clinical suspicion is high or the patient has significant cardiorespiratory compromise, venography or pulmonary angiography is indicated. Otherwise, serial venous ultrasonography is a reasonable alternative approach in patients with a low or moderate clinical probability of PE (29, 30).

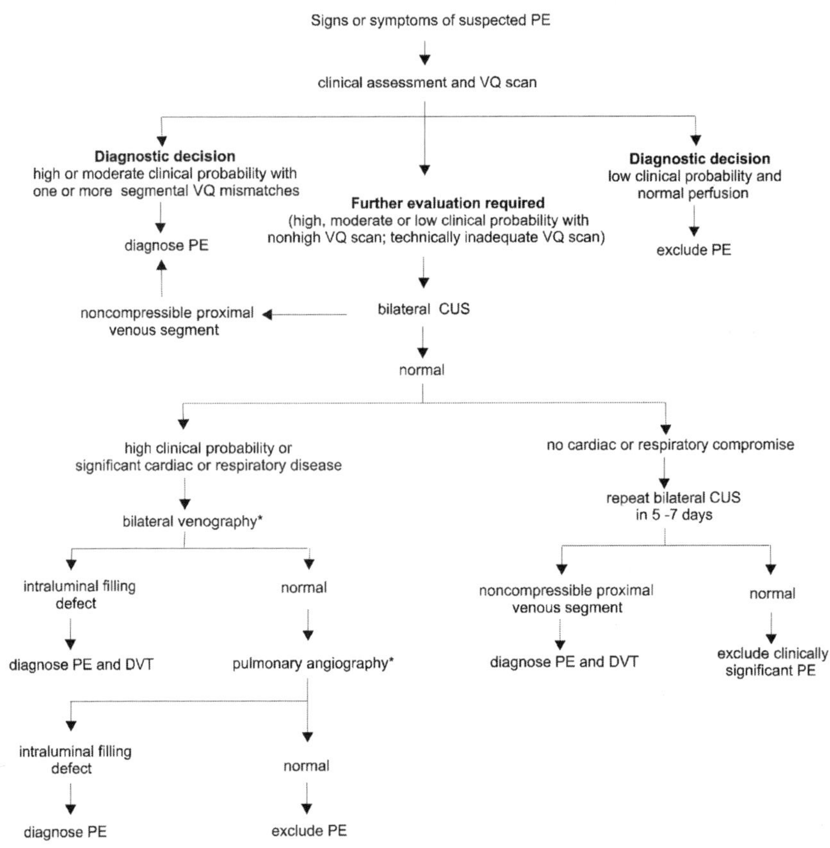

Figure 2 Diagnostic algorithms for diagnosing pulmonary embolism using either (*a*) ventilation-perfusion lung scanning or (*b*) spiral computed tomography as the initial screening test. "Central vessels" refers to main pulmonary arteries and lobar arteries.

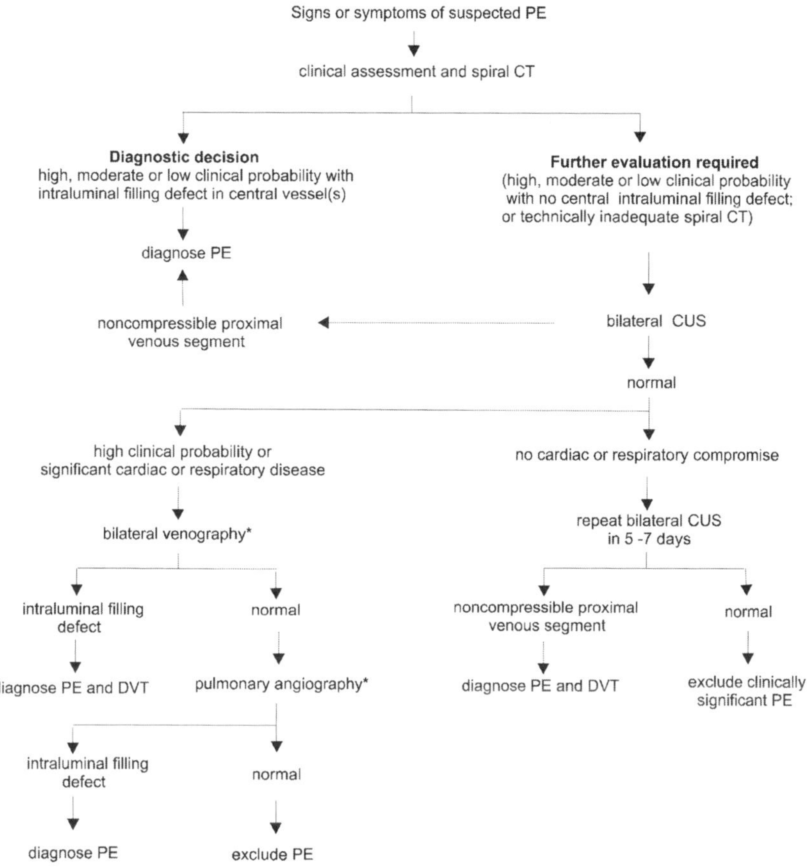

Figure 2   (*Continued*)

Spiral Computed Tomography

The limitations of pulmonary angiography and lung scanning have stimulated interest in the development of other imaging approaches. Spiral or helical CT is an angiography technique in which iodinated contrast is injected peripherally and images are taken by a rapidly rotating scanner, which is timed to capture the flow of contrast through the pulmonary arterial tree during a total acquisition time of less than 30 s. PE appears as complete or incomplete intraluminal filling defects in an arterial segment.

The accuracy of spiral CT was recently summarized in two systematic reviews including 15 different studies. The reported sensitivity ranges from 53% to 100%

and the specificity from 81% to 100% (31, 32). Spiral CT can make an alternative diagnosis in 33% of suspected cases (32), but it is not sufficiently sensitive or specific for detecting emboli involving subsegmental arteries or more distal segments (33, 34), which can occur in one third of patients with PE (35). False positive diagnoses can result from confusion with hilar lymphadenopathy, partial opacification of pulmonary veins, and circumferential perivascular edema in congestive heart failure (33, 36). A recent management study in 228 patients with suspected PE used a diagnostic algorithm incorporating spiral CT, D-dimer testing, lung scanning, and leg ultrasonography (37). The three-month risk of VTE in patients who were not diagnosed with PE initially and were not given anticoagulant therapy was 1.7%. In contrast, another study found that 5.4% of 112 patients with a normal spiral CT developed PE during three months of follow-up (38).

Because of the methodologic shortcomings of the studies performed to date, more rigorous studies are needed to evaluate spiral CT. Furthermore, withholding treatment in patients with a negative spiral CT scan has not been validated in adequate management studies.

Magnetic Resonance Angiography

Another method being evaluated for PE diagnosis is magnetic resonance angiography (MRA). Magnetic radiofrequencies are emitted and the received signals are transformed into images. Enchancement using gadolinium highlights the pulmonary vasculature, and an intravascular filling defect is considered diagnostic for PE. MRA provides high spatial resolution and does not expose patients to ionized radiation. It can be used in patients with iodine allergy and renal insufficiency (33, 36).

Based on a small study of 30 consecutive patients referred for angiography for suspected PE, MRA has a sensitivity of 100% and a specificity of 95% compared with conventional pulmonary angiography (39). The main disadvantage of MRA is its limited availability. Like other imaging studies used for diagnosing PE, it presents difficulties in detecting peripheral emboli because of potential confusion with peribronchial fat or slow flow in small vessels (40). However, with promising improvements in technology, MRA may prove to be the next reference standard for diagnosing PE.

D-Dimer Assay

D-dimer testing has been evaluated as an adjunct in noninvasive strategies to diagnose PE because it has a high negative predictive value for PE (41–43). Several management studies using D-dimer in combination with lung scan and venous ultrasound have suggested that a negative D-dimer test is useful and safe in excluding acute PE (14, 44). Another study reported that a negative D-dimer result in patients with a low clinical probability (based on a point-score clinical model) can safely exclude PE (45). However, other investigators have cautioned that D-dimer measurements were not helpful in excluding PE in hospitalized patients (46). Further management studies are ongoing to determine the role of this method in diagnosing PE.

DIAGNOSIS OF RECURRENT VENOUS THROMBOEMBOLISM

The difficulty in diagnosing recurrent DVT or PE is the lack of a reference standard. Although venography and pulmonary angiography, respectively, are considered the most reliable tests available, they are difficult to perform and impractical for repeated use. New intraluminal filling defects are accepted as diagnostic for recurrent thrombosis, but these may be difficult to detect or interpret if there are no previous studies or if the initial thrombosis was extensive.

As for DVT, venous ultrasonography is commonly used as the first investigation for recurrent DVT. However, since only about 50% of patients will have normalization of a positive ultrasound at one year from initial diagnosis (47), residual abnormalities will render the ultrasound nondiagnostic in many patients. As a result, a positive ultrasound can confirm recurrence only if the test result had reverted to normal and a previously compressible segment is now noncompressible. Some investigators have suggested that an increase of more than 4 mm in the compressed diameter of the involved vein provides strong evidence of recurrent thrombosis (48, 49), but this requires confirmation. In contrast, a negative ultrasound essentially excludes recurrent proximal but not distal DVT. Serial ultrasound testing over the next 7–10 days is recommended to exclude extension of a calf vein thrombus. When the ultrasound is nondiagnostic, venography should be done.

For diagnosing recurrent PE, clinical probability is an important part of the assessment, since none of the objective tests are definitive. The diagnostic approach is the same as in the initial episode of PE. New mismatched perfusion abnormalities on lung scan or intraluminal filling defects on contrast studies are accepted as evidence of acute recurrence.

It is likely that D-dimer testing will prove useful in diagnosing recurrent DVT or PE because it is sensitive to acute thrombin generation and fibrin breakdown (12, 50). However, the use of D-dimer in this setting has not been tested formally in clinical trials.

TREATMENT OF ACUTE VENOUS THROMBOEMBOLISM

The introduction of low-molecular-weight heparins (LMWHs) in the 1980s revolutionized the early treatment of VTE. Shown to be at least as effective and safe as heparin administered by monitored, continuous, intravenous infusion (51, 52), treatment with unmonitored, subcutaneous injections of LMWH is quickly replacing the old standard for initial therapy of acute VTE (53–55). In addition,

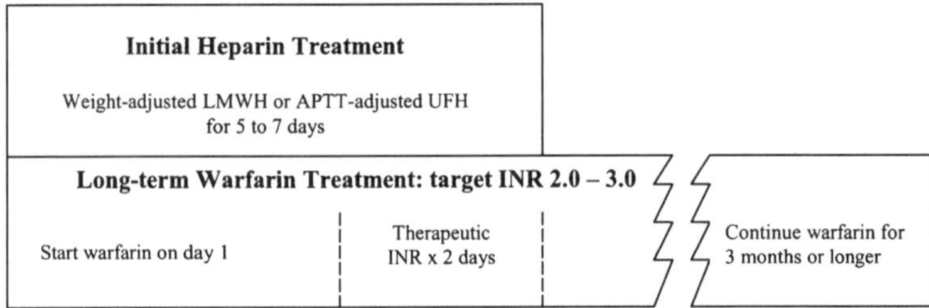

Figure 3   Treatment for acute venous thromboembolism.

LMWH is being evaluated for long-term treatment, and several new antithrombotic agents with potential advantages over current drugs are in advanced stages of development.

Initial Anticoagulant Therapy

Patients with acute VTE should receive heparin or LMWH (Figure 3). The standard intravenous loading dose for heparin of 5000 units should be followed by a continuous infusion of at least 30,000 units every 24 h, adjusted by a validated nomogram to maintain a therapeutic heparin level (56). The therapeutic activated partial thromboplastin time (APTT) range should correspond to a heparin level of 0.2 to 0.4 units/ml by protamine sulfate titration, or 0.4 to 0.7 units/ml by anti-factor Xa assay (56). Because APTT reagents vary in their responsiveness to heparin, an APTT of 1.5 times control is inadequate (57). In patients requiring large doses of heparin (greater than 40,000 units per 24 h), the heparin level should be monitored by anti-Xa assay or protamine sulfate titration. In these heparin-resistant patients, there is dissociation between the APTT and heparin concentration because of high levels of factor VIII and acute phase reactant proteins (58).

The major advantage of a heparin infusion is that rapid reversal of the anticoagulant effect can be achieved by stopping the infusion and by administering protamine sulfate, if necessary (56). The disadvantages include the cost and inconvenience of intravenous administration and frequent APTT monitoring, the lack of standardized assays, heparin resistance, and the risks of osteoporosis and heparin-induced thrombocytopenia (59).

In the majority of patients with confirmed VTE, LMWHs are now used for initial therapy. Their superior bioavailability and predictable pharmacokinetic properties allow weight-adjusted dosing without laboratory monitoring. Depending on the LMWH agent, a dose of 100 anti-Xa units/kg twice daily or 150 to 200 anti-Xa units/kg daily is given subcutaneously. There is also recent evidence that fixed-dose, weight-independent injections of a LMWH (certoparin, 8000 anti-Xa units twice daily) are as safe and efficacious as APTT-adjusted intravenous heparin (60). Although laboratory monitoring is not usually required with LMWHs, the anti-Xa level should be checked in patients who have advanced renal disease, are morbidly obese, or are pregnant, because the pharmacokinetic properties and efficacy and safety of LMWHs are not well-established in these patients. Although LMWHs are more expensive than heparin, the elimination of hospitalization and laboratory monitoring have made LMWH therapy more cost-effective (61, 62). Other potential advantages of LMWHs include a lower risk of bleeding, osteoporosis, and heparin-induced thrombocytopenia (63).

In uncomplicated acute thrombosis, heparin or LMWH should be continued for a minimum of five days and should not be stopped until therapeutic levels of the oral anticoagulant have been maintained for two consecutive days, as indicated by an international normalized ratio (INR) of 2.0 to 3.0 (56). For patients presenting with extensive disease, e.g., iliofemoral DVT, or life-threatening PE, a course of 7–10 days is indicated.

Long-Term Anticoagulant Therapy

Long-term anticoagulant therapy is necessary to prevent VTE recurrence. Warfarin, or other vitamin K antagonists, is the standard drug for long-term anticoagulant therapy. It can be started within the first 24 h of initial treatment at a dose of 5 mg for the first 2–3 days. Higher loading doses may be associated with a transient period of excessive anticoagulation without a corresponding antithrombotic effect and increase the risk of warfarin-induced skin necrosis in patients with protein C (64, 65). After the initial few doses, warfarin doses are adjusted to maintain the INR between 2.0 and 3.0. Once this target level is achieved, heparin or LMWH can be stopped, and warfarin is continued alone. The narrow therapeutic window of oral anticoagulant therapy mandates regular monitoring of the INR.

Until recently, secondary prophylaxis or long-term treatment has been limited to the use of oral coumarin derivatives. LMWHs are now a feasible alternative and have several advantages over oral anticoagulants. First, LMWH treatment does not require laboratory monitoring. Second, it achieves a more uniform antithrombotic response because diet and concomitant drugs do not influence its anticoagulant effect, whereas warfarin is sensitive to multiple interactions (66). Third, heparins and LMWHs are effective in patients with warfarin-resistant thrombosis, a condition that can occur in patients with advanced malignancy and possibly in patients with antiphospholipid antibody syndrome (67).

To date, several randomized controlled trials have compared LMWH with oral anticoagulant therapy for long-term treatment (68–70). In all of these studies, the incidence of recurrent thrombosis and major bleeding was similar in the two treatment groups. However, most of the studies were insufficiently powered to detect small but clinically important differences. The largest trial, in approximately 400 patients, was recently published in abstract form (70). After three months of follow-up, the rates of recurrent thrombosis and major bleeding were comparable in the two treatment groups.

Duration of Anticoagulant Therapy

The duration of anticoagulant therapy should be adjusted according to the competing risks of recurrence and bleeding. Patients with idiopathic (unprovoked) VTE, and those with activated protein C resistance or deficiencies of protein C or S, should be treated for at least six months (71–73). If treated for only three months, up to 27% of these patients may develop a recurrence within the first year of stopping warfarin (71). In contrast, patients with a reversible risk factor can be treated for three months, and patients with continuing strong risk factors, such as those with malignancy, recurrent VTE, a lupus anticoagulant, or a deficiency of antithrombin, should probably be treated with warfarin indefinitely. Treatment of symptomatic calf thrombosis for 6–12 weeks is probably sufficient if there is no ongoing risk factor.

Risk of Bleeding During Anticoagulant Therapy

The risk of bleeding during the initial period of anticoagulation with heparin or LMWHs is probably < 5%, whereas the estimated risk of major bleeding with oral anticoagulant therapy is about 3% per year (74, 75). About 20% of major bleeds are fatal. The risk is largely dependent on the intensity of anticoagulation, as well as patient-specific factors such as age (65 years or older), comorbid illness (e.g., myocardial infarction, renal failure, diabetes), and concomitant use of antiplatelet drugs (76, 77). One study reported the annual risk of major bleeding to be 3% in patients without risk factors, 12% in those with one or two risk factors, and 48% in those with three or more risk factors (78).

New Antithrombotic Agents

Unlike heparin and LMWHs, which indirectly inhibit thrombin by accelerating the action of antithrombin, many of the new antithrombotic agents target other steps in the coagulation cascade. Some are direct inhibitors of thrombin (e.g., hirudin, bivalirudin, argatroban, melagatran) whereas others block the activity of factor Xa (e.g., DX-9065, pentasaccharide), activated factor IX (e.g., IXai) or the activated factor VII/tissue factor complex (e.g., recombinant nematode anticoagulant protein c2) (79, 80).

For the prophylaxis and treatment of venous thrombosis, results from small or early-phase clinical trials have been published for recombinant hirudin, bivalirudin, napsagatran, melagatran and its oral precursor ximelagatran, and pentasaccharide. For treatment of heparin-induced thrombocytopenia, recombinant hirudins, danaparoid, and argatroban have been approved in some countries. Phase III trials are now evaluating the safety and efficacy of pentasaccharide and ximelagatran in the treatment of acute DVT and PE. Preliminary results appear promising (81, 82).

Other Treatment Options for Venous Thromboembolism

THROMBOLYSIS   Thrombolytic agents can produce rapid lysis of thromboemboli and potentially have advantages over standard anticoagulant therapy in the treatment of patients with PE or extensive iliofemoral DVT. In the acute period, rapid dissolution of pulmonary emboli can relieve symptoms and restore pulmonary perfusion and hemodynamic stability. Over the long term, complete clot resolution can also prevent further embolization and reduce the risk of chronic vascular obstruction that can lead to pulmonary hypertension and postphlebitic syndrome.

Despite these theoretical advantages, the indications for the use of thrombolytic agents in PE and DVT remain controversial (83). Studies using arteriographic and echocardiographic endpoints indicate that thrombolytic agents are more efficacious than heparin alone for the treatment of PE (84). Unfortunately, these surrogate outcomes have not translated into improved clinical outcomes, such as decreased mortality. In addition, major bleeding can occur in up to 30% of treated patients, a three-fold greater incidence than with heparin alone, and the risk of intracranial hemorrhage is approximately 2% (84–86).

Based on the available evidence, thrombolytic therapy is indicated for patients who present with hemodynamic instability with right heart failure or shock due to massive PE because thrombolysis is likely to reduce mortality in this setting. It remains unclear whether right ventricular dysfunction on echocardiography alone is a sufficient indication for thrombolysis. Thrombolytic therapy should be used only in selected patients having massive iliofemoral vein thrombosis with signs of phlegmasia or circulatory compromise. The various thrombolytic agents and regimens appear to have similar efficacy and safety profiles (84).

VENA CAVAL INTERRUPTION   The primary indications for placement of an intraluminal inferior vena caval filter are active bleeding, risk of serious bleeding that precludes the use of anticoagulant therapy, and failure of anticoagulant therapy. The use of filters remains controversial in other scenarios, e.g., to prevent embolization of "free-floating" thrombi in iliofemoral disease and as first-line treatment (alone) in patients with central nervous system malignancy (87, 88).

To date, only one randomized controlled trial has evaluated the use of caval filters. In this study, 400 patients with proximal DVT considered at high risk for PE were randomized to receive a vena caval filter or no filter (89). All patients received anticoagulant therapy for at least three months. The use of a filter reduced the occurrence of PE during the first 12 days, but after two years, this was counterbalanced by an increase in recurrent DVT, probably due to thrombosis at the filter site. At two years, there was no difference in mortality between the filter and no-filter groups.

SURGICAL THROMBOEMBOLECTOMY AND CATHETER-DIRECTED THROMBOFRAGMENTATION   Surgical thrombectomy for acute DVT or pulmonary embolectomy for acute PE is infrequently used. Thrombectomy is usually complicated by acute recurrence despite post operative anticoagulant therapy because it leaves a deendothelialized venous surface that is highly thrombogenic (90). More recently, mechanical thrombolysis using a rotational catheter tip or high-pressure saline jets to break up the thrombus have been introduced (91, 92). Although short-term success has been reported, most of the studies have been small and descriptive, without systematic long-term follow-up (93, 94).

Although these invasive procedures can be lifesaving in a patient with massive embolism, most hospitals do not have the resources to perform them. Further, the mortality rate remains high, and randomized controlled trials are unlikely to be done to compare these aggressive measures with more conservative approaches. However, elective pulmonary thromboendarterectomy can be very effective in selected patients with chronic large-vessel thromboembolic pulmonary hypertension (95).

SUMMARY

Diagnosis and treatment of venous VTE remain challenging in some patients. New technology and emerging therapies will undoubtedly improve the management of this common medical problem.

ACKNOWLEDGMENT

Dr. Lee is a recipient of a New Investigator Award from the Canadian Institutes of Health Research/Rx&D Research Program.

Visit the Annual Reviews home page at www.AnnualReviews.org

LITERATURE CITED

1. Silverstein MD, Heit JA, Mohr DN, et al. 1998. Trends in the incidence of deep vein thrombosis and pulmonary embolism. *Arch. Int. Med.* 158:585–93
2. Weinmann EE, Salzman EW. 1994. Deep-vein thrombosis. *N. Engl. J. Med.* 331: 1630–41
3. Wells PS, Hirsh J, Anderson DR, et al. 1995. Accuracy of clinical assessment of deep-vein thrombosis. *Lancet* 345:1326–30; erratum, *Lancet* 346:516
4. Wells PS, Anderson DR, Bormanis J, et al. 1999. Application of a diagnostic clinical model for the management of hospitalized patients with suspected deep-vein thrombosis. *Thromb. Haemost.* 81:493–97
5. Lensing AW, Buller HR, Prandoni P, et al. 1992. Contrast venography, the gold standard for the diagnosis of deep-vein thrombosis: improvement in observer agreement. *Thromb. Haemost.* 67:8–12
6. Kearon C, Ginsberg JS, Hirsh J. 1998. The role of venous ultrasonography in the diagnosis of suspected deep venous thrombosis and pulmonary embolism. *Ann. Intern. Med.* 129:1044–49
7. Anderson DR, Lensing AW, Wells PS, et al. 1993. Limitations of impedance plethysmography in the diagnosis of clinically suspected deep-vein thrombosis. *Ann. Intern. Med.* 118:25–30
8. Wells PS, Brill-Edwards P, Stevens P, et al. 1995. A novel and rapid whole-blood assay for D-dimer in patients with clinically suspected deep vein thrombosis. *Circulation* 91:2184–87
9. Ginsberg JS, Kearon C, Douketis J, et al. 1997. The use of D-dimer testing and impedance plethysmographic examination in patients with clinical indications of deep vein thrombosis. *Arch. Intern. Med.* 157: 1077–81

10. Raimondi P, Bongard O, de Moerloose P, et al. 1993. D-dimer plasma concentration in various clinical conditions: implication for the use of this test in the diagnostic approach of venous thromboembolism. *Thromb. Res.* 69:125–30

11. Becker DM, Philbrick JT, Bachhuber TL, Humphries JE. 1996. D-dimer testing and acute venous thromboembolism. A short-cut to accurate diagnosis? *Arch. Intern. Med.* 156:939–46

12. Lee AY, Ginsberg JS. 1998. Laboratory diagnosis of venous thromboembolism. *Baillieres Clin. Haematol.* 11:587–604

13. Bernardi E, Prandoni P, Lensing AW, et al. 1998. D-dimer testing as an adjunct to ultrasonography in patients with clinically suspected deep vein thrombosis: prospective cohort study. The Multicentre Italian D-dimer Ultrasound Study Investigators Group. *BMJ* 317:1037–40

14. Perrier A, Desmarais S, Miron MJ, et al. 1999. Non-invasive diagnosis of venous thromboembolism in outpatients. *Lancet* 353:190–95

15. Farrell S, Hayes T, Shaw M. 2000. A negative SimpliRED D-dimer assay result does not exclude the diagnosis of deep vein thrombosis or pulmonary embolus in emergency department patients. *Ann. Emerg. Med.* 35:121–25

16. Lee AY, Julian JA, Levine MN, et al. 1999. Clinical utility of a rapid whole-blood D-dimer assay in patients with cancer who present with suspected acute deep venous thrombosis. *Ann. Intern. Med.* 131:417–23

17. The PIOPED Investigators. 1990. Value of the ventilation/perfusion scan in acute pulmonary embolism. Results of the prospective investigation of pulmonary embolism diagnosis (PIOPED). *JAMA* 263:2753–59

18. Hull RD, Raskob GE, Carter CJ, et al. 1988. Pulmonary embolism in outpatients with pleuritic chest pain. *Arch. Intern. Med.* 148:838–44

19. Hull RD, Hirsh J, Carter CJ, et al. 1983. Pulmonary angiography, ventilation lung scanning, and venography for clinically suspected pulmonary embolism with abnormal perfusion lung scan. *Ann. Intern. Med.* 98:891–99

20. Girard P, Musset D, Parent F, et al. 1999. High prevalence of detectable deep venous thrombosis in patients with acute pulmonary embolism. *Chest* 116:903–8

21. Wells PS, Ginsberg JS, Anderson DR, et al. 1998. Use of a clinical model for safe management of patients with suspected pulmonary embolism. *Ann. Intern. Med.* 129:997–1005

22. Nilsson T, Carlsson A, Mare K. 1998. Pulmonary angiography: a safe procedure with modern contrast media and technique. *Eur. Radiol.* 8:86–89

23. Hudson ER, Smith TP, McDermott VG, et al. 1996. Pulmonary angiography performed with iopamidol: complications in 1,434 patients. *Radiology* 198:61–65

24. Stein PD, Athanasoulis C, Alavi A, et al. 1992. Complications and validity of pulmonary angiography in acute pulmonary embolism. *Circulation* 85:462–68

25. van Beek EJ, Reekers JA, Batchelor DA, et al. 1996. Feasibility, safety and clinical utility of angiography in patients with suspected pulmonary embolism. *Eur. Radiol.* 6:415–19

26. Kipper MS, Moser KM, Kortman KE, Ashburn WL. 1982. Long term follow-up of patients with suspected pulmonary embolism and a normal lung scan. Perfusion scans in embolic suspects. *Chest* 82:411–15

27. van Beek EJ, Kuyer PM, Schenk BE, et al. 1995. A normal perfusion lung scan in patients with clinically suspected pulmonary embolism. Frequency and clinical validity. *Chest* 108:170–73

28. Hull RD, Hirsh J, Carter CJ, et al. 1985. Diagnostic value of ventilation-perfusion lung scanning in patients with suspected pulmonary embolism. *Chest* 88:819–28

29. Hull RD, Raskob GE, Ginsberg JS, et al. 1994. A noninvasive strategy for the treatment of patients with suspected pulmonary embolism. *Arch. Intern. Med.* 154:289–97

30. Stein PD, Hull RD, Pineo G. 1995. Strategy that includes serial noninvasive leg tests for diagnosis of thromboembolic disease in patients with suspected acute pulmonary embolism based on data from PIOPED. *Arch. Intern. Med.* 155:2101–4

31. Rathbun SW, Raskob GE, Whitsett TL. 2000. Sensitivity and specificity of helical computed tomography in the diagnosis of pulmonary embolism: a systematic review. *Ann. Intern. Med.* 132:227–32

32. Mullins MD, Becker DM, Hagspiel KD, Philbrick JT. 2000. The role of spiral volumetric computed tomography in the diagnosis of pulmonary embolism. *Arch. Intern. Med.* 160:293–98

33. Gefter WB, Hatabu H, Holland GA, et al. 1995. Pulmonary thromboembolism: recent developments in diagnosis with CT and MR imaging. *Radiology* 197:561–74

34. Remy-Jardin M, Remy J, Wattinne L, Giraud F. 1992. Central pulmonary thromboembolism: diagnosis with spiral volumetric CT with the single-breath-hold technique—comparison with pulmonary angiography. *Radiology* 185:381–87

35. Oser RF, Zuckerman DA, Gutierrez FR, Brink JA. 1996. Anatomic distribution of pulmonary emboli at pulmonary angiography: implications for cross-sectional imaging. *Radiology* 199:31–35

36. Matsumoto AH, Tegtmeyer CJ. 1995. Contemporary diagnostic approaches to acute pulmonary emboli. *Radiol. Clin. N. Am.* 33:167–83

37. Lorut C, Ghossains M, Horellou MH, et al. 2000. A noninvasive diagnostic strategy including spiral computed tomography in patients with suspected pulmonary embolism. *Am. J. Respir. Crit. Care Med.* 162:1413–18

38. Ferretti GR, Bosson JL, Buffaz PD, et al. 1997. Acute pulmonary embolism: role of helical CT in 164 patients with intermediate probability at ventilation-perfusion scintigraphy and normal results at duplex US of the legs. *Radiology* 205:453–58

39. Meaney JF, Weg JG, Chenevert TL, et al. 1997. Diagnosis of pulmonary embolism with magnetic resonance angiography. *N. Engl. J. Med.* 336:1422–27

40. Loubeyre P, Revel D, Douek P, et al. 1994. Dynamic contrast-enhanced MR angiography of pulmonary embolism: comparison with pulmonary angiography. *Am. J. Roentgenol.* 162:1035–39

41. de Moerloose P, Desmarais S, Bounameaux H, et al. 1996. Contribution of a new, rapid, individual and quantitative automated D-dimer ELISA to exclude pulmonary embolism. *Thromb. Haemost.* 75:11–13

42. Duet M, Benelhadj S, Kedra W, et al. 1998. A new quantitative D-dimer assay appropriate in emergency: reliability of the assay for pulmonary embolism exclusion diagnosis. *Thromb. Res.* 91:1–5

43. Ginsberg JS, Wells PS, Kearon C, et al. 1998. Sensitivity and specificity of a rapid whole-blood assay for D-dimer in the diagnosis of pulmonary embolism. *Ann. Intern. Med.* 129:1006–11

44. Perrier A, Bounameaux H, Morabia A, et al. 1996. Diagnosis of pulmonary embolism by a decision analysis-based strategy including clinical probability, D-dimer levels, and ultrasonography: a management study. *Arch. Intern. Med.* 156:531–36

45. Wells PS, Anderson DR, Rodger M, et al. 2000. Derivation of a simple clinical model to categorize patients probability of pulmonary embolism: increasing the models utility with the SimpliRED D-dimer. *Thromb. Haemost.* 83:416–20

46. Miron MJ, Perrier A, Bounameaux H, et al. 1999. Contribution of noninvasive evaluation to the diagnosis of pulmonary embolism in hospitalized patients. *Eur. Respir. J.* 13:1365–70

47. Kearon C, Julian JA, Newman TE, Ginsberg JS. 1998. Noninvasive diagnosis of deep venous thrombosis. McMaster Diagnostic Imaging Practice Guidelines Initiative. *Ann. Intern. Med.* 128:663–77; erratum, *Ann. Intern. Med.* 129:425

48. Prandoni P, Cogo A, Bernardi E, et al.

1993. A simple ultrasound approach for detection of recurrent proximal-vein thrombosis. *Circulation* 88:1730–35

49. Koopman MM, Jongbloets J, Lensing A, et al. 1993. Clinical utility of a quantitative B-mode ultrasonography method in patients with suspected recurrent deep-vein thrombosis (DVT). *Thromb. Haemost.* 69:623 (Abstr.)

50. Bridey F, Philippoteau C, Simmoneau G, et al. 1991. Is D-dimer measurement a marker of recurrence of thromboembolic disease? *Thromb. Haemost.* 65:981 (Abstr.)

51. Gould MK, Dembitzer AD, Doyle RL, et al. 1999. Low-molecular-weight heparins compared with unfractionated heparin for treatment of acute deep venous thrombosis. A meta-analysis of randomized, controlled trials. *Ann. Intern. Med.* 130:800–9

52. Dolovich LR, Ginsberg JS, Douketis JD, et al. 2000. A meta-analysis comparing low-molecular-weight heparins with unfractionated heparin in the treatment of venous thromboembolism: examining some unanswered questions regarding location of treatment, product type, and dosing frequency. *Arch. Intern. Med.* 160:181–88

53. Kovacs MJ, Anderson D, Morrow B, et al. 2000. Outpatient treatment of pulmonary embolism with dalteparin. *Thromb. Haemost* 83:209–11

54. Wells PS, Kovacs MJ, Bormanis J, et al. 1998. Expanding eligibility for outpatient treatment of deep venous thrombosis and pulmonary embolism with low-molecular-weight heparin: a comparison of patient self-injection with homecare injection. *Arch. Intern. Med.* 158:1809–12

55. Harrison L, McGinnis J, Crowther M, et al. 1998. Assessment of outpatient treatment of deep-vein thrombosis with low-molecular-weight heparin. *Arch. Intern. Med.* 158:2001–3

56. Hirsh J, Warkentin TE, Raschke R, et al. 1998. Heparin and low-molecular-weight heparin: mechanisms of action, pharmacokinetics, dosing considerations, monitoring, efficacy, and safety. *Chest* 114:489S–510S

57. Brill-Edwards P, Ginsberg JS, Johnston M, Hirsh J. 1993. Establishing a therapeutic range for heparin therapy. *Ann. Intern. Med.* 119:104–9

58. Levine MN, Hirsh J, Gent M, et al. 1994. A randomized trial comparing activated thromboplastin time with heparin assay in patients with acute venous thromboembolism requiring large daily doses of heparin. *Arch. Intern. Med.* 154:49–56

59. Walenga JM, Bick RL. 1998. Heparin-induced thrombocytopenia, paradoxical thromboembolism, and other side effects of heparin therapy. *Med. Clin. N. Am.* 82:635–58

60. Riess H, Tolle A, Koppenhagen K, et al. 2000. Fixed-dose body weight-independent low-molecular-weight heparin (LMWH) certoparin is as efficacious as adjusted-dose intravenous unfractionated heparin (UFH) for the initial treatment of proximal deep venous thrombosis (DVT). *Blood* 96:449a (Abstr.)

61. Gould MK, Dembitzer AD, Sanders GD, Garber AM. 1999. Low-molecular-weight heparins compared with unfractionated heparin for treatment of acute deep venous thrombosis. A cost-effectiveness analysis. *Ann. Intern. Med.* 130:789–99

62. Hull RD, Raskob GE, Rosenbloom D, et al. 1997. Treatment of proximal vein thrombosis with subcutaneous low-molecular-weight heparin vs intravenous heparin. An economic perspective. *Arch. Intern. Med.* 157:289–94

63. Weitz JI. 1997. Low-molecular-weight heparins. *N. Engl. J. Med.* 337:688–98; erratum, *N. Engl. J. Med.* 337:1567

64. Harrison L, Johnston M, Massicotte MP, et al. 1997. Comparison of 5-mg and 10-mg loading doses in initiation of warfarin therapy. *Ann. Intern. Med.* 126:133–36

65. Sallah S, Thomas DP, Roberts HR. 1997. Warfarin and heparin-induced skin necrosis and the purple toe syndrome: infrequent

complications of anticoagulant treatment. *Thromb. Haemost.* 78:785–90

66. Wells PS, Holbrook AM, Crowther NR, Hirsh J. 1994. Interactions of warfarin with drugs and food. *Ann. Intern. Med.* 121:676–83

67. Eikelboom JW, Baker RI. 1998. Low-molecular-weight heparin for the treatment of venous thrombosis in patients with adenocarcinoma. *Am. J. Hematol.* 59:260–61

68. Veiga F, Escriba A, Maluenda MP, et al. 2000. Low molecular weight heparin (enoxaparin) versus oral anticoagulant therapy (acenocoumarol) in the long-term treatment of deep venous thrombosis in the elderly: a randomized trial. *Thromb. Haemost.* 84:559–64

69. Pini M, Aiello S, Manotti C, et al. 1994. Low molecular weight heparin versus warfarin in the prevention of recurrences after deep vein thrombosis. *Thromb. Haemost.* 72:191–97

70. Hull R, Pineo G, Mah A, et al. 2000. Long-term low molecular weight heparin treatment versus oral anticoagulant therapy for proximal deep vein thrombosis. *Blood* 96:449a (Abstr.)

71. Kearon C, Gent M, Hirsh J, et al. 1999. A comparison of three months of anticoagulation with extended anticoagulation for a first episode of idiopathic venous thromboembolism. *N. Engl. J. Med.* 340:901–7; erratum, *N. Engl. J. Med.* 341:298

72. Schulman S, Granqvist S, Holmstrom M, et al. 1997. The duration of oral anticoagulant therapy after a second episode of venous thromboembolism. The Duration of Anticoagulation Trial Study Group. *N. Engl. J. Med.* 336:393–98

73. Schulman S, Rhedin AS, Lindmarker P, et al. 1995. A comparison of six weeks with six months of oral anticoagulant therapy after a first episode of venous thromboembolism. Duration of Anticoagulation Trial Study Group. *N. Engl. J. Med.* 332:1661–65

74. Hirsh J, Dalen JE, Anderson DR, et al. 1998. Oral anticoagulants: mechanism of action, clinical effectiveness, and optimal therapeutic range. *Chest* 114:445S–69S

75. Levine MN, Raskob G, Landefeld S, Kearon C. 1998. Hemorrhagic complications of anticoagulant treatment. *Chest* 114:511S–23S

76. Landefeld CS, Beyth RJ. 1993. Anticoagulant-related bleeding: clinical epidemiology, prediction, and prevention. *Am. J. Med.* 95:315–28

77. Nieuwenhuis HK, Albada J, Banga JD, Sixma JJ. 1991. Identification of risk factors for bleeding during treatment of acute venous thromboembolism with heparin or low molecular weight heparin. *Blood* 78:2337–43

78. Beyth RJ, Quinn LM, Landefeld CS. 1998. Prospective evaluation of an index for predicting the risk of major bleeding in outpatients treated with warfarin. *Am. J. Med.* 105:91–99

79. Hirsh J, Weitz JI. 1999. New antithrombotic agents. *Lancet* 353:1431–36; erratum, *Lancet* 353:1804

80. Lee AY, Bates SM, Weitz JI. 1999. Direct thrombin inhibitors. *Curr. Opin. Cardiovasc. Pulm. Renal Drugs* 1:28–39

81. Eriksson H, Eriksson UG, Frison L, et al. 1999. Pharmacokinetics and pharmacodynamics of melagatran, a novel synthetic LMW thrombin inhibitor, in patients with acute DVT. *Thromb. Haemost.* 81:358–63

82. The Rembrandt Investigators. 2000. Treatment of proximal deep vein thrombosis with a novel synthetic compound (SR90107A/ORG31540) with pure antifactor Xa activity: a phase II evaluation. 2000. *Circulation* 102:2726–31

83. Rogers LQ, Lutcher CL. 1990. Streptokinase therapy for deep vein thrombosis: a comprehensive review of the English literature. *Am. J. Med.* 88:389–95

84. Arcasoy SM, Kreit JW. 1999. Thrombolytic therapy of pulmonary embolism: a comprehensive review of current evidence. *Chest* 115:1695–707

85. Levine MN, Goldhaber SZ, Gore JM, et al. 1995. Hemorrhagic complications of

thrombolytic therapy in the treatment of myocardial infarction and venous thromboembolism. *Chest* 108:291S–301S

86. Kanter DS, Mikkola KM, Patel SR, et al. 1997. Thrombolytic therapy for pulmonary embolism. Frequency of intracranial hemorrhage and associated risk factors. *Chest* 111:1241–45

87. Streiff MB. 2000. Vena caval filters: a comprehensive review. *Blood* 95:3669–77

88. Pacouret G, Alison D, Pottier JM, et al. 1997. Free-floating thrombus and embolic risk in patients with angiographically confirmed proximal deep venous thrombosis. A prospective study. *Arch. Intern. Med.* 157:305–8

89. Decousus H, Leizorovicz A, Parent F, et al. 1998. A clinical trial of vena caval filters in the prevention of pulmonary embolism in patients with proximal deep-vein thrombosis. Prevention du Risque d'Embolie Pulmonaire par Interruption Cave Study Group. *N. Engl. J. Med.* 338:409–15

90. Lansing AM, Davis WM. 1968. Five-year follow-up study of iliofemoral venous thrombectomy. *Ann. Surg.* 168:620–28

91. Schmitz-Rode T, Janssens U, Duda SH, et al. 2000. Massive pulmonary embolism: percutaneous emergency treatment by pigtail rotation catheter. *J. Am. Coll. Cardiol.* 36:375–80

92. Koning R, Cribier A, Gerber L, et al. 1997. A new treatment for severe pulmonary embolism: percutaneous rheolytic thrombectomy. *Circulation* 96:2498–500

93. Cho KJ, Dasika NL. 2000. Catheter technique for pulmonary embolectomy or thrombofragmentation. *Semin. Vasc. Surg.* 13:221–35

94. Goldhaber SZ. 1998. Integration of catheter thrombectomy into our armamentarium to treat acute pulmonary embolism. *Chest* 114:1237–38

95. Moser KM, Auger WR, Fedullo PF. 1990. Chronic major-vessel thromboembolic pulmonary hypertension. *Circulation* 81:1735–43

Annu. Rev. Med. 2002. 53:35–57

CYCLOOXYGENASE-2: A Therapeutic Target

Marco E. Turini[1] and Raymond N. DuBois[2]

[1]Department of Nutrition, Nestlé Research Center, CH-1000 Lausanne 26, Switzerland;
[2]Departments of Medicine/GI & Cell Biology, Vanderbilt University Medical Center,
Nashville, Tennessee 37232; e-mail: raymond.dubois@mcmail.vanderbilt.edu

Key Words   cyclooxygenase, prostaglandins, biology, disease, inflammation

■ **Abstract**   Cyclooxygenase (COX), also known as prostaglandin endoperoxide synthase, is the key enzyme required for the conversion of arachidonic acid to prostaglandins. Two COX isoforms have been identified, COX-1 and COX-2. In many situations, the COX-1 enzyme is produced constitutively (e.g., in gastric mucosa), whereas COX-2 is highly inducible (e.g., at sites of inflammation and cancer). Traditional non-steroidal anti-inflammatory drugs (NSAIDs) inhibit both enzymes, and a new class of COX-2 selective inhibitors (COXIBs) preferentially inhibit the COX-2 enzyme. This review summarizes our current understanding of the role of COX-1 and COX-2 in normal physiology and disease.

INTRODUCTION

Prostaglandin endoperoxide synthase, commonly called cyclooxygenase (COX), is the key enzyme required for the conversion of arachidonic acid to prostaglandins. The two known COX isoforms are referred to as COX-1 and COX-2 for the order in which they were discovered. Aspirin, which works by inhibiting COX activity, has been available to the public for over 100 years; in fact, extracts from willow bark and myrtle, containing salicylates or their precursors, were prescribed by physicians for pain and fever centuries ago. However, only since 1971 has our understanding of the role of the COX enzyme in biology and disease become more clear.

Despite the wide use of nonsteroidal anti-inflammatory drugs (NSAIDs) over the past century, their mechanism of action was not fully appreciated until Vane (1) published his seminal observations indicating that the ability of NSAIDs to suppress inflammation is probably due to their ability to inhibit the COX enzyme. This effectively limits the production of proinflammatory prostaglandins (PGs) at a site of injury. Following this discovery, scientists and clinicians have used NSAIDs to dissect the critical role of both the COX enzymes and the eicosanoids derived from this pathway in normal physiology and disease states. It is important to note that inhibition of the COX enzyme occurs at a drug concentration in the nanomolar to micromolar range. When NSAIDs and COX-2 selective inhibitors (COXIBs) are given at much higher doses, achieving concentrations of >100 μM, their effects are probably due to modulation of COX-independent signaling pathways.

Given the broad role of PGs in normal human physiology, it is not surprising that systemic suppression of PG synthesis through inhibition of COX can lead to unwanted side effects (Table 1). It is well-known that individuals taking NSAIDs for even short periods of time can experience severe gastrointestinal and renal side effects (2, 3), in addition to effects on other physiological systems. As many as 25% of individuals using NSAIDs experience some side effect and up to 5% develop serious health consequences.

The different effects of PGs can be explained by their varied chemistry, the diversity of PG receptors, and modulation of PG synthesis. The structural, cellular, and molecular biology of COX (4) and of prostanoid receptors (5) have recently been reviewed. Here, we focus on the role of COX-1 and COX-2 on the biology of different organ systems. Intensive research in the past 10 years has evaluated the relative contribution of each isoform. Because NSAIDs have proven efficacy in treating arthritis and pain yet can also cause deleterious side effects, a major goal of the pharmaceutical industry was to design an anti-inflammatory drug with a wider therapeutic window that lacked the serious side effects of non-selective NSAIDs. This led to the development of COXIBs, of which celecoxib (Celebrex) and rofecoxib (Vioxx) have dominated the U.S. market.

TABLE 1 Known and potential processes involved with COX-2 upregulation

Inflammation	Urogenital disease
Pain	Alzheimer's disease
Fever	Cancers:
Ovulation, pregnancy, and childbirth	Familial adenomatous polyposis
Renal function	Colorectal
Bone metabolism	Prostate
Tissue repair	Pancreatic
Myocardial infarction	Skin
Stroke	Head and neck
Atheroma	Esophagus
Diabetes	Breast
Diabetic retinopathy	Lung
Allograft rejection	

DISCOVERY OF AN INDUCIBLE CYCLOOXYGENASE

The COX-1 cDNA was initially isolated in 1988 from sheep, mouse, and human sources. The gene is 25 kb in size, is located on human chromosome 9q32–q33.3 (6), contains 11 exons (7), and produces a 2.8-kb mRNA (8) and a $\sim$68-kDa protein. Investigators evaluating a variety of signaling pathways identified a unique, inducible gene product that was homologous to the known COX-1 sequence (reviewed in 9). Others evaluating PG production in response to cytokines and other inflammatory mediators noted increases in COX activity probably due to increased expression of another COX (10). Immunoprecipitation of this COX variant with an anti-COX antibody, as well as the production of an antibody that precipitated only the COX-2 isoform, indicated the possibility of two different COX isoforms. Later, it was determined that the COX-1 and COX-2 proteins are derived from distinct genes that diverged well before birds and mammals (11). COX-2 is an 8-kb gene composed of 10 exons located on human chromosome 1q25.2–q25.3 (6). The mRNA is 4.1–4.5 kb (9) and encodes a protein of $\sim$68 kDa.

Both enzymes carry out essentially the same catalytic reaction and have similar tertiary structures (12), but the proinflammatory role appears to be mediated mainly by COX-2, whereas most of the "housekeeping" functions appear to be regulated by COX-1 (Figure 1). For the most part, each isoform's apparent function is consistent with its tissue expression pattern. Nearly all normal tissues express COX-1 with low to undetectable levels of COX-2, whereas COX-2 is constitutively expressed in the brain, pancreatic islet cells, ovary, uterus, and kidney (13). Other differences between COX-1 and COX-2 include differences in utilization of arachidonic acid substrate pools as well as in mRNA stability (14–16).

Joints

INFLAMMATION AND ARTHRITIS   Although the role of COX activity in the production of PGs has been known since 1967 (17), the inducibility of this activity and the central role of this induction in inflammation have been elucidated only recently (18). Studies from animal models of inflammatory arthritis strongly suggest that increased expression of COX-2 is responsible for the increased PG production seen in inflamed joint tissues (19). COX-2 induction has been observed in both human osteoarthritis-affected cartilage (20) and synovial tissue from rheumatoid arthritis patients (21). Cell culture experiments utilizing primary cells derived from human synovial tissue or other cells, such as monocytes, have advanced our understanding of the regulation of COX-2 expression. The proinflammatory agents IL-1,TNF-α, and lipopolysaccharide, as well as the growth factors TGF-β, EGF, PDGF, and FGF,[1] have all been shown to induce COX-2 expression in this

---

[1]IL, interleukin; TNF, tumor necrosis factor; TGF, transforming growth factor; EGF, epidermal growth factor; PDGF, platelet-derived growth factor; FGF, fibroblast growth factor.

system. On the other hand, the anti-inflammatory cytokines IL-4 and IL-13, as well as the immunosuppressive glucocorticoids, were shown to decrease COX-2 levels (22).

Although the synovial tissues of patients with osteoarthritis express lower amounts of COX-2, primary explant cultures of human osteoarthritis-affected cartilage have been found to contain significant levels of COX-2, which produces

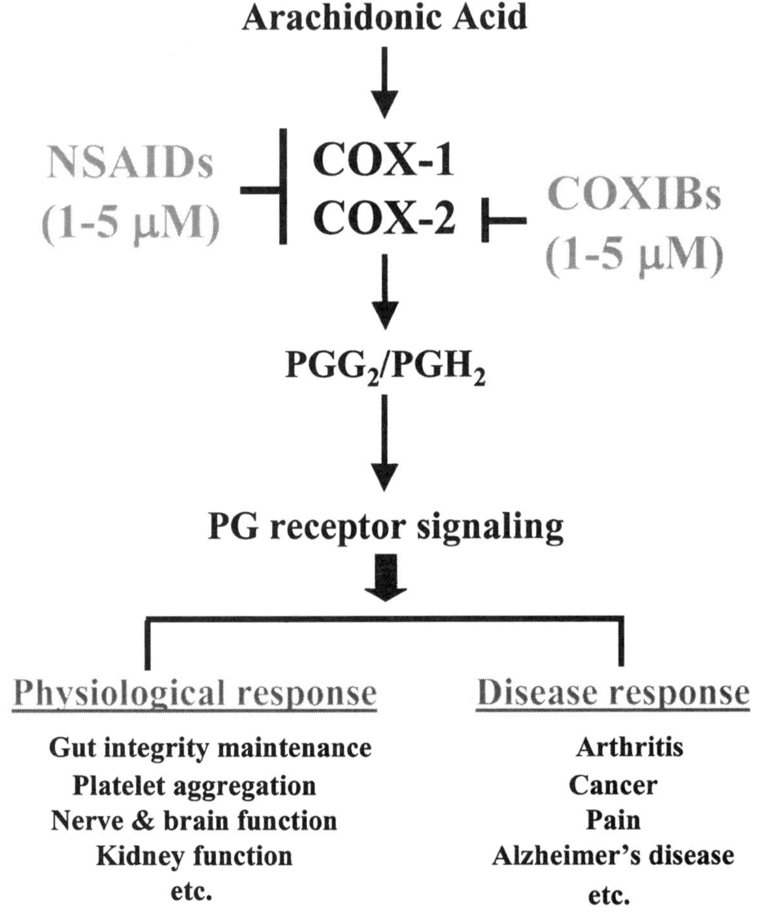

Figure 1   Schematic diagram of prostanoid signaling. COX-1 or COX-2 mediates the synthesis of PGG_2 and PGH_2 from arachidonic acid in a two-step reaction. PGH_2 is then metabolized by specific PG synthases to the 2-series prostanoids. Signaling through specific prostaglandin receptors mediates cellular responses in both physiological and disease states. Nonsteroidal anti-inflammatory drugs (NSAIDs) inhibit both COX-1 and COX-2, whereas specific COX-2 inhibitors (COXIBs) inhibit COX-2 with improved safety in the gut.

measurable quantities of PGs (20). Nitric oxide, another important inflammatory modulator, has been shown to regulate PG production in osteoarthritic cartilage, though not in synovial cells. Whether this modulation attenuates or enhances COX activity remains uncertain, although cross-talk between inducible nitric oxide synthase (iNOS) and COX-2 has been reported (23) and may be important in the development of osteoarthritis. Recently, investigators have shown that decreased production of nitric oxide through the selective inhibition of iNOS by N-iminoethyl-L-lysine significantly reduced the production of major catabolic factors such as metalloproteases, IL-1β, and peroxynitrite, as well as COX-2 expression (24, 25). More recent studies have shown that cells from iNOS$^{-/-}$ animals had a marked reduction in prostaglandin E$_2$ (PGE$_2$) formation compared with cells from control animals (26). However, COX-2 protein expression was not significantly different in cells from control versus knockout animals. Additionally, levels of PGE$_2$ in the urine of iNOS-deficient mice were decreased by 78% compared with control animals. These studies support the hypothesis that NO and/or NO-derived species modulate COX activity and eicosanoid production in vivo.

A better understanding of the role of COX-2 in inflammation led to drug discovery programs aimed at identifying new anti-inflammatory agents that selectively inhibit COX-2 activity (27). It appears that COX-2 specific inhibitors are useful alternatives for the treatment of osteoarthritis and rheumatoid arthritis, particularly in patients at high risk of developing gastrointestinal complications.

Celecoxib (Celebrex) is a COX inhibitor that exhibits relative in vitro and in vivo selectivity for COX-2 over COX-1. Celecoxib was found superior to placebo and has similar efficacy to that of conventional NSAIDs in reducing the signs and symptoms of osteoarthritis and rheumatoid arthritis, as indicated by randomized, double-blind, multicenter studies (reviewed in 28). This drug reduced pain and inflammation for up to 24 weeks of treatment in clinical trials. Another placebo-controlled, randomized, double-blind, multicenter trial demonstrated that celecoxib was effective in treating osteoarthritis, as measured by clinical improvement in signs and symptoms comparable to results seen in patients on naproxen for symptomatic osteoarthritis of the knee (29).

Rofecoxib (Vioxx) is another COX-2 selective inhibitor approved for use in humans. Phase II and phase III clinical trials evaluating the efficacy of rofecoxib demonstrated that a dose of 25 or 50 mg once daily was effective and generally well-tolerated in patients with rheumatoid arthritis (30), and its clinical efficacy was comparable to that of a daily dose of 150 mg of diclofenac over a one-year study period (31). Additionally, both 12.5 and 50 mg of rofecoxib daily demonstrated clinical efficacy for treatment of osteoarthritis that was comparable to a high dose of ibuprofen (32).

COX-2 is thought to be involved in the inflammatory process. Inhibition of its activity achieves the same therapeutic effect provided by less specific inhibitors that also target COX-1, and offers superior gastrointestinal safety. Based on animal and clinical data, rofecoxib is now commercially available in the United States and United Kingdom for the treatment of pain and osteoarthritis, and celecoxib has been approved in the United States and other countries for the treatment of rheumatoid arthritis and osteoarthritis.

PAIN   Local tissue injury and inflammatory diseases such as osteoarthritis are associated with elevated PG production and increased sensitization of pain receptors to PGs (33). Thus, the action of COX at the site of injury or inflammation is hyperalgesic, and local pain relief following NSAID treatment is easily explained by this mechanism. In addition, PGs are thought to act in the spinal cord to facilitate the transmission of pain responses, though little is known about the mechanism for this effect. NSAIDs can also act centrally (34–36).

COX-2 is induced in both local and central sites (37), and the question of whether COX-2 mediates pain reception or transmission is currently being investigated, primarily through the use of COXIBs. Intrathecal injection of both the COX-2 selective inhibitor NS-398 and the nonselective NSAID indomethacin suppressed a formalin-mediated pain response (which measures a central response), but neither inhibitor suppressed a high-temperature-induced pain response (a local response) (38). In contrast, meloxicam, when given systemically, suppressed the inflammatory pain response locally (39) without affecting central pain transmission. Meloxicam, at low doses, is more selective for COX-2 than COX-1. In neither of these studies was the drug introduced into both sites to allow an internal comparison, but collectively this work shows that COX-2 can act both locally and centrally to mediate pain. Short-term human studies showed that celecoxib and rofecoxib effectively suppress the pain associated with dental extractions, osteoarthritis, or rheumatoid arthritis without causing any significant gastroduodenal toxicity (40–44). Additionally, rofecoxib has been found to be effective for treatment of primary dysmenorrhea (45).

Central Nervous System and Brain

PHYSIOLOGICAL FUNCTION OF COX-2   COX-2 appears to play some role in the regulation of brain function. PGs have long been known as mediators of fever, of inflammatory reactions in neural tissue, and, more recently, of brain function. The recognition that each of these processes involves induction of PG synthesis has led to an appreciation of COX-2's role in the PG-mediated functions. Although NSAIDs are commonly used to control fever, the actual mechanism of fever induction has only recently been elucidated. Intraperitoneal injection with lipopolysaccharide causes a marked fever response in rats. In an elegant dissection of molecular and tissue interactions, Cao and colleagues have shown that COX-2 induction in brain endothelial cells temporally parallels the fever response (46, 47). This leads to the synthesis of PGs, which then act on temperature-sensing neurons in the preoptic area. In turn, COX-2 inhibition by an isoform-specific NSAID can effectively block the fever response (48). Communication between local inflammatory sites and the brain endothelium is mediated by cytokines such as IL-1, which can directly induce COX-2 expression in these cells

(49). These investigators have also shown induction of COX-2 expression in other parts of the brain, but these areas are not directly associated with the fever pathway.

A separate inflammatory pathway is mediated by microglial cells, a type of tissue-specific macrophage that lies dormant until needed for defense or tissue remodeling (50). Though known as a source of PGs during inflammation, the microglial cells do not induce COX-2 in response to cytokines, unlike other inflammatory cells. Instead, the microglial COX-2 response is limited to direct lipopolysaccharide exposure, which would occur only by direct bacterial infection of the brain. Thus, the microglial defensive response is segregated from systemic inflammation by its limited repertoire of inducers.

Recent studies suggest involvement of COX-2 in amyotrophic lateral sclerosis (ALS), a neurodegenerative process. COX-2 inhibition may have some promise as therapy for the treatment of ALS (51, 52). Further studies are needed to explore this issue.

ALZHEIMER'S DISEASE   The molecular and therapeutic mechanisms of Alzheimer's disease (AD) and inflammation have recently been reviewed (53–55). AD is characterized by progressive dementia and the extracellular deposition of β-amyloid fibrils within the brain. Subsequently, there is a phenotypic activation of microglial cells associated with the amyloid plaque. The amyloid-β peptide (Abeta) is a proteolytic fragment of the amyloid precursor protein (APP). Microglia activation results in a complex local proinflammatory response and secretion of inflammatory products.

Several epidemiological studies have indicated that patients taking NSAIDs for other diseases (e.g., rheumatoid arthritis) have a 50% lower risk of developing AD than those not taking NSAIDs (56–58). However, the precise pharmacological actions of anti-inflammatory drugs in the brain are still unclear. Several studies are attempting to identify a role for COX in the etiology of AD.

Cytokines such as IL-1 or IL-6, as well as acute-phase proteins such as α1-antichymotrypsin (ACT), participate in the etiopathology of AD. Tepoxalin, a novel NSAID, markedly inhibited IL-1β-induced IL-6 and ACT synthesis in astrocytes (59). Lipopolysaccharide-stimulated microglial cells treated with tepoxalin also exhibited decreased synthesis of IL-1β and IL-6 (59). This effect was mediated through inhibition of NF-κB via decreased IκB-α degradation. NF-κB is known to activate COX-2 expression under some circumstances. The β-amyloid-stimulated secretion of proinflammatory products by microglia and monocytes, mediating neurotoxicity and astrocyte activation, was also inhibited by NSAIDs, reportedly through PPAR$_\gamma$ activation (60).

Recognition of COX-2's key role in inflammation led to the hypothesis that it may represent a primary target for NSAIDs in AD, consistent with inflammatory processes occurring in AD brain (61, 62). Elevated CSF PGE$_2$ levels are observed in patients with probable AD (63). COX-2 was elevated in the hippocampal pyramidal layer in sporadic AD and was correlated with amyloid plaque density (64). In vitro studies using COX-2–overexpressing neurons derived from transgenic mice suggest that elevation of COX-2 may potentiate A-beta–mediated oxidative stress (64). Further analyses of 54 post-mortem brain specimens from patients with normal or impaired cognitive status suggested that neuronal COX-2 expression in subsets of hippocampal pyramidal neurons may be a marker of progression of dementia in early AD (65). IL-1β and synthetic β-amyloid peptides induced COX-2 expression and PGE_2 release in the human neuroblastoma cell line SK-N-SH (66, 67). As demonstrated in human breast cancer cells (68), neuroblastoma cells also exhibit increased COX-2 expression mediated by p38 mitogen-activated protein kinase (MAPK), suggesting p38 MAPK as a potential therapeutic target in AD (67).

However, COX-1 and COX-2 may be involved in different cellular processes in the pathogenesis of AD, as indicated by their different distribution profile. An overall increase of COX-1 expression in AD has also been suggested. COX-1 expression was detected in microglial cells, whereas COX-2 expression was found in neuronal cells (69). In AD brains, COX-1-positive microglial cells were primarily associated with the amyloid plaques, and AD fusiform cortex exhibited increased density of COX-1 immunopositive microglia (69, 70). Furthermore, more COX-2-positive neurons were detected in AD brains than in control brains (69). Although in vitro studies use astrocytes to investigate the role of COX in AD, no COX expression was detected in astrocytes in vivo. Therefore, COX-1 could also contribute to central nervous system pathology, which brings up the issue of whether nonselective inhibitors would be more effective.

The possible implication of COX-1 in AD is further substantiated by the Alzheimer's Disease Cooperative Study (ADCS) (71). A multicenter clinical trial found that a repressor of COX-2 expression, prednisone, neither prevented nor accelerated cognitive decline in AD, although interpretation of these data is complex because glucocorticoids are fairly nonspecific and affect many other pathways. Nevertheless, the ADCS has initiated a trial to compare a nonselective NSAID and a selective COX-2 inhibitor for effectiveness in slowing the rate of cognitive decline in AD. Indomethacin showed promising results in a pilot clinical trial (72). Whether COX-2 inhibitors will be more effective is uncertain, since the enzyme is constitutively expressed in neurons and may play some role in normal brain function (73). Animal experiments suggest that COX-2 may be responsible for the regulation of adaptive functions associated with normal neurons and protective functions associated with stressed neurons. Other mechanisms for NSAID neuroprotective potency unrelated to their ability to inhibit COX-1 or COX-2, such as inhibition of monocyte cytotoxicity, have been suggested based on in vitro neurotoxicity assays (74).

The antithrombotic activity of PGs may also be important for protection against AD. For example, de la Torre (75) hypothesizes that AD is caused by the development of tortuous and flow-impeded capillaries in the brain. This would presumably promote intravascular coagulation, leading to ischemic damage in the brain that could promote the development of AD. Platelets contain both APP and

A-beta, which may contribute to the perivascular amyloid deposition seen in AD. Skowronski et al. (76) provide evidence that in human platelets, protein kinase C (PKC) is involved in the secretory cleavage of APP, whereas COX plays only a minor role in this process.

The precise role of the COX isoenzymes in AD is not clear, but the use of NSAIDs that inhibit both COX-1 and COX-2 activity appears to be beneficial. Nonselective NSAIDs can reduce inflammation associated with activation of microglia, but they seem ineffective in reversing the degenerative process in AD. Nevertheless, the effects of NSAIDs are likely to be mediated through a combination of mechanisms. Although reduced microglial or monocyte activation has been shown to be effective in various cell culture and animal models, clinical studies have yet to be performed. Mechanistic studies already under way will provide insight and direction for further developments.

Kidney

RENAL FUNCTION   PGs are important physiologic modulators of vascular tone and salt and water homeostasis in the mammalian kidney. Their functions include modulation of glomerular hemodynamics, tubular reabsorption of salt and water, and regulation of renin secretion (77–79). While COX-1 has long been recognized to be involved in normal kidney function, COX-2 is thought to have a distinct role. Localization studies have found COX-2 in both the macula densa of the rat kidney (80) and the interstitial cells of the medulla (81). The macula densa plays an important role in mediating the interaction between glomerular filtration, proximal reabsorption, and regulation of renin release (82), which in turn is responsible for salt balance and fluid volume. Although PGE_2 has been reported to inhibit chloride reabsorption in the ascending limb of Henle, chronic salt deprivation was found to increase COX-2 levels in the region of the macula densa, and COX-2-generated prostanoids may be important mediators of renin production and tubuloglomerular feedback. The details of interactions between the COX-1- and COX-2-mediated systems in the kidney are not clear. Mapping of PG receptors in the kidney (83, 84) does show differential location of receptors specific for different PGs, indicating that differential synthesis of specific types of PGs may be responsible for the effects of COX-1 and COX-2. This topic has recently been reviewed (85).

In addition to the multiple roles of PGs in the adult kidney, the original strains of COX-2 null mice show severe disruption of kidney development (86, 87). Studies in COX-2$^{-/-}$ mice demonstrate that tissue-specific and time-dependent expression of COX-2 may be necessary for normal postnatal renal development and for maintenance of normal renal architecture and renal function (88). However, in later generations, the COX-2$^{-/-}$ mice demonstrate a much less severe phenotype with regard to renal function.

NSAIDs are known to have multiple effects on kidney function, and specific COX-2 inhibitors should be useful in dissecting the role of PGs generated from the

COX-2 pathway in normal renal physiology. However, caution is advised in clinical practice, since patients with chronic renal insufficiency taking COX-2 inhibitors may develop acute renal failure (89).

NEPHRITIS   Biopsies of patients with IgA nephritis showed higher expression of COX-1, relative to COX-2, in glomeruli, whereas COX-2 was strongly expressed in infiltrating interstitial cells (90). Both COX isoforms may thus play a role in human glomerular inflammation associated with IgA nephritis.

In a rat model of transient mesangioproliferative glomerulonephritis, a dramatic transient increase of COX-1 staining in diseased glomeruli, localized mainly to mesangial cells, coincided with cell proliferation (90). A transient increase in COX-2 expression occurred in the macula densa region, and glomerular cells did not exhibit significant upregulation of COX-2 at any time. It was concluded that glomerular COX-1, but not COX-2, mediated PG production, which may contribute to the resolution rather than to the progression of nephritis in this rat model. In addition, regulatory interactions between the arachidonic and nitric oxide pathways in glomerulonephritis have been reported (91).

GASTROINTESTINAL TRACT

Maintenance of Gastrointestinal Integrity

The intestinal epithelium undergoes constant regeneration and remodeling in response to both insult and normal use. The use of NSAIDs can cause a variety of problems in the gastrointestinal tract (92), including irritation and ulceration of the stomach lining (93). Radiation exposure leads to intestinal epithelial cell death, leaving crypt cells to regenerate the epithelial lining. In animal studies, COX-2 is not induced following exposure to radiation and is not essential for crypt cell survival under these circumstances (94). Following radiation treatment, COX-1 plays a major role in maintaining proper glandular architecture of the small intestine and in maintaining healthy gastric mucosa. For example, indomethacin, which effectively inhibits COX-1 and COX-2, suppressed crypt survival and PGE_2 production in the intestine following radiation damage (94).

The gastrointestinal epithelium is also the target of numerous infectious and parasitic organisms. In response to infection or invasion, COX-2 expression is induced in epithelial cells (95), which leads to increased PG production. The PGs then stimulate chloride and fluid secretion from the mucosa, which flushes bacteria from the intestine. In addition, COX-2 is expressed during inflammation and wound healing, and in animals, treatment with COX-2 inhibitors can exacerbate inflammation and inhibit healing (96–98). Nevertheless, COX-2 selective inhibitors appear to be associated with less gastrointestinal damage than conventional NSAIDs (99). Clinical trials evaluating agents that are highly selective for COX-2 have demonstrated that selective COX-2 inhibitors have a significantly better safety profile than nonselective NSAIDs (100, 101).

Cancer

Several population-based studies have detected a 40%–50% decrease in relative risk for colorectal cancer in persons who regularly use aspirin and other NSAIDs (102–106). Studies in a variety of colon cancer animal models (both genetic and carcinogen-induced) have also demonstrated a significant reduction in tumor multiplicity following NSAID treatment (107). In fact, some studies have shown as much as an 80%–90% reduction in tumor burden (108).

Initial attempts to determine the molecular basis for these observations revealed that the majority of both human and animal colorectal tumors express high levels of COX-2, whereas the surrounding tissue has low to undetectable COX-2 expression (14, 109–111). Although COX-2 appears to play a role in colon cancer, the molecular mechanisms are only partially understood. Processes recently recognized as important include the inhibition of tumor cell growth, prevention of angiogenesis, and induction of apoptosis in neoplastic cells (Figure 2).

Celecoxib has been shown to dramatically inhibit colon carcinoma growth in preclinical studies, both in vitro and in vivo, without toxicity to the gastrointestinal tract (112). These results support the need for additional clinical studies of celecoxib for treatment and/or prevention of colorectal cancer in humans. Other work in cell culture models has shown that COX-2 expression contributes significantly to the tumorigenic potential of epithelial cells by increasing adhesion to extracellular matrix and making cells resistant to apoptosis (113). These phenotypic changes are reversed by treatment with a highly selective COX-2 inhibitor. Immunohistochemistry and RT-PCR measurements of COX-2 in sporadic colorectal cancers, including adenomas, carcinomas, hyperplastic lesions, and normal tissues suggested that enhanced expression of COX-2 occurs early during colorectal carcinogenesis and may contribute to tumor progression (114). In this regard, a number of *cis* regulatory elements are present within the COX-2 promoter that may be involved in its upregulation during progression to neoplasia (Table 2).

TABLE 2   Identified regulators of COX-1 and COX-2 gene expression

COX-1 Upregulators	COX-2 Upregulators		COX-2 Downregulators
iNOS	iNOS	EGF	p53
Estrogen	IL-1α	TGF-β	Fish oil
	Wnt-1	TNF-α	Antioxidants
	Wnt-3	UVB	
	Src	Estrogen	
	Ras	Androgen	
	Benzo[α] Pyrene		

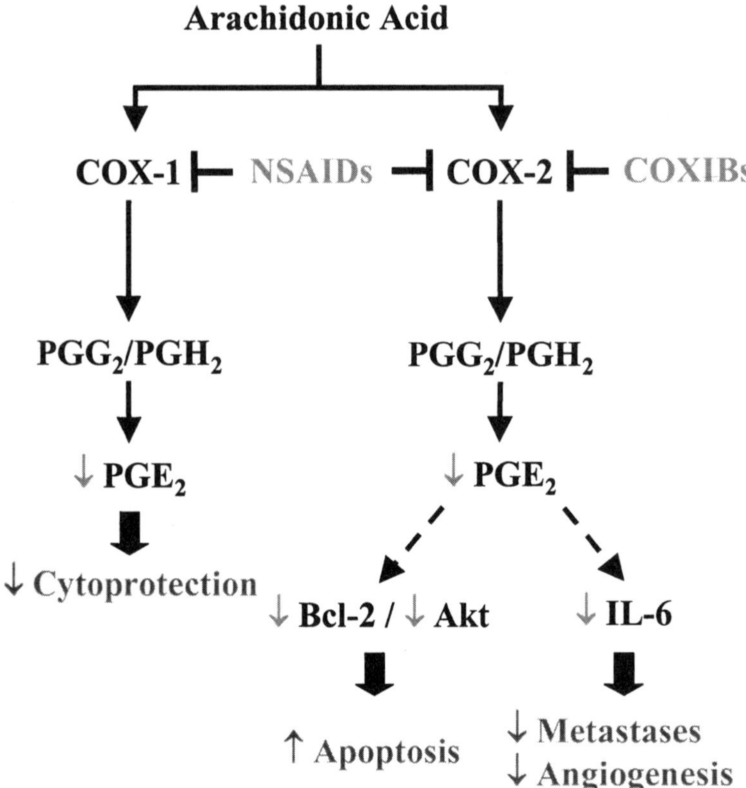

Figure 2 Potential mechanism of COX-2 inhibitors in neoplasia. COX-2 produces prostaglandins that inhibit apoptosis and stimulate angiogenesis and invasion. Prostaglandin synthesis can be reduced by selective COX-2 inhibitors to restore apoptosis and inhibit cancer cell proliferation. These effects may be mediated through the inhibition of IL-6 production and the downregulation of Bcl-2 and Akt.

Several studies indicate that COX-independent pathways are also important in the cancer chemopreventive properties of NSAIDs, and it is likely that both COX-dependent and COX-independent effects are involved (115–117). For example, certain NSAIDs induce apoptosis and alter expression of cell cycle regulatory genes in some cell lines when administered at relatively high concentrations (200–1000 μM) (115, 118). By using COX-deficient cell lines or drug metabolites lacking COX-inhibitory activity, these studies rule out the involvement of COX in the growth-inhibitory effect (112). Certainly, this class of drugs can affect biochemical pathways unrelated to COX, and these effects appear to be dose-dependent (some effects occurring only at toxic doses). He et al. (119) have implicated a direct effect of sulindac (another NSAID) on inhibition of PPAR$_\delta$-directed transcription in cell culture models, but only at drug concentrations above the 100-μM range.

More recently, this group has shown that sulindac has similar effects on cells that completely lack the $PPAR_\delta$ gene (120), indicating that other targets are probably responsible for this effect. The specific mechanisms of these COX-independent effects and their therapeutic implications are not yet well understood. However, most of the studies demonstrating effects on COX-independent pathways utilize concentrations of NSAID (100–1000 μM) that are difficult to achieve in living organisms without severe toxic side effects.

Familial Adenomatous Polyposis

Clinical trials with NSAIDs in patients with familial adenomatous polyposis (FAP) have clearly demonstrated that NSAID treatment results in regression of preexisting adenomas (121). Genetic evidence supporting a role for COX-2 in the development of intestinal neoplasia has also been reported. Oshima et al. (122) assessed the development of intestinal adenomas in $Apc^{\Delta716}$ mice (a model in which a targeted truncation deletion in the tumor suppresser gene APC causes intestinal polyposis) in a wild-type and homozygous null COX-2 genetic background. The number and size of polyps were reduced six- to eight-fold in the COX-2 null mice compared with COX-2 wild-type mice. In addition, a COX-2 inhibitor, Merck Frosst (MF) tricyclic, reduced polyp number in the $Apc^{\Delta716}$ mice more significantly than the nonselective NSAID, sulindac (122). Jacoby et al. (123) provided further support for a role of COX-2 by demonstrating that celecoxib was effective for the prevention and regression of adenomas in the adenomatous polyposis coli (APC) mutant Min mouse model. These and other studies (124) support ongoing clinical trials of COX-2 selective inhibitors in humans with FAP. Treatment twice daily for six months with celecoxib (400 mg) resulted in a significant reduction in the number of colorectal polyps in patients with FAP (125), leading to U.S. Food and Drug Administration (FDA) provisional approval of this drug for use in FAP patients.

Angiogenesis

Angiogenesis, the formation of new capillaries, is essential not only for the growth and metastasis of solid tumors but also for wound and ulcer healing. Blood flow for oxygen and nutrient delivery to the healing site cannot be restored without angiogenesis. Angiogenesis and suppressed cell-mediated immunity are central to the development and progression of malignant disease (reviewed in 126). Recent work indicates that COX may play a very important role in the regulation of angiogenesis associated with neoplastic tumor cells (127).

NSAIDs, such as aspirin, have antiangiogenic and immunomodulatory properties. COX-2 contributes to tumor angiogenesis through various mechanisms (reviewed in 128). Key mechanisms appear to involve the increased expression of the proangiogenic growth factor VEGF (129); the production of the eicosanoid products thromboxane (TX) A_2 (130), PGE_2, and PGI_2, which can directly stimulate endothelial cell migration and growth factor–induced angiogenesis; and, potentially, the inhibition of endothelial cell apoptosis by induction of Bcl-2 expression or Akt activation.

Both selective and nonselective NSAIDs inhibit angiogenesis through direct effects on endothelial cells (131). This effect is mediated through inhibition of MAPK (ERK2) activity and interference with ERK nuclear translocation but is independent of protein kinase C. It also involves prostaglandin-independent and prostaglandin-dependent components. In some circumstances, both COX-1 and COX-2 appear to be regulators of angiogenesis (132).

Other Cancers

Overexpression of COX-2 may not be unique to colon cancer and does occur in other epithelial tumors. Elevated COX-2 expression was reported in human breast cancers (133), lung cancer (134), uterine carcinoma (135), and carcinoma of the cervix (136). In vitro and animal experiments also suggest a role of COX-2 in bladder cancer (137, 138) and skin cancer (139, 140). A possible therapeutic effect of COX inhibition has also been suggested for head and neck cancers (141, 142) and esophageal cancer (143, 144).

Inflammatory Bowel Disease

Inflammatory bowel disease (IBD) is known to be associated with increased local production of prostanoids (145). Chronic intestinal inflammation (especially long-standing pancolitis) is directly linked to an increased lifetime risk for colorectal cancer.

Animal studies investigating the role of COX-2 in IBD have yielded conflicting results. Karmeli et al. (146) reported beneficial effects of COX-2 inhibitors on the extent and severity of experimental colitis in two rat models. Colitis was induced by intracaecal administration of 2 ml 5% acetic acid or intracolonic administration of 0.1 ml 3% iodoacetamide. On the other hand, three highly selective COX-2 inhibitors, NS-398, SC-58125, and PD-138387, did not exhibit any beneficial effect in the trinitro-benzene sulfonic acid (TNBS) model of colitis in rats (147). In agreement with the latter study is the report of PGD_2-mediated downregulation of granulocyte infiltration into the colonic mucosa, probably through the DP receptor in the same TNBS model of colitis (148). The increase in PGD_2 synthesis was abolished by treatment with a selective COX-2 inhibitor and resulted in a concomitant doubling of granulocyte infiltration. On the other hand, aspirin, a COX-1–preferential inhibitor, was more effective than selective COX-2 inhibitors at inhibiting granuloma dry weight, vascularity, and COX activity in the murine chronic granulomatous tissue air-pouch model of chronic inflammation (149).

In IBD patients, a relationship between endoscopic activity and relative levels of COX-2 mRNA has been reported (150). Whereas COX-2 was undetectable in normal ileum or colon, it was induced in apical epithelial cells of inflamed foci and in mononuclear cells of the colonic lamina propria of biopsies from IBD patients (151). COX-1 expression in inflamed tissue was similar to that of normal tissue

(150–152). Differences in the effects of inhibitors in experimental colitis may be due to differences in the animal models and in the COX inhibitors used. However, the ability of NSAIDs and COX-2 inhibitors to exacerbate IBD (148, 153) suggests that PGs are important anti-inflammatory mediators in this context, or that COX inhibition results in shunting of the arachidonic acid substrate to other pathways such as lipoxygenase for production of proinflammatory leukotrienes (e.g. LTB_4). Whether inhibition of COX-2 would improve symptoms in patients suffering from chronic IBD is presently unclear. To our knowledge, no studies evaluating the effect of COXIBs in IBD patients have been reported.

CONCLUSIONS

The COX isoenzymes and their eicosanoid products play functional roles in many physiological systems. NSAIDs such as aspirin, indomethacin, and ibuprofen are the most widely used drugs for pain, arthritis, and cardiovascular diseases and now are under consideration for the prevention of colon cancer and AD. COX-2 selective agents appear to be an improvement over conventional NSAIDs for patients with pain, rheumatoid arthritis, and osteoarthritis, which has resulted in their widespread use in medical practice.

The ability of NSAIDs to exacerbate IBD in both humans and animals suggests that prostanoids are important anti-inflammatory mediators in this context. In addition, specific COX-2 inhibitors have been reported to exacerbate chronic inflammation in animals. Because of the adverse effects reported in animal studies, a trial testing the efficacy of COX-2 inhibitors in IBD patients is unlikely.

Constitutive COX-2 expression has been detected in the stomach, kidney, pancreatic islet cells, and central nervous system, suggesting a homeostatic role for COX-2 in certain tissues. In addition, both COX isoenzymes play an important role in tissue repair. The safety of COX-2 inhibitors in patients with active ulcers or with cardiovascular or renal disease requires further investigation.

Arachidonic acid metabolism through the COX and lipoxygenase pathways generates an array of bioactive eicosanoids. The mechanisms by which this biosynthetic pathway can mediate such diverse functions are largely unknown and likely to remain so until the various PG synthases and receptors downstream of COX are more fully characterized. The production of leukotrienes and their role in inflammation and cancer should not be overlooked.

Advancements in NSAID research have enabled the development of the COXIBs, a new class of NSAIDs that have quickly moved into clinical use. The quest for new drugs may lead to the development of additional compounds targeted toward specific eicosanoids (such as TXA_2), their synthetic enzymes, or their specific receptors to allow for the normal physiologic effect of eicosanoids without a pathologic response. Specific pathways, downstream of the COX/lipoxygenase enzymes involved in pathogenesis, theorically could be modulated with minimal alterations in the production of eicosanoids necessary to maintain homeostasis. This may result in more effective therapies for an array of diseases.

A little more than a century after the discovery of aspirin, the potential clinical indications for NSAIDs are widening from their original use as analgesics. Ongoing studies to more clearly delineate the role of each COX isoform in both health and disease will be crucial in defining additional applications for these drugs in the next century and in determining their ultimate safety.

Visit the Annual Reviews home page at www.AnnualReviews.org

LITERATURE CITED

1. Vane JR. 1971. Inhibition of prostaglandin synthesis as a mechanism of action for aspirin-like drugs. *Nature* 231:232–35

2. Murray MD, Brater DC. 1993. Renal toxicity of the nonsteroidal anti-inflammatory drugs. *Annu. Rev. Pharmacol. Toxicol.* 33:435–65

3. Davies NM. 1995. Toxicity of nonsteroidal anti-inflammatory drugs in the large intestine. *Dis. Colon Rectum* 38:1311–21

4. Smith WL, Dewitt DL, Garavito RM. 2000. Cyclooxygenases: structural, cellular, and molecular biology. *Annu. Rev. Biochem.* 69:145–82

5. Narumiya S, Sugimoto Y, Ushikubi F. 1999. Prostanoid receptors: structures, properties, and functions. *Physiol. Rev.* 79:1193–226

6. Kosaka T, Miyata A, Ihara H, et al. 1994. Characterization of the human gene (PTGS2) encoding prostaglandin-endoperoxide synthase 2. *Eur. J. Biochem.* 221:889–97

7. Kraemer SA, Meade EA, DeWitt DL. 1992. Prostaglandin endoperoxide synthase gene structure: identification of the transcriptional start site and 5′-flanking regulatory sequences. *Arch. Biochem. Biophys.* 293:391–400

8. Otto JC, Smith WL. 1995. Prostaglandin endoperoxide synthases-1 and -2. *J. Lipid Mediat. Cell Signal.* 12:139–56

9. Herschman HR. 1996. Prostaglandin synthase 2. *Biochim. Biophys. Acta* 1299:125–40

10. Raz A, Wyche A, Siegel N, et al. 1988. Regulation of fibroblast cyclooxygenase synthesis by interleukin-1. *J. Biol. Chem.* 263:3022–28

11. Reed DW, Bradshaw WS, Xie W, et al. 1996. In vivo and in vitro expression of a non-mammalian cyclooxygenase-1. *Prostaglandins* 52:269–84

12. Smith W, Garavito R, DeWitt D. 1996. Prostaglandin endoperoxide H synthases (cyclooxygenases)-1 and 2. *J. Biol. Chem.* 271:33157–60

13. Fosslien E. 2000. Biochemistry of cyclooxygenase (COX)-2 inhibitors and molecular pathology of COX-2 in neoplasia. *Crit. Rev. Clin. Lab. Sci.* 37:431–502

14. Kutchera W, Jones DA, Matsunami N, et al. 1996. Prostaglandin H synthase-2 is expressed abnormally in human colon cancer: evidence for a transcriptional effect. *Proc. Natl. Acad. Sci. USA* 93:4816–20

15. Reddy ST, Herschman HR. 1996. Transcellular prostaglandin production following mast cell activation is mediated by proximal secretory phospholipase A_2 and distal prostaglandin synthase 1. *J. Biol. Chem.* 271:186–91

16. Shao J, Sheng H, Inoue H, et al. 2000. Regulation of constitutive cyclooxygenase-2 expression in colon carcinoma cells. *J. Biol. Chem.* 275:33951–56

17. Lands WE. 1979. The biosynthesis and metabolism of prostaglandins. *Annu. Rev. Physiol.* 41:633–52

18. Needleman P, Isakson P. 1997. The discovery and function of COX-2. *J. Rheumatol.* 24:6–8

19. Anderson GD, Hauser SD, McGarity

KL, et al. 1996. Selective inhibition of cyclooxygenase (COX)-2 reverses inflammation and expression of COX-2 and interleukin 6 in rat adjuvant arthritis. *J. Clin. Invest.* 97:2672–79

20. Amin AR, Attur M, Patel RN, et al. 1997. Superinduction of cyclooxygenase-2 activity in human osteoarthritis-affected cartilage: influence of nitric oxide. *J. Clin. Invest.* 99:1231–37

21. Kang RY, Freire-Moar J, Sigal E, et al. 1996. Expression of cyclooxygenase-2 in human and an animal model of rheumatoid arthritis. *Br. J. Cancer* 35:711–18

22. Crofford LJ. 1997. COX-1 and COX-2 tissue expression: implications and predictions. *J. Rheumatol.* 24:15–19

23. Clancy R, Varenika B, Huang W, et al. 2000. Nitric oxide synthase/COX crosstalk: nitric oxide activates COX-1 but inhibits COX-2-derived prostaglandin production. *J. Immunol.* 165:1582–87

24. Manfield L, Jang D, Murrell GA. 1996. Nitric oxide enhances cyclooxygenase activity in articular cartilage. *Inflamm. Res.* 45:254–58

25. Pelletier JP, Lascau-Coman V, Jovanovic D, et al. 1999. Selective inhibition of inducible nitric oxide synthase in experimental osteoarthritis is associated with reduction in tissue levels of catabolic factors. *J. Rheumatol.* 26:2002–14

26. Marnett LJ, Wright TL, Crews BC, et al. 2000. Regulation of prostaglandin biosynthesis by nitric oxide is revealed by targeted deletion of inducible nitric-oxide synthase. *J. Biol. Chem.* 275:13427–30

27. Penning T, Talley J, Bertenshaw S, et al. 1997. Synthesis and biological evaluation of the 1,5-diarylpyrazol class of cyclooxygenase-2 inhibitors: identification of 4-[5-(4-methylphenyl)-3 (trifluoromethyl)-1Hpyrazol-1-yl] benzenesulfonamide (SC-58635, celecoxib). *J. Med. Chem.* 440:1347–65

28. Clemett D, Goa KL. 2000. Celecoxib: a review of its use in osteoarthritis, rheumatoid arthritis and acute pain. *Drugs* 59:957–80

29. Bensen WG, Fiechtner JJ, McMillen JI, et al. 1999. Treatment of osteoarthritis with celecoxib, a cyclooxygenase-2 inhibitor: a randomized controlled trial. *Mayo Clin. Proc.* 74:1095–105

30. Schnitzer TJ, Truitt K, Fleischmann R, et al. 1999. The safety profile, tolerability, and effective dose range of rofecoxib in the treatment of rheumatoid arthritis. Phase II Rofecoxib Rheumatoid Arthritis Study Group. *Clin. Ther.* 21:1688–702

31. Cannon GW, Caldwell JR, Holt P, et al. 2000. Rofecoxib, a specific inhibitor of cyclooxygenase 2, with clinical efficacy comparable with that of diclofenac sodium: results of a one-year, randomized, clinical trial in patients with osteoarthritis of the knee and hip. Rofecoxib Phase III Protocol 035 Study Group. *Arthritis Rheumatol.* 43:978–87

32. Day R, Morrison B, Luza A, et al. 2000. A randomized trial of the efficacy and tolerability of the COX-2 inhibitor rofecoxib vs ibuprofen in patients with osteoarthritis. Rofecoxib/Ibuprofen Comparator Study Group. *Arch. Intern. Med.* 160:1781–87

33. Dray A, Urban L. 1996. New pharmacological strategies for pain relief. *Annu. Rev. Pharmacol. Toxicol.* 36:253–80

34. Cashman JN, McAnulty G. 1995. Nonsteroidal antiinflammatory drugs in perisurgical pain management. Mechanisms of action and rationale for optimum use. *Drugs* 49:51–70

35. Cashman JN. 1996. The mechanisms of action of NSAIDs in analgesia. *Drugs* 52:13–23

36. Cherng CH, Wong CS, Ho ST. 1996. Spinal actions of nonsteroidal anti-inflammatory drugs. *Acta Anaesthesiol. Sinica* 34:81–88

37. Beiche F, Scheuerer S, Brune K, et al. 1996. Up-regulation of cyclooxygenase-2 mRNA in the rat spinal cord following peripheral inflammation. *FEBS Lett.* 390:165–69

38. Yamamoto T, Nozaki-Taguchi N. 1996. Analyses of the effects of cyclooxygenase (COX)-1 and COX-2 in spinal nociceptive transmission using indomethacin, a nonselective inhibitor. *Brain Res.* 739:104–10

39. Laird JMA, Herrero JF, Garcia de la Rubia P, et al. 1997. Analgesic activity of the novel COX-2 preferring NSAID, meloxicam, in mono-arthritic rats: central and peripheral components. *Inflamm. Res.* 46:203–10

40. Seibert K, Zhang Y, Leahy K, et al. 1994. Pharmacological and biochemical demonstration of the role of cyclooxygenase 2 in inflammation and pain. *Proc. Natl. Acad. Sci. USA* 91:12013–17

41. Lane NE. 1997. Pain management in osteoarthritis: the role of COX-2 inhibitors. *J. Rheumatol.* 24:20–24

42. Morrison BW, Fricke J, Brown J, et al. 2000. The optimal analgesic dose of rofecoxib: overview of six randomized controlled trials. *J. Am. Dent. Assoc.* 131:1729–37

43. Chang DJ, Christensen KS, Bulloch SE, et al. 2001. Superior efficacy of rofecoxib compared to codeine with acetaminophen for the treatment of acute pain. *Acad. Emerg. Med.* 8:429

44. Reicin A, Brown J, Jove M, et al. 2001. Efficacy of single-dose and multidose rofecoxib in the treatment of post-orthopedic surgery pain. *Am. J. Orthop.* 30:40–48

45. Morrison BW, Daniels SE, Kotey P, et al. 1999. Rofecoxib, a specific cyclooxygenase-2 inhibitor, in primary dysmenorrhea: a randomized controlled trial. *Obstet. Gynecol.* 94:504–8

46. Cao C, Matsumara K, Watanabe Y. 1997. Involvement of cyclooxygenase-2 in LPS-induced fever and regulation of its mRNA by LPS in the brain. *Am. J. Physiol. Regulatory Integrative Comp. Physiol.* 272:R1712–R1725

47. Matsumura K, Cao C, Wantanabe Y. 1997. Possible role of cyclooxygenase-2 in the brain vasculature in febrile response. *Ann. NY Acad. Sci.* 813:302–6

48. Taniguchi Y, Yokoyama K, Inui K, et al. 1997. Inhibition of brain cyclooxygenase-2 activity and the antipyretic action of nimesulide. *Eur. J. Pharmacol.* 330:221–29

49. Cao C, Matsumara K, Watanabe Y. 1997. Induction of cyclooxygenase-2 in the brain by cytokines. *Ann. NY Acad. Sci.* 813:309

50. Bauer MK, Lieb K, Schultze-Osthoff K, et al. 1997. Expression and regulation of cyclooxygenase-2 in rat microglia. *Eur. J. Biochem.* 243:726–31

51. Drachman DB, Rothstein JD. 2000. Inhibition of cyclooxygenase-2 protects motor neurons in an organotypic model of amyotrophic lateral sclerosis. *Ann. Neurol.* 48:792–95

52. Almer G, Guegan C, Teismann P, et al. 2001. Increased expression of the pro-inflammatory enzyme cyclooxygenase-2 in amyotrophic lateral sclerosis. *Ann. Neurol.* 49:176–85

53. Halliday G, Robinson SR, Shepherd C, et al. 2000. Alzheimer's disease and inflammation: a review of cellular and therapeutic mechanisms. *Clin. Exp. Pharmacol. Physio.* 27:1–8

54. Hull M, Lieb K, Fiebich BL. 2000. Anti-inflammatory drugs: a hope for Alzheimer's disease? *Expert Opin. Investig. Drugs* 9:671–83

55. Lukiw WJ, Bazan NG. 2000. Neuroinflammatory signaling upregulation in Alzheimer's disease. *Neurochem. Res.* 25:1173–84

56. Andersen K, Launer LJ, Ott A, et al. 1995. Do nonsteroidal anti-inflammatory drugs decrease the risk of Alzheimer's disease? The Rotterdam study. *Neurology* 45:1441–45

57. McGeer PL, Schulzer M, McGeer EG 1996. Arthritis and anti-inflammatory agents as possible protective factors for Alzheimer's disease: a review of 17 epidemiologic studies. *Neurology* 47:425–32

58. Stewart WF, Kawas C, Corrada M, et al. 1997. Risk of Alzheimer disease and duration of NSAID use. *Neurology* 48:626–32

59. Fiebich BL, Hofer TJ, Lieb K, et al. 1999. The non-steroidal anti-inflammatory drug tepoxalin inhibits interleukin-6 and alpha1-anti-chymotrypsin synthesis in astrocytes by preventing degradation of IkappaB-alpha. *Neuropharmacology* 38:1325–33

60. Combs CK, Johnson DE, Karlo JC, et al. 2000. Inflammatory mechanisms in Alzheimer's disease: inhibition of beta-amyloid-stimulated proinflammatory responses and neurotoxicity by PPARgamma agonists. *J. Neurosci.* 20:558–67

61. Breitner J, Welsh K, Helms M, et al. 1995. Delayed onset of Alzheimer's disease with nonsteroidal anti-inflammatory and histamine H2 blocking drugs. *Neurobiol. Aging* 16:523–30

62. Breitner J. 1996. Inflammatory processes and antiinflammatory drugs in Alzheimer's disease: a current appraisal. *Neurobiol. Aging* 17:789–94

63. Ho L, Luterman JD, Aisen PS, et al. 2000. Elevated CSF prostaglandin E2 levels in patients with probable AD. *Neurology* 55:323

64. Ho L, Pieroni C, Winger D, et al. 1999. Regional distribution of cyclooxygenase-2 in the hippocampal formation in Alzheimer's disease. *J. Neurosci. Res.* 57:295–303

65. Ho L, Purohit D, Haroutunian V, et al. 2001. Neuronal cyclooxygenase 2 expression in the hippocampal formation as a function of the clinical progression of Alzheimer disease. *Arch. Neurol.* 58:487–92

66. Pasinetti GM, Aisen PS. 1998. Cyclooxygenase-2 expression is increased in frontal cortex of Alzheimer's disease brain. *Neuroscience* 87:319–24

67. Fiebich BL, Mueksch B, Boehringer M, et al. 2000. Interleukin-1beta induces cyclooxygenase-2 and prostaglandin E(2) synthesis in human neuroblastoma cells: involvement of p38 mitogen-activated protein kinase and nuclear factor-kappaB. *J. Neurochem.* 75:2020–28

68. Wollheim FA. 1999. New functions for COX-2 in health and disease: report of "The Third International Workshop on Cox-2." *Arthritis Res.* 1:45–49

69. Hoozemans JJ, Rozemuller AJ, Janssen I, et al. 2001. Cyclooxygenase expression in microglia and neurons in Alzheimer's disease and control brain. *Acta Neuropathol. (Berl.)* 101:2–8

70. Yermakova AV, Rollins J, Callahan LM, et al. 1999. Cyclooxygenase-1 in human Alzheimer and control brain: quantitative analysis of expression by microglia and CA3 hippocampal neurons. *J. Neuropathol. Exp. Neurol.* 58:1135–46

71. Aisen PS, Davis KL, Berg JD, et al. 2000. A randomized controlled trial of prednisone in Alzheimer's disease. Alzheimer's Disease Cooperative Study. *Neurology* 54:588–93

72. Rogers J, Kirby LC, Hempelman SR, et al. 1993. Clinical trial of indomethacin in Alzheimer's disease. *Neurology* 43:1609–11

73. O'Banion MK. 1999. Cyclooxygenase-2: molecular biology, pharmacology, and neurobiology. *Crit. Rev. Neurobiol.* 13:45–82

74. Klegeris A, Walker DG, McGeer PL. 1999. Toxicity of human THP-1 monocytic cells towards neuron-like cells is reduced by non-steroidal anti-inflammatory drugs (NSAIDs). *Neuropharmacology* 38:1017–25

75. de la Torre JC. 1997. Cerebromicrovascular pathology in Alzheimer's disease compared to normal aging. *Gerontology* 43:26–43

76. Skovronsky DM, Lee VM, Pratico D. 2001. Amyloid precursor protein and amyloid beta peptide in human platelets: role of cyclooxygenase and protein kinase C. *J. Biol. Chem.* 276:17036–43

77. Dunn MJ, Hood VL. 1977. Prostaglandins and the kidney. *Am. J. Physiol.* 233:169–84

78. Pugliese F, Ciabattoni G. 1984. The role of prostaglandins in the control of renal function: renal effects of nonsteroidal anti-inflammatory drugs. *Clin. Exp. Rheumatol.* 2:345–52

79. Breyer MD, Breyer RM. 2000. Prostaglandin receptors: their role in regulating renal function. *Curr. Opin. Nephrol. Hypertens.* 9:23–29

80. Harris RC, McKanna JA, Akai Y, et al. 1994. Cyclooxygenase-2 is associated with the macula densa of rat kidney and increases with salt restriction. *J. Clin. Invest.* 94:2504–10

81. Guan Y, Chang M, Cho W, et al. 1997. Cloning, expression and regulation of rabbit cyclooxygenase-2 in renal medullary interstitial cells. *Am. J. Physiol. Renal Physiol.* 273:F18–F26

82. Stokes JB. 1979. Effect of prostaglandin E2 on chloride transport across the rabbit thick ascending limb of Henle. *J. Clin. Invest.* 64:495–502

83. Breyer MD, Jacobson HR, Breyer RM. 1996. Functional and molecular aspects of renal prostaglandin receptors. *J. Am. Soc. Nephrol.* 7:8–17

84. Breyer MD, Davis L, Jacobson HR, et al. 1996. Differential localization of prostaglandin E receptor subtypes in human kidney. *Am. J. Phys. Renal Physiol.* 270:F912–F918

85. Breyer M, Breyer R. 2001. G protein-coupled prostanoid receptors and the kidney. *Annu. Rev. Physiol.* 63:579–605

86. Dinchuk JE, Car BD, Focht RJ, et al. 1995. Renal abnormalities and an altered inflammatory response in mice lacking cyclooxygenase II. *Nature* 378:406–9

87. Morham SG, Langenbach R, Loftin CD, et al. 1995. Prostaglandin synthase 2 gene disruption causes severe renal pathology in the mouse. *Cell* 83:473–82

88. Norwood VF, Morham SG, Smithies O. 2000. Postnatal development and progression of renal dysplasia in cyclooxygenase-2 null mice. *Kidney Int.* 58:2291–300

89. Perazella MA, Eras J. 2000. Are selective COX-2 inhibitors nephrotoxic? *Am. J. Kidney Dis.* 35:937–40

90. Hartner A, Pahl A, Brune K, et al. 2000. Upregulation of cyclooxygenase-1 and the PGE_2 receptor EP2 in rat and human mesangioproliferative glomerulonephritis. *Inflamm. Res.* 49:345–54

91. Lianos EA, Guglielmi K, Sharma M. 1998. Regulatory interactions between inducible nitric oxide synthase and eicosanoids in glomerular immune injury. *Kidney Int.* 53:645–53

92. Scheiman JM. 1996. NSAIDs, gastrointestinal injury and cytoprotection. *Gastroenterol. Clin. North Am.* 25:279–98

93. Roth SH. 1996. NSAID gastropathy. A new understanding. *Arch. Int. Med.* 156:1623–28

94. Cohn SM, Schloemann S, Tessner T, et al. 1997. Crypt stem cell survival in the mouse intestinal epithelium is regulated by prostaglandins synthesized through cyclooxygenase-1. *J. Clin. Invest.* 99:1367–79

95. Eckmann L, Stenson WF, Savidge TC, et al. 1997. Role of intestinal epithelial cells in the host secretory response to infection by invasive bacteria. Bacterial entry induces epithelial prostaglandin H synthase-2 expression and prostaglandin E2 and F2 alpha production. *J. Clin. Invest.* 100:296–309

96. Hull MA, Thomson JL, Hawkey CJ. 1999. Expression of cyclooxygenase 1 and 2 by human gastric endothelial cells. *Gut* 45:529–36

97. Brzozowski T, Konturek PC, Konturek SJ, et al. 2000. Involvement of cyclooxygenase (COX)-2 products in acceleration of ulcer healing by gastrin and hepatocyte growth factor. *J. Physiol. Pharmacol.* 51:751–73

98. Sun WH, Tsuji S, Tsujii M, et al. 2000. Induction of cyclooxygenase-2 in rat gastric mucosa by rebamipide, a mucoprotective agent. *J. Pharmacol. Exp. Ther.* 295:447–52

99. Simon LS. 1997. Biologic effects of

nonsteroidal anti-inflammatory drugs. *Curr. Opin. Rheumatol.* 9:178–82

100. Bombardier C, Laine L, Reicin A, et al. 2000. Comparison of upper gastrointestinal toxicity of rofecoxib and naproxen in patients with rheumatoid arthritis. VIGOR Study Group. *N. Engl. J. Med.* 343:1520–28

101. Silverstein FE, Faich G, Goldstein JL, et al. 2000. Gastrointestinal toxicity with celecoxib vs nonsteroidal anti-inflammatory drugs for osteoarthritis and rheumatoid arthritis: the CLASS Study: a randomized controlled trial. *JAMA* 284:1247–55

102. Thun MJ, Namboodiri MM, Heath CW Jr. 1991. Aspirin use and reduced risk of fatal colon cancer. *N. Engl. J. Med.* 325:1593–96

103. Thun MJ, Namboodiri MM, Calle EE, et al. 1993. Aspirin use and risk of fatal cancer. *Cancer Res.* 53:1322–27

104. Giovannucci E, Rimm EB, Stampfer MJ, et al. 1994. Aspirin use and the risk for colorectal cancer and adenoma in male health professionals. *Ann. Intern. Med.* 121:241–46

105. Giovannucci E, Egan KM, Hunter DJ, et al. 1995. Aspirin and the risk of colorectal cancer in women. *N. Engl. J. Med.* 333:609–14

106. Smalley W, DuBois RN. 1997. Colorectal cancer and nonsteroidal anti-inflammatory drugs. *Adv. Pharmacol.* 39:1–20

107. Williams CS, Mann M, DuBois RN. 1999. The role of cyclooxygenases in inflammation, cancer and development. *Oncogene* 18:7908–16

108. Kawamori T, Rao CV, Seibert K, et al. 1998. Chemopreventive activity of celecoxib, a specific cyclooxygenase-2 inhibitor, against colon carcinogenesis. *Cancer Res.* 58:409–12

109. Eberhart CE, Coffey RJ, Radhika A, et al. 1994. Up-regulation of cyclooxygenase-2 gene expression in human colorectal adenomas and adenocarcinomas. *Gastroenterology* 107:1183–88

110. Kargman S, O'Neill G, Vickers P, et al. 1995. Expression of prostaglandin G/H synthase-1 and -2 protein in human colon cancer. *Cancer Res.* 55:2556–59

111. Sano H, Kawahito Y, Wilder RL, et al. 1995. Expression of cyclooxygenase-1 and -2 in human colorectal cancer. *Cancer Res.* 55:3785–89

112. Williams CS, Watson AJM, Sheng H, et al. 2000. Celecoxib prevents tumor growth in vivo without toxicity to normal gut: lack of correlation between in vitro and in vivo models. *Cancer Res.* 60:6045–51

113. Tsujii M, DuBois RN. 1995. Alterations in cellular adhesion and apoptosis in epithelial cells overexpressing prostaglandin endoperoxide synthase-2. *Cell* 83:493–501

114. Hao X, Bishop AE, Wallace M, et al. 1999. Early expression of cyclo-oxygenase-2 during sporadic colorectal carcinogenesis. *J. Pathol.* 187:295–301

115. Piazza GA, Rahm AL, Krutzsch M, et al. 1995. Antineoplastic drugs sulindac sulfide and sulfone inhibit cell growth by inducing apoptosis. *Cancer Res.* 55:3110–16

116. Hanif R, Pittas A, Feng Y, et al. 1996. Effects of nonsteroidal anti-inflammatory drugs on proliferation and on induction of apoptosis in colon cancer cells by a prostaglandin-independent pathway. *Biochem. Pharmcol.* 52:237–45

117. Thompson HJ, Jiang C, Lu JX, et al. 1997. Sulfone metabolite of sulindac inhibits mammary carcinogenesis. *Cancer Res.* 57:267–71

118. Piazza GA, Rahm AK, Finn TS, et al. 1997. Apoptosis primarily accounts for the growth-inhibitory properties of sulindac metabolites and involves a mechanism that is independent of cyclooxygenase inhibition, cell cycle arrest, and p53 induction. *Cancer Res.* 57:2452–59

119. He TC, Chan TA, Vogelstein B, et al. 1999. PPARδ is an APC-regulated target

of nonsteroidal anti-inflammatory drugs. *Cell* 99:335–45

120. Park BH, Vogelstein B, Kinzler KW. 2001. Genetic disruption of PPARdelta decreases the tumorigenicity of human colon cancer cells. *Proc. Natl. Acad. Sci. USA* 98:2598–603

121. Giardiello FM, Offerhaus GJA, DuBois RN. 1995. The role of nonsteroidal anti-inflammatory drugs in colorectal cancer prevention. *Eur. J. Cancer* 31A:1071–76

122. Oshima M, Dinchuk JE, Kargman SL, et al. 1996. Suppression of intestinal polyposis in APC$^{\Delta 716}$ knockout mice by inhibition of prostaglandin endoperoxide synthase-2 (COX-2). *Cell* 87:803–9

123. Jacoby RF, Seibert K, Cole CE, et al. 2000. The cyclooxygenase-2 inhibitor celecoxib is a potent preventive and therapeutic agent in the min mouse model of adenomatous polyposis. *Cancer Res.* 60:5040–44

124. Oshima M, Murai N, Kargman S, et al. 2001. Chemoprevention of intestinal polyposis in the Apcdelta716 mouse by rofecoxib, a specific cyclooxygenase-2 inhibitor. *Cancer Res.* 61:1733–40

125. Steinbach G, Lynch PM, Phillips RK, et al. 2000. The effect of celecoxib, a cyclooxygenase-2 inhibitor, in familial adenomatous polyposis. *N. Engl. J. Med.* 342:1946–52

126. O'Byrne KJ, Dalgleish AG, Browning MJ, et al. 2000. The relationship between angiogenesis and the immune response in carcinogenesis and the progression of malignant disease. *Eur. J. Cancer* 36:151–69

127. Masferrer JL, Leahy KM, Koki AT. 2000. Role of cyclooxygenases in angiogenesis. *Curr. Med. Chem.* 7:1163–70

128. Gately S. 2000. The contributions of cyclooxygenase-2 to tumor angiogenesis. *Cancer Metastasis Rev.* 19:19–27

129. Williams CS, Tsujii M, Reese J, et al. 2000. Host cyclooxygenase-2 modulates carcinoma growth. *J. Clin. Invest.* 105:1589–94

130. Daniel TO, Liu H, Morrow JD, et al. 1999. Thromboxane A$_2$ is a mediator of cyclooxygenase-2-dependent endothelial migration and angiogenesis. *Cancer Res.* 59:4574–77

131. Jones MK, Wang H, Peskar BM, et al. 1999. Inhibition of angiogenesis by nonsteroidal anti-inflammatory drugs: insight into mechanisms and implications for cancer growth and ulcer healing. *Nat. Med.* 5:1418–23

132. Tsujii M, Kawano S, Tsuji S, et al. 1998. Cyclooxygenase regulates angiogenesis induced by colon cancer cells. *Cell* 93:705–16

133. Hwang D, Scollard D, Byrne J, et al. 1998. Expression of cyclooxygenase-1 and cyclooxygenase-2 in human breast cancer. *J. Natl. Cancer Inst.* 90:455–60

134. Wolff H, Saukkonen K, Anttila S, et al. 1998. Expression of cyclooxygenase-2 in human lung carcinoma. *Cancer Res.* 58:4997–5001

135. Tong BJ, Tan J, Tajeda L, et al. 2000. Heightened expression of cyclooxygenase-2 and peroxisome proliferator-activated receptor-δ in human endometrial adenocarcinoma. *Neoplasia* 2:483–90

136. Gaffney DK, Holden J, Davis M, et al. 2001. Elevated cyclooxygenase-2 expression correlates with diminished survival in carcinoma of the cervix treated with radiotherapy. *Int. J. Radiat. Oncol. Biol. Phys.* 49:1213–17

137. Grubbs CJ, Lubet RA, Koki AT, et al. 2000. Celecoxib inhibits N-butyl-N-(4-hydroxybutyl)-nitrosamine-induced urinary bladder cancers in male B6D2F1 mice and female Fischer-344 rats. *Cancer Res.* 60:5599–602

138. Grossman EM, Longo WE, Panesar N, et al. 2000. The role of cyclooxygenase enzymes in the growth of human gall bladder cancer cells. *Carcinogenesis* 21:1403–9

139. Buckman SY, Gresham A, Hale P, et al. 1998. COX-2 expression is induced by

UVB exposure in human skin: implications for the development of skin cancer. *Carcinogenesis* 19:723–29

140. Denkert C, Kobel M, Berger S, et al. 2001. Expression of cyclooxygenase 2 in human malignant melanoma. *Cancer Res.* 61:303–8

141. Mestre JR, Chan G, Zhang F, et al. 1999. Inhibition of cyclooxygenase-2 expression. An approach to preventing head and neck cancer. *Ann. NY Acad. Sci.* 889:62–71

142. Gallo O, Franchi A, Magnelli L, et al. 2001. Cyclooxygenase-2 pathway correlates with VEGF expression in head and neck cancer. Implications for tumor angiogenesis and metastasis. *Neoplasia* 3: 53–61

143. Zimmermann KC, Sarbia M, Weber AA, et al. 1999. Cyclooxygenase-2 expression in human esophageal carcinoma. *Cancer Res.* 59:198–204

144. Shamma A, Yamamoto H, Doki Y, et al. 2000. Up-regulation of cyclooxygenase-2 in squamous carcinogenesis of the esophagus. *Clin. Cancer Res.* 6:1229–38

145. Eberhart CE, DuBois RN. 1995. Eicosanoids and the gastrointestinal tract. *Gastroenterology* 109:285–301

146. Karmeli F, Cohen P, Rachmilewitz D. 2000. Cyclo-oxygenase-2 inhibitors ameliorate the severity of experimental colitis in rats. *Eur. J. Gastroenterol. Hepatol.* 12:223–31

147. Lesch CA, Kraus ER, Sanchez B, et al. 1999. Lack of beneficial effect of COX-2 inhibitors in an experimental model of colitis. *Methods Find. Exp. Clin. Pharmacol.* 21:99–104

148. Ajuebor MN, Singh A, Wallace JL. 2000. Cyclooxygenase-2-derived prostaglandin D(2) is an early anti-inflammatory signal in experimental colitis. *Am. J. Physiol. Gastrointest. Liver Physiol.* 279:G238–G244

149. Gilroy DW, Tomlinson A, Willoughby DA. 1998. Differential effects of inhibition of isoforms of cyclooxygenase (COX-1, COX-2) in chronic inflammation. *Inflamm. Res.* 47:79–85

150. Hendel J, Nielsen OH. 1997. Expression of cyclooxygenase-2 mRNA in active inflammatory bowel disease. *Am. J. Gastroenterol.* 92:1170–73

151. Singer II, Kawka DW, Schloemann S, et al. 1998. Cyclooxygenase 2 is induced in colonic epithelial cells in inflammatory bowel disease. *Gastroenterology* 115: 297–306

152. Muller-Decker K, Albert C, Lukanov T, et al. 1999. Cellular localization of cyclooxygenase isozymes in Crohn's disease and colorectal cancer. *Int. J. Colorectal Dis.* 14:212–18

153. Felder JB, Korelitz BI, Rajapakse R, et al. 2000. Effects of nonsteroidal antiinflammatory drugs on inflammatory bowel disease: a case-control study. *Am. J. Gastroenterol.* 95:1949–54

Annu. Rev. Med. 2002. 53:59–74

NEW THERAPEUTICS FOR CHRONIC HEART FAILURE

Douglas L. Mann[1], Anita Deswal[1], Biykem Bozkurt[1], and Guillermo Torre-Amione[2]

[1]*Winters Center for Heart Failure Research, Department of Medicine, Baylor College of Medicine, 6565 Fannin Street, Houston, Texas 77030; and Houston Veterans Administration Medical Center, 2002 Holcombe Blvd., Houston, Texas 77030;* [2]*The Methodist Hospital, 6565 Fannin Street, Houston, Texas 77030*

Key Words   left ventricular remodeling, renin angiotensin system, cyokines, adrenergic nervous system

■ **Abstract**   Traditionally, clinicians have viewed heart failure either as a problem of excessive salt and water retention caused by abnormalities of renal blood flow, or as a hemodynamic problem associated with a reduced cardiac output and excessive peripheral vasoconstriction. Recently, clinicians have begun to adopt a neurohormonal model in which heart failure progresses because of the toxic effects of endogenous biological systems that become activated in heart failure. We review the rationale for existing heart failure therapies and discuss the reasoning behind the development of some emerging therapies.

INTRODUCTION

Thus far, all attempts to develop a unifying hypothesis that explains the clinical syndrome of heart failure have fallen short when tested in large-scale clinical trials. Whereas clinicians initially viewed heart failure as a problem of excessive salt and water retention caused by abnormalities of renal blood flow [the cardiorenal model (1)], as physicians began to perform careful hemodynamic measurements, it also became apparent that heart failure was associated with a reduced cardiac output and excessive peripheral vasoconstriction. This latter realization led to the development of the cardiocirculatory or hemodynamic model for heart failure (1), wherein heart failure was thought to arise largely from abnormalities of the pumping capacity of the heart and excessive peripheral vasoconstriction. However, although both the cardiorenal and cardiocirculatory models for heart failure explained the excessive salt and water retention that heart failure patients experience, neither model explained the relentless disease progression that occurs in this syndrome. That is, although the cardiorenal model provided the rational basis for the use of diuretics to control the volume status of patients with heart failure, and the cardiocirculatory model provided the rational basis for the use of inotropes and intravenous vasodilators to augment cardiac output, these therapeutic strategies have not prevented heart failure from progressing, nor have they prolonged life for patients with moderate to severe heart failure (1, 2).

Figure 1 provides a general conceptual framework for discussing the development and progression of heart failure. As shown, heart failure may be viewed as a progressive disorder that is initiated after an index event either damages the heart muscle, with a resultant loss of functioning cardiac myocytes, or disrupts the ability of the myocardium to generate force, thereby preventing the heart from contracting normally. This index event may have an abrupt onset, as in the case of a myocardial infarction; it may have a gradual or insidious onset, as in the case hemodynamic pressure or volume overloading; or it may be hereditary, as in the case of genetic cardiomyopathies. All index events produce a decline in the pumping capacity of the heart. In most instances, patients remain asymptomatic

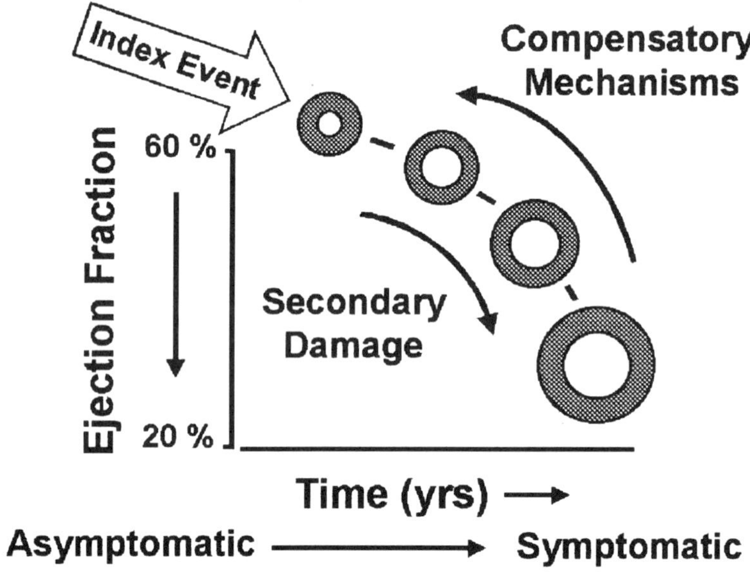

Figure 1   Pathogenesis of heart failure. Heart failure begins after an index event produces an initial decline in the pumping capacity of the heart. Following this initial decline, several compensatory mechanisms are activated, including the adrenergic nervous system, the renin angiotensin system, and the cytokine system. In the short term, these systems restore cardiovascular function to a normal homeostatic range, so the patient remains asymptomatic. However, with time, the sustained activation of these systems can lead to secondary end-organ damage within the ventricle, with worsening left ventricular (LV) remodeling and subsequent cardiac decompensation. As a result, patients undergo the transition from asymptomatic to symptomatic heart failure. (Adapted with permission from Reference 14.)

or minimally symptomatic following the initial decline in pumping capacity of the heart, or will develop symptoms only after the dysfunction has been present for some time. Thus, when viewed within this conceptual framework, left ventricular (LV) dysfunction is necessary but not sufficient for the development of the syndrome of heart failure.

Although it is not clear why patients with LV dysfunction remain asymptomatic, one potential explanation is that compensatory mechanisms that become activated in cardiac injury are able to sustain and modulate LV ventricular function for a period of days, months, or years. Known compensatory mechanisms include early activation of the sympathetic nervous system and salt- and water-retaining systems in order to preserve cardiac output (3), as well as activation of a family of vasodilatory molecules, including natriuretic peptides, prostaglandins (PGE_2 and $PGEI_2$), and nitric oxide (4). However, as discussed below, our understanding of the family of molecules that may be involved in this process is far from complete. Moreover, we have very little information about the impact of genetic background, gender, age, or environment on these compensatory mechanisms.

As shown in Figure 1, the compensatory mechanisms activated following the initial decline in the pumping capacity of the heart are able to modulate LV function within a physiological/homeostatic range, such that the functional capacity of the patient is preserved or is depressed only minimally. Thus, patients may remain asymptomatic or minimally symptomatic for years. However, at some point patients will become overtly symptomatic, with a resultant striking increase in morbidity and mortality. Why this transition to symptomatic heart failure occurs, exactly how it occurs, and whether it occurs in all patients with LV ventricular dysfunction, remain unknown and represent an important area of discovery in heart failure. What is known, however, is that the transition to symptomatic heart failure is accompanied by further activation of neurohormonal and cytokine systems, as well as a series of adaptations within the myocardium, collectively referred to as LV ventricular remodeling. Although there are further modest declines in the overall pumping capacity of the heart during the transition to symptomatic heart failure, the weight of experimental and clinical evidence suggests that heart failure progression occurs independently of the hemodynamic status of the patient. Accordingly, it becomes difficult to ascribe the transition to symptomatic heart failure to worsening LV function alone. Thus, one important question that arises from the above discussion is why heart failure progresses.

PROGRESSIVE MODEL OF HEART FAILURE

Neurohormonal Mechanisms

It has been suggested that heart failure should be viewed as a neurohormonal model, in which heart failure progresses as a result of the overexpression of biologically active molecules that exert toxic effects on the heart and circulation (1, 5). Thus far, a variety of proteins including norepinephrine, angiotensin II, endothelin-1

(ET-1), aldosterone, and tumor necrosis factor (TNF) have been implicated as potentially biologically active molecules whose biochemical properties are sufficient to contribute to disease progression in the failing heart. It bears emphasis that "neurohormone" is largely a historical term, reflecting the original observation that many of the molecules elaborated in heart failure were produced by the neuroendocrine system and thus acted on the heart in an endocrine manner. However, it has since become apparent that a great many of the so-called classical neurohormones, such as norepinephrine and angiotensin II, are synthesized directly within the myocardium and act in an autocrine and paracrine manner. Furthermore, molecules such as angiotensin II, endothelin, and TNF are peptide growth factors and/or cytokines that are produced by a variety of nucleated cell types within the heart, including cardiac myocytes, and thus do not necessarily have a neuroendocrine origin.

The important unifying concept that arises from the neurohormonal model is that the overexpression of portfolios of biologically active molecules can contribute to disease progression independently of the hemodynamic status of the patient, by virtue of the direct toxic effects that these molecules exert on the heart and circulation. Supporting evidence is derived from two lines of investigation. First, several experimental models have shown that pathophysiologically relevant concentrations of neurohormones are sufficient to mimic some aspects of the heart failure phenotype (6, 7). Second, clinical studies have shown that antagonizing neurohormone systems, such as the renin angiotensin system (RAS) and the adrenergic system, leads to clinical improvement for patients with heart failure (8–10). Thus, one logical explanation for why heart failure progresses is that long-term activation of a variety of neurohormonal mechanisms produces direct end-organ damage within the heart and circulation. This, in turn, provides the current rationale for antagonizing RAS with angiotensin-converting enzyme (ACE) inhibitors and the adrenergic system with β-blockers.

Are Current Neurohormonal Models Adequate to Explain the Progression of Heart Failure?

Despite the many strengths of the neurohormonal model in explaining disease progression, and the many insights that neurohormonal models have contributed to drug development for heart failure, increasing clinical evidence suggests that the current neurohormonal explanation of disease progression in heart failure is incomplete. This is illustrated by the differences in the Kaplan-Meier curves observed in lipid lowering trials for patients with coronary artery disease and for neurohormonal antagonism in patients with heart failure. Figure 2a illustrates a Kaplan-Meier curve for death or nonfatal myocardial infarction among patients randomized to receive placebo or pravastatin in the West of Scotland Coronary Prevention Study (11). As shown, the Kaplan-Meier curves begin to diverge at one year. They continue to diverge over the next five years, which implies that pravastatin has in some way altered the underlying mechanism of the disease process, presumably through lipid lowering. In contrast, Figure 2b illustrates Kaplan-Meier

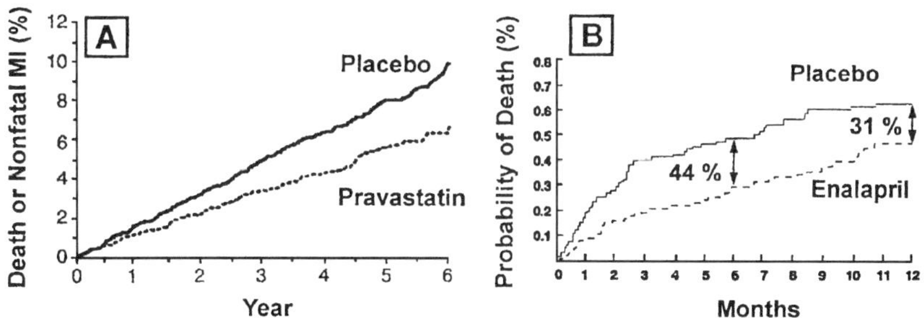

Figure 2   Kaplan-Maier curves in lipid lowering and heart failure trials. (*a*) Kaplan-Maier curves for death or nonfatal myocardial infarction among patients randomized to receive placebo or pravastatin in the West of Scotland Coronary Prevention Study (11). (*b*) Kaplan-Maier curves for death among patients randomized to placebo or enalapril in the CONSENSUS I Study (12). [Figure 2*a* (11) and Figure 2*b* (8) were adapted with permission from the *New England Journal of Medicine*.]

curves for death among patients randomized to placebo or enalapril in the treatment arm of the Cooperative North Scandanavian Enalapril Survival Study (CONSENSUS I) (12). The curves begin to diverge at six months, suggesting that enalapril has at least initially altered the underlying mechanism of the disease process, presumably by preventing disease progression. However, the Kaplan-Meier curves for the placebo and enalapril arms begin to collapse and come closer together between 6 and 12 months. Interestingly, similar patterns exist in the Kaplan-Meier curves for patients randomized to receive both β-blockers and ACE inhibitors (10). The convergence of event curves following neurohormonal antagonism suggests possible attenuation or loss of effectiveness of neurohormonal antagonism as heart failure progresses.

Although the precise mechanism(s) for this attenuation or loss of effectiveness of neurohormonal antagonism is not known, at least four potential explanations warrant a brief discussion. One obvious explanation is that it may not be possible to achieve complete inhibition of the renin angiotensin system or the adrenergic system in heart failure because of dose-limiting side effects of ACE inhibitors and β-blockers. A second explanation is that there may be alternative metabolic pathways for neurohormones that are not antagonized by conventional treatment strategies. For example, as shown in Figure 3, angiotensin II synthesis in the heart may follow several pathways that are not antagonized by conventional ACE inhibitors. Recent studies have focused on heart chymase, a chymostatin-sensitive angiotensin II–forming serine protease that can convert angiotensin I to angiotensin II (13). Therefore, ACE inhibitors do not completely antagonize the renin angiotensin system. Third, the currently available portfolio of neurohormonal antagonists, namely ACE inhibitors and β-blockers, may not antagonize all of the biologically active systems that become activated in heart failure (e.g., endothelin, aldosterone, and TNF). As shown in Table 1, there is a great deal of redundancy within the spectrum of toxic effects that these biologically active molecules exert on the heart and

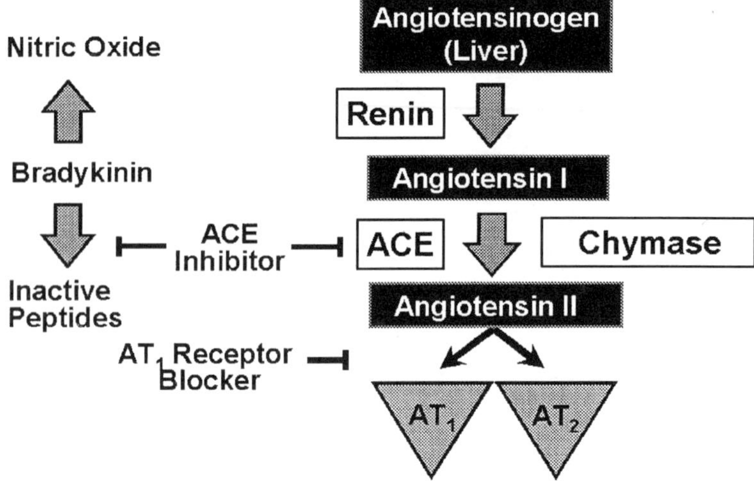

Figure 3 Activation of the renin-angiotensin system (RAS). Angiotensinogen is converted to angiotensin I by renin. Angiotensin I can be converted to angiotensin II through angiotensin converting enzyme (ACE) and chymase-dependent pathways. Angiotensin II exerts its biological effects by binding to a type 1 (AT_1) and type 2 (AT_2) angiotensin receptor. ACE inhibitors block ACE-dependent conversion of angiotensin I to angiotensin II, but have no effect on chymase-dependent conversion of angiotensin I to angiotensin II. ACE inhibitors also prevent the catabolism of bradykinin, which can lead to an increase in the local generation of nitric oxide.

circulation. This in turn has provided the rationale (see below) for antagonizing these systems in clinical trials. A fourth, albeit speculative, explanation for the loss of effectiveness of neurohormonal antagonism is that, at some point in time, heart failure may progress independently of the neurohormonal status of the patient (reviewed in 14).

ALTERNATIVE APPROACHES TOWARD ANTAGONISM OF THE RENIN ANGIOTENSIN SYSTEM

Based on the critical importance of RAS activation in the pathogenesis of heart failure, as well as the inherent limitations of ACE inhibitors, several approaches have been taken to antagonize RAS more effectively in the setting of heart failure.

Angiotensin Receptor Blockade

One logical approach to circumvent the problem of ACE-independent conversion of angiotensin I to angiotensin II is to directly block the effects of angiotensin

TABLE 1 Redundant biological effects of neurohormones

	Angiotensin II	Norepinephrine	ET-1[a]	TNF[b]
Myocyte apoptosis	Yes	Yes	Yes	Yes
Myocyte necrosis	Yes	Yes	Yes	Yes
Myocyte hypertrophy	Yes	Yes	Yes	Yes
Activation of fetal gene program	Yes	Yes	Yes	Yes
Alterations in extracellular matrix	Yes	Yes	Yes	Yes
Uncoupling of β-adrenoceptor	No	Yes	No	Yes

[a]ET-1, endothelin-1.

[b]TNF, tumor necrosis factor.

II at the receptor level. In the Evaluation of Losartan in the Elderly (ELITE-II), investigators compared the effects of enalapril, an ACE inhibitor, with losartan. This double-blind, randomized, controlled trial of 3152 patients with New York Heart Association (NYHA) class II–IV heart failure showed no significant differences in all-cause mortality (11.7% vs. 10.4% average annual mortality rate) or sudden death or resuscitated arrests (9.0% vs. 7.3%) between the two treatment groups (15). Thus, in this study, blocking the angiotensin I type 1 receptor was not superior to ACE inhibition; indeed, ACE inhibitors appeared marginally superior to angiotensin receptor blockers. This latter observation has suggested the interesting possibility that one of the beneficial effects of ACE inhibitors, in addition to blocking the conversion of angiotensin I to angiotensin II, may be to block the catabolism of bradykinin (Figure 3), which may increase generation of nitric oxide (which has vasodilatory and antioxidant properties).

A slightly different approach was taken in the Valsartan in Heart Failure Trial (Val-HeFT), in which 5010 patients with NYHA class II–IV heart failure were randomized to conventional therapy (digoxin, diuretics, ACE inhibitors, β-blockers) or conventional therapy plus valsartan, an angiotensin I receptor blocker (16). In Val-HeFT, the combination of valsartan plus an ACE inhibitor conferred no survival benefit relative to placebo (19.7% vs. 19.4%, respectively; $p = 0.80$); however, the combination of valsartan with conventional therapy resulted in significant ($p = 0.009$) 13.3% relative risk reduction in all-cause morbidity and mortality relative to patients receiving conventional therapy alone.

Thus, at the time of this writing, angiotensin receptor blockers do not appear to confer a survival benefit compared with traditional ACE inhibitors. Nonetheless, the addition of an angiotensin receptor blocker to conventional ACE inhibitors may retard the progression of heart failure more effectively than ACE inhibitors alone. Moreover, the encouraging results of these recent studies argue strongly for the widespread use of angiotensin receptor blockers in patients who are ACE-intolerant. However, it is unclear whether the effects of angiotensin receptor blockers represent a class effect or whether there are properties that are unique to individual angiotensin receptor blockers.

Neutral Endopeptidase Inhibition

A second, novel approach to RAS antagonism has been the development of a unique class of compounds that block the conversion of angiotensin I to angiotensin II, as well as block the catabolism of natriuretic and/or vasodilatory peptides, such as bradykin, atrial natriuretic peptide (ANP), and brain natriuretic peptide (BNP). Neutral endopeptidase (NEP) is an enzyme that inactivates several biologically active peptides, including bradykinin and natriuretic peptides. Simultaneous inhibition of NEP and ACE increases natriuretic and vasodilatory peptides (including ANP and BNP) and increases the half-life of other vasodilator peptides including bradykinin and adrenomedullin (17). Theoretically, inhibition of NEP and ACE would be expected to have greater beneficial effects in heart failure than ACE inhibition alone. Omapatrilat is a vasopeptidase inhibitor that inhibits both NEP and ACE. Thus far, experience with omapatrilat in heart failure has been promising. In the Inhibition of Metaloprotease by Omapatrilat in a Randomized Exercise and Symptoms Trial (IMPRESS) (18), treatment with omapatrilat for 24 weeks was superior to ACE inhibition (lisinopril) alone in improving the exercise tolerance and morbidity in 573 patients with NYHA class II–IV congestive heart failure. Although there was no significant improvement in the primary endpoint of maximal exercise treadmill test time at week 12, all the individual secondary clinical endpoints related to survival or any comorbid event for worsening heart failure favored omapatrilat. Similar results were observed in a longer-term safety study with omapatrilat, in which this agent improved the combined endpoint of death or hospitalization for heart failure (19). When the data from the above two trials were combined, there was a statistically significant reduction in the combined endpoint with omapatrilat. Whether omapatrilat is really superior to ACE inhibitors in heart failure will be tested in the ongoing large-scale trial, Omapatrilat versus Enalapril Randomized Trial of Utility in Reducing Events (OVERTURE).

Aldosterone Antagonism

One of the mechanisms for the toxic effects of sustained RAS activation is through increased production of aldosterone. Given that angiotensin II stimulates the release of aldosterone, it has always been assumed that treatment with ACE inhibitors would suffice to block both angiotensin II and aldosterone. However, aldosterone production may "escape" through non–angiotensin II–dependent mechanisms (20). Aldosterone escape has several important consequences, including worsening sodium retention, potassium and magnesium loss, myocardial collagen production, ventricular hypertrophy, myocardial norepinephrine release, and endothelial dysfunction. Given this background, investigators have begun to study aldosterone antagonists in the setting of heart failure. In the Randomized Aldactone Evaluation Study (RALES) 1663 patients with NYHA functional class IIIb and IV heart failure were randomized to receive conventional therapy (ACE inhibitor, loop diuretic, and digoxin) or conventional therapy plus spironolactone (aldactone), an aldosterone antagonist. This double-blind, placebo-controlled study was stopped prematurely because of the striking 30% reduction in the primary endpoint, which was death from all causes (21). Although spironolactone acts functionally as a competitive inhibitor of the mineralocorticoid (aldosterone) receptor, this agent has unwanted progestational and antiadrogenic side effects that limit its use in the chronic treatment of disease. Based on the striking results of the RALES trial, newer mineralocorticoid receptor antagonists [e.g., epoxymexrenone (eplerenone)] are being developed as more selective aldosterone antagonists (22).

NEW THERAPEUTIC TARGETS IN THE TREATMENT OF HEART FAILURE

Recent studies have highlighted the importance of a second class of biologically active molecules, termed cytokines, in the pathogenesis of heart failure. As noted above, cytokines exert similar toxic effects on the heart and circulation as do angiotensin II and norepinephrine. This forms the logical basis for antagonizing these molecules in patients with heart failure. Thus far, two major classes of cytokines have been identified in heart failure: vasconstrictor cytokines, such as endothelin and its precursor, big-endothelin; and vasodepressor proinflammatory cytokines, such as tumor necrosis factor (TNF) and interleukin-6 (IL-6).

Endothelin Antagonism

Endothelin-1 (ET-1) is a member of the endothelin family of genes, which includes three peptide ligands encoded for by separate genes: ET-1, ET-2, and ET-3. ET-1 plays a minor role in normal cardiovascular function, but in pathophysiologic states such as heart failure, ET-1 assumes a larger role in the regulation of peripheral hemodynamics, as well as LV function and LV remodeling. The myocardium contains several sources of ET, including the vascular endothelial cells, endocardium, and myocytes. Moreover, the myocardium expresses both ET receptors subtypes: ET_A and ET_B. Although the limited expression of ET-1 within the myocardium may be thought of initially as an adaptive response to stress, providing increased inotropic support for the cardiac myocyte and increasing the rate of myocyte protein synthesis, overexpression of ET-1 may eventually become maladaptive by producing focal vasospasm, myocyte necrosis, and increased myocardial fibrosis (23).

Both mature ET-1 and its precursor, big ET-1, have been identified in experimental and clinical heart failure and are elaborated in the peripheral circulation in relation to the hemodynamic and functional severity of heart failure (24), as well as patient prognosis (25). The effects of ET-1 antagonism in heart failure have been addressed in several recent studies (26).

In the Research on Endothelin Antagonism in Chronic Heart Failure Study (REACH-1), 370 patients with NYHA class IIIb or IV heart failure were randomized to receive conventional therapy alone or with bosentan, a nonselective ET_A and ET_B antagonist, for six months. Initiation of bosentan therapy was associated with an increased risk of worsening heart failure. However, long-term therapy with bosentan may have improved symptoms and favorably altered the progression of heart failure. More recently, enrasenten, a similar dual ET_A and ET_B antagonist, also resulted in a threefold increase in hospitalizations, raising the question of the utility of dual ET_A/AT_B receptor antagonism versus selective ET_A antagonism in heart failure. For acute heart failure, the only drug available is tezosentan, a nonselective ET-1 antagonist that has been shown to exert beneficial hemodyamic effects, including an increase in cardiac index and a decrease in pulmonary capillary wedge pressure and pulmonary and systemic vascular resistance, with no change in heart rate (27). Thus, although data on dual ET-1 antagonism in chronic heart failure have been disappointing thus far, the results of studies with dual ET-1 antagonism in acute heart failure appear more promising, particularly with regard to the treatment of pulmonary hypertension.

Antagonism of Proinflammatory Cytokines

The current interest in understanding the role of proinflammatory cytokines, such as TNF, in heart failure relates to the observation that many aspects of the syndrome of heart failure can be explained by the known biological effects of TNF. Simply stated, when expressed at sufficiently high concentrations, TNF mimics some aspects of the so-called heart failure phenotype, including (but not limited to) progressive LV dysfunction, pulmonary edema, LV remodeling, fetal gene expression, and cardiomyopathy. Accordingly, the elaboration of TNF, much like the elaboration of neurohormones, may represent a biological mechanism that is responsible for producing symptoms in patients with heart failure.

One of the first successful attempts to use a cytokine antagonist in the setting of human heart failure was performed by Sliwa and associates (28), who studied the effects of pentoxifylline in patients with dilated cardiomyopathy and NYHA class II–III heart failure. After six months, they noted an improvement in functional class in the pentoxifylline group, whereas functional deterioration occurred in the placebo group. At that time they also found a significant increase in the ejection fraction in the pentoxifylline group, whereas no significant change occurred in the placebo group. An important observation was that TNF levels fell significantly in the pentoxifylline group, whereas no significant change occurred in TNF levels in the placebo group. Thus, it appears that modulation of TNF levels via agents that alter intracellular cAMP levels, and therefore block the transcriptional activation of TNF, may be a useful strategy for altering cytokine levels in heart failure. An alternative strategy to suppressing cytokine production is to attempt to neutralize the biological effects of TNF using soluble TNF receptors as decoys in order to prevent TNF from binding to its cognate receptors on cell surface membranes. The strategy thus far has been to use a soluble TNF antagonist consisting of the extracellular domains of the type 2 TNF receptor fused in duplicate to the Fc portion of the IgG_1 molecule. Although the soluble TNF antagonist (etanercept; ENBREL®) was shown to be effective in two small phase I clinical studies (29, 30), two large-scale clinical trials of etanercept in patients with NYHA class II–IV heart failure were stopped because of lack of efficacy. Thus, although the results of large clinical trials with soluble TNF antagonists have been disappointing, agents that block the transcriptional activation of TNF appear to be the most useful strategy for altering cytokine levels in heart failure.

LEFT VENTRICULAR REMODELING AS A THERAPEUTIC TARGET IN HEART FAILURE

An increasing body of evidence suggests that the process of LV remodeling can contribute to disease progression in heart failure independently of the neurohormonal status of the patient (reviewed in 14). Thus, several approaches have been taken to arrest or reverse LV remodeling. The most obvious clinical example of reversal of LV remodeling following a surgical intervention is the striking changes that occur in the dilated cardiomyopathic ventricle following implantation of a LV assist device (LVAD). These changes include increased LV wall thickness, decreased LV volume, and a favorable leftward shift in the LV pressure-volume curve (31).

In addition to LVADs, several other surgical approaches have been tried to prevent and/or retard LV remodeling, including surgical myoplasty, which has largely been abandoned (32), mitral valve surgery (33), and volume reduction surgery (34). Perhaps the most widely heralded approach has been partial left ventriculectomy (the so-called Batista procedure) (34). Although appealing at first glance, the concept that progressive LV remodeling can be prevented or treated by surgically removing a segment of the myocardium in order to reduce LV wall stress has not been borne out by organized clinical studies, wherein patients have been treated with optimal medical therapy (35). As a result, this therapeutic modality has been abandoned in most large medical centers.

Currently, a more promising surgical approach, termed endoventricular circular patch plasty (the so-called Dor procedure), is under active investigation for the treatment of LV aneurysms. The akinetic and/or dyskinetic myocardium is excluded from the LV and a tight circumferential suture is placed around the base of the aneurysm to reduce LV volume, as well as to return the contour of the LV to a more normal shape (36). Two other novel surgical approaches deserve mention. The first is the cardiac assist support device (Acorn jacket), in which a synthetic surgical sleeve is placed around the heart in order to prevent progressive cardiac dilation. In preclinical and clinical studies, this procedure appears to improve ejection fraction and decrease LV end-diastolic volume and pressure (37). A second novel approach is the myosplint procedure, in which synthetic rods are surgically placed through the middle of the LV in order to reduce the radius of curvature (and hence wall stress) of the dilated LV. Both of these novel surgical approaches are currently being investigated clinically.

A promising approach to the problems engendered by LV remodeling is biventricular pacing, in which patients with a dilated LV and a widened QRS complex undergo simultaneous pacing from the right ventricular apex and the lateral wall of the ventricle, thus allowing a more synchronous contraction of the ventricle. This so-called re-synchronization therapy has been shown to lead to short-term gains in functional capacity (6-min walk distance), improvement in NYHA functional class, and quality of life in the Multisite Stimulation in Cardiomyopathies trial (MUSTIC) (38), as well as the recently completed Multicenter InSync Randomized Clinical Evaluation (MIRACLE) trial. Ongoing large-scale morbidity/mortality trials are now comparing re-synchronization therapy with conventional medical therapy.

CLINICAL IMPLICATIONS

This review has described the clinical syndrome of heart failure in terms of three different clinical model systems: a cardiorenal model, a hemodynamic model, and a neurohormonal model. As shown in Figure 4, therapeutic strategies stemming

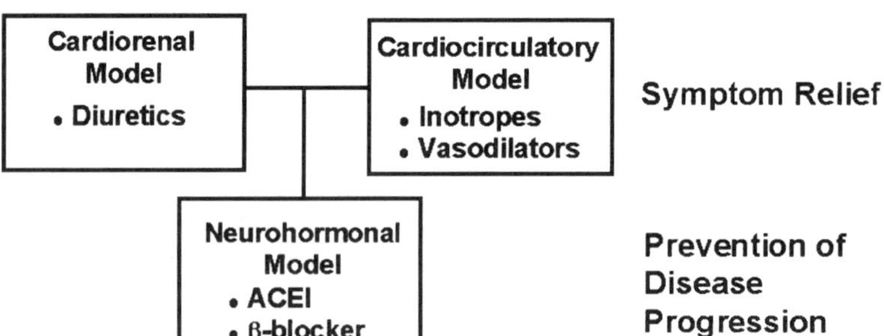

Figure 4   Current treatment of chronic heart failure. The combination of cardiorenal and cardiocirculatory models is extremely useful for developing short-term strategies to treat symptoms related to volume overload and/or acute cardiac decompensation. Accordingly, the use of diuretics (cardiorenal model) is warranted to treat congestive symptoms, whereas the use of short-term inotropic support and/or intravenous vasodilators (cardiocirculatory model) is warranted during periods of extreme cardiac decompensation. However, diuretics and inotropes/vasodilators will not prevent disease progression. Therefore, long-term treatment strategies should include the use of neurohormonal antagonists known to attenuate disease progression. Patients with asymptomatic and symptomatic LV dysfunction should receive both ACE inhibitors and β-blockers in order to antagonize the renin-angiotensin and the adrenergic systems, respectively. (ACEI, angiotensin converting enzyme inhibitor; ARB, angiotensin receptor blocker.) (Adapted with permission from Reference 14).

from the cardiorenal and cardiocirculatory models provide symptom relief, whereas therapeutic strategies that stem from neurohormonal models prevent disease progression.

We have also discussed the point of view that current neurohormonal strategies do not completely prevent disease progression in heart failure. Thus, our current therapy for heart failure should be viewed as a work in progress. Although it is not known why heart failure progresses in patients who are receiving optimal therapy with ACE inhibitors and β-blockers, one explanation is that these agents do not directly and/or sufficiently antagonize all the biologically active systems that become activated in heart failure.

Accordingly, one logical direction for future heart failure therapies will be to develop therapeutic strategies that more effectively antagonize the neurohormonal systems we believe to be deleterious. As shown in Figure 5, these new neurohormonal treatment strategies will probably be adjunctive to existing clinical strategies

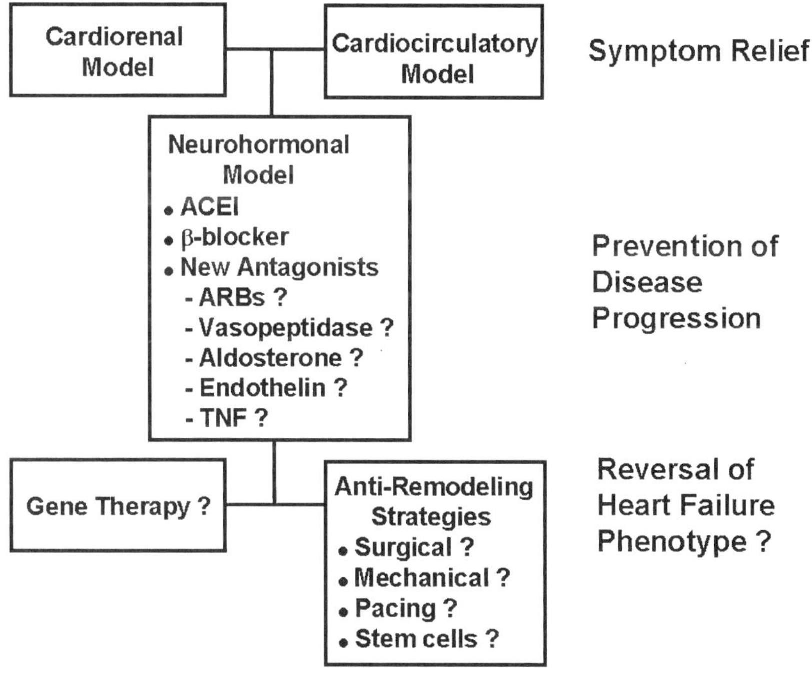

Figure 5 Future treatment strategies for chronic heart failure are likely to either antagonize known neurohormonal systems more effectively or to antagonize other biologically active systems that are believed to be important (aldosterone, endothelin, and TNF). Moreover, it is possible that antiremodeling and/or gene-therapeutic strategies may be combined with existing strategies. (ACEI, angiotensin converting enzyme inhibitor; ARB, angiotensin receptor blocker.)

for relieving symptoms and preventing disease progression. However, it may not be possible and/or feasible to antagonize all of the biologically active systems that become activated in heart failure. Accordingly (Figure 5), it is possible that future therapeutic targets will extend beyond antagonizing neurohormonal systems and may instead begin to address remodeling as a new therapeutic target. In addition, recent advances in the delivery of gene constructs into the vasculature and/or the myocardium raise the important possibility that gene therapy may one day be used to attenuate disease progression in heart failure. Conceivably, these newer strategies would also be adjunctive to and/or synergistic with existing therapies. Whether a combinatorial approach that incorporates antiremodeling strategies along with existing strategies will ever completely prevent disease progression in heart failure remains unknown, but the possibility represents a potentially important area of theoretical and therapeutic discovery in the new millennium.

ACKNOWLEDGMENTS

We would like to thank Dr. Andrew I. Schafer for his past and present guidance and support. This work was supported, in part, by research funds from the N.I.H. (P50 HL-O6H and RO1 HL58081-01, RO1 HL61543-01, HL-42250-10/10). Dr. Deswal is a recipient of the Clinical Research Career Development Award (CRCD #712B) from the Veterans Cooperative Studies Program. Dr. Bozkurt is a recipient of the Research Career Development Award from the Veterans Administration.

Visit the Annual Reviews home page at www.AnnualReviews.org

LITERATURE CITED

1. Packer M. 1992. The Neurohormonal Hypothesis: a theory to explain the mechanism of disease progression in heart failure. *J. Am. Coll. Cardiol.* 20:248–54

2. Massie BM. 1998. 15 years of heart-failure trials: What have we learned? *Lancet* 352 (Suppl. 1):29–33

3. Eichhorn EJ, Bristow M. 1997. Medical therapy can improve the biological properties of the chronically failing heart: a new era in the treatment of heart failure. *Circulation* 94:2285–96

4. Dzau VJ, Packer M, Lilly LS, et al. 1984. Prostaglandins in severe congestive heart failure: relation to activation of the renin-angiotensin system and hyponatremia. *N. Engl. J. Med.* 310:347–52

5. Bristow MR. 1984. The adrenergic nervous system in heart failure. *N. Engl. J. Med.* 311:850–51

6. Tan LB, Jalil JE, Pick R, et al. 1991. Cardiac myocyte necrosis induced by angiotensin II. *Circ. Res.* 69:1185–95

7. Mann DL, Kent RL, Parsons B, Cooper G IV. 1992. Adrenergic effects on the biology of the adult mammalian cardiocyte. *Circulation* 85:790–804

8. The SOLVD Investigators. 1991. Effect of enalapril on survival in patients with reduced left ventricular ejection fractions and congestive heart failure. *N. Engl. J. Med.* 325:293–302

9. Bristow MR, Gilbert EM, Abraham WT, et al. 1996. Carvedilol produces dose-related improvements in left ventricular function and survival in subjects with

chronic heart failure. *Circulation* 94:2807–16

10. Packer M, Bristow MR, Cohn JN, et al. 1996. The effect of carvedilol on morbidity and mortality in patients with chronic heart failure. *N. Engl. J. Med.* 334:1350–55

11. Shepherd J, Cobbe SM, Ford I, et al. 1995. Prevention of coronary heart disease with pravastatin in men with hypercholesterolemia. West of Scotland Coronary Prevention Study Group. *N. Engl. J. Med.* 333:1301–7

12. CONSENSUS Trial Study Group. 1987. Effects of enalapril on mortality in severe congestive heart failure: results of the cooperative North Scandanavian enalapril survival study. *N. Engl. J. Med.* 316:1429–35

13. Urata H, Kinoshita A, Misono KS, et al. 1990. Identification of a highly specific chymase as the major angiotensin II–forming enzyme in the human heart. *J. Biol. Chem.* 265:22348–57

14. Mann DL. 1999. Mechanisms and models in heart failure: a combinatorial approach. *Circulation* 100:999–1088

15. Pitt B, Poole-Wilson PA, Segal R, et al. 2000. Effect of losartan compared with captopril on mortality in patients with symptomatic heart failure: randomised trial—the Losartan Heart Failure Survival Study ELITE II. *Lancet* 355:1582–87

16. Cohn JN. 1999. Improving outcomes in congestive heart failure: Val-HeFT. Valsartan in Heart Failure Trial. *Cardiology* 91 (Suppl. 1):19–22

17. Burnett JC Jr. 1999. Vasopeptidase inhibition: a new concept in blood pressure management. *J. Hypertens. Suppl.* 17:S37–S43

18. Rouleau JL, Pfeffer MA, Stewart DJ, et al. 2000. Comparison of vasopeptidase inhibitor, omapatrilat, and lisinopril on exercise tolerance and morbidity in patients with heart failure: IMPRESS randomised trial. *Lancet* 356:615–20

19. Kostis JB, Rouleau JL, Pfeffer MA, et al. 2000. Beneficial effects of vasopeptidase inhibition on mortality and morbidity in heart failure: evidence from the omapatrilat

heart failure program. *J. Am. Coll. Cardiol.* 35(Suppl. 1):1–704

20. Pitt B. 1995. "Escape" of aldosterone production in patients with left ventricular dysfunction treated with an angiotensin converting enzyme inhibitor: implications for therapy. *Cardiovasc. Drugs Ther.* 9:145–49

21. Pitt B, Zannad F, Remme WJ, et al. 1999. The effect of spironolactone on morbidity and mortality in patients with severe heart failure. Randomized Aldactone Evaluation Study Investigators. *N. Engl. J. Med.* 341:709–17

22. Delyani JA. 2000. Mineralocorticoid receptor antagonists: the evolution of utility and pharmacology. *Kidney Int.* 57:1408–11

23. Sakai S, Miyauchi T, Kobayashi M, et al. 1996. Inhibition of myocardial endothelin pathway improves long-term survival in heart failure. *Nature* 384:353–55

24. Tsutamoto T, Wada A, Maeda Y, et al. 1994. Relation between endothelin-1 spillover in the lungs and pulmonary vascular resistance in patients with chronic heart failure. *J. Am. Coll. Cardiol.* 23:1427–33

25. Wei CM, Lerman A, Rodeheffer RJ, et al. 1994. Endothelin in human congestive heart failure. *Circulation* 89:1580–86

26. Packer M, Avraham C, Charlon V, et al. 1998. Circulation 98(Suppl. I):12 (Abstr.)

27. Torre-Amione G, Young JB, Durand JB, et al. 2001. Hemodynamic effects of tezosentan, an intravenous dual endothelin receptor antagonist, in patients with class III to IV congestive heart failure. *Circulation* 103:973–80

28. Sliwa K, Skudicky D, Candy G, et al. 1998. Randomized investigation of effects of pentoxifylline on left ventricular performance in idiopathic dilated cardiomyopathy. *Lancet* 351:1091–93

29. Deswal A, Bozkurt B, Seta Y, et al. 1999. A phase I trial of tumor necrosis factor receptor (p75) fusion protein (TNFR:Fc) in patients with advanced heart failure. *Circulation* 99:3224–26

30. Bozkurt B, Torre-Amione G, Warren MS, et al. 2001. Result of targeted anti-tumor

necrosis factor therapy with etanercept (ENBREL) in patients with advanced heart failure. *Circulation* 103:1044–47

31. Mann DL, Willerson JT. 1998. Left ventricular assist devices and the failing heart: a bridge to recovery, a permanent assist device, or a bridge too far? *Circulation* 98:2367–69

32. Patel HJ, Polidori DJ, Pilla JJ, et al. 1997. Stabilization of chronic remodeling by asynchronous cardiomyoplasty in dilated cardiomyopathy: effects of a conditioned muscle wrap. *Circulation* 96:3665–71

33. Bolling SF, Deeb GM, Brunsting LA, Bach DS. 1995. Early outcome of mitral valve reconstruction in patients with end-stage cardiomyopathy. *J. Thorac. Cardiovasc. Surg.* 109:676–82

34. Batista RJ, Verde J, Nery P, et al. 1997. Partial left ventriculectomy to treat end-stage heart disease. *Ann. Thorac. Surg.* 64:634–38

35. Starling RC, McCarthy PM, Buda T, et al. 2000. Results of partial left ventriculectomy for dilated cardiomyopathy: hemodynamic, clinical and echocardiographic observations. *J. Am. Coll. Cardiol.* 36:2098–103

36. Doenst T, Ahn-Veelken L, Schlensak C, et al. 2001. Endoventricular patch plasty in patients with idiopathic dilated cardiomyopathy: an alternative to heart transplantation? *Z. Kardiol.* 90 (Suppl. 1):38–44

37. Konertz W, Rombeck B, Hotz H, et al. 2000. Short-term safety of the Acorn cardiac support device in patients with advanced heart failure. *J. Am. Coll. Cardiol.* 35:182a (Abstr.)

38. Cazeau S, Leclercq C, Lavergne T, et al. 2001. Effects of multisite biventricular pacing in patients with heart failure and intraventricular conduction delay. *N. Engl. J. Med.* 344:873–80

Annu. Rev. Med. 2002. 53:75–88

THROMBOTIC THROMBOCYTOPENIC PURPURA:
The Systemic Clumping "Plague"

Joel L. Moake

*Hematology/Oncology Section, Department of Medicine, Baylor College of Medicine
and Bioengineering Laboratory, Rice University, Houston, Texas 77030;
e-mail: jmoake@rice.edu*

Key Words   microvascular platelet aggregation, von Willebrand factor,
vWf-cleaving metalloprotease

■ **Abstract**   In thrombotic thrombocytopenic purpura (TTP), a multimeric form
of von Willebrand factor (vWf) that is larger than ordinarily found in the plasma
causes systemic platelet aggregation under the high-shear conditions of the microcirculation. A divalent cation–activated, vWf-cleaving metalloprotease that metabolizes
large vWf multimers to smaller forms in normal plasma is severely reduced or absent in most patients with TTP. The vWf-cleaving metalloprotease either is not produced or is defective in children with chronic relapsing TTP. When the enzyme is
provided by the infusion of normal plasma, these patients remain free of TTP symptoms for about three weeks. An IgG autoantibody to the vWf-cleaving metalloprotease is found transiently in many adult patients with acute idiopathic, recurrent, and
ticlopidine/clopidogrel-associated TTP. These patients require plasma exchange, i.e.,
concurrent replacement of the inhibited vWf-cleaving metalloprotease by plasma infusion and plasmapheresis. The vWf-cleaving metalloprotease is present in fresh-frozen
plasma, in cryoprecipitate-depleted plasma (cryosupernatant), and in plasma that has
been treated with solvent and detergent. The pathophysiology of platelet aggregation in
bone marrow transplantation/chemotherapy–associated thrombotic microangiopathy,
and in the hemolytic-uremic syndrome, is not established. In neither condition is there
a severe decrease in plasma vWf–cleaving metalloprotease activity.

INTRODUCTION

Thrombotic thrombocytopenic purpura (TTP), originally described by
Moschcowitz in 1924 (1), is the most dangerous intravascular platelet aggregation disorder. For unknown reasons, this once rare disease has become an "orphan
disease epidemic" in recent years. The several thousand new cases of acute idiopathic TTP that now occur annually in the United States and Canada represent more
than increased recognition of a disorder with clinical and laboratory characteristics
unchanged for decades.

CLINICAL AND LABORATORY ABNORMALITIES

Severe thrombocytopenia, hemolytic anemia with many fragmented red cells (schistocytes) on blood films, and global or focal ischemic neurological signs comprise a common clinical triad. A minority of patients also has fever or severe renal dysfunction. Clinical evidence of ischemia in the abdominal, coronary, retinal, or pulmonary circulation may appear. Abdominal signs, including pancreatic involvement, are becoming more frequently recognized either at presentation or during the course of TTP episodes (2).

The severity of thrombocytopenia in TTP reflects the extent of microvascular platelet aggregation. Platelet counts below $20,000/\mu l$ are common during acute episodes. Erythrocyte fragmentation presumably reflects the mechanical stress on red cells attempting to pass at high flow rates through and around the microvascular platelet clumps. Hemolysis is predominantly intravascular and contributes to the increased serum levels of lactic acid dehydrogenase (LDH). Recently it has been appreciated that most of the LDH is derived from ischemic, injured tissue cells rather than from red cells (3).

Coagulation studies are usually normal in the early stages of a TTP episode. If tissue necrosis is severe or protracted, however, secondary disseminated intravascular coagulation (DIC) may occur. This is probably the result of excessive exposure of tissue factor on injured tissue cells, followed by factor VII binding and activation.

TYPES OF THROMBOTIC THROMBOCYTOPENIC PURPURA

Acute, idiopathic TTP in adults may occur as a single episode or may subsequently recur at irregular intervals (10%–30% of patients) (4–6). The structurally similar platelet adenosine diphosphate-blocking drugs, ticlopidine (Ticlid) (7, 8) and clopidogrel (Plavix) (9), which are used to suppress arterial thrombosis, have been associated with acute episodes of TTP in a fraction of exposed patients. TTP may occur in pregnancy, especially during the last trimester, or in the peripartum period. Occasionally, patients with HIV-1 infection develop TTP. Chronic relapsing TTP, the rarest type, is characterized by episodes at approximately three-week intervals that usually begin in infancy (10, 11).

Mitomycin C, cyclosporin, FK506 (tacrolimus), chemotherapeutic agents in combination, and total body irradiation have been associated with the subsequent development of thrombotic microangiopathy (12–16). The syndrome often more closely resembles the hemolytic-uremic syndrome (HUS) than TTP and usually occurs weeks to months after exposure (15–17). Bone marrow transplant recipients make up a relatively large subgroup (17), although thrombotic microangiopathy has also been reported after kidney, liver, heart, and lung transplants (16).

ETIOLOGY AND PATHOPHYSIOLOGY

Most patients who develop TTP episodes are 20–60 years old, with women more susceptible than men. TTP during pregnancy or the peripartum period accounts for a small percentage of cases, as does exposure to ticlopidine or clopidogrel. Abnormal immune modulation or macrophage/lymphocyte activation (18–20) may contribute to etiology in some of these patients. Elevated levels of interleukin (IL)-1, IL-6, the soluble IL-2 receptor, TNF-α, and transforming growth factor-β (TGF-β) have all been reported in TTP (18, 19). Individuals lacking the class II HLA antigen, DR53, may be more susceptible to thrombotic microangiopathy (21).

Acute episodes of TTP have occurred occasionally in diseases characterized by autoimmune or other types of abnormal immune responses, including systemic lupus erythromatosus (SLE) (22), autoimmune "idiopathic" thrombocytopenic purpura (ITP) (23, 24), and the acquired immunodeficiency syndrome (AIDS) (24–26).

VON WILLEBRAND FACTOR

The vascular occlusive lesions in TTP consist almost exclusively of platelet thrombi with little or no fibrin and without perivascular inflammation or detectable endothelial cell damage (27). Microvascular thrombi can occur in any organ but are most frequent in the brain, heart, spleen, kidneys, pancreas, and adrenals.

TTP is likely to be the result of the abnormal presence in the circulation of a platelet-aggregating agent (6, 28, 29). Organ ischemia and thrombocytopenia in TTP may be caused by direct, potentially reversible, platelet aggregation in the microcirculation that is not preceded by endothelial cell desquamation and platelet-subendothelial adherence (10, 30–32). Immunohistochemical studies of TTP thrombi (33) reveal an abundance of von Willebrand factor (vWf) with little fibrinogen/fibrin, implying that vWf is involved in the systemic platelet aggregation. The opposite findings are characteristic of thrombotic lesions in DIC (33). vWf multimers within these thrombi may function as polymeric bridges promoting platelet-platelet cohesion (aggregation). The relative predominance of platelets (rather than fibrin) as the occlusive component in microvessels, as well as the paucity of laboratory coagulation abnormalities, also distinguish TTP from DIC.

vWf monomers (280 kDa) are linked by disulfide bonds into multimers of varying sizes that range into the millions of Daltons (34). vWf multimers are produced within megakaryocytes and endothelial cells and are stored within the α-granules of platelets and the Weibel-Palade bodies of endothelial cells. Endothelial cells are the predominant sources of plasma vWf multimers. Both cell types produce vWf multimeric forms that are even larger in size than those found in normal plasma [unusually large (UL)vWf multimers] (28, 30, 35). ULvWf forms may be more effective than the largest plasma vWf forms at binding under the influence of elevated fluid shear stresses to the GPIbα component of platelet GPIbα-IX-V receptors, and to activated platelet GPIIb-IIIa complexes, resulting in aggregation (30).

vWf-cleaving metalloprotease activity in normal plasma degrades vWf multimers by cleaving the 842Tyr-843Met peptide bond of vWf monomeric subunits (36, 37). This cleavage occurs in vitro if the vWf multimers are partially unfolded mechanically (as by shear stress) or chemically (as by guanidine-HCl) (36, 38). The vWf-cleaving metalloprotease activity in vitro is also accentuated by low ionic strength buffer, urea, and the presence of divalent cations (especially Ba^{2+}) (37). Enzyme function is inhibited by ethylene diamine tetraacetic acid (EDTA). The conditions for activating the vWf-cleaving metalloprotease in vitro are artificial. Nevertheless, the enzyme has a role in normal physiology, because cleavage in vitro of vWf and ULvWf multimers results in the generation of 176-kDa and 140-kDa vWf fragments identical to those found in normal plasma (37).

Serial studies of plasma samples from patients during single episodes of TTP often demonstrate either the presence of ULvWf multimers or, alternatively, absence of the largest plasma vWf forms (28, 39). The presence of ULvWf forms in TTP patient plasma may reflect failure to process adequately the ULvWf multimers released from endothelial cells (28, 29). The disappearance of large plasma vWf forms in some TTP patient plasma samples during acute TTP episodes may be predominantly because these ULvWf forms, along with the largest plasma vWf multimers, bind to platelets and cause aggregation (28, 39, 40).

Serial flow cytometry studies of EDTA–whole blood samples from patients with TTP indicate that the amount of vWf bound to single platelets is significantly increased during relapses relative to remission periods in patients with acute idiopathic single-episode, recurrent, ticlopidine- or clopidogrel-associated, or chronic relapsing types of TTP (8, 9, 40). Evidence suggests that the vWf bound to platelets in TTP is likely to be from plasma rather than from platelet α-granules (40).

Almost all reported acute idiopathic single-episode and recurrent TTP patients have had extremely low levels (<10%) of plasma vWf-cleaving metalloprotease activity during, but not after, TTP episodes (41–43). An IgG antibody inhibiting the vWf-cleaving metalloprotease activity was detected in many of the patients studied in detail (41–43). The cause of this transient (or recurrent) defect of immune regulation is unknown, as is the reason why the vWf-cleaving metalloprotease is selectively targeted for autoantibody attack. The few ticlopidine- or clopidogrel-associated TTP patients studied also had antibodies against the vWf-cleaving metalloprotease during their TTP episodes (8, 9) (Table 1).

Chronic relapsing TTP patients almost always have unusually large vWf multimers in their plasma, especially between episodes when these huge multimeric forms may be less actively attaching to platelets (28, 39). Chronic absence (or a severely low level) of the plasma vWf-cleaving metalloprotease, without the presence of an inhibiting autoantibody, characterizes chronic relapsing TTP (11, 44) (Table 1). In this autosomal recessive disorder, which begins in childhood, there is a congenital defect in the production, structure, or survival of the vWf-cleaving metalloprotease. [vWf-cleaving metalloprotease values have been found to be

TABLE 1   vWf-cleaving metalloprotease and factor H in thrombotic microangiopathies

	vWf-cleaving metalloprotease		
	Severely reduced or absent	**Inhibiting antibodies may be present**	**Factor H deficiency**
Thrombotic thrombocytopenic purpura			
Chronic relapsing	Yes	No	No
Acute idiopathic	Yes	Yes	No
Recurrent	Yes	Yes	No
Ticlopidine/clopidogrel-associated	Yes	Yes	No
Hemolytic uremic syndrome			
Acquired	No	No	No
Familial	No	No	Yes
Thrombotic microangiopathy associated with transplantation-chemotherapy-irradiation	No	No	No

reduced to about 50% of normal in patients with decompensated liver cirrhosis, suggesting that the liver is an important site of synthesis of the protease (45).]

What is the result of a failure to eliminate unusually large vWf multimers after their secretion from endothelial cells into the plasma? In children with chronic relapsing TTP, the unusually large vWf multimers are associated with periodic platelet aggregation that may be triggered by elevated shear stresses in the microcirculation (10). Elevated fluid shearing forces induce platelet aggregation in vitro by stimulating the binding of large or unusually large vWf multimers to platelet glycoprotein Ibα-IX-V and activated IIb-IIIa receptors (30–32). In chronic relapsing TTP, the slow accumulation of ULvWf forms in the bloodstream may exceed a threshold level about every three weeks that is required to initiate ULvWf-induced intravascular platelet aggregation under the high shear conditions of the microcirculation (10).

The pathophysiology of platelet aggregation in bone marrow transplantation–associated microangiopathy, and in the hemolytic-uremic syndrome, is not established (12–17, 46). In neither condition is there a severe deficiency or inhibition of vWf-cleaving metalloprotease activity, as there is in TTP (41, 43).

Other Observations

Five patients with a TTP-like illness were reported in 1997 to have rod-shaped, *Bartonella bacilliformis*–like organisms adherent to 0.1%–2% of circulating erythrocytes during disease episodes (47). Four of the five patients survived, and two of these four were treated with the tetracycline derivative, doxycycline, instead of plasma exchange.

It has also been reported (48) that the serum of some TTP or hemolytic-uremic syndrome (HUS) patients induces apoptosis in cultured microvascular endothelial cells but not in macrovascular human umbilical vein endothelial cells (HUVECs). The mechanism of this in vitro phenomenon is unknown. Either a Ca^{2+}-dependent cysteine protease (calpain) (49) or a lysosomal-derived non–Ca^{2+}-dependent cathepsin-type cysteine protease (50) may be present in patient plasma during TTP episodes, perhaps derived from injured or apoptotic cells.

Differential Diagnosis

The combination of thrombocytopenia, hemolysis, and schistocytosis also occurs (usually to a less extreme extent than in TTP) in the following disorders: DIC; pre-eclampsia/eclampsia; the HELLP syndrome (pre-eclampsia–associated hemolytic anemia with elevated liver enzymes and low platelets); malignant hypertension; severe vasculitis; scleroderma with associated hypertension and renal failure; Evans syndrome (concurrent autoimmune thrombocytopenia and direct Coomb's test–positive autoimmune hemolysis); and malfunctioning prosthetic cardiac valves. Of these, the most frequently troublesome diagnostic dilemma is between TTP or HUS and DIC.

Platelet aggregates in the microcirculation in TTP produce fluctuating ischemia or infarction in various organs, including the brain in 50%–71% of episodes (4, 5). In the closely related HUS, initially reported by Gasser and colleagues in 1955 (51), the ischemia is predominantly renal. Thrombocytopenia, erythrocyte fragmentation, and increased serum levels of LDH are less extreme in many HUS patients. The variability of organ dysfunction in TTP (including renal abnormalities in 50%–75% of episodes) (4, 5) and the extrarenal manifestations in some HUS patients can make the two syndromes difficult to distinguish (4, 5, 46, 52, 53).

In contrast to most TTP patients, renal dysfunction is severe in HUS. Oliguria, anuria, chronic renal failure, and hypertension may be complications. These problems are uncommon in patients who recover from episodes of TTP.

Truly recurrent TTP (as opposed to a single protracted episode with brief intervening periods of incomplete remission) (5) occurs in at least 11%–28% of TTP patients (4, 5). HUS usually occurs as a single episode, often associated with gastroenteritis caused by cytotoxin-producing serotypes of *Escherichia coli* (e.g., 0157:H7) or *Shigella* species (54). Rarely, children have a familial, recurrent type of HUS associated with a low level of the plasma complement control protein, factor H (55) (Table 1). Complement component 3 (C3) is, apparently, excessively activated whenever the alternative complement pathway is stimulated (55). An HUS-like syndrome may also follow transplantation or the use of quinine, mitomycin, cyclosporin, total body irradiation, or multiple chemotherapeutic agents (6, 12–17, 46).

TTP and HUS are clinical diagnoses. A biopsy of bone marrow, gingiva, or kidney may be obtained at a moment when few platelet thrombi are present in the microvessels of the tissue sampled (56). Biopsy samples are usually unnecessary for diagnosis, and the procedures are often unsafe in severely thrombocytopenic patients.

TTP and HUS are both manifestations of microvascular platelet aggregation. If the platelet aggregation is systemic and extensive, and especially if the central nervous system is involved, the disorder is called TTP. If platelet aggregation predominantly involves the kidneys, the patient is considered to have HUS. Severe renal involvement in a "TTP" patient, or extra-renal manifestations in a patient with "HUS," can blur the clinical boundaries between the two syndromes (4, 5, 46, 52, 53). Some patients diagnosed with TTP have severely reduced or absent plasma vWf-cleaving metalloprotease activity (11, 41–44). In contrast, the plasma activity was normal, or only moderately reduced, in other patients considered to have familial or acquired HUS (41) (Table 1). If these findings are confirmed in large clinical studies, assay of plasma vWf-cleaving metalloprotease may, ultimately, provide the basis for a more precise distinction between TTP and HUS. The results may also elucidate the reason that plasma therapy, usually so effective in TTP, is often disappointing in acquired HUS. The vWf-cleaving metalloprotease assay is not yet available widely or rapidly enough to influence emergency clinical decisions. If the differential diagnosis in an adult patient is between TTP and HUS, then the patient should be presumed to have TTP and therapy should commence immediately (6, 53).

TREATMENT

Nearly 90% of adults with acute TTP episodes will respond to daily plasma exchanges (4, 5), i.e., the combination of plasmapheresis and plasma infusion with normal platelet-poor fresh-frozen plasma (FFP) (3–4 liters). Skipping even one day prior to complete remission may lead to rapid relapse. More than one exchange per day has not been demonstrated to be beneficial. Cryoprecipitate-poor plasma (cryosupernatant) is at least as effective as FFP in plasma-exchange procedures (57, 58). Cryosupernatant is relatively deficient in the largest plasma vWf multimers, as well as fibrinogen and fibronectin, compared with FFP. Solvent- and detergent-treated plasma (for inactivation of the lipid-envelope viruses HIV-1 and hepatitis B and C) also lacks the large vWf multimers found in normal plasma and is effective in treating TTP episodes (10). Transfusions or exchange transfusions with fluids other than plasma, cryosupernatant, or solvent/detergent-treated plasma (e.g., albumin alone or concentrated immunoglobulin) are usually ineffective (6, 59, 60).

The infusion of normal plasma or cryosupernatant provides supplemental quantities of the vWf-cleaving metalloprotease that is inhibited by autoantibodies in some adult TTP patients (41–43). However, the effectiveness of plasmapheresis in removing plasma ULvWf multimers or autoantibodies against the vWf-cleaving metalloprotease has not been shown conclusively.

Relapses in children (or rare adults) with true chronic relapsing TTP usually respond to, or are prevented by, the infusion of normal FFP, cryosupernatant, or solvent/detergent-treated plasma alone (in quantities varying from one to several units) without the need for concurrent plasmapheresis (10). These observations are compatible with reports that inadequate or defective production of plasma vWf-cleaving metalloprotease causes chronic relapsing TTP (11, 44).

Older children or adolescents with an initial episode of TTP may require plasma exchange, perhaps because TTP in this age group is caused by autoantibody inhibition of vWf-cleaving metalloprotease (as in adults), rather than a congenital deficiency of the enzyme (as in infants and young children).

Infusion of normal FFP at the rate of about 30 ml/kg/day can be used initially in an adult TTP patient until plasma exchanges are arranged. This should be within a few hours (usually no more than 24 h) in most circumstances. Plasma infusion alone is less effective than plasma exchange (4) and may result in volume overload. Ticlopidine, clopidogrel, quinine, mitomycin, cyclosporin, or tacrolimus should be discontinued.

It is prudent to institute glucocorticoid therapy (e.g., intravenous prednisolone at 200 mg/day) in association with plasma exchange in all adult patients with initial or recurrent TTP episodes, unless there is a strong contraindication (5). Glucocorticoids may suppress the production of autoantibodies against the vWf-cleaving metalloprotease. Red blood cell transfusions may be required to counter bleeding and mechanical hemolysis. If the platelet count is very low and bleeding is a primary problem, or if intracranial bleeding is demonstrated by computerized tomography, then transfusion of platelets at a slow rate (to minimize the risk of microvascular occlusion) will be necessary. It is otherwise better to withhold platelet transfusions because they have been temporally associated with exacerbation of ischemia from the formation of platelet thrombi in the microcirculation, especially in the central nervous system (27, 61).

In order to achieve a sustained remission, plasma exchange should be continued for more than three days after patients attain complete remission (i.e., a normal neurological status, a platelet count of 150–200,000/μl, a rising hemoglobin value, and a normal serum lactic acid dehydrogenase level) (5). Some centers perform at least five additional postremission exchanges. Schistocytes in declining numbers often persist for many days on peripheral blood films, so they are not a reliable marker for remission. Plasma exchange should then be stopped and glucocorticoids tapered over days to weeks. Platelet counts should be monitored regularly in order to detect nascent relapse. If TTP does recur quickly, then the same treatment should be repeated. If a patient with TTP responds minimally within the first few days of therapy, or deteriorates, cryosupernatant should be substituted for FFP in the plasma-exchange procedures (57, 58).

Aspirin therapy for TTP is controversial (62, 63). If shear stress–induced, vWf-mediated platelet aggregation in vivo is important in the pathogenesis of platelet aggregation, then aspirin would not be expected to be helpful. Blockade of cyclooxygenase-mediated platelet thromboxane A2 generation by aspirin does not inhibit shear-induced aggregation in vitro (64). Aspirin may exacerbate hemorrhagic complications in severely thrombocytopenic patients (62).

Patients who achieve only a partial response or worsen during therapy may have concurrent heparin-associated thrombocytopenia (HIT). This is especially likely if LDH values have decreased progressively toward normal during therapy. In the latter situation, all exposure to heparin should be eliminated (including via keep-open intravenous lines or indwelling catheters, during dialysis, and in the tips of Swan-Ganz catheters).

Currently available treatment is ineffective in some patients with acute TTP episodes. vWf-cleaving metalloprotease autoantibodies may be produced for longer periods in higher titer in these refractory patients. Other therapeutic options include vincristine (65), which depolymerizes platelet microtubules and may alter the exposure of platelet GPIbα-IX-V or activated GPIIb-IIIa receptors that bind vWf onto platelet surfaces; or azathioprine (Imuran) (66), other immunosuppressive agents, or splenectomy (67) to suppress or remove immunological cells producing vWf-cleaving metalloprotease autoantibodies. Frequent or prolonged TTP relapses in some adult patients may also be controlled by splenectomy (68).

If the explanation for TTP in most adults proves to be the production of vWf-cleaving metalloprotease autoantibodies of IgG type, some form of therapeutic protein-A column immunoadsorption might be reconsidered. A retrospective study contended that column treatment was effective in 7 of 10 patients who had not responded optimally to plasma exchange (69). Each column procedure removes only a small percentage of circulating IgG, however, and IgG has an extensive extravascular distribution. A convincing prospective demonstration of any consistent therapeutic effect of ex vivo protein-A immunoadsorption in TTP using presently available columns is not available.

The binding of ULvWf or large vWf forms to platelet GPIbα, followed by vWf binding to adenosine diphosphate (ADP)-activated GPIIb-IIIa complexes, is required for platelet aggregation in fluid shear fields (30–32, 70–73). It is possible that compounds capable of interfering with shear-induced platelet aggregation could be useful in the treatment of refractory TTP or the prophylaxis of relapsing TTP. Agents in this category, presently used to prevent coronary thrombosis or restenosis after angioplasty, include (*a*) 7E3 Fab, or ReoPro®, an intravenous chimeric mouse/human monoclonal antibody fragment directed against platelet GPIIb-IIIa, which inhibits the attachment of large vWf multimers to GPIIb-IIIa under conditions of abnormally high shear stess (74); and (*b*) a cyclic heptapeptide, integrilin, containing the lysine-glycine-aspartate (KGD) sequence that is also capable of blocking the binding of vWf to platelet GPIIb-IIIa under high shear (75). Substances under development include ADP purinoceptor blockers (76), and recombinant fragments of the human vWf monomer that contain the platelet GPIbα-binding site, bind to the GPIbα component of platelet GPIbα-IX-V in the absence of any modulator, and block the binding of large vWf multimers to platelet GPIbα (77–79). Hemorrhage is a risk of using these compounds in severely thrombocytopenic patients, so any initial trials will probably be confined to patients with refractory TTP or other thrombotic microangiopathies unresponsive to conventional therapy.

Additional new therapeutic stagies in refractory TTP may target the production of autoantibodies against vWf-cleaving metalloprotease in these patients. For example, anti-CD20 (Rituximab) (80) is a chimeric mouse/human monoclonal antibody directed against CD20 antigens predominantly expressed on B-lymphocytes.

It is likely that purified (or recombinant) preparations of vWf-cleaving metalloprotease will replace plasma products in the therapy of TTP within a few years. Because only about 5% of the normal plasma level of vWf-cleaving metalloprotease is necessary to prevent TTP, gene therapy may eventually be used to provide more durable remissions in children with chronic relapsing TTP.

Visit the Annual Reviews home page at www.AnnualReviews.org

LITERATURE CITED

1. Moschcowitz E. 1924. Hyaline thrombosis of the terminal arterioles and capillaries: a hitherto undescribed disease. *Proc. NY Pathol. Soc.* 24:21–24

2. Baker KR, Moake JL. 2000. Thrombotic thrombocytopenic purpura and the hemolytic-uremic syndrome. *Curr. Opin. Pediatr.* 12:23–28

3. Cohen JA, Brecher ME, Bandarenko N. 1998. Cellular source of serum lactate dehydrogenase elevation in patients with thrombotic thrombocytopenic purpura. *J. Clin. Apheresis* 13:16–19

4. Rock G, Sumak K, Buskard N, et al. 1991. Comparison of plasma exchange with plasma infusion in the treatment of thrombotic thrombocytopenic purpura. *N. Engl. J. Med.* 325:393–97

5. Bell WR, Braine HG, Ness PM, et al. 1991. Improved survival in thrombotic thrombocytopenic purpura–hemolytic-uremic syndrome: clinical experience in 108 patients. *New Engl. J. Med.* 325:398–403

6. Byrnes JJ, Moake JL. 1986. Thrombotic thrombocytopenic purpura and the hemolytic-uremic syndrome: evolving concepts of pathogenesis and therapy. *Clin. Haematol.* 15:413–42

7. Bennett CL, Weinberg PD, Rozenberg B-DK, et al. 1998. Thrombotic thrombocytopenic purpura associated with ticlopidine: a review of 60 cases. *Ann. Int. Med.* 128:541–44

8. Tsai H-M, Rice L, Sarode R, et al. 2000. Antibody inhibitors to von Willebrand factor metalloproteinase and increased von Willebrand factor–platelet binding in ticlopidine-associated thrombotic thrombocytopenic purpura. *Ann. Int. Med.* 132:794–99

9. Bennett CL, Connors JM, Carwile JM, et al. 2000. Thrombotic thrombocytopenic purpura associated with clopidogrel. *New Engl. J. Med.* 342:1773–77

10. Moake J, Chintagumpala M, Turner N, et al. 1994. Solvent/detergent-treated plasma suppresses shear-induced platelet aggregation and prevents episodes of thrombotic thrombocytopenic purpura. *Blood* 84:490–97

11. Furlan M, Robles R, Solenthaler M, et al. 1997. Deficient activity of von Willebrand factor–cleaving protease in chronic relapsing thrombotic thrombocytopenic purpura. *Blood* 89:3097–103

12. Rabadi SJ, Khandekar JD, Miller HJ. 1982. Mitomycin-induced hemolytic uremic syndrome: case presentation and

review of the literature. *Cancer Treat. Rep.* 66:1244–47

13. Atkinson K, Biggs JC, Hayes J, et al. 1983. Cyclosporin A associated nephrotoxicity in the first 100 days after allogeneic bone marrow transplantation: three distinct syndromes. *Br. J. Haematol.* 54:59–67

14. Mach-Pascual S, Samii K, Beris P. 1996. Microangiopathic hemolytic anemia complicating FK506 (tacrolimus) therapy. *Am. J. Hematol.* 52:310–12

15. Charba D, Moake JL, Harris MA, et al. 1993. Abnormalities of von Willebrand factor multimers in drug-associated thrombotic microangiopathies. *Am. J. Hematol.* 42:268–77

16. Singh N, Gayowski T, Marino IR. 1996. Hemolytic uremic syndrome in solid-organ transplant recipients. *Transpl. Int.* 9:68–75

17. Moake JL, Byrnes JJ. 1996. Thrombotic microangiopathies associated with drugs and bone marrow transplantation. *Hematol. Oncol. Clin. North Am.* 10:485–97

18. Zauli G, Gugliotta L, Catani L, et al. 1993. Increased serum levels of transforming growth factor beta-1 in patients affected by thrombotic thrombocytopenic purpura (TTP): its implications on bone marrow haematopoiesis. *Br. J. Haematol.* 84:381–86

19. Wada H, Kaneko T, Ohiwa M, et al. 1992. Plasma cytokine levels in thrombotic thrombocytopenic purpura. *Am. J. Hematol.* 40:167–70

20. Neame PD. 1980. Immunologic and other factors in thrombotic thrombocytopenic purpura (TTP). *Semin. Thromb. Hemost.* 6:416–29

21. Joseph G, Smith KJ, Hadley TJ, et al. 1994. HLA-DR53 protects against thrombotic thrombocytopenic purpura/adult hemolytic uremic syndrome. *Am. J. Hematol.* 47:189–93

22. Nesher G, Hanna VE, Moore TL, et al. 1994. Thrombotic microangiopathic hemolytic anemia in systemic lupus erythematosus. *Semin. Arthritis Rheum.* 24:175–72

23. Zacharski LR, Lustad D, Glick JL. 1976. Thrombotic thrombocytopenic purpura in a previously splenectomized patient. *Am. J. Med.* 60:1061–63

24. Yospur LS, Sun NC, Figueroa P, et al. 1996. Concurrent thrombotic thrombocytopenic pupura and immune thrombocytopenic purpura in an HIV-positive patient: case report and review of the literature. *Am. J. Hematol.* 51:73–78

25. Leaf AN, Laubenstein LJ, Raphael B, et al. 1988. Thrombotic thrombocytopenic purpura associated with immunodeficiency virus type I (HIV-1) infection. *Ann. Intern. Med.* 109:194–97

26. Nair JM, Bellevue R, Bertoni M, et al. 1988. Thrombotic thrombocytopenic purpura in patients with the acquired immunodeficiency syndrome (AIDS)-related complex: a report of two cases. *Ann. Intern. Med.* 109:209–12

27. Harkness D, Byrnes JJ, Lian EC-Y, et al. 1981. Hazard of platelet transfusion in thrombotic thrombocytopenic purpura. *JAMA* 246:1931–33

28. Moake J, Rudy C, Troll J, et al. 1982. Unusually large plasma factor VIII: von Willebrand factor multimers in chronic relapsing thrombotic thrombocytopenic purpura. *N. Engl. J. Med.* 307:1432–35

29. Moake JL, Byrnes JJ, Troll JH, et al. 1985. Effects of fresh-frozen plasma and its cryosupernatant fraction on von Willebrand factor multimeric forms in chronic relapsing thrombotic thrombocytopenic purpura. *Blood* 65:1232–36

30. Moake JL, Turner NA, Stathopoulos NA, et al. 1986. Involvement of large plasma von Willebrand factor (vWF) multimers and unusually large vWF forms derived from endothelial cells in shear stress-induced platelet aggregation. *J. Clin. Invest.* 78:1456–61

31. Moake JL, Turner NA, Stathopoulos NA, et al. 1988. Shear-induced platelet aggregation can be mediated by vWF released from platelets, as well as by exogenous large or unusually large vWF multimers, requires

adenosine diphosphate, and is resistant to aspirin. *Blood* 71:1366–74

32. Peterson DM, Stathopoulos NA, Giorgio TD, et al. 1987. Shear-induced platelet aggregation requires von Willebrand factor and platelet membrane glycoproteins Ib and IIb-IIIa. *Blood* 69:625–28

33. Asada Y, Sumiyoshi A, Hayashi T, et al. 1985. Immunochemistry of vascular lesions in thrombotic thromocytopenic purpura, with special reference to factor VIII related antigen. *Thromb. Res.* 38:469–79

34. Ruggeri ZM. 2000. Developing basic and clinical research on von Willebrand factor and von Willebrand disease. *Thromb. Haemost.* 84:147–49

35. Moake JL. 1989. Insolubilized von Willebrand factor and the initial events in hemostasis. *J. Lab. Clin. Med.* 114:1–3

36. Tsai HM. 1996. Physiologic cleavage of von Willebrand factor by a plasma protease is dependent on its confirmation and requires calcium ion. *Blood* 87:4235–44

37. Furlan M, Robles R, Lammle B. 1996. Partial purification and characterization of a protease from human plasma cleaving von Willebrand factor to fragments produced by in vivo proteolysis. *Blood* 87:4223–34

38. Tsai HM, Sussman II, Nagel RL. 1994. Shear stress enhances the proteolysis of von Willebrand factor in normal plasma. *Blood* 83:2171–79

39. Moake JL, McPherson PD. 1989. Abnormalities of von Willebrand factor multimers in thrombotic thrombocytopenic purpura and hemolytic-uremic syndrome. *Am. J. Med.* 87(3N):9N–15N

40. Chow TW, Turner NA, Chintagumpala M, et al. 1998. Increased von Willebrand factor binding to platelets in single episode and recurrent types of thrombotic thrombocytopenic purpura. *Am. J. Hematol.* 57:293–302

41. Furlan M, Robles R, Galbusera M, et al. 1998. von Willebrand factor–cleaving protease in thrombotic thrombocytopenic purpura and hemolytic-uremic syndrome. *N. Engl. J. Med.* 339:1578–84

42. Furlan M, Robles R, Solenthaler M, et al. 1998. Acquired deficiency of von Willebrand factor–cleaving protease in a patient with thrombotic thrombocytopenic purpura. *Blood* 91:2839–46

43. Tsai HM, Lian EC-Y. 1998. Antibodies of von Willebrand factor cleaving protease in acute thrombotic thrombocytopenic purpura. *N. Engl. J. Med.* 339:1585–94

44. Furlan M, Robles R, Morselli B, et al. 1999. Recovery and half-life of von Willebrand factor–cleaving protease after plasma therapy in patients with thrombotic thrombocytopenic purpura. *Thromb. Haemost.* 81:8–13

45. Moake JL, Sadler JE, Mannucci P, Ganguly P. 2001. Report on the Workshop: von Willebrand factor and thrombotic thrombocytopenic purpura. *Am. J. Hematol.* 68:122–26

46. Moake JL. 1994. Haemolytic-uremic syndrome: basic science. *Lancet* 343:393–97

47. Tarantolo SR, Landmark JD, Iwen PC. 1997. Bartonella-like erythrocyte inclusions in thrombotic thrombocytopenic purpura. *Lancet* 350:1602

48. Laurence J, Mitra D, Steiner M, et al. 1996. Plasma from patients with idiopathic and human immunodeficiency virus-associated thrombotic thrombocytopenic purpura induced apoptosis in microvascular endothelial cells. *Blood* 87:3245–54

49. Moore JC, Murphy WG, Kelton JG. 1990. Calpain proteolysis of von Willebrand factor enhances its binding to platelet membrane glycoprotein IIb/IIIa: an explanation for platelet aggregation in thrombotic thrombocytopenic purpura. *Br. J. Haematol.* 74:457–64

50. Consonni R, Falanga A, Barbui T. 1994. Further characterization of platelet-aggregating cysteine proteinase activity in thrombotic thrombocytopenic purpura. *Br. J. Haematol.* 87:321–24

51. Gasser C, Gautier E, Steck A, et al. 1955. Hamolytisch-uramische syndrome: bilaterale nierenrindennekrosen bei akuten

erworbenen hamolytischen anamien. *Schweizer. Med. Wochenschr.* 85:905–9

52. Kaplan BS, Proesmans W. 1987. The hemolytic uremic syndrome of childhood and its variants. *Semin. Hematol.* 24:1480–88

53. George JN. 2000. How I treat patients with thrombotic thrombocytopenic purpura–hemolytic uremic syndrome. *Blood* 96:1223–29

54. Karmali MA, Petric M, Lim C, et al. 1985. The association between idiopathic hemolytic uremic syndrome and infection by verotoxin-producing *Escherichia coli. J. Infect. Dis.* 151:775–82

55. Warwicker P, Goodship THJ, Donne RL, et al. 1998 Genetic studies into inherited and sporadic hemolytic uremic syndrome. *Kidney Int.* 53:836–44

56. Goodman A, Ramos R, Petrelli M, et al. 1978. Gingival biopsy in thrombotic thrombocytopenic purpura. *Ann. Int. Med.* 89:501–4

57. Byrnes JJ, Moake JL, Panpit K, et al. 1990. Effectiveness of the cryosupernatant fraction of plasma in the treatment of refractory thrombotic thrombocytopenic purpura. *Am. J. Hematol.* 34:169–74

58. Rock G, Shumack KH, Sutton DM, et al. 1996. Cyrosupernatant as a replacement fluid for plasma exchange in thrombotic thrombocytopenic purpura. *Br. J. Haematol.* 94:383–86

59. Byrnes JJ, Khurana M. 1977. Treatment of thrombotic thrombocytopenic purpura with plasma. *N. Engl. J. Med.* 297:1386–89

60. Bukowski RM, Hewlett JS, Reime RR, et al. 1981. Therapy of thrombotic thrombocytopenic purpura: an overview. *Semin. Thromb. Hemost.* 7:1–8

61. Gordon LI, Kwaan HC, Rossi EC. 1987. Deleterious effects of platelet transfusions and recovery thrombocytosis in patients with thrombotic microangiopathy. *Semin. Hematol.* 24:194–201

62. Rosove MH, Ho WG, Goldfinger D. 1982. Ineffectiveness of aspirin and dipyridamole in the treatment of thrombotic thrombo-

cytopenic purpura. *Ann. Int. Med.* 96:27–33

63. del Zoppo GJ. 1987. Antiplatelet therapy in thrombotic thrombocytopenic purpura. *Semin. Hematol.* 24:130–39

64. Hardwick RA, Hellums JD, Moake JL, et al. 1980. Effects of antiplatelet agents on platelets exposed to shear stress. *Trans. Am. Soc. Artif. Intern. Organs* 26:179–84

65. Gutterman LA, Stevenson TD. 1982. Treatment of thrombotic thrombocytopenic purpura with vincristine. *JAMA* 247:1433–36

66. Moake JL, Rudy CK, Troll JH, et al. 1985. Therapy of chronic relapsing thrombotic thrombocytopenic purpura with prednisone and azathioprine. *Am. J. Hematol.* 20:73–79

67. Thompson CE, Damon LE, Ries CA, Linker CA. 1992. Thrombotic microangiopathies in the 1980s: clinical features, response to treatment, and the impact of the human immunodeficiency virus epidemic. *Blood* 80:1890–95

68. Crowther MA, Heddle N, Hayward CPM, et al. 1996. Splenectomy done during hematologic remission to prevent relapse in patients with thrombotic thrombocytopenic purpura. *Ann. Int. Med.* 125:294–96

69. Gaddis TG, Guthrie TH, Drew MJ. 1997. Treatment of plasma refractory thrombotic thrombocytopenic purpura with protein A immunoabsorption. *Am. J. Hematol.* 55:55–58

70. Chow TW, Hellums JD, Moake JL, Kroll MH. 1992. Shear stress-induced von Willebrand factor binding to platelet glycoprotein Ib initiates calcium influx associated with aggregation. *Blood* 80:113–20

71. McCrary JK, Nolasco LH, Hellums JD, et al. 1995. Direct demonstration of radiolabeled von Willebrand factor binding to platelet glycoprotein Ib and IIb-IIIa in the presence of shear stress. *Ann. Biomed. Eng.* 23:787–93

72. Goto S, Salomon DR, Ikeda Y, et al. 1995. Characterization of the unique mechanism

mediating the shear-dependent binding of soluble von Willebrand factor to platelets. *J. Biol. Chem.* 270:23,352–61

73. Konstantopoulos K, Chow TW, Turner NA, et al. 1997. Shear stress-induced binding of von Willebrand factor to platelets. *Biorheology* 34:57–71

74. Turner NA, Moake JL, Kamat SG, et al. 1995. Comparative real-time effects on platelet adhesion and aggregation under flowing conditions of in vivo aspirin, heparin, and monoclonal antibody fragment against glycoprotein IIb-IIIa. *Circulation* 91:1354–62

75. Kamat SG, Turner NA, Konstantopoulos K, et al. 1997. Effects of Integrelin on platelet function in flow models of arterial thrombosis. *J. Cardiovasc. Pharmacol.* 29:156–63

76. Turner NA, Moake JL, Turner JD, et al. 2001. Blockade of both ADP receptors, $P2Y_{12}$ and $P2Y_1$, is necessary for effective inhibition of platelet aggregation under flow. *Blood.* In press

77. Sugimoto M, Ricca G, Hrinda ME, et al. 1991. Functional modulation of the isolated glycoprotein Ib-binding domain of von Willebrand factor expressed in *Escherichia coli*. *Biochemistry* 30:5202–9

78. Kasiewski C, Crook J, Hrinda M, et al. 1991. Inhibition of thrombus formation in monkeys by RG 12986, a recombinant von Willebrand factor fragment. *Circulation* 84(Suppl. II):II–247

79. Yao SK, Ober JC, Garfinkel LI, et al. 1994. Blockade of platelet membrane glycoprotein Ib receptors delays intracoronary thrombogenesis, enhances thrombolysis, and delays coronary artery reocclusion in dogs. *Circulation* 89:2822–28

80. Reff M, Carner K, Chambers K, et al. 1994. Depletion of B cells in vivo by a chimeric mouse human monoclonal antibody to CD20. *Blood* 83:435–45

Annu. Rev. Med. 2002. 53:89–112

POSITRON EMISSION TOMOGRAPHY SCANNING:
Current and Future Applications

Johannes Czernin and Michael E. Phelps

Department of Molecular and Medical Pharmacology, Ahmanson Biological Imaging Clinic, UCLA School of Medicine, 10833 LeConte Avenue, Los Angeles, California 90095-6942; e-mail: jczernin@mednet.ucla.edu

Key Words   whole-body PET, FDG, oncology, clinical applications

■ **Abstract**   Whole-body positron emission tomography (PET) imaging with ^{18}F deoxyglucose (FDG) is a molecular imaging modality that detects metabolic alterations in tumor cells that are common to neoplastic cells. FDG-PET has recently been approved by the Health Care Finance Administration for Medicare reimbursement for diagnosing, staging, and restaging lung cancer, colorectal cancer, lymphoma, melanoma, head and neck cancer, and esophageal cancer. This review discusses the scientific evidence that led to the emergence of PET imaging as an accepted clinical tool in patients with solitary pulmonary nodules, lung cancer, colorectal cancer, melanoma, lymphoma, breast cancer, and other cancers. When possible, we compare the performance of PET to that of anatomical imaging. We discuss future clinical applications of this imaging modality.

INTRODUCTION

In 1924, German biochemist Otto Warburg published his observations on the metabolism of cancer cells (1). He posed the fundamental questions of the metabolism of tumors as follows: "If the carcinoma problem is attacked in its relation to the physiology of metabolism, the first question is: In what way does the metabolism of growing tissue differ from the metabolism of resting tissue?" Using a previously established rat model (2), Warburg observed that of 13 sugar molecules metabolized, only one was oxidized while the remainder was "fermented." From these and other observations, he concluded that the predominant form of glucose metabolism in rat tumor cells is glycolysis. He subsequently confirmed these findings in a variety of human cancer cells.

These early studies identified what is well-known today: Tumor cells rely on ATP generated from glycolysis to meet the energy requirements of rapidly replicating tissue. That is, neoplastic degeneration of tumor cells is associated with a loss of efficient production of ATP by the Krebs cycle. This results in a 19-fold increase in glucose consumption per mole of ATP produced. Further increases in glycolysis occur because of activation of the hexose monophosphate pathway, which provides the carbon backbone for DNA and RNA synthesis in growing tumors (3, 4). Glucose transporter proteins in tumor cell membranes and expression of hexokinase are also increased to meet the greater glycolytic demand (5). These alterations of cellular metabolism are common to neoplastic cells. Cancer is now understood as a systemic disease resulting from alterations in the interactions between oncogenes and tumor suppressor genes, which under physiological condition control cell replication and migration.

Prior to the emergence of clinical whole-body positron emission tomography (PET), the clinical armamentarium for diagnosing, staging, and restaging of cancer was carried out primarily by anatomic imaging with computed tomography (CT), magnetic resonance imaging (MRI), and ultrasound. Although these imaging technologies can detect lesions, they cannot reliably distinguish between benign and malignant tumors or between pre- and post-therapeutic anatomical alterations such as scarring, inflammation, or necrosis and neoplastic processes. Further, these techniques do not address cancer as a systemic disease of the whole human organism.

The understanding of the nature of tumor cells from more than 70 years of research, along with the development of PET (6), has resulted in the emergence of biological whole-body imaging of cancer with PET and the glucose analogue ^{18}F deoxyglucose (FDG) as a clinical tool (7–11). After intravenous injection, FDG is taken up by tumor cells and phosphorylated by hexokinase to FDG-6-PO4 in proportion to the glycolytic rates (Figure 1, upper panel). Unlike glucose-6-PO4, FDG-6-PO4 is not metabolized in the glycolytic pathway and remains trapped intracellularly because tumor cells do not contain sufficient amounts of glucose-6-phosphatase to reverse this reaction during the imaging procedure. Thus, the trapped FDG-6-PO4 provides a record of glycolysis in cells throughout the body that is imaged 45 to 60 min after the injection of FDG.

This chapter provides a brief overview of the clinical role and accuracy of FDG-PET for diagnosing, staging, and restaging the most important cancers, placing FDG-PET in the context of other diagnostic imaging modalities. An extensive tabulation of sensitivity, specificity, and accuracy of PET derived from more than 26,000 patients has been published recently (12). When possible, we review the prognostic value, cost-effectiveness, and impact on patient management of PET. Finally, we discuss novel approaches to cancer imaging using PET.

CURRENT CLINICAL APPLICATIONS
OF PET IN ONCOLOGY

Characterization of Solitary Pulmonary Nodules

The conventional work-up of indeterminate solitary pulmonary nodules includes chest CT, bronchoscopy, transthoracic needle biopsy, and sometimes thoracotomy. Several morphological criteria have been used in an attempt to characterize these

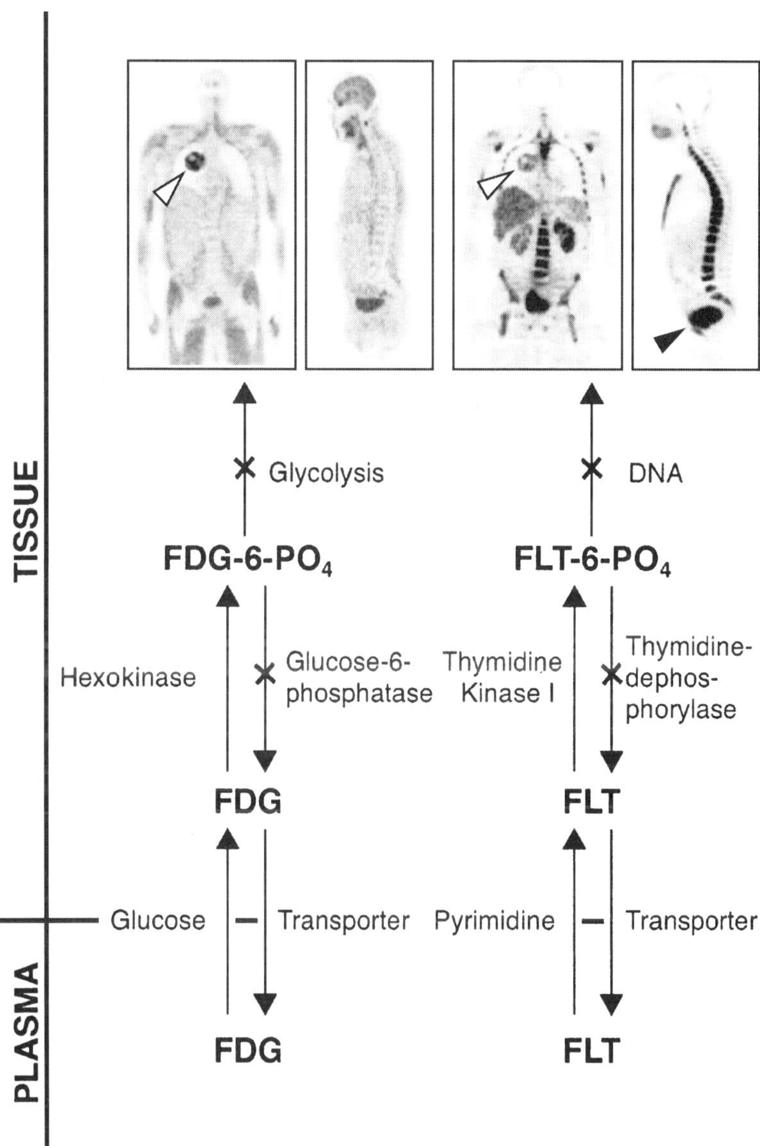

Figure 1 *Top*: FDG is phosphorylated to FDG-6-PO$_4$ by hexokinase. Since the activity of glucose-6-phosphatase is negligible, FDG-6-phosphate is essentially trapped in tumor cells (arrow). *Bottom*: Fluorothymidine is phosphorylated by thymidine kinase to FLT-6-PO$_4$ and accumulates in tumor cells.

TABLE 1   Characterizing solitary pulmonary nodules with FDG-PET

	Sens[a] (%)	Spec[a] (%)	PPV[a] (%)	NPV[a] (%)	Acc[a] (%)
	95[c]	83	93	98	90
95% CI[b]	93–97	80–86	89–95	95–100	85–95
Patients (N)	560	560	141	141	137

[a]Sens = Sensitivity, Spec = Specificity, PV = Positive Predictive Value, NPV = Negative Predictive Value, Acc = Accuracy.

[b]Confidence Interval.

[c]Weighted mean values and 95% Confidence Intervals were calculated from references 14, 15, 17, 18, 20, 22 and 23.

lesions as malignant or benign. However, even sophisticated image analysis leaves many lung lesions indeterminate (13). PET characterizes solitary pulmonary nodules quite accurately and cost-effectively (14–22) (Table 1). Major clinical trials (23, 24) have established a high sensitivity of PET for detecting malignancy that ranged from 92%–96%. Thus, PET misses only a small number of lung cancers in solitary pulmonary nodules. The specificity of PET ranged from 78% to 96% in these studies because the prevalence of benign conditions, such as granuloma, pneumonia, benign tumors, and inflammation, varies geographically. However, the incidence of false positive PET results is lower than the false positive rate of CT. Prior to the emergence of PET, most patients with solitary pulmonary nodules underwent a diagnostic biopsy for tissue characterization. Thus, even with FDG-PET's false positive rate of 5%–20%, most unnecessary biopsies will be avoided. Because of its high diagnostic accuracy, FDG-PET has been incorporated into the diagnostic work-up of solitary pulmonary nodules (25).

We currently recommend performing FDG-PET in every patient with an indeterminate solitary pulmonary nodule. Although PET might detect 4–5-mm lesions, referring physicians should be cautioned about negative PET findings if the lung nodule is smaller than 1 cm. Because the sensitivity of this test is less than 100%, each negative PET study must be followed by reevaluation with CT within three months to detect changes in nodule morphology. Conversely, because of the relatively high specificity of FDG-PET, each positive scan must be considered suspicious for malignancy until proven otherwise by biopsy.

Diagnosing, Staging, and Restaging of Lung Cancer

Lung cancer is the most common cancer in the world and its incidence is increasing (26). The five-year survival rate of lung cancer patients remains disappointingly low at 13%. Surgical removal of the tumor represents the only curative treatment.

A considerable number of patients are understaged based on anatomic imaging, as is revealed by surgery (27). It is important to note that the size of lymph nodes is not a reliable predictor of the presence of cancer metastases in lymph nodes (28, 29). The Radiologic Diagnostic Oncology Group reported disappointing findings for mediastinal staging with CT and MRI. Sensitivity and specificity of these two imaging modalities were 52% and 69% for CT and 48% and 64% for MRI (30). Histopathological findings obtained through mediastinoscopy are frequently used as the gold standard for staging of the mediastinum. Dillemans et al. (31) questioned the validity of this approach in a study of 569 patients with presumed resectable non–small-cell lung cancers. Using a cut-off point of 1.5 cm for defining lymph nodes as malignant, these authors reported sensitivity, specificity, and accuracy of 69%, 71%, and 71% for CT, and corresponding values of 72%, 100%, and 89% for mediastinoscopy. Thus, a considerable number of abnormal mediastinal lymph nodes are missed by mediastinoscopy.

MEDIASTINAL LYMPH NODE STAGING WITH PET   FDG-PET stages mediastinal involvement more accurately than conventional imaging with CT (17, 32–40) (Table 2). Pieterman et al. (39) prospectively compared the standard CT approach for staging of the mediastinum to one involving PET in 102 patients prior to surgical resection. The sensitivity and specificity of PET for the detection of mediastinal metastases were 91 (95% confidence interval: 81%–100%) and 86% (95% CI: 78%–94%), which was significantly more accurate than CT [sensitivity and specificity of 75% (95% CI: 60%–90%) and 66% (95% CI: 55%–77%)]. As an additional advantage, PET identified unknown distant metastases in about 10% of the patients. These authors concluded that PET "improves the rate of detection of local and distant metastases in patients with non–small-cell lung cancer."

An additional gain in diagnostic accuracy might arise from the fusion of anatomic and metabolic images (41, 42). Vansteenkiste et al. (43) found PET + CT more accurate than CT alone (87% vs. 59%). Based on the high positive and negative predictive value of PET for mediastinal lymph node involvement, these authors demonstrated that mediastinoscopy could have been omitted in 29 of their 68 patients. To avoid the consequences of false positive PET findings, however, they advocated performing a mediastinoscopy after a positive PET to confirm mediastinal lymph node involvement and recommended that a negative mediastinal PET be followed by thoracotomy without prior mediastinoscopy. These and other

TABLE 2   PET and CT for staging of the mediastinum

	Sens[a] (%)		Spec[a] (%)		PPV[a] (%)		NPV[a] (%)		Acc[a] (%)	
	PET	CT	PET	CT	PET	CT	PET	CT	PET	CT
	89[c]	67	94	73	77	62	89	87	86	68
95% CI[b]	86–91	63–71	91–96	69–77	66–88	49–74	77–100	75–99	82–90	61–74
Patients (N)	528	528	528	528	57	57	30	30	231	231

[a]Sens = Sensitivity, Spec = Specificity, PV = Positive Predictive Value, NPV = Negative Predictive Value.
[b]Confidence Interval.
[c]Weighted mean and 95% Confidence Intervals were calculated from references 32, 33, 35–37, 39, 41, 42 and 46.

findings have led to the development of imaging devices that combine functional molecular (PET) and anatomic imaging (CT) into a single device (44, 45), which will improve staging of the mediastinum.

STAGING FOR DISTANT DISEASE   Unsuspected distant metastatic disease was identified by PET in 11% (46) to 15% (47) of lung cancer patients. The sensitivity of PET for distant metastases was 100% with a specificity of 91%. By contrast, conventional imaging had a sensitivity of 80% and a specificity of 90% (47). Thus, PET alone provided equivalent or better staging information than all conventional imaging modalities combined (Figure 2).

IMPACT OF PET ON MANAGEMENT OF LUNG CANCER PATIENTS   PET improves the cost-effectiveness of staging and managing lung cancer patients (48–51). In their study of 97 patients, Saunders et al. (48) reported that PET corrected the clinical stage in 27% and detected distant unknown metastases in 13%. Lewis et al. (49) reported management changes in 41% of their 34 patients as a result of PET. In a survey of more than 350 referring physicians (52), PET changed the clinical stage in 43% of the 583 patients enrolled. PET resulted in treatment changes in more than 40% of these patients.

These and other data provide convincing evidence that PET should be considered the diagnostic imaging modality of choice for the presurgical staging of patients with lung cancer.

Diagnosis, Staging, and Restaging of Colorectal Cancer

FDG-PET imaging has not been examined systematically for its ability to detect primary colorectal cancer. Rather, reported studies have focused on staging and restaging the disease before and after therapeutical interventions.

INITIAL STAGING OF COLORECTAL CANCER   Abdel-Nabi et al. (53) correlated the presurgical PET findings with histopathological results and CT results in 48 patients with biopsy-proven or -suspected colorectal cancer. The sensitivity of PET for primary tumors was 95%. However, the specificity was only 40% owing to several false positive PET findings caused by inflammatory bowel disease and postsurgical inflammation, both of which can be associated with markedly increased glucose metabolic activity (54, 55). The positive and negative predictive value of PET were high (90% and 100%, respectively) (53). PET was more sensitive than CT for detecting liver metastases (88% vs. 38%), with no significant difference in specificity (100% vs. 97%).

RESTAGING OF COLORECTAL CANCER   A recent meta-analysis of 11 research articles (56–59) evaluated the use of FDG-PET in the detection of recurrent colorectal cancer, using quality criteria established a priori (60). This analysis yielded a sensitivity of 97% (95% CI: 95%–99%) and specificity of 76% (95% CI: 64%–88%)

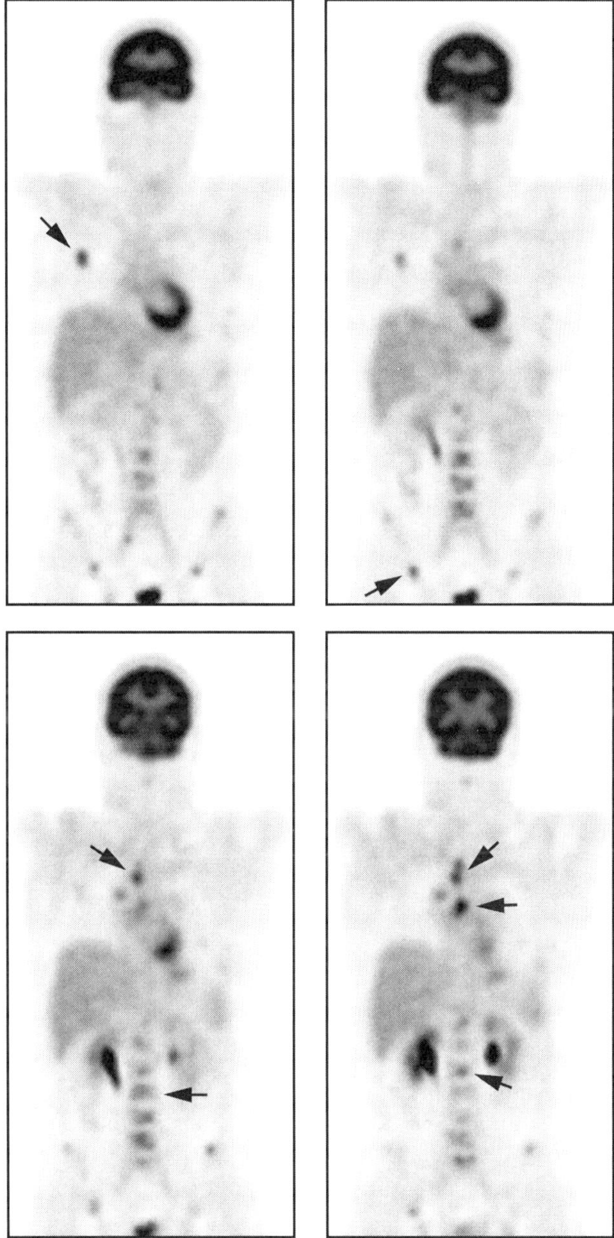

Figure 2 75-year-old patient with known non–small-cell lung cancer. Whole-body PET uncovered extensive bone metastases involving ribs, vertebrae bodies, sacrum, iliac wings, and other sites (arrows). Thus, the patient was upstaged from resectable to nonsectable.

TABLE 3   PET and CT for restaging of colorectal cancer

	Sens[a] (%)		Spec[a] (%)		Acc[a] (%)	
	PET	**CT**	**PET**	**CT**	**PET**	**CT**
	93[c]	70	93	84	93	61
95% CI[b]	89–96	64–77	89–96	79–89	90–96	55–67
Patients (N)	192	192	192	192	274	274

[a]Sens = Sensitivity, Spec = Specificity, Acc = Accuracy.

[b]Confidence Interval.

[c]Weighted mean and 95% Confidence Intervals were calcutaed from references 56–59, 61 and 62.

for recurrent disease. Further, FDG-PET affected clinical management in 29% (95% CI: 25%–34%) of the patients (Table 3).

Valk et al. (61) compared PET with CT in a trial using histological diagnosis, serial CT imaging, and clinical follow-up as reference standards. In these patients, PET sensitivity and specificity were 93% and 98%, respectively, compared with 69% and 96% for CT. The sensitivity of both modalities varied with anatomic site of recurrence. These authors also analyzed cost-effectiveness based on discussions with referring physicians and on the assumption that patients with more than one metastatic lesion were no longer surgical candidates. The costs of surgical procedures that were avoided because of PET were then compared to the cost of PET imaging. The authors reported that unnecessary surgery would have been avoided in 32% of the patients with recurrent colorectal cancer and concluded that $3000/patient could have been saved if PET had been included in the management algorithm. Delbeke et al. (62) and Meta et al. (63) provided similar estimates regarding the impact of PET.

Thus, PET is superior to anatomical imaging for restaging of metastatic and recurrent colorectal cancer and has a considerable and cost-effective impact on patient management.

Diagnosis, Staging, and Restaging of Lymphoma

Correct staging is important in selecting the appropriate treatment for lymphoma patients. In addition to history, physical examination, and laboratory data, staging depends on imaging studies such as CT, MRI, and ^{67}Ga scintigraphy. Imaging studies are also important in restaging after treatment and in the detection of recurrent disease.

STAGING OF LYMPHOMA WITH PET   Hoh and colleagues (64) compared the accuracy of PET for staging of lymphoma to that of conventional imaging, which included bone scans, CT, chest films, and other methods. In this small pilot study, PET staged lymphoma with similar or even higher accuracy. These authors also

TABLE 4   FDG-PET versus CT for staging and restaging of lymphoma

	Sens[a] (%)		Spec[a] (%)		PPV[a] (%)		NPV[a] (%)	
	PET	**CT**	**PET**	**CT**	**PET**	**CT**	**PET**	**CT**
	93[c]	85	91	39	83	33	90	87
95% CI[b]	89–98	78–91	86–96	30–47	76–91	23–43	83–96	78–96
Patients (N)	128	128	128	128	88	88	88	88

[a]Sens = Sensitivity, Spec = Specificity, PV = Positive Predictive Value, NPV = Negative Predictive Value.
[b]Confidence Interval.
[c]Weighted mean values and 95% Confidence Intervals were calculated from references 66, 71–73.

suggested considerable cost savings if lymphoma staging is based on whole-body PET findings. The high accuracy of PET for lymphoma staging was subsequently confirmed in larger study groups (65, 66) (Table 4).

PET also identified marrow involvement with high diagnostic accuracy (65, 67).

MONITORING TREATMENT AND PROGNOSTIC IMPLICATIONS   Okada et al. (68) studied 21 untreated patients with lymphoma of the head and neck region with FDG-PET and ^{67}Ga SPECT to evaluate the prognostic significance of the degree of tumor tracer uptake. They reported that patients whose tumors had high rates of glucose metabolic activity tended to have a poor prognosis. The same group evaluated the relationship between tumor glucose metabolic activity and proliferative tumor activity by immunohistological staining techniques (69). Tumors with a high mitotic count tended to be associated with higher indices of glucose metabolic activity.

Using FDG-PET, Römer et al. (70) assessed the effects of chemotherapy on changes in tumor glucose metabolic activity in patients with non-Hodgkin's lymphoma. Long-term prognosis was best assessed when PET was performed after two full cycles of chemotherapy (six weeks after initiation of chemotherapy). Jerusalem et al. (71) compared the predictive value of a residual mass on CT to that of metabolic activity by PET in the post-treatment evaluation of 54 patients with Hodgkin's disease and non-Hodgkin's lymphoma. These authors reported similar negative predictive values of PET and CT of 83% and 87% for disease recurrence but found CT's positive predictive value significantly lower than PET's (40% vs. 100%). Others confirmed these findings (72, 73). These observations emphasize the major limitation of anatomical imaging, i.e., its inability to discriminate post-therapeutic anatomical alterations such as necrosis, scarring, or inflammation from residual/recurrent disease.

IMPACT ON MANAGEMENT   The impact of PET on managing patients with lymphoma was investigated by Yap et al. (74) in 46 patients. PET changed stage in 46% of the patients and management in 48%.

Thus, the literature provides scientific evidence that FDG-PET stages and restages lymphoma with high diagnostic accuracy and provides better prognostic information than that obtained by anatomical imaging.

Whole-Body PET Imaging in Patients with Melanoma

STAGING AND RESTAGING   Melanoma, the most aggressive of all skin cancers, causes more than 75% of all skin cancer deaths. Early and accurate staging is therefore of paramount importance to initiate the appropriate therapeutic approach. Traditionally, patients with melanoma are staged with a combination of standard imaging techniques such as CT, ultrasound, MRI, and X-ray.

Schwimmer et al. (75) used a priori quality criteria to perform a meta-analysis of published research articles addressing the role of PET in the management of melanoma patients. This analysis showed an overall sensitivity of 92% (95% CI: 88%–96%) and an overall specificity of 90% (95% CI: 83%–96%) of FDG-PET for detecting recurrent melanoma (Figure 3).

IMPACT ON MANAGEMENT   Because of its high diagnostic accuracy and because it examines all organ systems of the body, PET can reliably identify patients with solitary metastatic lesions who would benefit from surgery. Eigtved et al. (76) reported that 34% of their 38 patients would have been staged incorrectly by conventional methods, possibly resulting in unnecessary surgery. In a retrospective study, PET enabled avoidance of unnecessary surgery in 8% of patients (77). Wong et al. (78) examined the impact of PET on staging and managing 51 patients with melanoma from the referring physician's point of view. FDG-PET changed the clinical stage and management in 29% of these melanoma patients.

Diagnosis, Staging, and Restaging of Breast Cancer

CHARACTERIZATION OF PRIMARY BREAST LESIONS   In 1989, Kubota et al. (79) presented a case report of focally increased FDG uptake in one breast cancer patient. In a subsequent pilot study in 12 patients (80), PET correctly detected all primary tumors with a median tumor-to-background ratio of 8:1. Importantly, PET detected two primary breast cancers that had been missed on mammography in two patients with dense breasts. Others confirmed a high accuracy of FDG-PET for characterizing breast lesions in larger populations of selected patients (81–88) (Table 5). In 93 patients studied by Rostom et al. (88), PET had a sensitivity of 90.7%, specificity of 83.3%, and accuracy of 89.2% for detection of breast cancer. Four of the six patients with false negative scans had carcinoma in situ, a fifth had Paget's disease of the nipple, and the remaining patient had a tumor of 0.5 cm. The overall accuracy of PET determined in 86 patients was better than that of mammography (89.5% vs. 72.1%; $p < 0.0003$).

Novel approaches that combine mammography and PET or utilize a dedicated small high-resolution PET imaging system might further enhance the diagnostic

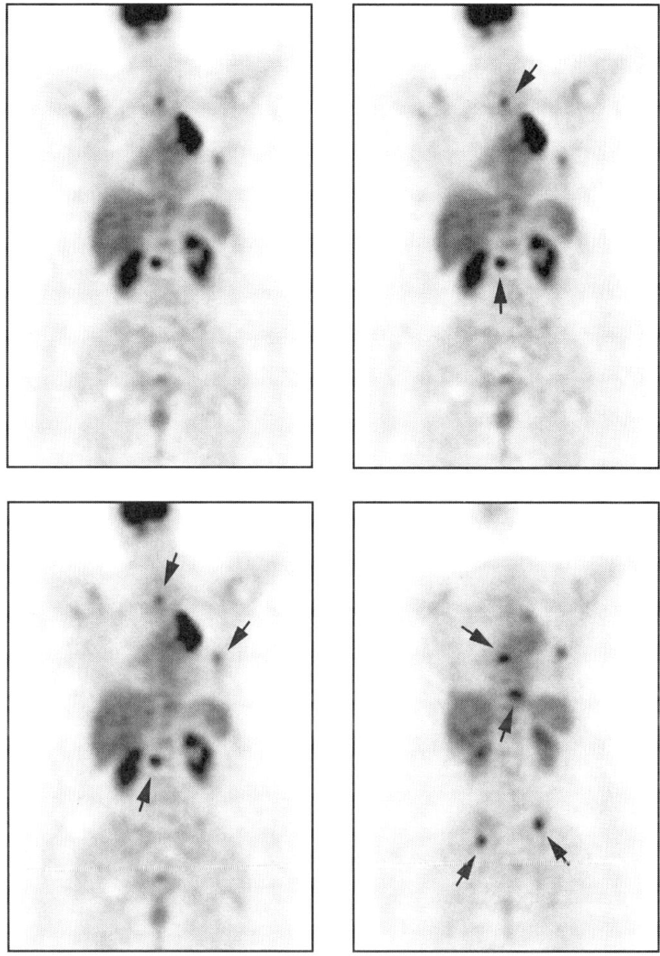

Figure 3   28-year-old man with melanoma. Whole-body PET revealed multiple metastatic lesions involving skeleton, right hilar, and right sub-carinal region (arrows).

accuracy of PET for primary breast tumors (89). These developments might further enrich the diagnostic armamentarium for characterizing primary breast lesions.

STAGING FOR AXILLARY LYMPH NODE INVOLVEMENT AND DISTANT DISEASE   Accurate staging of breast cancer patients is the prerequisite for optimal management. FDG-PET stages axillary lymph node involvement with high diagnostic accuracy (84, 86, 90–92) (Table 6; Figure 4). Adler et al. (83) reported a sensitivity and specificity of PET for detecting axillary lymph node involvement of 90% and 100%,

TABLE 5   Characterization of breast masses by FDG-PET

	Sens[a] (%)	Spec[a] (%)	Acc[a] (%)
	93[c]	93	92
95% CI[b]	90–95	90–96	89–96
Patients (N)	424	284	260

[a]Sens = Sensitivity, Spec = Specificity, Acc = Accuracy.
[b]Confidence Interval.
[c]Weighted means values and 95% Confidence Intervals were calculated from references 83–88, 92 and 94.

respectively. However, the number of tumor-involved lymph nodes could not be reliably assessed (93). The same group expanded their study and prospectively enrolled 50 patients prior to axillary lymph node dissections (93). In this study, the sensitivity of PET was 95%. The specificity, however, was lower (75%) because of several false positive findings later explained by sinus histiocytosis, mild plasmacytosis, and hemosiderin-laden macrophages that are known to have increased rates of glucose utilization.

The largest prospective study addressing the accuracy of PET for determining axillary lymph node involvement included 124 patients with a diagnosis of breast cancer (85). In this study, PET correctly identified all 44 tumor-involved lymph nodes, resulting in a sensitivity of 100%. Further, in 60 patients, all lymph nodes, pathologically proven normal, had normal PET findings. In 20 additional patients, however, PET showed increased FDG uptake that remained unexplained by pathology in 18. Scheidhauer et al. (94) examined 30 patients with inconclusive breast findings by ultrasonography and mammography using FDG-PET. PET correctly detected all eight distant metastatic lesions without false positive findings. The authors suggested that FDG-PET provided important diagnostic and staging information in addition to that obtained through other imaging approaches. Other investigators presented similar findings (88, 92, 95, 96).

TABLE 6   Axillary lymph node staging by FDG-PET

	Sens[a] (%)	Spec[a] (%)	Acc[a] (%)
	89[c]	87	88
95% CI[b]	86–92	84–90	84–92
Patients (N)	495	495	281

[a]Sens = Sensitivity, Spec = Specificity, Acc = Accuracy.
[b]Confidence Interval.
[c]Weighted means values and 95% Confidence Intervals were calculated from references 85, 86, 88, 90, 92, 93 and 96.

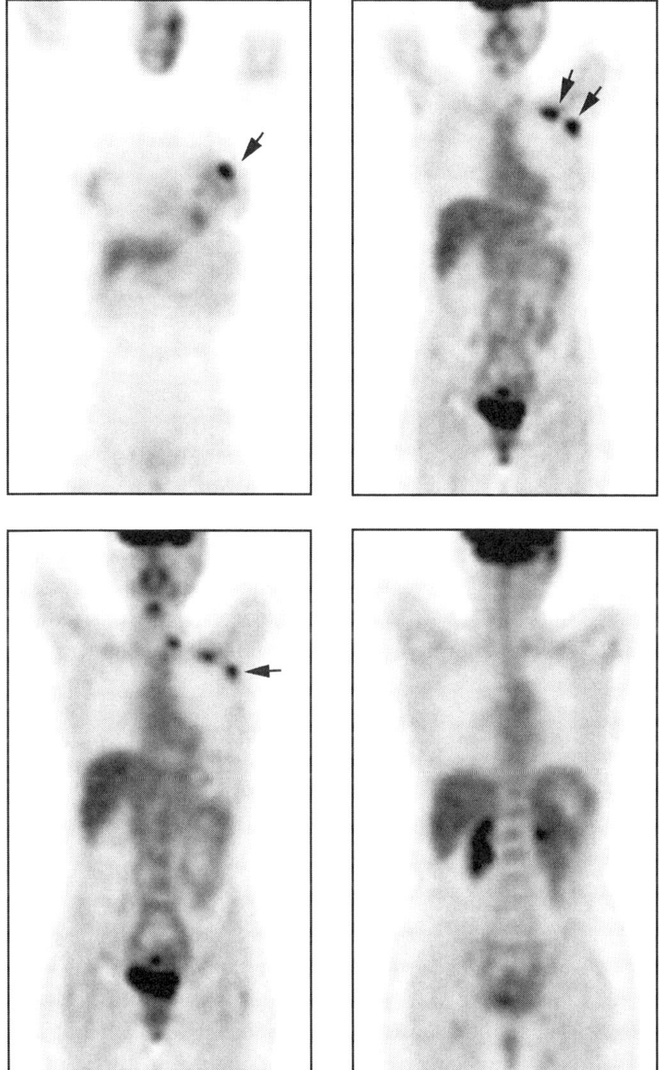

Figure 4 44-year-old woman with equivocal mammogram and normal MRI of the left axilla is restaged after radiation and chemotherapy for breast cancer. PET revealed unsuspected tumor recurrence in the left breast as well as lymph node involvement in the left axilla and left supraclavicular region (arrows).

MONITORING TREATMENT   Wahl et al. (97) demonstrated that in treatment responders, FDG uptake declined to 78% of baseline eight days after initiation of chemotherapy. After nine weeks, tumor FDG uptake was reduced to 52% of the baseline value. No such decline was observed in nonresponders. Further, conventional imaging failed to discriminate treatment responders from nonresponders. Similar observations were made by Bassa et al. (84). Dehdashti et al. (98) reported the unusual finding that patients who responded to tamoxifen treatment had increases in FDG uptake after treatment, referred to as a flare phenomenon. Nonresponders with estrogen-receptor–positive breast cancer did not exhibit this phenomenon.

FDG-PET was used to monitor therapy responses in 22 patients with breast cancer (99). This study included only patients with locally advanced disease who underwent combination chemotherapy prior to surgery. Using ROC analysis, a tumor FDG uptake of <55% of baseline best distinguished responders from nonresponders. This resulted in a sensitivity of 100% and a specificity of 85% for predicting treatment response. The predictive accuracy was 88%. After the second treatment course, the predictive accuracy was 91% when the threshold of 55% of baseline tumor FDG uptake was used as a cutoff point. The authors concluded that monitoring treatment with FDG-PET was useful to predict responses early in treatment. Similar observations were made by Smith et al. (100).

The role of PET for diagnosing and staging of breast cancer is evolving. However, PET imaging has a theoretical advantage over mammography, ultrasound, and MRI: It permits not only the accurate characterization of primary tumors and the staging of axillary and mediastinal lymph node involvement but also the detection of distant metastases, all in a single whole-body examination. With regard to monitoring the effects of chemotherapy, FDG-PET seems well-suited to predict therapy outcome in patients with locally advanced breast cancer.

PET in Head and Neck Cancer

The diagnosis of recurrent/residual head and neck cancers after surgical treatment, chemotherapy, or radiation is difficult using conventional anatomic imaging. This difficulty arises from the complex anatomy of the head and neck region as well as from the high incidence of inflammatory changes with subsequent lymph node enlargement in the oro- and nasopharyngeal space. Nonspecific post-therapeutic changes and anatomic distortions due to scarring, inflammation, and necrosis render the differentiation between benign and malignant alterations difficult.

DIAGNOSIS, STAGING, AND RESTAGING OF HEAD AND NECK CANCER   Head and neck cancers exhibit markedly increased glucose metabolic activity (101–104). FDG-PET can be used to accurately detect primary and recurrent head and neck cancers (105). PET correctly identified the primary tumor in 29 of 30 patients, superior to MRI, which identified 23 of 30 primary tumors. Further, PET correctly detected tumor recurrence in 9 of 10 patients, whereas MRI detected only 6 of 10. PET and

MRI correctly confirmed the presence or absence of lymph node involvement in 32 and 31 of 34 patients (106).

STAGING OF LYMPH NODE INVOLVEMENT   Adam et al. (107) evaluated the accuracy of FDG-PET for lymph node staging relative to that of conventional imaging in 60 patients with histologically proven squamous cell cancer of the head and neck. In this study, the sensitivity (90%), specificity (94%), positive (58%) and negative (99%) predictive value, and accuracy (93%) of PET were superior to those of CT, MRI, and ultrasound. Similar results were provided by Benchaou et al. (108).

MONITORING OF TREATMENT   The effects of chemotherapy on tumor glucose metabolism provide important clinical information. In a study by Lowe et al. (109), the positive and negative predictive values of PET for treatment response were 95% and 71%. The overall accuracy of PET was 89%. The same group evaluated prospectively the ability of FDG-PET (110) to detect recurrence of head and neck cancer in 44 patients with advanced disease. PET detected residual/recurrent disease with a sensitivity and specificity of 100% and 93%, whereas conventional imaging had a low sensitivity of 38% and a specificity of 85%. FDG-PET was also useful to predict the response to radiation therapy (111).

The available literature suggests that PET is highly accurate for detecting primary head and neck tumors, staging lymph node involvement, and monitoring the effects of radiation or chemotherapy. Recent technological advances, such as the PET/CT device, are likely to further improve the management of this patient group.

FDA APPROVAL AND REIMBURSEMENT

Because of the high accuracy of FDG-PET as a molecular imaging technique of disease biology, the U.S. Food and Drug Administration (FDA) has approved PET-FDG for all cancers. In addition, the Health Care Finance Administration approved Medicare reimbursement for diagnosing, staging, and restaging of lung cancer, colorectal cancer, lymphoma, melanoma, head and neck cancers, and esophageal cancer. Over 500 private insurance companies now provide reimbursement for FDG-PET in various cancers. A summary of the data from published papers involving over 26,000 patients studied with PET has been recently published (12). This publication includes many cancers that are accurately diagnosed and staged with PET but are not covered in this chapter.

FUTURE APPLICATIONS OF PET IMAGING

PET technology is rapidly advancing (11). Among the most exciting developments is the emergence of combined PET/CT imaging devices (44). The combination of molecular and anatomic imaging has several advantages: First, biological and anatomical whole-body staging can be performed in one examination. Second, because of limited patient motion due to the nearly simultaneous acquisition of PET and CT images, nearly ideal fusion of biological and anatomical images can be achieved. Third, anatomical landmarks provided by CT will greatly facilitate the assignment of biological abnormalities to anatomical structures. Finally and importantly, difficult-to-image regions of the body such as head and neck, mediastinum and postsurgical abdomen will be evaluated with high diagnostic accuracy thanks to improved anatomical assignment of biologically identified disease. The first commercial PET/CT devices will be available for clinical testing in the later part of 2001. The combination of PET and CT will dramatically change the planning of radiation therapy and the monitoring of surgical, medical, and radiation treatments.

The development of new tracers that target specifically biological properties of cancer cells is another important line of current research. Several new tracers are currently being tested for their clinical usefulness in cancer patients. For instance, ^{11}C acetate and ^{18}F choline are being tested to identify lipid synthesis that is increased tenfold in prostate cancer (50). FDG-PET detects distant prostate cancer metastases with high diagnostic accuracy in patients with moderately to severely elevated prostate-specific antigen levels (see Figure 5). However, FDG undergoes renal clearance and accumulates in the urinary bladder, which tends to obscure the prostate bed. Although this can be reduced by catheterization and irrigation of the bladder, this complicates the procedure and limits its usefulness for assessing primary and locally recurrent prostate cancer. Renal clearance of activity is eliminated in the case of ^{11}C acetate because the ^{11}C label is in the acid (COOH) group of acetate. Thus, when ^{11}C acetate is metabolized, the labeled product is ^{11}C-CO_2, which is diluted through the body in the bicarbonate pool and therefore does not undergo renal clearance. The labeled product is retained in tissue in the form of labeled lipids that are rapidly synthesized in prostate cancer cells. This represents a strategy of placing a positron label in a specific location in the molecular imaging probe to improve its diagnostic accuracy.

A different strategy is used with ^{18}F choline. It has been shown that the synthetic reaction involving choline in prostate cancer is faster than the renal clearance of the tracer. Thus, the prostate bed can be imaged before tracer accumulation in the bladder occurs. Initial studies with ^{11}C acetate by Seltzer et al. (50) and with ^{18}F methyl choline by DeGrado et al. (112) suggest that these tracers detect primary and recurrent prostate cancer with good diagnostic accuracy.

Shields et al. (113) used ^{18}F fluoro-thymidine (FLT) to image cell replication and proliferation of tumors in vivo. This tracer is retained in proliferating tissues through the enzyme thymidine kinase 1 (Figure 1, lower panel). The authors obtained high target-to-background images of tumor proliferation in human subjects. A similar approach using ^{11}C-thymidine was used to monitor the tumor response to chemotherapy (114).

The novel and elegant concept of in vivo imaging of gene expression with PET was recently introduced by Tjuvajev et al. (115), Gambhir et al. (116), and MacLaren et al. (117). Gambhir et al. (116) employed a PET reporter-gene/

FDG

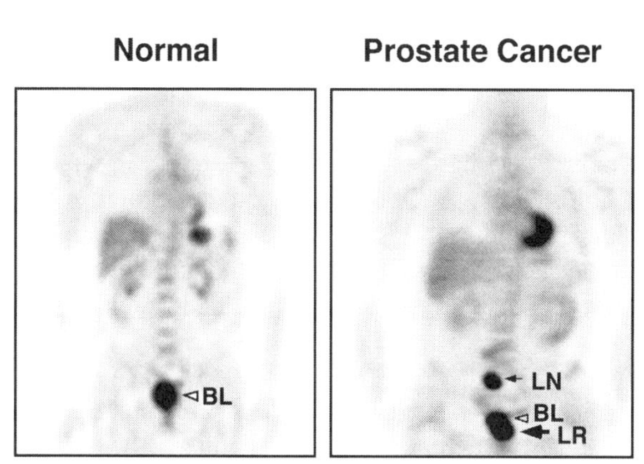

C-11 Acetate

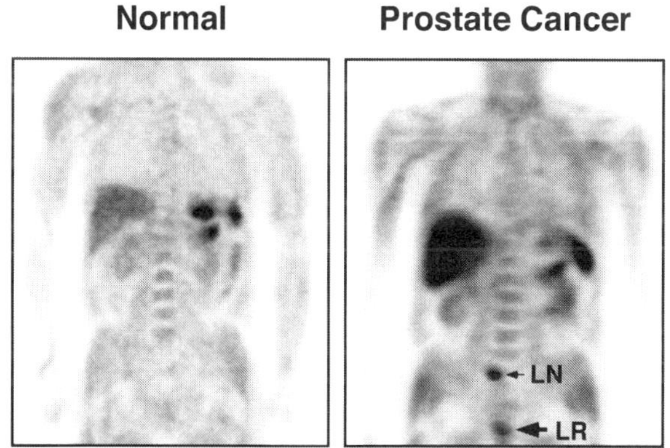

Figure 5   Patient with prostate cancer is studied with FDG (*top*) and C-acetate (*bottom*). Because of intense FDG accumulation in the bladder (BL), local tumor recurrence (LR) was detected only by ^{11}C acetate, whereas lymph node involvement (LN) was detected by both tracers.

reporter-probe imaging approach using the herpes simplex type 1 virus thymidine kinase (HSV1-tk) gene; MacLaren et al. (117) used the dopamine type 2-receptor (D2R) gene as a reporter gene for imaging gene expression in vivo. In this approach, a PET reporter gene is connected to another gene (e.g., a therapy gene), and this genetic construct is administered to the subject via a viral vector. The reporter gene product is a protein. This protein is the target of the PET reporter probe, which can be administered at any time to image the location and degree of the reporter gene expression and therefore the expression of the other gene attached to it. This allows in vivo monitoring of gene therapy dosing at the site of action within cells of the target organs. The approach can also be used to image the expression of endogenous genes as they initiate disease processes (11, 118).

In addition, a new high-resolution PET technology, microPET (119), has been developed for imaging genetically engineered and human disease cell transplant models of disease in mice. This technology provides the means to perform modern biological and genetic experiments in the living mouse by assessing such processes as metabolism, cell communication, and gene expression. The microPET technology will also enable dramatic improvement in the resolution of clinical PET scanners.

In summary, molecular imaging with PET and FDG has arrived as a clinical tool for diagnosing, staging, and restaging most cancers. PET radio-pharmacies have been set up throughout the United States to provide FDG and other imaging probes to hospitals and private radiology groups. PET also represents the entry of molecular imaging of the fundamental biology of disease as a paradigm shift in diagnostic imaging (12). In this way, the importance of PET reaches far beyond characterizing the glucose metabolism of tumors, as important as this is in its own right. New molecular imaging probes, as well as technological advances, will provide a powerful armamentarium for specifically characterizing and targeting the biological properties and genetics of tumor cells in vivo, monitoring the response to treatment, and establishing prognostic information. PET will play an important role in molecular medicine in the post-genome era and will allow biologically directed and monitored therapeutic interventions to correct the molecular errors of disease.

Visit the Annual Reviews home page at www.AnnualReviews.org

LITERATURE CITED

1. Warburg O, Posener K, Negelein E VIII. 1924. The metabolism of cancer cells. *Biochem. Zeitschr.* 152:129–69

2. Flexnor S, Jobling S. 1910. Studies upon a tranplantable rat tumour. In *Monographs on Medical and Allied Subjects*, pp. 1–51. New York: Rockefeller Inst. Med. Res.

3. Weber G. 1977. Enzymology of cancer cells (Part 1). *N. Engl. J. Med.* 296: 541–55

4. Weber G. 1977. Enzymology of cancer cells (Part 2). *N. Engl. J. Med.* 296: 541–55

5. Flier J, Mueckler M, Usher P, Lodish H. 1987. Elevated levels of glucose transport and transporter messenger RNA are induced by ras and sarc oncogenes. *Science* 235:1492–95

6. Phelps M, Hoffmann E, Mullani N, Ter-Pogossian M. 1975. Application of annihilation coincidence detection to transaxial reconstruction tomography. *J. Nucl. Med.* 16:210–24

7. Valk PE, Pounds TR, Tesar RD, et al. 1996. Cost-effectiveness of PET imaging in clinical oncology. *Nucl. Med. Biol.* 23:737–43

8. Silverman D, Hoh C, Seltzer M, et al.

1998. Evaluating tumor biology and oncological disease with positron emission tomography. *Sem. Rad. Oncol.* 8:183–96

9. Conti PS, Lilien DL, Hawley K, et al. 1996. PET and 18-F-FDG in oncology: a clinical update. *Nucl. Med. Biol.* 23:717–35

10. Rigo P. 1997. Positron emission tomography using 18F-fluorodeoxyglucose in oncology. *Bull.et Memoires de L'Academie Royale de Medicine de Belgique* 152:353–61

11. Phelps M. 2000. Positron emission tomography provides molecular imaging of biological processes. *Proc. Natl. Acad. Sci. USA* 97:9226–33

12. Gambhir S, Czernin J, Schwimmer J, et al. 2001. A tabulated summary of the FDG-PET literature. *J. Nucl. Med.* 42 (5 Suppl.):1S–93S

13. Siegelman S, Zerhouni E, Leo R, et al. 1980. CT of the solitary pulmonary nodule. *Am. J. Roentgenol.* 135:1–13

14. Kubota K, Matsuzawa T, Fujiwara T, et al. 1990. Differential diagnosis of lung tumor with positron emission tomography: a prospective study. *J. Nucl. Med.* 31:1927–33

15. Dewan N, Gupta N, Redepennig L, et al. 1993. Diagnostic efficacy of PET-FDG imaging in solitary pulmonary nodules; potential role in evaluation and management. *Chest* 104:997–1002

16. Patz E, Lowe V, Hoffman J, et al. 1993. Focal pulmonary abnormalities: evaluation with F-18 fluorodeoxyglucose PET scanning. *Radiology* 188:487–90

17. Duhaylongsod F, Lowe V, Patz E, et al. 1995. Detection of primary and recurrent lung cancer by means of F-18 fluorodeoxyglucose positron emission tomography. *J. Thorac. Cardiovasc. Surg.* 110:130–40

18. Gupta N, Maloof J, Gunel E. 1996. Probability of malignancy in solitary pulmonary nodule using fluorine-18-FDG and PET. *J. Nucl. Med.* 37:943–48

19. Knight S, Delbeke D, Stewart J, Sandler M. 1996. Evaluation of pulmonary lesions with FDG-PET: comparison of findings in patients with and without a history of prior malignancy. *Chest* 109:982–88

20. Bury T, Dowlati A, Paulus P, et al. 1996. Evaluation of the solitary pulmonary nodule by positron emission tomography imaging. *Eur. Respir. J.* 9:410–14

21. Worsely D, Celler A, Adam M, et al. 1996. Pulmonary nodules: differential diagnosis using 18F-fluorodeoxyglucose single photon emission tomography. *AJR* 168:771–74

22. Lowe V, Duhaylongsod F, Patz E, et al. 1997. Pulmonary abnormalities and PET data analysis: a retrospective study. *Radiology* 202:435–39

23. Lowe V, Fletcher J, Gobar L, et al. 1998. Prospective investigation of positron emission tomography in lung nodules. *J. Clin. Oncol.* 16:1075–84

24. Dewan N, Shehan C, Reeb S, et al. 1997. Likelihood of malignancy in a solitary pulmonary nodule: comparison of Bayesian analysis and results of FDG-PET scan. *Chest* 112:416–22

25. Gambhir SS, Shepherd JE, Shah BD, et al. Analytical decision model for the cost-effective management of solitary pulmonary nodules. *J. Clin. Oncol.* 16:2113–25

26. American Cancer Society AC. 1996. Cancer facts and figures.

27. Mountain C. 1989. Value of the new TNM staging system for lung cancer. *Chest* 97:935

28. McKenna R, Libshitz H, Mountain C, McMurtey M. 1985. Roentgenographic evaluation of mediastinal lymph nodes for pre-operative assessment in lung cancer. *Chest* 88:206–10

29. Arita T, Kuramitsu T, Kawamura M. 1995. Bronchogenic carcinoma: incidence of metastases to normal sized lymph nodes. *Thorax* 50:1267–69

30. Webb R, Gatsonis C, Zerhouni E, et al. 1991. CT and MRI imaging in staging

non-small cell bronchogenic carcinoma: report of the radiologic diagnostic oncology group. *Radiology* 178:705–13

31. Dillemans B, Deneffe G, Verschakelen J, Decramer M. 1994. Value of computed tomography and mediastinoscopy in pre-operative evaluation of mediastinal nodes in non-small cell lung cancer. *Eur. J. Cardio-thorac. Surg.* 8:37–42

32. Sasaki M, Ichiya Y, Kuwabara Y, et al. 1996. The usefulness of FDG positron emission tomography for the detection of mediastinal lymph node metastases in patients with non-small cell lung cancer: a comparative study with X-ray computed tomography. *Eur. J. Nucl. Med.* 23:741–47

33. Scott W, Schwabe J, Gupta N, et al. 1994. Positron emission tomography of lung tumors and mediastinal lymph nodes using [18F]fluorodeoxyglucose. *Ann. Thorac. Surg.* 58:698–703

34. Scott WJ, Shepherd J, Gambhir SS. 1998. Cost-effectiveness of FDG-PET for staging non-small cell lung cancer: a decision analysis. *Ann. Thorac. Surg.* 66:1876–83; discussion 1883–85

35. Patz E, Lowe V, Goodman P, Herndon J. 1995. Thoracic nodal staging with PET imaging with 18FDG in patients with bronchogenic carcinoma. *Chest* 108:1617–21

36. Sazon D, Santiago S, Soo Hoo G, et al. 1996. Fluorodeoxyglucose-positron emission tomography in the detection and staging of lung cancer. *Am. J. Respir. Crit. Care Med.* 153:417–21

37. Steinert H, Hauser M, Aleman F, et al. 1997. Non-small cell lung cancer: nodal staging with FDG-PET versus correlative lymph node mapping and sampling. *Radiology* 202:441–46

38. Marom E, McAdams H, Erasmus J, et al. 1999. Staging non-small cell lung cancer with whole body PET. *Radiology* 212:803–9

39. Pieterman R, van Putten J, Meuzelaar J, et al. 2000. Preoperative staging of non-small-cell lung cancer with positron-emission tomography. *N. Engl. J. Med.* 343:254–61

40. Dwamena B, Sonnad S, Angobaldo J, Wahl R. 1999. Metastases from non-small cell lung cancer: mediastinal staging in the 1990s—meta-analytic comparison of PET and CT. *Radiology* 213:530–36

41. Wahl RL, Quint L, Greenough R, et al. 1994. Staging of mediastinal non-small cell lung cancer with FDG-PET, CT, and fusion images: preliminary prospective evaluation. *Radiology* 191:371–77

42. Chin R, Ward R, Keyes J, et al. 1995. Mediastinal staging of non-small-cell lung cancer with positron emission tomography. *Am. J. Respir. Crit. Care Med.* 152:2090–96

43. Vansteenkiste J, Stroobants S, De Leyn P, et al. 1998. Lymph node staging in non-small-cell lung cancer with FDG-PET scan: a prospective study on 690 lymph node stations from 68 patients. *J. Clin. Oncol.* 16:2142–49

44. Beyer T, Townsend D, Brun T, et al. 2000. A combined PET/CT scanner for clinical oncology. *J. Nucl. Med.* 41:1369–79

45. Patton J, Delbeke D, Sandler M. 1996. Image fusion using an integrated, dual-head coincidence camera with X-ray tube-based attenuation maps. *J. Nucl. Med.* 41:1364–68

46. Valk P, Pounds T, Hopkins D, et al. 1995. Staging non-small cell lung cancer by whole body positron emission tomographic imaging. *Ann. Thorac. Surg.* 60:1573–82

47. Bury T, Dowlati A, Paulus P, et al. 1997. Whole-body 18FDG positron emission tomography in the staging of non-small cell lung cancer. *Eur. Respir. J.* 10:2529–34

48. Saunders C, Dussek J, O'Doherty J. 1999. Evaluation of fluorine-18-fluorodeoxyglucose whole body positron emission tomography imaging in the staging of lung cancer. *Ann. Thorac. Surg.* 67:790–97

49. Lewis P, Griffin S, Marsden P, et al. 1994. Whole-body 18F-fluorodeoxyglucose positron emission tomography in preoperative evaluation of lung cancer. *Lancet* 344:1265–66

50. Seltzer M, Barbaric Z, Belldegrun A, et al. 1999. Comparison of helical computerized tomography, positron emission tomography and monoclonal antibody scans for evaluation of lymph node metastases in patients with prostate specific antigen relapse after treatment for localized prostate cancer. *J. Urol.* 162:1322–28

51. Gambhir SS, Hoh CK, Phelps ME, et al. 1996. Decision tree sensitivity analysis for cost-effectiveness of FDG-PET in the staging and management of non-small-cell lung carcinoma. *J. Nucl. Med.* 37:1428–36

52. Seltzer M, Valk P, Wong C, et al. 2000. Prospective survey of referring physicians to determine the impact of whole body FDG-PET on management of cancer patients. 2000. *J. Nucl. Med.* 41(5 Suppl.): 108P

53. Abdel-Nabi H, Doerr RJ, Lamonica DM, et al. 1998. Staging of primary colorectal carcinomas with fluorine-18 fluorodeoxyglucose whole-body PET: correlation with histopathologic and CT findings. *Radiology* 206:755–60

54. Meyer M. 1995. Diffusely increased colonic F-18 FDG uptake in acute enterocolitis. *Clin. Nucl. Med.* 20:434–35

55. Hannah A, Scott AM, Akhurst T, et al. 1996. Abnormal colonic accumulation of fluorine-18-FDG in pseudomembranous colitis. *J. Nucl. Med.* 37:1683–85

56. Falk P, Gupta N, Thorson A, et al. 1994. Positron emission tomography for preoperative staging of colorectal carcinoma. *Dis. Colon Rectum* 37:153–56

57. Schiepers C, Penninckx F, De Vadder N, et al. 1995. Contribution of PET in the diagnosis of recurrent colorectal cancer: comparison with conventional imaging. *Eur. J. Surg. Oncol.* 21:517–22

58. Ito K, Nakata K, Watanabe T, et al. 1997. Diagnosis of local recurrence of colorectal cancer, using PET and immunoscintigraphy by means of ^{131}I or ^{111}In anti-CEA monoclonal antibody. *J. Jpn. Surg. Soc.* 98:373–79

59. Vitola JV, Delbeke D, Sandler MP, et al. 1996. Positron emission tomography to stage suspected metastatic colorectal carcinoma to the liver. *Am. J. Surg.* 171:21–26

60. Huebner R, Park K, Shepherd J, et al. 2000. A meta-analysis of the literature for whole-body FDG PET detection of recurrent colorectal cancer. *J. Nucl. Med.* 41:1177–89

61. Valk P, Abella-Columna E, Haseman M, et al. 1999. Whole-body PET imaging with [18F]Fluorodeoxyglucose in management of recurrent colorectal cancer. *Arch. Surg.* 134:503–11

62. Delbeke D, Vitola JV, Sandler MP, et al. 1997. Staging recurrent metastatic colorectal carcinoma with PET. *J. Nucl. Med.* 38:1196–1201

63. Meta J, Seltzer MA, Schiepers C, et al. 2001. Impact of ^{18}F-FDG PET on managing patients with colorectal cancer: the referring physician's perspective. *J. Nucl. Med.* 42:586–90

64. Hoh C, Glaspy J, Rosen P, et al. 1997. Whole-body FDG-PET imaging for staging of Hodgkin's disease and lymphoma. *J. Nucl. Med.* 38:343–48

65. Moog F, Kotzerke J, Reske S. 1999. FDG PET can replace bone scintigraphy in primary staging of malignant lymphoma. *J. Nucl Med.* 40:1407–13

66. Stumpe K, Urbinelli M, Steinert H, et al. 1998. Whole-body positron emission tomography using fluorodeoxyglucose for staging of lymphoma: effectiveness and comparison with computed tomography. *Eur. J. Nucl. Med.* 25:721–28

67. Carr R, Barrington S, Madan B, et al. 1998. Detection of lymphoma in bone marrow by whole-body positron emission tomography. *Blood* 91:3340–46

68. Okada J, Yoshikawa K, Imazeki K, et al. 1991. The use of FDG-PET in the detection and management of malignant lymphoma: correlation of uptake with prognosis. *J. Nucl. Med.* 32:686–91

69. Okada J, Yoshikawa K, Itami M, et al. 1992. Positron emission tomography using fluorine-18-fluorodeoxyglucose in malignant lymphoma: a comparison with proliferative activity. *J. Nucl. Med.* 33:325–29

70. Römer W, Avril N, Dose J, et al. 1997. Metabolic characterization of ovarian tumors with positron-emission tomography and F-18 fluorodeoxyglucose. *Rofo. Fortschr. Verfahr.* 166:62–68

71. Jerusalem G, Beguin Y, Fasotte M, et al. 1999. Whole body positron emission tomography using 18F-fluorodeoxyglucose for post-treatment evaluation in Hodgkin's disease and non-Hodgkin's lymphoma has higher diagnostic and prognostic value than classical computed tomography scan imaging. *Blood* 94:429–33

72. de Witt M, Bumann D, Herbst K, et al. 1997. Whole body positron emission tomography for diagnosis of residual mass in patients with lymphoma. *Ann. Oncol.* 8:S57–S60

73. Zinzani P, Magagnoli M, Chierichetti F, et al. 1999. The role of positron emission tomography (PET) in the management of lymphoma patients. *Ann. Oncol.* 10:1181–84

74. Schoder H, Meta J, Yap C, et al. 2001. Effect of whole-body 18F-FDG PET imaging on clinical staging and management of patients with malignant lymphoma. *J. Nucl. Med.* 42:1139–43

75. Schwimmer J, Essner R, Patel A, et al. 2000. A review of the literature for whole-body FDG PET in the management of patients with melanoma. *Q. J. Nucl. Med.* 44:153–67

76. Eigtved A, Andersson A, Dahlstrom K, et al. 2000. Use of fluorine-18 fluorodeoxyglucose positron emission tomography in the detection of silent metastases from malignant melanoma. *Eur. J. Nucl. Med.* 27:70–75

77. Jadvar H, Johnson D, Segall G. 2000. The effect of fluorine-18 fluorodeoxyglucose positron emission tomography on the management of cutaneous malignant melanoma. *Clin. Nucl. Med.* 25:48–51

78. Wong C, Valk P, Ariannejad M, et al. 2000. Impact of FDG-PET on management of patients with melanoma. *J. Nucl. Med.* (5 Suppl.):282P

79. Kubota K, Matsuzawa T, Amemiya A, et al. 1989. Imaging of breast cancer with [F18]fluorodeoxyglucose and positron emission tomography. *J. Comput. Assist. Tomogr.* 13:1097

80. Wahl R, Cody R, Hutchins G, Mudgett E. 1991. Primary and metastatic breast carcinoma: initial clinical evaluation with the radiolabeled glucose analogue 2-[F-18]-fluoro-2-deoxy-D-glucose. *Radiology* 179:765–70

81. Tse N, Hoh C, Hawkins R, et al. 1992. The application of positron emission tomographic imaging with fluorodeoxyglucose to the evaluation of breast disease. *Ann. Surg.* July:27–34

82. Nieweg O, Kim E, Wong W, et al. 1993. Positron emission tomography with fluorine-18-deoxyglucose in the detection and staging of breast cancer. *Cancer* 71:3920–25

83. Adler L, Crowe J, al-Kaisi NK, Sunshine J. 1993. Evaluation of breast masses and axillary lymph nodes with [F-18] 2 deoxy-2-fluoro-D-glucose PET. *Radiology* 187:743–50

84. Bassa P, Kim E, Inoue T, et al. 1996. Evaluation of pre-operative chemotherapy using PET with fluorine-18-fluorodeoxyglucose in breast cancer. *J. Nucl. Med.* 37:931–38

85. Utech C, Young C, Winter P. 1996. Prospective evaluation of fluorine-18 fluorodeoxyglucose positron emission tomography in breast cancer for staging of the axilla related to surgery and immunocytochemistry. *Eur. J. Nucl. Med.* 23:1588–93

86. Noh D, Yun I, Kim S, et al. 1998. Diagnostic value of positron emission tomography for detecting breast cancer. *World J. Surg.* 22:223–28

87. Avril N, Dose J, Jänicke F, et al. 1996. Metabolic characterization of breast tumors with positron emission tomography using F-18 fluorodeoxyglucose. *J. Clin. Oncol.* 14:1848–57

88. Rostom A, Powe J, Kandil A, et al. 1999. Positron emission tomography in breast cancer: a clinicopathological correlation of results. *Br. J. Radiol.* 72:1064–68

89. Murthy K, Aznar M, Thompson C, et al. 2000. Results of preliminary clinical trials of the positron emission mammography system PEM-1: a dedicated breast imaging system producing glucose metabolic images using FDG. *J. Nucl. Med.* 41:1851–58

90. Crippa F, Agresti R, Seregni E, et al. 1998. Prospective evaluation of fluorine-18-FDG PET in pre-surgical staging of the axilla in breast cancer. *J. Nucl. Med.* 39:4–8

91. Crippa F, Agresti R, Delle Donne V, et al. 1997. The contribution of positron emission tomography (PET) with 18F-fluorodeoxyglucose (FDG) in the pre-operative detection of axillary metastases of breast cancer: the experience of the national cancer institute of Milan. *Tumori* 83:542–43

92. Schirrmeister H, Kühn T, Guhlman A, et al. 2001. Fluorine-18 2-deoxy-2-fluoro-D-glucose PET in the preoperative staging of breast cancer: comparison with the standard staging procedures. *Eur. J. Nucl. Med.* 28:351–58

93. Adler L, Faulhaber P, Schnur K, et al. 1997. Axillary lymph node metastases: screening with [F18] 2-deoxy-2-D-glucose (FDG) PET. *Radiology* 203:323–27

94. Scheidhauer K, Scharl A, Pietrzyk U, et al. 1996. Qualitative [18F] FDG positron emission tomography in primary breast cancer: clinical relevance and practicability. *Eur. J. Nucl. Med.* 23:618–23

95. Moon D, Maddahi J, Silverman D, et al. 1998. Accuracy of whole-body fluorine-18-FDG PET for the detection of recurrent or metastatic breast carcinoma. *J. Nucl. Med.* 39:431–35

96. Smith I, Ogston K, Whitford P, et al. 1998. Staging of the axilla in breast cancer: accurate in vivo assessment using positron emission tomography with 2-(fluorine-18)-fluoro-2-deoxy-D-glucose. *Ann. Surg.* 228:220–27

97. Wahl RL, Zasadny KR, Helvie M, et al. 1993. Metabolic monitoring of breast cancer chemohormonotherapy using positron emission tomography: initial evaluation. *J. Clin. Oncol.* 11:2101–11

98. Dehdashti F, Flanagan FL, Mortimer J, et al. 1998. Positron emission tomographic assessment of "metabolic flare" to predict response of metastatic breast cancer to anti-estrogen therapy. *Eur. J. Nucl. Med.* 26:51–56

99. Schelling M, Avril N, Nährig J, et al. 2000. Positron emission tomography using [(18)F]Fluorodeoxyglucose for monitoring primary chemotherapy in breast cancer. *J. Clin. Oncol.* 18:1689–95

100. Smith I, Welch A, Hutcheon A, et al. 2000. Positron emission tomography using [18F]-fluorodeoxy-D-glucose to predict the pathologic response of breast cancer to primary chemotherapy. *J. Clin. Oncol.* 18:1676–88

101. Minn H, Paul R, Ahonen A. 1989. Evaluation of treatment response to radiotherapy in head and neck cancer with fluorine-18 fluorodeoxyglucose. *J. Nucl. Med.* 29:1521–25

102. Lowe V, Kim H, Boyd J, et al. 1999. Primary and recurrent early stage laryngeal cancer: preliminary results of 2-[fluorine 18]fluoro-2-deoxy-D-glucose PET imaging. *Radiology* 212:799–802

103. Hubner K, Thie J, Smith G, et al. 2000. Clinical utility of FDG-PET in detecting

head and neck tumors: a comparison of diagnostic methods and modalities. *Clin. Positron Imag.* 3:7–16

104. Lapela M, Grenman R, Kurki T, et al. 1995. Head and neck cancer: detection of recurrence with PET and 2-[F-18]fluoro-2-deoxy-D-glucose. *Radiology* 197:205–11

105. Jabour B, Choi Y, Hoh C, et al. 1993. Extracranial head and neck: PET imaging with 2-[F-18]fluoro-2-deoxy-D-glucose and MR imaging correlation. *Radiology* 186:27–35

106. Rege S, Maas A, Chaiken L, et al. 1994. Use of positron emission tomography with fluorodeoxyglucosein patients with extracranial head and neck cancers. *Cancer* 73:3047–58

107. Adam S, Baum R, Stuckensen T, et al. 1998. Prospective comparison of 18F-FDG PET with conventional imaging modalities (CT, MRI, US) in lymph node staging of head and neck cancer. *Eur. J. Nucl. Med.* 25:1255–60

108. Benchaou M, Lehmann W, Slosman D et al. 1996. The role of FDG-PET in the preoperative assessment of N-staging in head and neck cancer. *Acta Otolaryngol. (Stockh.)* 116:332–35

109. Lowe V, Dunphy F, Varvares M, et al. 1997. Evaluation of chemotherapeutic response in patients with advanced head and neck cancer using [F-18] fluorodeoxyglucose positron emission tomography. *Head & Neck* 19:666–74

110. Lowe V, Boyd J, Dunphy F, et al. 2000. Surveillance for recurrent head and neck cancer using positron emission tomography. *J. Clin. Oncol.* 18:651–58

111. Sakamoto H, Nakai Y, Ohaqshi Y, et al. 1998. Monitoring of response to radio-therapy with fluorine-18 deoxyglucose PET of head and neck squamous cell carcinomas. *Acta Otolaryngol. (Stockh.)* 538:254–60

112. DeGrado T, Coleman R, Wang S, et al. 2001. Synthesis and evaluation of 18F-labeled choline as an oncologic tracer for positron emission tomography: initial findings in prostate cancer. *Cancer Res.* 6:110–17

113. Shields A, Grierson J, Dohmen B, et al. 1998. Imaging proliferation in vivo with [F-18]FLT and positron emission tomography. *Nat. Med.* 4:1334–36

114. Shields A, Mankoff D, Link J, et al. 1998. Carbon-11-thymidine and FDG to measure therapy response. *J. Nucl. Med.* 39:1757–62

115. Tjuvajev J, Chen S, Joshi A, et al. 1999. Imaging adenoviral-mediated herpes virus thymidine kinase gene transfer and expression in vivo. *Cancer Res.* 59:5186–93

116. Gambhir S, Barrio J, Wu L, et al. 1998. Imaging of adenoviral-directed herpes simplex virus type 1 thymidine kinase reporter gene expression in mice with radiolabeled ganciclovir. *J. Nucl. Med.* 39:2003–11

117. MacLaren D, Toyokuni T, Cherry S, et al. 2000. PET imaging of transgene expression. *Biol. Psychiatry* 48:337–48

118. Gambhir S, Herschman H, Cherry S, et al. 2000. Imaging transgene expression with radionuclide imaging technologies. *Neoplasia* 2:118–38

119. Chatziioannou A, Cherry S, Shao Y, et al. 1999. Performance evaluation of microPET: a high resolution lutetium oxyorthosilicate PET scanner for animal imaging. *J. Nucl. Med.* 40:1164–75

Annu. Rev. Med. 2002. 53:113–31

ATTENTION DEFICIT/HYPERACTIVITY DISORDER ACROSS THE LIFESPAN

Timothy E. Wilens, Joseph Biederman, and Thomas J. Spencer

Clinical Research Program in Pediatric Psychopharmacology, Massachusetts General Hospital and Harvard Medical School, 15 Parkman Street, Boston, Massachusetts 02114; e-mail: wilens@helix.mgh.harvard.edu; biederman@helix.mgh.harvard.edu; spencer@helix.mgh.harvard.edu

Key Words   ADHD, ADD, comorbidity, stimulants, antidepressants

■ **Abstract**   Attention deficit/hyperactivity disorder (ADHD) is the most common neurobehavioral disorder presenting for treatment in youth. ADHD is often chronic with prominent symptoms and impairment spanning into adulthood. ADHD is often associated with co-occurring anxiety, mood, and disruptive disorders, as well as substance abuse. The diagnosis of ADHD by careful review of symptoms and impairment is both reliable and valid. Recent genetic, imaging, neurochemistry, and neuropsychological data support the biological underpinning of the disorder. All aspects of an individual's life must be considered in the diagnosis and treatment of ADHD. Pharmacotherapy, including stimulants, antidepressants, and antihypertensives, plays a fundamental role in the management of ADHD across the lifespan.

INTRODUCTION AND OVERVIEW

Introduction

Attention deficit/hyperactivity disorder (ADHD) is the most common emotional, cognitive, and behavioral disorder treated in youth (1, 2). (The term ADHD in this report refers to previously used definitions including hyperkinesis, minimal brain dysfunction, and ADD with or without hyperactivity.) Epidemiologic studies indicate that ADHD is a prevalent disorder, affecting 4% to 5 % of children in the United States, New Zealand/Australia, Germany, and Brazil (3). Although it was previously thought to remit largely in adolescence, a growing literature supports the persistence of the disorder and/or associated impairment into adulthood in a majority of cases. It is a major clinical and public health problem because of its associated morbidity and disability in children, adolescents, and adults (2). Data from cross-sectional, retrospective, and follow-up studies indicate that youth with ADHD are at risk for developing other psychiatric difficulties in childhood,

0066-4219/02/0218-0113$14.00

adolescence, and adulthood including delinquent, mood, anxiety, and substance-use disorders (4).

Diagnostic Considerations

The diagnosis of ADHD is made by careful clinical history (5). A child with ADHD is characterized by a considerable degree of inattentiveness, distractibility, impulsivity, and often hyperactivity that is inappropriate for the developmental stage of the child. Other common symptoms include low frustration tolerance, shifting activities frequently, difficulty organizing, and daydreaming. These symptoms are usually pervasive; however, they may not all occur in all settings. Children whose predominant symptom is inattention may have more difficulties in school and in completing homework but not manifest difficulties with peers or family. Conversely, children with excessive hyperactive or impulsive symptoms may do relatively well in school but have difficulties at home or in situations of less guidance and structure.

Adults must have childhood-onset, persistent, and current symptoms of ADHD to be diagnosed with the disorder. Adults with ADHD often present with marked inattention, distractibility, organization difficulties, and poor efficiency reflected in life histories of academic and occupational failure (4, 6).

Rating scales such as the Conners and Brown scales are available for all age groups and can be useful in assessing and monitoring home, academic, and occupational performance (7, 8). Although neuropsychological testing is not relied on to diagnose ADHD, it may serve to identify particular weaknesses within ADHD (9) or specific learning disabilities co-occurring with ADHD (for review see 5).

Our concept of the disorder has undergone a number of changes over the past several decades. Whereas ADHD was initially characterized as a disorder of hyperkinesis or overactivity, both inattention and hyperactivity are now equally emphasized as important core features. Three subtypes of ADHD are currently recognized: predominantly inattentive, predominantly hyperactive-impulsive, and a combined subtype (Figure 1). The combined subtype is the most commonly represented subgroup, accounting for 50% to 75% of all ADHD individuals, followed by the inattentive subtype (20% to 30%) and the hyperactive-impulsive subtype (less than 15%) (6, 10–12). Children, adolescents, and adults with the inattentive subtype of ADHD have fewer other emotional or behavioral problems than individuals with the other subtypes. Youth with prominent inattentive problems as part of their ADHD (combined or inattentive subtype) have greater academic impairment than those with predominant hyperactivity/impulsivity. The combined-type ADHD individuals have more co-occurring psychiatric and substance-abuse disorders and are the most impaired overall.

Follow-up studies of ADHD children into adolescence and early adulthood indicate that the disorder frequently persists and is associated with significant psychopathology and dysfunction in later life. The ADHD adolescent and young adult is at risk for school failure, emotional difficulties, poor peer relationships,

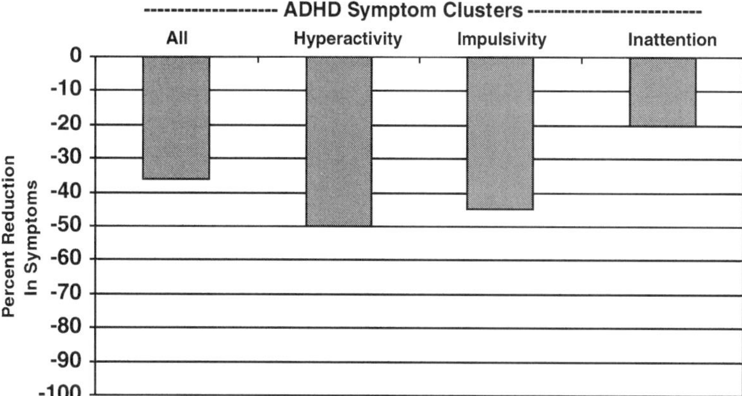

Figure 1   As observed in an ongoing longitudinal study of ADHD youth, assessed off medication, the reduction in ADHD symptom clusters is depicted from age 6 to 19 years (adapted from Reference 12a). A greater reduction in the hyperactive and impulsive symptoms was noted relative to inattentive symptoms from early childhood into young adulthood.

and trouble with the law (13, 14). Factors identifiable in younger youth that predict the persistence of ADHD into adulthood include family history of ADHD and psychiatric comorbidity—particularly aggression or delinquency problems (13, 15–17).

Prospective, longitudinal follow-up studies provide compelling evidence of the continuation of ADHD into adulthood, though the rate at which this occurs remains unclear. Partly because of methodological differences, prior longitudinal studies found highly variable rates of persistence of ADHD symptoms into adolescence (50%–75%) (18–20) and adulthood (4%–60%) (21, 22). More recent studies based in DSM IIIR nomenclature and mindful of the cognitive features of the disorder have indicated higher persistence rates of 75% into young adulthood (23, 24). These studies showed that the persistence of ADHD into adulthood included symptoms of inattention, disorganization, distractibility, and impulsivity, along with academic and occupational failure. In support of this, we reported that over 90% of ADHD adults presenting for treatment endorsed functionally impairing inattentive symptomatology (6).

PSYCHIATRIC COMORBIDITY

During the past decade, epidemiological studies have documented high rates of concurrent psychiatric and learning disorders among individuals with ADHD (25, 26). Most commonly, comorbidity with ADHD in youth includes oppositional, conduct, mood, and anxiety disorders (4).

Conduct Disorder

Conduct disorder is the best-established comorbid condition of childhood ADHD and has been widely reported in epidemiological (26), clinical (28), follow-up (13–15, 29), and family genetic studies. Consistent with childhood studies, recent studies of referred and nonreferred ADHD adults have found high rates of childhood conduct disorder as well as adult antisocial disorders in these subjects (30).

Depression

The comorbidity of ADHD and mood disorders has been controversial. However, reviews of ADHD studies (28) and reviews of depression studies (31) agree that ADHD and depression co-occur beyond what one would expect by chance. Follow-up studies provide additional evidence for major depression as an outcome of childhood hyperactivity. For example, Mannuzza et al. (22) found that 23% of their hyperkinetic children had a lifetime diagnosis of depression in adulthood. This rate is similar to that reported among ADHD children and adults (28, 30). To what extent depression develops as a result of ADHD or independently remains to be seen.

Bipolar Disorder

The overlap of ADHD and bipolar disorder is of recent clinical and scientific interest. Winokur et al. (32) showed that traits of hyperactivity in childhood were elevated among bipolar adults and their bipolar relatives. Similarly, many reports of bipolar children have noted the co-occurrence of mania and ADHD, and there are case reports of hyperactive children developing manic-depressive illness (33). Prior systematic studies of children and adolescents found rates of ADHD ranging from 57% to 98% in bipolar children and rates of bipolar disorder of 22% in ADHD inpatients (34). Family studies suggest a familial link between ADHD and bipolar disorder. Using pooled data from five studies, Faraone et al. (34) showed significantly elevated rates of ADHD in children of bipolar parents and significantly elevated rates of bipolar disorder among families of ADHD children.

Despite an emerging literature from convergent sources, there continues to be much controversy about the validity of the concurrent diagnoses of ADHD and bipolar disorder. Overlap of symptoms does not account for spurious diagnosis of either bipolar disorder or ADHD (35). Whereas ADHD is characterized by cognitive and hyperactive/impulsive features, bipolar disorder is characterized by mood instability, pervasive irritability, grandiosity, psychosis, cyclicity, and lack of response to structure. When youth experience both sets of symptoms, they may suffer from both ADHD and bipolar disorder.

Substance-Use Disorders

Combined data from retrospective accounts of adults and prospective observations of youth indicate that juveniles with ADHD are at increased risk for cigarette smoking and substance abuse during adolescence. In particular, ADHD youth with bipolar or conduct disorder are at risk for very early (i.e., <16 years of age) cigarette use and substance-use disorders, whereas the typical age of risk for the onset of substance use accounted for by ADHD itself is probably between 17 and 22 years of age (36). Recent work suggests that ADHD youth disproportionately become involved with cigarettes, alcohol, and then drugs (37, 38). ADHD adolescents and adults become addicted to cigarette smoking at twice the rate of non-ADHD individuals. Moreover, ADHD substance abusers tend to prefer drugs other than alcohol with no evidence of a preference for a specific type of drug (39): Data indicate that cocaine and stimulant abuse are not overrepresented in ADHD; in fact, as among non-ADHD abusers, marijuana is the most commonly abused agent (39). Individuals with ADHD, independent of comorbidity, tend to maintain their addiction longer than do their non-ADHD peers (40).

Based largely on some preclinical animal studies (41), concerns about the later abuse liability and potential kindling of specific types of drug abuse secondary to early stimulant exposure in ADHD children have been raised. However, the preponderance of clinical data and consensus in the field do not appear to support such concerns. For example, in a prospective study of ADHD youth, a significant reduction in the risk for substance abuse was reported in treated versus untreated ADHD youth followed into midadolescence (42). Moreover, of five studies evaluating substance-use disorder risk in treated and untreated ADHD individuals, both studies with follow-up in adolescents (Figure 2) and two of three studies with follow-up in adults indicated a significant reduction in the risk for substance abuse in the treated ADHD group (T. E. Wilens, unpublished data). Clearly, further work is needed in this important area.

GENDER AND ADHD

Although little doubt remains that ADHD affects both genders, the literature on ADHD in females is limited (43). It indicates that ADHD females share with their male counterparts prototypical features of the disorder (e.g., inattention, impulsivity, and hyperactivity), high rates of school failure, comorbidity, and high levels of familiality (44–46). For instance, in the largest study of girls with ADHD, girls had rates of mood, anxiety, and learning disorders paralleling findings in boys. Girls with ADHD had lower rates of conduct and oppositional disorders than boys, which may account for the up to 10:1 overrepresentation of males over females in clinical samples of children with ADHD. The preponderance of males is much less dramatic in epidemiological and adult samples, in which the ratio approximates 2:1 (6). This suggests that ADHD may be underidentified in girls. If confirmed, the underidentification and undertreatment of females with ADHD would have substantial clinical and educational implications, depriving girls of effective treatment programs aimed at improving ADHD-associated impairments.

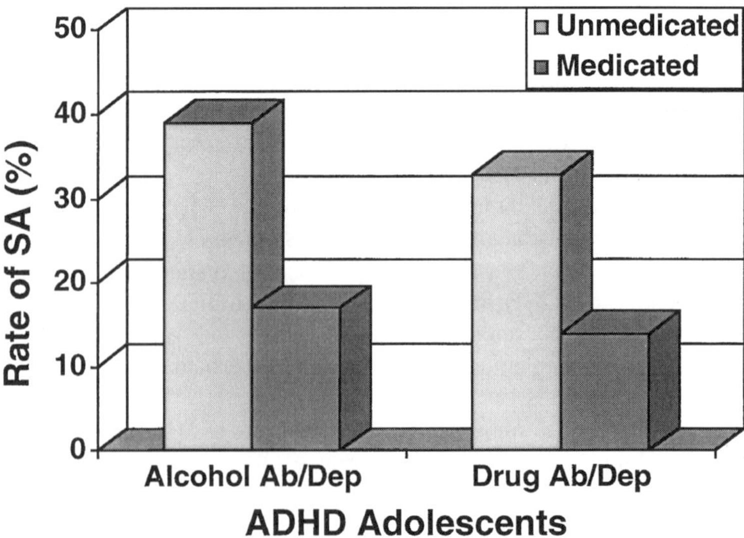

Figure 2 The effect of pharmacotherapy in ADHD children on the development of later substance abuse (SA)—alcohol or drug abuse (Ab) or dependence (Dep). These data represent studies of youth followed for five years (mean age of adolescents is 16 years). ADHD pharmacotherapy (almost ubiquitously with stimulants) was strongly associated with a reduction in the risk for substance abuse. Note that the unmedicated ($N = 198$) and medicated ($N = 118$) groups were similar in severity of ADHD and associated comorbidity at baseline.

PATHOPHYSIOLOGY AND GENETICS

Neurobiology

Although the precise neural and pathophysiological substrate of ADHD remains unknown, an emerging neuropsychological and neuroimaging literature suggests the presence of abnormalities in frontal and/or frontostriatal networks (47–49). As reviewed by Zametkin & Liotta (50), a number of brain structural and functional imaging studies have demonstrated differences between ADHD individuals and matched controls. Structural magnetic resonance imaging (MRI) studies in boys and girls with ADHD have generally shown reduced total brain, corpus callosum, caudate, and/or cerebellar volumes (47, 51, 52). Positron emission tomography (PET) research has demonstrated reduced prefrontal cortex metabolism in ADHD adults and reduced global metabolism in adolescent girls (53). No differences in brain structure related to stimulant exposure have been reported (52). Despite robust changes in behavioral ratings with stimulants, imaging studies have failed to demonstrate reversal in baseline abnormalities in ADHD (54, 55).

More recently, using single photon emission computed tomography (SPECT) scanning, adults with ADHD were found to have increased binding at the dopamine transporter protein (56, 57). In one study (56), the binding of I^{123}-altropane to the dopamine transporter in patients with ADHD did not overlap with, and was twofold higher than, that in age-matched controls, suggesting the potential utility of developing SPECT or related imaging techniques for diagnostic purposes.

Neurochemical studies continue to point to the centrality of catecholamine dysregulation in the pathophysiology of ADHD (50). Dopaminergic dysfunction, in particular, and norepinephrine, indirectly, appear to be important in the underlying pathophysiology of ADHD. Although serotonin and the inhibitory neurotransmitters glycine and GABA are apparently not central to ADHD, reports of alterations of serotonin in aggressive individuals have been reported. Pharmacological agents affecting catecholamine neurotransmission appear useful for ADHD, whereas those affecting serotonin are not (58).

Given the previously mentioned overlap of nicotine use with ADHD, there has been interest in the interface of the cholinergic and catecholaminergic-dopaminergic systems (59). Nicotine is known to improve cognition and heighten attention (59). Data from laboratory studies showed that nicotine stimulates dopaminergic neurotransmission, whereas nicotinic receptor antagonism results in diminished dopamine release (60).

Genetics of ADHD

As recently highlighted in the special issue of *Science* dedicated to the Human Genome Project, ADHD is among the most recognized genetic-based disorders in psychiatry (61). Family studies of ADHD have shown that the relatives of ADHD children are at high risk for ADHD, comorbid psychiatric disorders, school failure, learning disability, and impairments in intellectual functioning (62). Additional lines of evidence from twin, adoption, and segregation analysis studies suggest that the familial aggregation of ADHD has a substantial genetic component. Twin studies find greater similarity for ADHD and components of the syndrome between monozygotic twins than between dizygotic twins (63, 64). Their results suggest that the heritability of ADHD ranges from 0.88 to 1.0, suggesting a substantial role for genetic factors in its etiology.

Molecular genetic studies have implicated the dopamine D4 and the dopamine transporter as candidate genes (65–67). Of these candidate genes, multiple groups have independently reported on associations between ADHD and the postsynaptic D4 receptor in both children and adults with ADHD (67). The occurrence of the postsynaptic D4 polymorphism in ADHD youth is higher than would be expected by chance. In addition, ADHD youth with the polymorphism have more severe symptomatology and impairment than those without it. The D4 polymorphism is related to a deficiency in the third cytoplasmic loop of the receptor resulting in an incomplete receptor coupling to the G-protein system. It is of interest that the D4 receptor has affinity for both dopamine and norepinephrine, and its response to dopamine appears to be blunted in the affected state. Clearly, more work is necessary to disentangle the relationship of candidate genes to ADHD, as well as patients' response to pharmacological and nonpharmacological treatments.

TREATMENT

The management of ADHD includes consideration of two major areas: nonpharmacological therapy (educational remediation, individual and family psychotherapy) and pharmacotherapy.

Nonpharmacological Therapy

Support groups for ADHD are a valuable and inexpensive manner for families to learn about ADHD and resources available for their children or themselves. Support groups can be accessed through a large organization such as Children and Adults with ADD (CHADD, http://www.chadd.org) or the National Alliance for the Mentally Ill (NAMI, http://www.nami.org).

Specialized educational planning based on the child's difficulties is necessary in most cases (68). Because learning disorders co-occur in one third of ADHD youth, ADHD individuals should be screened and appropriate remediation plans developed. Parents should be encouraged to work closely with the child's school guidance counselor, who can provide direct contact with the child and serve as a valuable liaison with teachers and school administration. The school's psychologist can provide cognitive testing and assist in the development and implementation of the individualized education plan, commonly referred to as an IEP. Educational adjustments should be considered in ADHD youth with difficulties in behavioral or academic performance. Increased structure, predictable routine, learning aids, resource room time, and checked homework are among typical educational considerations in these youth. Similar modifications in the home environment should be undertaken to optimize the child's ability to complete homework. Frequent parental communication with the school about the child's progress is essential.

Focused therapies incorporating cognitive-behavioral features have been reportedly effective in children, adolescents, and adults with ADHD (68); however, the benefit of these treatments independent of pharmacotherapy has yet to be determined (69, 70). Behavioral modification for the child and parents is useful in cases of co-occurring disruptive behaviors, inflexibility, anxiety, or outbursts. More traditional insight-oriented psychotherapy should be considered in ADHD cases with evidence of self-esteem issues, adjustment problems, or depression. Social-skills remediation for improving interpersonal interactions, and coaching for improving organization and study skills, are useful adjuncts to treatment.

Pharmacotherapy

Medications remain a mainstay of treatment for children, adolescents, and adults with ADHD (Table 1). In fact, recent multisite studies suggest that medication

TABLE 1   Medications used in the treatment of ADHD

Generic class (Brand name)	Daily dose (mg/kg)	Daily dosage schedule	Typical dosing schedule**	Common adverse effects
Stimulants				
Amphetamine	0.3–1.5			Insomnia
Short-acting (Dexedrine tablets)		Twice or three times	5–30 mg BID to TID	Decreased appetite, weight loss
				Tic exacerbation
				Depression, anxiety
Intermediate-acting (Adderall, Dexedrine spansules)		Once or twice	5–30 mg BID	Rebound phenomena (short-acting preparations only)
Extended-release (Adderall-LA)		Once	10–30 mg QD	
Methylphenidate	0.5.0–2.0			
Short-acting (Ritalin, Metadate, Ritadex)		Twice to four times	5–40 mg BID to QID	Insomnia
				Decreased appetite, weight loss
Intermediate-acting (Ritalin SR, Metadate SR)		Once or twice	10–60 mg QD to BID	Tic exacerbation
				Depression, anxiety
				Rebound phenomena (short-acting preparations only)
Extended-release (Concerta, Ritalin LA,* Metadate CD)		Once	18–108 mg QD	
Magnesium Pemoline (Cylert)	1.0–3.0	Once	37.5–150 mg QD	Same as other stimulants
				Hepatitis
Antidepressants				
Tricyclics (TCAs) e.g., Imipramine, Desipramine, Nortriptyline (NT)	2.0–5.0 (1.0–3.0 for NT)	Once or twice	25–300 mg QD (25–150 mg QD for NT)	Dry mouth, constipation
				Weight change
				Vital sign and ECG changes
Bupropion (Wellbutrin, short-acting and sustained-release—SR)	1.0–6.0	Once to three times	75–100 mg TID (short) 150–200 BID (SR)	Irritability, insomnia
				Risk of seizures
				Contraindicated in bulimics
Venlafaxine (Effexor)	0.5–3	Twice	75–150 mg BID	Nausea, GI distress
				Agitation
Antihypertensives				
Clonidine (Catapress)	3–10 mcg/kg	Twice or three times	0.05–0.1 mg TID	Sedation, dry mouth, depression
				Confusion (with high dose)
				Rebound hypertension
Guanfacine (Tenex)	30–100 mcg/kg	Twice	0.5–1 mg TID	Similar to clonidine but less sedation
				Insomnia, irritability reported

* Not FDA approved at time of publication.

**Denotes typical clinical dosing of these compounds; not reflective of FDA-approved indications or dosing.

management of ADHD is the most important variable in outcome in the context of multimodal treatment (70, 71). For example, in the largest prospective and randomized long-term study of ADHD youth, those receiving stimulants alone showed similar improvement in multiple domains at 14 months follow-up compared to those receiving stimulants plus behavior modification (70). Both medicated groups had a better overall outcome than those receiving extensive behavior modification without stimulants.

Stimulants, antidepressants, and antihypertensives comprise the available agents for ADHD. Stimulants and antidepressants have been demonstrated to have similar pharmacological responsivity across the lifespan, including school-aged children, adolescents, and adult groups with ADHD.

STIMULANTS   The stimulants are considered first-line agents for children and adults with ADHD based on their extensive efficacy and safety data (72). Although there are more than 250 controlled studies of stimulants with more than 6000 children, adolescents, and adults, the vast majority of the studies are limited to latency-age, Caucasian boys treated for no longer than two months (73). The most commonly used compounds for this class include methylphenidate (Ritalin, Concerta, Metadate, and others), amphetamine (Dexedrine, Adderall), and pemoline (Cylert). Stimulants are sympathomimetic drugs that increase intrasynaptic catecholamines (mainly dopamine) by inhibiting the presynaptic reuptake mechanism and releasing presynaptic catecholamines (74). Whereas methylphenidate and pemoline are specific for blockade of the dopamine transporter protein, amphetamines, in addition to blocking the dopamine transporter protein, also release dopamine stores and cytoplasmic dopamine directly into the synaptic cleft (for review see 75). Moreover, amphetamines release serotonin and norepinephrine to a greater extent than other stimulants. Recent data suggest that acute tolerance to stimulants may develop rapidly (76).

Methylphenidate and D-amphetamine are both short-acting compounds, with an onset of action within 30 to 60 min and a peak clinical effect usually seen between 1 and 2 h after administration lasting 2 to 5 h. The amphetamine compounds (e.g., Adderall) and sustained-release preparations of methylphenidate and dextroamphetamine are intermediate-acting compounds, with an onset of action within 60 min and duration of 6 to 8 h (72, 77).

Given the need to additionally treat ADHD outside of school (e.g., social settings and homework) and to reduce the need for in-school dosage and likelihood for diversion, there has been great interest in extended-release preparations of the stimulants. Extended-release preparations greatly reduce untoward peak adverse effects of stimulants, such as headaches and moodiness, as well as essentially eliminating afternoon wearoff and rebound. Recently released preparations of methylphenidate, Concerta and Metadate CD, have an immediate onset of action with a duration of 8 to 10 h (78). Other preparations of methylphenidate (Ritalin LA as well as a pure D-isomer, Ritadex) and amphetamine (Adderall long-acting) are soon to be released with an extended-release profile of 8 to 12 h.

Although methylphenidate is by far the best-studied stimulant (72, 77), the literature suggests more similarities than differences in response to the various available stimulants. However, based on marginally different mechanisms of action, some patients who lack a satisfactory response or manifest adverse effects to one stimulant may respond favorably to another. Stimulants should be initiated at the lowest available dose once daily and increased every three to four days until a response is noted or adverse effects emerge. Typically, parameters for upward daily dosage of the stimulants are 1 mg/kg/day for the amphetamines, 2 mg/kg/day for methylphenidate, and 3 mg/kg/day for pemoline (77).

Stimulants appear to work in all age groups. Seven studies in preschoolers report improvement in structured tasks as well as mother-child interaction; however, the response is less robust with a higher side-effect burden than in other age groups (for review see 77, 79). In adolescents, response has been reported as moderate to robust, with no abuse or tolerance noted (80). There has been a great interest in the use of stimulant treatment in adults with ADHD. Fourteen studies of stimulants have demonstrated moderate reductions in ADHD symptoms with associated overall improvement in ADHD and general functioning, particularly when aggressive dosing (i.e., 20 mg TID of methylphenidate or 30 mg BID of Adderall) is employed (81).

Predictable short-term adverse effects include reduced appetite, insomnia, edginess, and gastrointestinal upset (82). In adults, elevated vital signs may emerge, necessitating baseline and on-drug monitoring. Stimulant-induced hypertension appears particularly problematic in adults with baseline borderline hypertension (i.e., $\geq 140/80$). Pemoline may rarely cause hepatitis; hence, patient education about the symptoms of early hepatic dysfunction and frequent liver function tests are advised.

There are several controversial issues related to chronic stimulant use. Although stimulants may produce anorexia and weight loss, their effect on ultimate height remains less certain. Although initial reports suggested a persistent stimulant-associated decrease in growth in height in children (83), other reports have failed to substantiate this finding (84), and still others raise the possibility that growth deficits may represent maturational delays related to ADHD itself rather than to stimulant treatment (85). Stimulants may precipitate or exacerbate tic symptoms in ADHD children. Recent work suggests that the majority of ADHD youth with tics can tolerate stimulant medications (86); however, up to one third of children with tics may have worsening of their tics with stimulant exposure (87). In those cases, alternative medications for ADHD should be considered. Current consensus suggests that stimulants can be used in youth with comorbid ADHD plus tics with careful monitoring for stimulant-induced tic exacerbation.

Despite case reports of stimulant misuse (88), there is a paucity of scientific evidence that stimulant-treated ADHD individuals abuse their medication (42); however, data suggest that diversion of stimulants to non-ADHD youth continues to be a concern. Families should closely monitor stimulant medication, and college students receiving stimulants should be advised to store their medication carefully.

Despite the findings on efficacy of the stimulants, studies have also reported consistently that typically one third of ADHD individuals do not respond to or cannot tolerate this class of agents.

ANTIDEPRESSANTS   The antidepressants are generally considered second-line drugs of choice for ADHD. The tricyclic antidepressants (TCAs)—imipramine (Tofranil), desipramine (Norpramine), and nortriptyline (Pamelor, Aventyl)—block the reuptake of neurotransmitters, including norepinephrine. TCAs are effective in controlling abnormal behaviors and improving cognitive impairments associated with ADHD, but less so than the stimulants (73). The TCAs are particularly useful in stimulant failures, or when oppositionality, anxiety, tics, or depressive symptoms co-occur within ADHD. Doses of the TCAs start with 25 mg daily and are titrated upward slowly to a maximum of 5 mg/kg/day (2 mg/kg/day for nortriptyline) (89). Although relief can be immediate, a lag of two to four weeks to maximal effect is common (73).

Unwanted side effects may emerge from activity at histaminic sites (sedation, weight gain), cholinergic sites (dry mouth, constipation), α-adrenergic sites (postural hypotension), and serotonergic sites (sexual dysfunction). In general, the secondary amines are more selective (noradrenergic) and have fewer side effects, an important consideration in sensitive juvenile populations. Four deaths of ADHD children treated with desipramine have been reported (90); however, independent evaluation of these cases has failed to support a causal link. Because minor increases in heart rate and electrocardiogram (ECG) intervals are predictable with TCAs, ECG monitoring at baseline and at therapeutic dose is suggested, but not mandatory.

Bupropion (Wellbutrin, Zyban) is an antidepressant with indirect dopamine and noradrenergic effects. Bupropion has been shown effective for ADHD in controlled trials of children (91) and adults (92) and in open trials in adults with ADHD and bipolar disorder. Given its utility in reducing cigarette smoking and improving mood, its lack of monitoring requirements, and its paucity of adverse effects, bupropion is often used as an initial agent for complex ADHD patients with substance abuse or a mood disorder. For example, a recent open report suggested the utility of bupropion in adolescents with comorbid ADHD and depression (93). Based on anecdotal reports of anti-ADHD effectiveness at low doses in a minority of patients, it is recommended that the treatment be initiated at 37.5 mg and titrated upward every three to four days up to 300 mg in younger children and 450 mg in older children or adults. Adverse events include activation, irritability, insomnia, and (rarely) seizures.

Although the serotonin reuptake inhibitors (e.g., Prozac) are not useful for ADHD, venlafaxine (Effexor), because of its noradrenergic reuptake inhibition, may have mild efficacy for ADHD (94). Monoamine oxidase inhibitors (MAOIs) have been shown effective in juvenile and adult ADHD. The response to treatment is rapid, and standard antidepressant doses are often necessary. A major limitation to the use of MAOIs is the potential for hypertensive crisis associated with dietetic transgressions with tyramine-containing foods, such as most cheeses, and interactions with prescribed, illicit, and over-the-counter drugs (pressor amines, most cold medicines, and amphetamines).

ANTIHYPERTENSIVES   The antihypertensives clonidine (Catapress) and guanfacine (Tenex) are α-adrenergic agonists that have been primarily used in the treatment of hypertension. These compounds are typically used to treat the hyperactive-impulsive symptoms of ADHD. Clonidine is a relatively short-acting compound with a plasma half-life ranging from ~6 h (in children) to 9 h (in adults) (95). Usual daily doses range from 0.05 mg to 0.4 mg. Guanfacine is longer-acting and less potent than clonidine, with usual daily doses ranging from 0.5 mg to 3 mg. The antihypertensives have been used for the treatment of ADHD as well as associated tics, aggression, and sleep disturbances, particularly in younger children.

Although sedation is more commonly seen with clonidine, both agents may cause depression and rebound hypertension. Recent reports have implicated the combination of clonidine plus methylphenidate in the deaths of four children; however, the presence of many mitigating and extenuating circumstances makes these cases uninterpretable (96). Cardiovascular monitoring (vital signs, ECG) remains optional.

TREATMENT-REFRACTORY AND COMPLEX CASES   A number of individuals either do not respond to or are intolerant of the adverse effects of medications used to treat their ADHD. Youth who are nonresponders to one stimulant should be considered for another stimulant trial. If two stimulant trials are unsuccessful, bupropion and the TCAs are reasonable second-line agents. Antihypertensives may be useful for younger children or those with prominent hyperactivity, impulsivity, and aggressiveness. MAOIs and cognitive activators such as donepezil (Aricept) may be considered for refractory youth.

Combined pharmacological approaches can be used for the treatment of co-morbid ADHD, as augmentation strategies for patients with insufficient response to a single agent, and for the management of treatment-emergent adverse effects. Examples include the use of an antidepressant plus a stimulant for ADHD and comorbid depression [fluoxetine (Prozac) plus methylphenidate] (97), bupropion plus a stimulant for ADHD individuals with moodiness, clonidine to ameliorate stimulant-induced insomnia (98), and a mood stabilizer plus an anti-ADHD agent to treat ADHD comorbid with bipolar disorder (99).

SUMMARY

ADHD is a prevalent, worldwide, heterogeneous disorder that frequently persists into adulthood. The diagnosis of ADHD is made by careful history; neuropsychological testing is helpful in confirming the diagnosis or mapping out co-occurring learning problems. The scope of co-occurring disorders has expanded to include not only conduct and oppositional defiant disorders but also mood, anxiety, and substance-use disorders as well. ADHD is increasingly being recognized in girls and in those with the inattentive subtype of the disorder. ADHD in adults entails significant impairment in occupational, academic, social, and intrapersonal domains, necessitating treatment. Converging data strongly support a neurobiological and genetic basis for ADHD, with catecholaminergic dysfunction as a central finding.

Psychosocial interventions such as educational remediation, structure/routine, and cognitive-behavioral therapy should be considered in the management of ADHD. An extensive literature supports the effectiveness of pharmacotherapy, not only for the core behavioral symptoms of ADHD but also for linked impairments including cognition, social skills, and family function. ADHD treatment may translate into reduced risk for the development of sequelae such as substance abuse. Data suggest a similar positive response of individuals with ADHD to treatment from age 6 to 60 years. The stimulant medications are the most effective agents for ADHD with ~80% of individuals responding favorably, followed by the TCAs (65%), bupropion (55%), and antihypertensives (55%). Similarities between juveniles and adults in the presentation, characteristics, neurobiology, and pharmacological responsivity of ADHD support the continuity of the disorder across the lifespan.

Visit the Annual Reviews home page at www.AnnualReviews.org

LITERATURE CITED

1. Jensen P, Kettle L, Roper M, et al. 1999. Are stimulants overprescribed? Treatment of ADHD in four U.S. communities. *J. Am. Acad. Child Adolesc. Psychiatry* 38:797–804

2. Goldman L, Genel M, Bezman R, et al. 1998. Diagnosis and treatment of attention-deficit/hyperactivity disorder in children and adolescents. *JAMA* 279:1100–7

3. Szatmari P. 1992. The epidemiology of attention-deficit hyperactivity disorders. In *Attention-Deficit Hyperactivity Disorder*, ed. G Weiss, pp. 361–71. Philadelphia: Saunders

4. Biederman J, Newcorn J, Sprich S. 1991. Comorbidity of attention deficit hyperactivity disorder with conduct, depressive, anxiety, and other disorders. *Am. J. Psychiatry* 148:564–77

5. Barkley R. 1998. *Attention-Deficit/Hyperactivity Disorder: A Handbook for Diagnosis and Treament*. New York: Guilford. 628 pp. 2nd ed.

6. Millstein RB, Wilens TE, Biederman J, et al. 1997. Presenting ADHD symptoms and subtypes in clinically referred adults with ADHD. *J. Attent. Disord.* 2:159–66

7. Brown T. 1996. *Brown Attention Deficit Disorder Scales*. San Antonio, TX: Psychol. Corp.

8. Conners C, Jett J. 1999. *Attention Deficit Hyperactivity Disorder (in Adults and Children): The Latest Assessment and Treatment Strategies*. Salt Lake City, UT: Compact Clinicals. 121 pp.

9. Seidman LJ, Biederman J, Faraone SV, et al. 1997. Toward defining a neuropsychology of ADHD: performance of children and adolescents from a large clinically referred sample. *J. Consult. Clin. Psychol.* 65:150–60

10. Morgan A, Hynd G, Riccio C, et al.

1996. Validity of DSM-IV ADHD predominantly inattentive and combined types: relationship to previous DSM diagnoses/subtype differences. *J. Am. Acad. Child Adolesc. Psychiatry* 35:325–33

11. Paternite C, Loney J, Roberts M. 1995. External validation of oppositional disorder and attention deficit disorder with hyperactivity. *J. Abnorm. Child Psychol.* 23:453–71

12. Wolraich M, Hannah J, Pinnock T, et al. 1996. Comparison of diagnostic criteria for attention-deficit hyperactivity disorder in a county-wide sample. *J. Am. Acad. Child Adolesc. Psychiatry* 35:319–24

12a. Biederman J, Faraone S, Mick E. 2000. Age dependent decline of ADHD symptoms revisited: impact of remission definition and symptom subtype. *Am. J. Psychiatry* 157:816–17

13. Gittelman R, Mannuzza S, Shenker R, et al. 1985. Hyperactive boys almost grown up. I. Psychiatric status. *Arch. Gen. Psychiatry* 42:937–47

14. Hechtman L, Weiss G. 1986. Controlled prospective fifteen year follow-up of hyperactives as adults: non-medical drug and alcohol use and anti-social behaviour. *Can. J. Psychiatry* 31:557–67

15. Loney J, Kramer J, Milich RS. 1981. The hyperactive child grows up: predictors of symptoms, delinquency and achievement at follow-up. In *Psychosocial Aspects of Drug Treatment for Hyperactivity*, ed. KD Gadow, J Loney, pp. 381–416. Boulder, CO: Westview

16. Taylor E, Sandberg S, Thorley G, et al. 1991. *The Epidemiology of Childhood Hyperactivity*. New York: Oxford Univ. Press. 158 pp.

17. Hart E, Lahey B, Loeber R, et al. 1995. Developmental change in attention-deficit hyperactivity disorder in boys: a four-year longitudinal study. *J. Abnorm. Child Psychol.* 23:729–49

18. Klein RG, Mannuzza S. 1991. Long-term outcome of hyperactive children: a review.

J. Am. Acad. Child Adolesc. Psychiatry 30:383–87

19. Thorley G. 1984. Review of follow-up and follow-back studies of childhood hyperactivity. *Psychol. Bull.* 96:116–32

20. Weiss G, Hechtman LT. 1986. *Hyperactive Children Grown Up*. New York: Guilford. 367 pp.

21. Hechtman L. 1992. Long-term outcome in attention-deficit hyperactivity disorder. *Psychiatr. Clin. North Am.* 1:553–65

22. Mannuzza S, Klein RG, Bessler A, et al. 1993. Adult outcome of hyperactive boys: educational achievement, occupational rank and psychiatric status. *Arch. Gen. Psychiatry* 50:565–76

23. Biederman J, Faraone S, Milberger S, et al. 1996. Predictors of persistence and remission of ADHD into adolescence: results from a four-year prospective follow-up study. *J. Am. Acad. Child Adolesc. Psychiatry* 35:343–51

24. Fischer M. 1997. Persistence of ADHD into adulthood: it depends on whom you ask. *ADHD Rep.* 5:8–10

25. Anderson JC, Williams S, McGee R, et al. 1987. DSM-III disorders in preadolescent children: prevalence in a large sample from the general population. *Arch. Gen. Psychiatry* 44:69–76

26. Bird HR, Gould MS, Staghezza BM. 1993. Patterns of psychiatric comorbidity in a community sample of children aged 9 through 16 years. *J. Am. Acad. Child Adolesc. Psychiatry* 32:361–68

27. Deleted in proof

28. Biederman J, Newcorn J, Sprich S. 1991. Comorbidity of attention deficit hyperactivity disorder with conduct, depressive, anxiety, and other disorders. *Am. J. Psychiatry* 148:564–77

29. Biederman J, Faraone S, Kiely K. 1996. Comorbidity in outcome of attention-deficit hyperactivity disorder. In *Do They Grow Out of It? Long Term Outcome of Childhood Disorders*, ed. L Hechtman, pp. 39–76. Washington, DC: Am. Psychiatr. Press

30. Biederman J, Faraone SV, Spencer T, et al. 1993. Patterns of psychiatric comorbidity, cognition, and psychosocial functioning in adults with attention deficit hyperactivity disorder. *Am. J. Psychiatry* 150:1792–98

31. Angold A, Costello EJ. 1993. Depressive comorbidity in children and adolescents: empirical, theoretical and methodological issues. *Am. J. Psychiatry* 150:1779–91

32. Winokur G, Coryell W, Endicott J, et al. 1993. Further distinctions between manic-depressive illness (bipolar disorder) and primary depressive disorder (unipolar depression). *Am. J. Psychiatry* 150:1176–81

33. Biederman J, Faraone SV, Mick E, et al. 1996. Attention deficit hyperactivity disorder and juvenile mania: an overlooked comorbidity? *J. Am. Acad. Child Adolesc. Psychiatry* 35:997–1008

34. Faraone SV, Biederman J, Wozniak J, et al. 1997. Is comorbidity with ADHD a marker for juvenile onset mania? *J. Am. Acad. Child Adolesc. Psychiatry* 36:1046–55

35. Milberger S, Biederman J, Faraone SV, et al. 1995. Attention deficit hyperactivity disorder and comorbid disorders: issues of overlapping symptoms. *Am. J. Psychiatry* 152:1793–800

36. Wilens TE, Biederman J, Mick E, et al. 1997. Attention deficit hyperactivity disorder (ADHD) is associated with early onset substance use disorders. *J. Nerv. Ment. Dis.* 185:475–82

37. Biederman J, Wilens T, Mick E, et al. 1998. Does attention-deficit hyperactivity disorder impact the developmental course of drug and alcohol abuse and dependence? *Biol. Psychiatry* 44:269–73

38. Milberger S, Biederman J, Faraone S, et al. 1997. ADHD is associated with early initiation of cigarette smoking in children and adolescents. *J. Am. Acad. Child Adolesc. Psychiatry* 36:37–43

39. Biederman J, Wilens T, Mick E, et al. 1995. Psychoactive substance use disorder in adults with attention deficit hyperactivity disorder: effects of ADHD and psychiatric comorbidity. *Am. J. Psychiatry* 152:1652–58

40. Wilens T, Biederman J, Mick E. 1998. Does ADHD affect the course of substance abuse? Findings from a sample of adults with and without ADHD. *Am. J. Addict.* 7:156–63

41. Drug Enforcement Administration. 1995. *Methylphenidate Review Document*, Off. Diversion Control, Drug and Chem. Eval. Sect., Washington, DC

42. Biederman J, Wilens T, Mick E, et al. 1999. Pharmacotherapy of attention-deficit/hyperactivity disorder reduces risk for substance use disorder. *Pediatrics* 104: e20

43. Gaub M, Carlson CL. 1997. Gender differences in ADHD: a meta-analysis and critical review. *J. Am. Acad. Child Adolesc. Psychiatry* 36:1036–45

44. Faraone SV, Biederman J, Mick E, et al. 2000. Family study of girls with attention deficit hyperactivity disorder. *Am. J. Psychiatry* 157:1077–83

45. Gaub M, Carlson CL. 1997. Gender differences in ADHD: a meta-analysis and critical review. *J. Am. Acad. Child Adolesc. Psychiatry* 36:1036–45

46. Pelham WE, Walker JL, Sturges J, et al. 1989. Comparative effects of methylphenidate on ADD girls and ADD boys. *J. Am. Acad. Child Adolesc. Psychiatry* 28:773–76

47. Giedd JN, Castellanos FX, Casey BJ, et al. 1994. Quantitative morphology of the corpus callosum in attention deficit hyperactivity disorder. *Am. J. Psychiatry* 151:665–69

48. Hynd GW, Hern KL, Novey ES, et al. 1993. Attention deficit-hyperactivity disorder and asymmetry of the caudate nucleus. *J. Child Neurol.* 8:339–47

49. Zametkin AJ, Nordahl TE, Gross M, et al. 1990. Cerebral glucose metabolism in adults with hyperactivity of childhood onset. *N. Engl. J. Med.* 323:1361–66

50. Zametkin A, Liotta W. 1998. The neurobiology of attention-deficit/hyperactivity disorder. *J. Clin. Psychiatry* 59:17–23

51. Hynd GW, Semrud-Clikeman M, Lorys AR, et al. 1991. Corpus callosum morphology in attention-deficit hyperactivity disorder: morphometric analysis of MRI. *J. Learn. Disabil.* 24:141–46

52. Castellanos FX, Giedd JN, Berquin P, et al. 2001. Quantitative brain magnetic resonance imaging in girls with ADHD. *Arch. Gen. Psychiatry* 58:289–95

53. Ernst M, Liebenauer L, King A, et al. 1994. Reduced brain metabolism in hyperactive girls. *J. Am. Acad. Child Adolesc. Psychiatry* 33:858–68

54. Matochik JA, Nordahl TE, Gross M, et al. 1993. Effects of acute stimulant medication on cerebral metabolism in adults with hyperactivity. *Neuropsychopharmacol.* 8:377–86

55. Matochik J, Liebenauer L, King A, et al. 1994. Cerebral glucose metabolism in adults with attention deficit hyperactivity disorder after chronic stimulant treatment. *Am. J. Psychiatry* 51:658–64

56. Dougherty D, Bonab A, Spencer T, et al. 1999. Dopamine transporter density in patients with attention deficit hyperactivity disorder. *Lancet* 354:2132–33

57. Krause K, Dresel SH, Krause J, et al. 2000. Increased striatal dopamine transporter in adult patients with attention deficit hyperactivity disorder: effects of methylphenidate as measured by single photon emission computed tomography. *Neurosci. Lett.* 285:107–10

58. Spencer T, Biederman J, Wilens T, et al. 1996. Pharmacotherapy of attention deficit disorder across the life cycle. *J. Am. Acad. Child Adolesc. Psychiatry* 35:409–32

59. Levin E. 1992. Nicotinic systems and cognitive function. *Psychopharmaology* 108:417–31

60. Westfall T, Grant H, Perry H. 1983. Release of dopamine and 5-hydroxytryptamine from rat striatal slices following activation of nicotinic cholinergic receptors. *Gen. Pharmacol.* 14:321–25

61. McGuffin P, Riley B, Plomin R. 2001. Toward behavioral genomics. *Science* 291:1232–49

62. Faraone S, Biederman J. 1994. Genetics of attention-deficit hyperactivity disorder. *Child Adolesc. Psychiatr. Clin. N. Am.* 3:285–302

63. Goodman R, Stevenson J. 1989. A twin study of hyperactivity. I. An examination of hyperactivity scores and categories derived from Rutter teacher and parent questionnaires. *J. Child Psychol. Psychiatry* 30:671–89

64. Levy F, Hay D, McStephen M, et al. 1997. Attention-deficit hyperactivity disorder: a category or a continuum? Genetic analysis of a large-scale twin study. *J. Am. Acad. Child Adolesc. Psychiatry* 36:737–44

65. Cook EH, Stein MA, Krasowski MD, et al. 1995. Association of attention deficit disorder and the dopamine transporter gene. *Am. J. Hum. Genet.* 56:993–98

66. LaHoste GJ, Swanson JM, Wigal SB, et al. 1996. Dopamine D4 receptor gene polymorphism is associated with attention deficit hyperactivity disorder. *Mol. Psychiatry* 1:121–24

67. Faraone SV, Doyle A, Mick E, Biederman J. 2001. Meta-analysis of the association between the 7-repeat allele of the dopamine D4 receptor gene and ADHD. *Am. J. Psychiatry* 158:1052–57

68. Pelham W, Wheeler T, Chronis A. 1998. Empirically supported psychosocial treatments for attention deficit hyperactivity disorder. *J. Clin. Child. Psychol.* 27:190–205

69. Abikoff H. 1991. Cognitive training in ADHD children: less to it than meets the eye. *J. Learn. Disabil.* 24:205–9

70. The MTA Cooperative Group. 1999. A 14-month randomized clinical trial of treatment strategies for attention-deficit/hyperactivity disorder. Multimodal Treatment Study of Children with ADHD. *Arch. Gen. Psychiatry* 56:1073–86

71. Abikoff H, Hechtman L. 1995. *Advanced topics in psychopharmacology: multimodal treatment.* Presented at Annu. Meet. Am. Acad. Child Adolesc. Psychiatry, 42nd, New York, Oct. 1995

72. Greenhill L, Osman B. 1999. *Ritalin: Theory and Practice.* New York: Mary Ann Liebert. 443 pp.

73. Spencer T, Biederman J, Wilens T. 1998. Pharmacotherapy of attention-deficit/ hyperactivity disorder: a life span perspective. In *Review of Psychiatry*, ed. L Dickstein, M Riba, J Oldham, pp. IV-87–IV-127. Washington, DC: Am. Psychiatr. Press

74. Elia J. 1991. Stimulants and antidepressant pharmacokinetics in hyperactive children. *Psychopharmacol. Bull.* 27:411–15

75. Wilens T, Spencer T. 1998. Pharmacology of amphetamines. In *Handbook of Substance Abuse: Neurobehavioral Pharmacology*, ed. R Tarter, R Ammerman, P Ott, pp. 501–13. New York: Plenum

76. Swanson J, Gupta S, Guinta D, et al. 1999. Acute tolerance to methylphenidate in the treatment of attention deficit hyperactivity disorder in children. *Clin. Pharmacol. Ther.* 66:295–305

77. Wilens TE, Spencer TJ. 2000. The stimulants revisited. *Child Adolesc. Psychiatr. Clin. N. Am.* 9:573–603, viii

78. Wolraich M, Swanson J, Greenhill L, et al. 2001. Controlled clinical trial of an extended release form of methylphenidate in children with ADHD. *Pediatrics* 108: In press

79. Greenhill LL. 1998. The use of psychotropic medication in preschoolers: indications, safety, and efficacy. *Can. J. Psychiatry* 43:576–81

80. Varley CK. 1983. Effects of methylphenidate in adolescents with attention deficit disorder. *J. Am. Acad. Child Psychiatry* 22:351–54

81. Spencer T, Wilens TE, Biederman J, et al. 1995. A double blind, crossover comparison of methylphenidate and placebo in adults with childhood onset attention deficit hyperactivity disorder. *Arch. Gen. Psychiatry* 52:434–43

82. Barkley RA, McMurray MB, Edelbrock CS, et al. 1990. Side effects of methylphenidate in children with attention deficit hyperactivity disorder: a systemic, placebo-controlled evaluation. *Pediatrics* 86:184–92

83. Safer D, Allen R, Barr E. 1972. Depression of growth in hyperactive children on stimulant drugs. *N. Engl. J. Med.* 287:217–20

84. Kramer JR, Loney J, Ponto LB, et al. 2000. Predictors of adult height and weight in boys treated with methylphenidate for childhood behavior problems. *J. Am. Acad. Child Adolesc. Psychiatry* 39:517–24

85. Spencer T, Biederman J, Wilens T. 1998. Growth deficits in ADHD children. *Pediatrics* 102(Suppl. 2):501–6

86. Gadow K, Sverd J, Sprafkin J, et al. 1999. Long-term methylphenidate therapy in children with comorbid attention-deficit hyperactivity disorder and chronic multiple tic disorder. *Arch. Gen. Psychiatry* 56:330–36

87. Castellanos FX, Giedd JN, Elia J, et al. 1997. Controlled stimulant treatment of ADHD and comorbid Tourette's syndrome: effects of stimulant and dose. *J. Am. Acad. Child Adolesc. Psychiatry* 36:1–8

88. Jaffe SL. 1991. Intranasal abuse of prescribed methylphenidate by an alcohol and drug abusing adolescent with ADHD. *J. Am. Acad. Child Adolesc. Psychiatry* 30:773–75

89. Prince JB, Wilens TE, Biederman J, et al. 2000. A controlled study of nortriptyline in children and adolescents with attention deficit hyperactivity disorder. *J. Child Adolesc. Psychopharmacol.* 10:193–204

90. Riddle M, Geller B, Ryan N. 1993. Another sudden death in a child treated with desipramine. *J. Am. Acad. Child Adolesc. Psychiatry* 32:792–97

91. Conners CK, Casat CD, Gualtieri CT,

et al. 1996. Bupropion hydrochloride in attention deficit disorder with hyperactivity. *J. Am. Acad. Child Adolesc. Psychiatry* 35:1314–21

92. Wilens TE, Spencer TJ, Biederman J, et al. 2001. A controlled clinical trial of bupropion for attention deficit hyperactivity disorder in adults. *Am. J. Psychiatry* 158:282–88

93. Daviss WB, Bentivoglio P, Racusin R, et al. 2001. Bupropion SR in adolescents with combined attention-deficit/hyperactivity disorder and depression. *J. Am. Acad. Child Adolesc. Psychiatry* 40:307–14

94. Reimherr FW, Hedges DW, Strong RE, et al. 1995. *An open trial of venlafaxine in adult patients with attention deficit hyperactivity disorder.* Presented at Annu. Meet. New Clin. Drug Eval. Unit Program, 35th, Orlando, FL, June 1995

95. Hunt RD, Minderaa RB, Cohen DJ. 1985. Clonidine benefits children with attention deficit disorder and hyperactivity: report of a double-blind placebo-crossover therapeutic trial. *J. Am. Acad. Child Adolesc. Psychiatry* 24:617–29

96. Wilens TE, Spencer TJ, Swanson JM, et al. 1999. Combining methylphenidate and clonidine: a clinically sound medication option. *J. Am. Acad. Child Adolesc. Psychiatry* 38:614–9; discussion 19–22

97. Gammon GD, Brown TE. 1993. Fluoxetine and methylphenidate in combination for treatment of attention deficit disorder and comorbid depressive disorder. *J. Child Adolesc. Psychopharmacol.* 3:1–10

98. Prince J, Wilens T, Biederman J, et al. 1996. Clonidine for sleep disturbances associated with attention-deficit hyperactivity disorder: a systematic chart review of 62 cases. *J. Am. Acad. Child Adolesc. Psychiatry* 35:599–605

99. Biederman J, Mick E, Prince J, et al. 1999. Systematic chart review of the pharmacologic treatment of comorbid attention deficit hyperactivity disorder in youth with bipolar disorder. *J. Child Adolesc. Psychopharmacol.* 9:247–56

Annu. Rev. Med. 2002. 53:133–47

WILL THE PIG SOLVE THE TRANSPLANTATION BACKLOG?

David K. C. Cooper, Bernd Gollackner, and David H. Sachs
*Transplantation Biology Research Center, Massachusetts General
Hospital/Harvard Medical School, Boston, Massachusetts 02129;
e-mail: David.Cooper@tbrc.mgh.harvard.edu*

Key Words   antibodies, complement, primate, rejection, xenotransplantation

■ **Abstract**   The increasing shortage of human cadaveric organs for purposes of transplantation has become the critical limiting factor in the number of transplants performed each year. Some of this deficit is being met by the use of organs or partial organs from living donors, but this source is insufficient. Xenotransplantation—the transplantation of organs between species, namely from the pig to human—could provide a solution if immunologic and other associated problems could be solved. When a pig organ is transplanted into a primate, hyperacute rejection, induced by anti-pig antibody and mediated by complement and the coagulation system, develops rapidly. This immediate problem can now be overcome, but the return or persistence of anti-pig antibody leads to a delayed form of humoral rejection, acute humoral xenograft rejection, which leads to destruction of the organ within days or weeks. We review the various approaches being investigated to overcome this barrier. Whether they will also prevent subsequent acute cellular rejection remains unknown. Brief mention is made of the potential physiologic incompatibilities between pig and human organs, as well as the microbiologic safety aspects of xenotransplantation. Finally, the question of patient and societal acceptance of xenotransplantation is discussed.

THE SHORTAGE OF HUMAN ORGANS
FOR TRANSPLANTATION

The transplantation of human organs has been one of the success stories of the latter part of the twentieth century. The percentages of patients with an organ transplant who survive for 1, 5, and 10 years are currently approximately 85%, 65%, and 50%. The very success of allotransplantation, however, has led to increasing numbers of

---

Abbreviations used in this review: AHXR, acute humoral xenograft rejection; CRP, complement-regulatory protein; DIC, disseminated intravascular coagulation; Gal, galactose α1-3galactose; HAR, hyperacute rejection; hDAF, human decay accelerating factor; HERV, human endogenous retrovirus; Nabs, natural antibodies; PERV, porcine endogenous retrovirus; XTx, xenotransplantation.

patients being referred for organ transplantation and has created a crisis in donor organ availability.

In the United States, the number of patients waiting for an organ transplant more than tripled between 1990 and 1999 (from 21,914 to 72,110) (1). During this period, however, the number of organ transplants performed, using both cadaveric and living donors, increased by just 6066 (from 15,009 to 21,175). Much of this increase was attributed to the use of marginal cadaveric donors and to an increase in the number of living donors. This trend is not without risk to the patient, since the use of marginal cadaveric donors is associated with higher patient mortality. The increase has also entailed risk for the living donors, of whom a small number, particularly those donating partial livers, have died as a consequence.

Despite intense educational efforts appealing to altruism, cadaveric organ donation has not increased substantially during the past several years. Public education media campaigns have generally been unsuccessful. In some countries, however, the introduction of presumed-consent laws has increased the cadaveric donation rate to some extent. For example, Austria and Belgium/Luxembourg have recently reported 87 and 70 transplants per million inhabitants, respectively, whereas in Germany and the Netherlands, which have no presumed-consent law, the equivalent numbers are 41 and 31 per million. However, even if presumed consent were accepted universally, the number of donor organs would remain insufficient.

Living unrelated kidney donors represent the fastest-growing donor source in the United States and provide excellent long-term results. Transplants of the liver, lung, pancreas, and small intestine can also be carried out successfully in a living-donor setting. A marked increase in the number of living donors who come forward could certainly reduce the number of patients awaiting kidney transplantation. Furthermore, an increased permanent use of left ventricular assist devices could reduce the number of patients awaiting heart transplantation.

Despite the increased number of living donors, 6100 patients died in the United States during the year 2000 because organs were not available in time. Whereas about 60 patients receive an organ transplant each day, an additional 17 patients die on the waiting list. Because of the extreme inadequacy of the number of organs available for transplantation in the western world, increasing attention is being paid to other sources of organs suitable for transplantation into humans. In particular, xenotransplantation is being intensively investigated at several centers with an aim of using the pig as an organ source.

XENOTRANSPLANTATION

Xenotransplantation (XTx) refers to the transplantation of organs across species barriers, e.g., from pig to primate. "Xeno" is the Greek work for "foreign" or "strange." As originally proposed by Calne, donor-recipient combinations in which the recipient rejects an organ from a different species in a rapid (or "hyperacute") manner are termed discordant, whereas combinations in which organs are rejected with a tempo similar to that of allotransplants are called concordant. This difference is related to the levels of preformed antibodies in the recipient against the donor species, which are much higher in discordant species.

HISTORICAL ATTEMPTS AT XENOTRANSPLANTATION IN HUMANS

Clinical attempts at XTx go back to the early seventeenth century, when blood transfusions from animals to humans were carried out in England and France. In the nineteenth century, tissues, particularly skin, were transplanted from a variety of animals into humans. Throughout the twentieth century, attempts were made to transplant animal organs into humans (Table 1) (2, 3), but succeeded on only one or two occasions.

The most notable attempts were by Reemtsma and colleagues (4), who transplanted a series of chimpanzee kidneys into humans at a time when dialysis was not commonly available and human organ donors were scarce. Survival of their patients ranged from 11 days to two months, except for one patient who survived for almost nine months and died of what was believed to be an electrolyte disturbance, demonstrating no sign of rejection of the chimpanzee kidneys. This was particularly remarkable in that the patient was treated with primitive immunosuppressive therapy, consisting only of azathioprine and steroids. During this study, Reemtsma et al. demonstrated that acute cellular rejection of a chimpanzee kidney could be reversed by a course of increased steroid therapy.

The first heart transplant performed in a human (by Hardy in Mississippi in 1964) involved a chimpanzee donor, but the heart proved too small to support the circulation. Starzl and colleagues performed several kidney and liver transplants from nonhuman primates to humans between the 1960s and 1990s. The most notable attempts used baboons as donors in two orthotopic liver transplants, where patient survival was 70 and 26 days, respectively. Nonprimate mammals have been used as the source of organs on rare occasions, without success, organ survival sometimes being measured in hours rather than days (Table 1).

TABLE 1   World experience with clinical organ xenotransplantation

Donor	(*n*)	Survival
Kidney primate	30	1 day–9 months
nonprimate	3	3–9 days
Heart primate	5	<1–20 days
nonprimate	4	<1 day
Liver primate	11	<1–70 days
nonprimate	1	<2 days

Apart from whole-organ XTx, there have been notable attempts at the XTx of porcine pancreatic islet cells in diabetic patients and porcine neural cells in patients with conditions such as Parkinson's and Huntington's diseases. Pig livers have also been used for ex vivo liver hemoperfusion for temporary support of patients with fulminant hepatic failure. Extracorporeal liver assist devices, containing pig hepatocytes, have also been used for this purpose.

WHY THE PIG?

Although, from an immunologic perspective, nonhuman primates would be preferable sources of organs for humans, virtually all of these species are either endangered or are too small to provide organs suitable for transplantation into large adult humans. Furthermore, concerns have been raised about the transmission of infectious agents from nonhuman primates to humans, particularly since most nonhuman primates are either wild-caught or have been housed under colony conditions for relatively few generations. The time and expense of breeding these animals in captivity are also prohibitive, as is a lack of experience in genetically modifying them.

Most investigators now expect the pig to be the species most likely to be the source of organs for XTx (Table 2), and research efforts have been directed in recent years toward pig-to-primate transplantation (5, 6). In our own laboratories, we have focused on the use of partially inbred miniature swine. These animals, produced by a selective breeding program over the past 25 years, have a variety of advantages as a potential source of xenograft organs (7). Furthermore, there is considerable experience with techniques of transgenesis in pigs that allow insertion of new genes (8). Although it has not yet been possible to "knock out" a gene in pigs, the recent demonstration of the feasibility of nuclear transfer in swine should make it possible to knock out endogenous genes and thus modify the pig to make it more appropriate as an organ source. This would almost certainly represent an important advance and would obviate the need for some of the investigative approaches described in this brief review.

When considering whether the pig will solve the transplantation backlog, four major topics require consideration: (*a*) the immunologic barriers to discordant XTx, (*b*) the potential for physiologic incompatibilities between the two species, (*c*) the potential microbiologic safety hazards that might ensue, and (*d*) the attitude of potential patients and of society at large toward this radical therapeutic step forward.

IMMUNOLOGIC BARRIERS

Innate humoral responses involve preexisting or so-called natural antibodies (NAbs), which exist in the absence of any known exposure to antigen, whereas acquired humoral responses result from exposure to antigen (e.g., following organ

TABLE 2 Characteristics of pigs as sources of organs for transplantation into humans

Property	Domestic swine	Inbred miniature swine
Availability	Unlimited	Unlimited
Reproductive potential	Outstanding	Good
Time to reproductive maturity	4–8 months	4–8 months
Gestation	114 days	114 days
Offspring per litter	5–12	4–8
Growth	Rapid (>300 lb. at one year)	Moderate (130 lb. at one year)
Adult size	>1000 lb.	200–300 lb.
Similarity to humans	Good	Excellent
Anatomy	Close except size	Close
Physiology	Close	Close
Immunologic compatibility	Discordant	Discordant
Genetic characterization	Outbred	Inbred
MHC	Heterozygous, polymorphic	Homozygous, 3 alleles and 5 recombinant alleles available
Blood types	A and O	O
Infectious risk	Low	Low
Known pathogens	Can be bred specific-pathogen-free	Can be bred specific-pathogen-free
PERVs	Transmission to human cells detected only in vitro	No transmission to human cells detected in vitro from one inbred line
Cost	Low	Low
Public opinion about use	Favorable	Favorable

transplantation). In allotransplantation, only the acquired immune mechanisms need be overcome (except with regard to ABO incompatibility between recipient and donor), whereas in discordant XTx both the innate and acquired responses need to be suppressed or avoided. The innate xenograft response is proving more difficult to control than the acquired allograft response.

As a probable result of microbiologic colonization of the gastrointestinal tract, which begins during the first few weeks of life, humans develop NAbs against galactoseα1-3galactose (Gal) epitopes that are present on various bacteria, viruses, and parasites (9). These anti-Gal NAbs cross-react with Gal epitopes on the surface of certain pig cells, which include all of the vascular endothelium of pigs (10). The Gal epitope shows many structural similarities to the human B blood group epitope and can loosely be considered the pig blood group antigen. The binding of NAbs to the Gal epitope initiates complement activation, leading to rapid destruction of the transplanted organ or cells.

Although this mechanism was clearly demonstrated in the mid-1960s by Perper & Najarian (11) and others, it was not until the 1990s that the major target for anti-pig NAbs, namely the Gal epitope, was identified by Good and colleagues (12, 13).

Hyperacute Rejection

Rapid graft destruction, known as hyperacute rejection (HAR), is characterized histologically by vascular thrombi and congestion, disruption of the vascular endothelium, interstitial hemorrhage, and edema within the graft (14). The leakage of blood and fluid through the capillary walls is followed by necrosis of the endothelial cells. Immunohistologic examination reveals deposition of IgM, IgG, IgA, and complement on the graft endothelium.

Evidence that this process is initiated by xenoreactive NAbs comes from the fact that depletion of NAbs from the primate recipient prolongs pig graft survival even when the complement system remains intact (15, 16). Furthermore, XTx of a porcine organ into a newborn baboon that lacks xenoreactive NAbs but has an intact complement system does not result in rapid graft destruction (17). There is evidence that some human sera (though not baboon sera) may contain NAbs toward other, as yet undetermined, oligosaccharide epitopes on pig tissues (18). These NAbs appear to be less cytotoxic than anti-Gal NAbs but, nevertheless, may need to be removed when clinical XTx is initiated.

The important role of complement in HAR is supported by the detection of complement components in the grafted tissues and the fact that complement depletion with cobra venom factor or soluble complement receptor I, or the use of rodent recipients with genetic complement deficiencies, result in prolonged survival of xenografts.

In the experimental pig-to-nonhuman primate (baboon or cynomolgus monkey) model, HAR can now be routinely prevented by therapeutic measures (19). These include the extracorporeal immunoadsorption of anti-Gal NAbs from the recipient circulation, complement depletion or inhibition, and the use of organs from pigs transgenic for human complement regulatory proteins, such as human decay accelerating factor (hDAF). When these procedures or approaches are combined with intensive pharmacologic immunosuppressive therapy, a transplanted pig kidney or heart may continue functioning for several weeks.

Acute Humoral Xenograft Rejection

When HAR is prevented, although rejection is delayed, other mechanisms (still not fully understood) eventually destroy the graft, a process known as acute humoral xenograft rejection (AHXR) (20). Despite most pharmacologic immunosuppressive regimens, an induced antibody response appears, initially as IgM before converting to IgG, and includes induction not only of greater amounts (>100-fold) of anti-Gal antibody but also of new antibody against non-Gal porcine targets.

Although a pathogenic role for antibodies in AHXR is likely, possibly through antibody-dependent cell-mediated cytotoxicity (ADCC) or other mechanisms, there is controversy as to the extent of complement's involvement.

Antibodies, alone or in association with certain complement fractions, may be able to induce changes in the endothelial cells that are typical of those in an activation state, contributing to the development of AXHR. Activation of cytokine genes, expression of adhesion molecules, and changes from an anticoagulant to a procoagulant phenotype on the endothelial cell surface may all play a role. Binding of antibody to epitopes on the vascular endothelium may direct various killer cells, with Fc receptors for IgG, to exert their cytolytic potential on the cells. There are as yet no clinical laboratory data that are diagnostic of the development of AHXR, although it can be associated with an increasing thrombocytopenia due to consumption of platelets in the graft, and/or disturbance of coagulation parameters, in particular a fall in fibrinogen to below detectable levels (21).

The main histopathologic features of AHXR are endothelial swelling or disruption, vascular thrombosis with blood extravasation, interstitial edema, and features of tissue injury (22, 23). Deposition of immunoglobulins (IgM and IgG) and complement along the vascular endothelium, although generally present, may be minimal. In some cases, cellular infiltration [e.g., neutrophils, macrophages, T cells, and/or natural killer (NK) cells] can be seen, but this too is variable. Whether the cellular infiltration is entirely due to AHXR or also involves cellular responses (as seen in allotransplantation) remains unclear.

To date, no therapeutic regimen has been successful in preventing AHXR unless the therapy is so intensive that it leads to recipient mortality from complications such as infection. There is increasing evidence, however, that costimulatory blockade with an anti-CD154 monoclonal antibody, possibly in combination with pharmacologic agents, inhibits the induced antibody response in many cases, although it does not suppress the baseline production of anti-Gal NAbs (24, 25). The presence of NAbs alone, particularly IgM, appears to be sufficient to induce a procoagulant state even when the histopathologic features of AHXR are minimal, leading to the development of disseminated intravascular coagulation (DIC) (21, 26). This complication appears to be associated with XTx of a pig kidney but is either absent or much less marked following XTx of a pig heart (C. Knosalla, manuscript in progress). Emergency excision of the transplanted pig kidney may rapidly reverse DIC, strongly suggesting that the initiating factor is within the graft.

Preventing Antibody-Mediated Xenograft Rejection

In the absence of a pig that does not express Gal antigens, attention has been directed toward modification of the recipient's immune response. Extracorporeal immunoadsorption of primate plasma through an immunoaffinity column of a synthetic Gal oligosaccharide is successful in depleting anti-Gal antibodies (16, 27–30) but cannot be repeated indefinitely. An alternative or additional approach is the continuous infusion of soluble synthetic Gal sugars into the blood, which are bound by anti-Gal antibodies, thus protecting a transplanted pig organ from the effect of these antibodies (27). Recent work in our own laboratory with the continuous intravenous infusion of bovine serum albumin conjugated to multiple Gal molecules has resulted in a virtual absence of anti-Gal antibody for periods of over one month (31). However, a similar approach by other groups, using the continuous intravenous infusion of a polymeric form of Gal trisaccharide (GAS 914), has not greatly prolonged pig xenograft survival.

Much work has concentrated on suppression of B cell activity in order to suppress antibody production. Alwayn et al. (32) demonstrated that, even in the absence of measurable B cells in blood, bone marrow, and lymph nodes [as a result of a combination of anti-CD20 monoclonal antibody (mAb) therapy and whole-body irradiation], anti-Gal NAbs were still produced and remained at almost normal levels. This strongly suggested that the differentiated plasma cell, which is not susceptible to anti-CD20 mAb therapy nor to irradiation, is the probable source of anti-Gal NAbs. Our current attention is therefore directed toward means of depleting plasma cells or inhibiting their function.

The genetic modification of pigs to introduce a human gene for one or more complement-regulatory proteins (CRPs) has proved an advance in preventing HAR of a transplanted pig organ. Many studies, particularly by White and colleagues in the United Kingdom, have demonstrated that the presence of hDAF is generally efficient in preventing HAR, though not in every case (reviewed in 19). Other studies, however, suggest that the species specificity of the CRP may not be as important as overexpression of the CRP (33). Therefore, an abundance of pig CRP may be as protective as the expression of a human CRP.

Cellular Xenograft Rejection

Innate cellular responses include those mediated by NK cells, macrophages, certain T cell subsets, and neutrophils. Acquired cellular responses are those mediated by T cells. There has been little investigation of the mechanism of the cellular response in the pig-to-primate model, but in vitro evidence indicates that the T cell response is likely to be as strong as, if not stronger than, the response to an allograft (34), and that adhesive and costimulatory interactions between humans and pigs are effective.

Chronic Xenograft Rejection

Chronic rejection, such as graft atherosclerosis, is poorly understood even in allotransplantation, and we know virtually nothing about it in XTx. It appears, however, that chronic rejection is likely following pig organ transplantation in a primate—possibly in an accelerated form—unless every immune mechanism has been overcome. This would probably only be possible by the induction of immunologic tolerance. Certainly, with long-term pharmacologic immunosuppressive therapy, the incidence of chronic rejection increases as the years go by, and this is likely to be the case following XTx.

Induction of Immunologic Tolerance

In allotransplantation, it is now possible to induce a state of T cell tolerance in the recipient by various immune manipulations (35). At our center, Cosimi and associates induce tolerance to an allotransplanted kidney in monkeys by inducing a state of mixed hematopoietic chimerism at the time of the transplant (36). Even the relatively transient (a few weeks) engraftment of donor-specific bone marrow or mobilized peripheral blood hematopoietic progenitor cells can induce a state of tolerance in which the transplanted organ is not rejected after discontinuation of pharmacologic immunosuppressive therapy. Two patients at the Massachusetts General Hospital have undergone major histocompatibility complex (MHC)-matched bone marrow and donor-specific renal allotransplantation using this approach, and they remain well on no immunosuppressive therapy several months to years later.

We have attempted to induce this state in the pig-to-baboon organ transplantation model, to date without long-term success (20). In this model, it is necessary to achieve not only T cell tolerance, i.e., tolerance at a cellular level, but also B cell tolerance, i.e., the permanent suppression of antibody production directed to pig antigens. The presence of NAbs, which are T cell–independent, is a major factor that has prevented us from achieving this state, but there appear to be other factors involved, since pig cell chimerism has proved difficult to achieve even in species whose serum contains no anti-Gal antibodies. If production of NAbs could be suppressed by, for example, temporary depletion of plasma cells, then the transplantation of Gal-expressing pig cells and organs might lead to the deletion of maturing Gal-reactive B cells.

Other approaches include what has been termed molecular chimerism, whereby the gene for the enzyme that produces Gal (α1,3 galactosyltransferase) is transduced into baboon bone marrow cells and these autologous cells are infused back into the baboon after lethal irradiation. Engraftment of Gal-positive bone marrow cells should theoretically lead to deletion of those B cells that make anti-Gal antibody. Although this approach has been successful in Gal-knockout mice (37), it has not been successful in the pig-to-baboon model, largely because of difficulty in adequately transducing sufficient numbers of baboon bone marrow cells.

Another approach to the induction of T cell tolerance involves the transplantation of pig thymic tissue into the recipient primate. At present, we believe it is important that the thymic tissue should be vascularized at the time of XTx. This can be achieved by injecting autologous thymic tissue under the renal capsule of the donor pig. After some weeks, when renal vessels have vascularized the thymic tissue, the "thymokidney" is transplanted into the baboon host. Reeducation of the recipient's developing T cells in the pig thymus should lead to deletion of T cells reactive with pig tissues. This approach has proved successful in a pig-to-mouse xenograft model (38) and in a fully allogeneic pig model (39), but it has been only partially successful in the pig-to-baboon model, largely because of the destructive effects of anti-Gal NAbs. However, long-term porcine thymic engraftment has been achieved in Gal-knockout mice that have low levels of anti-Gal antibody, and, in the pig-to-primate model, evidence of donor-specific T cell unresponsiveness has been documented in two cases (R. Barth, manuscript in preparation).

PHYSIOLOGIC COMPATIBILITY

If the immunologic problems can be overcome and long-term function of a pig organ in a primate is obtainable, detailed studies of the function of pig organs will become possible. The crucial questions are whether the pig organ will be physiologically compatible in the human environment in the long term and whether it will fulfill the requirements of a human organ. Anatomic and physiologic differences between pig and human may result in inadequate function (40). As one small example, the pig body temperature is normally approximately 103°F and the metabolism of pig cells may be less than optimal at the human body temperature of 98.6°F. Nonetheless, despite these differences, pig kidneys have successfully supported the lives of monkeys for more than two months, and a pig orthotopic heart transplant has functioned satisfactorily for well over one month. There is therefore optimism that these organs will function adequately in humans for prolonged periods.

As pig insulin has been used in humans for many years in the treatment of diabetes, it is likely that pig pancreatic islet cells will produce insulin that functions adequately. Similarly, dopamine-producing pig cells implanted into human brains are likely to produce dopamine that will function satisfactorily. The liver, however, produces over 2000 proteins, and it is likely that many of these will be different when produced by a porcine liver than by a human liver. It is therefore likely that some of them will not function satisfactorily in the human environment. It is already known that there are significant differences in coagulation factors between the species (26). Whether, for example, human growth hormone will function adequately on a transplanted pig organ in an infant or child remains unknown.

It has been suggested that a whole new field of science will evolve, "xenoincompatibility," in which these various discrepancies will be identified and investigated. Some of these inadequacies, however, may well be resolved by transgenic manipulation of the pig, for example, by introducing a human gene to synthesize a human protein in the pig liver.

MICROBIOLOGIC SAFETY

With human cadaveric organ transplantation, an infectious agent, such as a cytomegalovirus or Epstein-Barr virus, is often knowingly transplanted with the organ. With the XTx of a pig organ, it may be possible to avoid transfer of any significant microorganisms. Using gnotobiotic techniques of delivery of piglets, early weaning from the sow, and excellent housing and handling techniques, it is possible for pigs to be bred and maintained without significant microorganisms that might be a problem after transplantation (41). The pig organ, therefore, should be a safer organ to transplant than a human organ. Nevertheless, there will always remain the risk of the transfer of a hitherto unknown microbiologic agent, although many of the techniques used to breed and maintain pigs free of known infectious agents should also keep them free of unidentified agents.

Concern has been raised, however, with regard to the transfer of porcine endogenous retroviruses (PERVs) (42–44). These retroviruses, which make up approximately 1% of the genome of every pig cell, are similar to human endogenous retroviruses (HERVs), which are present in all human cells. Although there is no evidence that PERVs or HERVs cause significant health problems in the pig or the human, respectively, concern has been raised that the transfer of a PERV (which will inevitably be transplanted with the pig organ) may cause health problems in the human recipient. Potentially, a PERV may mutate or PERV elements may combine with HERV elements to form a new virus that may be pathogenic to humans and/or pigs. The only data available from a study of human patients who have been transiently exposed to various pig cells under varying states of immunosuppression, however, have indicated no definitive evidence of PERV infection (45).

Although a PERV or a recombinant virus might cause problems in the recipient, the development of a disease process may take many years. This risk may be fully acceptable to the recipient, who would have died had a pig organ not been available for XTx. However, if there is a risk that the recipient could transfer the pathogenic virus to other members of the community, e.g., family, friends, and hospital staff, then this risk would have to be weighed against the benefit of XTx to the individual patient.

One recent observation suggesting that this scenario can be prevented is that the PERVs found in one strain of pig developed at our center appear unable to infect human cells when cultured with human cells in vitro (C. Patience, unpublished). The reason for this lack of infectivity remains uncertain, but if it is supported by further studies, this strain of pig may resolve this potential problem. Organs transplanted from pigs of this strain may not carry a risk of transfer of PERVs to the human recipient or to third parties.

Most of the efforts at regulating clinical XTx by government agencies, e.g., the U.S. Food and Drug Administration, are being directed toward its microbiologic safety.

PATIENT AND SOCIETAL ACCEPTANCE OF XENOTRANSPLANTATION

If the immunobiologic, physiologic, and microbiologic problems (or potential problems) can be resolved, then it is likely that both patients and society at large will accept XTx. In 1966, Sir Peter Medawar stated, "The transplantation of organs will be assimilated into ordinary clinical practice . . . for the single and sufficient

reason that people are so constituted that they would rather be alive than dead."
For the same reason, XTx is likely to be acceptable to the patient with end-stage
organ failure, and, if there is no inordinate perceived risk to public health, to the
majority of the public.

As 100 million pigs are killed in the United States each year for food, it seems
unlikely that there will be widespread ethical reservations about using them as a
source of life-saving organs. As stated bluntly by Robert Lanza, a scientist working
in this field, "If it is acceptable to kill pigs to make sausages, surely it is acceptable
to kill them to save lives." However, some will argue that a pig containing one or
more human genes, e.g., the gene for hDAF, is entitled to some human legal rights
(46).

The ready availability of pig organs could greatly change the way organs are
distributed to potential transplant recipients. The need for elaborate systems to
ensure fairness and efficient distribution, such as the United Network for Organ
Sharing in the United States, may disappear. Pig organs would almost certainly
be obtained on a commercial basis, as are surgical devices such as left ventricular
assist devices, drugs, and hospital equipment, involving private companies in the
process.

COMMENT

Significant barriers to successful clinical XTx remain. With the current rapid pace
of development in biologic sciences and biotechnology, however, the immunologic
hurdles are likely to be overcome in the near future. This will provide the opportunity to investigate potential physiologic incompatibilities, although currently
these are not considered significant enough to prevent XTx of kidneys or hearts.
The microbiologic safety concerns may be largely resolved by the demonstration
of an absence of trans-species infections in well-controlled studies and/or by the
identification of a strain of pigs incapable of transferring PERV into human cells.
Public acceptance of XTx is likely if it can be demonstrated to be both life-saving
and sufficiently safe. The development of successful techniques for clinical XTx
would prove a major advance in the management of patients with end-stage organ
failure and various cellular deficiencies, overcoming what has become the main
limitation to progress in the field of transplantation today.

ACKNOWLEDGMENTS

We thank our many colleagues at the Transplantation Biology Research Center and
at Immerge BioTherapeutics who have contributed to some of the work reviewed
in this paper, and Y.-G. Yang and R. Barth for reviewing the manuscript. Work
in our laboratory is supporterd by NIH Program Project 1PO1AI45897 and by
a Sponsored Research Agreement between Massachusetts General Hospital and
Immerge BioTherapeutics.

Visit the Annual Reviews home page at www.AnnualReviews.org

LITERATURE CITED

1. United Network for Organ Sharing. 2000. Annual Report. Richmond, Virginia
2. Taniguchi S, Cooper DKC. 1997. Clinical xenotransplantation—past, present and future. *Ann. R. Coll. Surg. Engl.* 79:13–19
3. Cooper DKC, Lanza RP. 2000. *Xeno—The Promise of Transplanting Animal Organs into Humans.* New York: Oxford Univ. Press. 274 pp.
4. Reemtsma K, McCracken BH, Schlegel JU, et al. 1964. Renal heterotransplantation in man. *Ann. Surg.* 160:384–410
5. Cooper DKC, Ye Y, Rolf LL Jr., Zuhdi N. 1991. The pig as potential organ donor for man. In *Xenotransplantation*, ed. DKC Cooper, E Kemp, K Reemtsma, DJG White DJG, pp. 481–500. Heidelberg: Springer
6. Sachs DH. 1994. The pig as a potential xenograft donor. *Vet. Immunol. Immunopathol.* 43:185–91
7. Sachs DH. 1992. MHC homozygous miniature swine. In *Swine as Models in Biomedical Research*, ed. MM Swindle, DC Moody, LD Phillips, pp. 3–15. Ames: Iowa State Univ. Press
8. Cozzi E, White DJG. 1995. The generation of transgenic pigs as potential organ donors for humans. *Nat. Med.* 1:964–66
9. Galili U, Mandrell RE, Hamadeh RM, et al. 1998. The interaction between the human natural anti-α-galactosyl IgG (anti-Gal) and bacteria of the human flora. *Infect. Immun.* 57:1730–37
10. Oriol R, Ye Y, Koren E, Cooper DKC. 1993. Carbohydrate antigens of pig tissues reacting with human natural antibodies as potential targets for hyperacute vascular rejection in pig-to-man organ xenotransplantation. *Transplantation* 56:1433–42
11. Perper RJ, Najarian JS. 1966. Experimental renal transplantation. 1. In widely divergent species. *Transplantation* 4:377–88
12. Good AH, Cooper DKC, Malcolm AJ, et al. 1992. Identification of carbohydrate structures which bind human anti-porcine antibodies: implications for discordant xenografting in man. *Transplant. Proc.* 24:559–62
13. Cooper DKC, Koren E, Oriol R. 1994. Oligosaccharides and discordant xenotransplantation. *Immunol. Rev.* 141:31–58
14. Rose AG, Cooper DKC. 2000. Venular thrombosis is the key event in the pathogenesis of antibody-mediated cardiac rejection. *Xenotransplantation* 7:31–41
15. Cooper DKC, Human PA, Lexer G, et al. 1998. Effects of cyclosporine and antibody adsorption on pig cardiac xenograft survival in the baboon. *J. Heart Transplant.* 7:238–46
16. Sablinski T, Latinne D, Gianello P, et al. 1995. Xenotransplantation of pig kidneys to nonhuman primates: development of the model. *Xenotransplantation* 2:264–70
17. Minanov OP, Itescu S, Neethling FA, et al. 1997. Anti-Gal IgG antibodies in sera of newborn humans and baboons and its significance in pig xenotransplantation. *Transplantation* 63:182–86
18. Zhu A. 2000. Binding of natural antibodies to non alpha Gal xeno-antigens on porcine erythrocytes. *Transplantation* 69:2422–28
19. Lambrigts D, Sachs DH, Cooper DKC. 1998. Discordant organ xenotransplantation in primates—world experience and current status. *Transplantation* 66:547–61
20. Sachs DH, Sykes M, Robson SC, Cooper DKC. 2001. Xenotransplantation. *Adv. Immunol.* In press
21. Buhler L, Basker M, Alwayn IPJ, et al. 2000. Coagulation and thrombotic disorders associated with pig organ and hematopoietic cell transplantation in nonhuman primates. *Transplantation* 70:1323–31
22. Shimizu A, Meehan SM, Kozlowski T,

et al. 2000. Acute humoral xenograft rejection: destruction of the microvascular capillary endothelium in pig-to-nonhuman primate renal grafts. *Lab Invest.* 80:815–30

23. Pino-Chavez G. 2001. Differentiating acute humoral from acute cellular rejection histopathologically. *Graft* 4:60–62

24. Buhler L, Awwad M, Basker M, et al. 2000. High-dose porcine hematopoietic cell transplantation combined with CD40 ligand blockade in baboons prevents an induced anti-pig humoral response. *Transplantation* 69:2296–304

25. Alwayn IPJ, Basker M, Buhler L, Cooper DKC. 1999. The problem of anti-pig antibodies in pig-to-primate xenografting: current and novel methods of depletion and/or suppression of production of anti-pig antibodies. *Xenotransplantation* 6:157–68

26. Robson SC, Cooper DKC, d'Apice AJF. 2000. Disordered regulation of coagulation and platelet activation in xenotransplantation. *Xenotransplantation* 7:166–76

27. Ye Y, Neethling FA, Niekrasz M, et al. 1994. Evidence that intravenously administered α-galactosyl carbohydrates reduce baboon serum cytotoxicity to pig kidney cells (PK15) and transplanted pig hearts. *Transplantation* 58:330–37

28. Taniguchi S, Neethling FA, Korchagina EY, et al. 1996. *In vivo* immunoadsorption of anti-pig antibodies in baboons using a specific Galα1-3Gal column. *Transplantation* 62:1379–84

29. Kozlowski T, Ierino FL, Lambrigts D, et al. 1998. Depletion of anti-Galα1-3Gal antibody in baboons by specific alpha-Gal immunoaffinity columns. *Xenotransplantation* 5:122–31

30. Xu Y, Lorf T, Sablinski T, et al. 1998. Removal of anti-porcine natural antibodies from human and nonhuman primate plasma *in vitro* and *in vivo* by a Galα1-3Galβ1-4βGlc-X immunoaffinity column. *Transplantation* 65:172–79

31. Teranishi K, Gollackner B, Buhler L, et al. 2001. Depletion of anti-Gal antibodies in baboons by intravenous therapy with bovine serum albumin conjugated to Gal oligosaccharides. *Transplantation* In press

32. Alwayn IPJ, Xu Y, Basker M, et al. 2001. Effects of specific anti–B and/or anti–plasma cell immunotherapy on antibody production in baboons: depletion of CD20/CD22-positive B cells does not result in significant decreased production of anti-αGal antibody. *Xenotransplantation* 8:157–71

33. van den Berg CW, Morgan BP. 2001. Understanding the immune protection afforded by endogenous complement regulatory molecules. *Graft* 4:63–65

34. Yamada K, Auchincloss H. 1999. Cell-mediated xenograft rejection. *Curr. Opin. Organ Transplant.* 4:90–94

35. Sachs DH. 2000. Mixed chimerism as an approach to transplantation tolerance. *Clin. Immunol.* 95:S63–S68

36. Kawai T, Cosimi AB, Colvin RB, et al. 1995. Mixed allogeneic chimerism and renal allograft tolerance in cynomolgus monkeys. *Transplantation* 59:256–62

37. Bracy JL, Sachs DH, Iacomini J. 1998. Inhibition of xenoreactive natural antibody production by retroviral gene therapy. *Science* 281:1845–47

38. Zhao Y, Swenson K, Sergio JJ, et al. 1996. Skin graft tolerance across a discordant xenogeneic barrier. *Nat. Med.* 2:1211–16

39. Yamada K, Shimizu A, Utsugi R, et al. 2000. Thymic transplantation in miniature swine. II. Induction of tolerance by transplantation of composite thymokidneys to thymectomized recipients. *J. Immunol.* 164:3079–86

40. Hammer C. 1997. Evolution: its complexity and impact on xenotransplantation. In *Xenotransplantation*, ed. DKC Cooper, E Kemp, JL Platt, DJG White, pp. 716–35. Heidelberg: Springer. 2nd ed.

41. Onions D, Cooper DKC, Alexander TJL, et al. 2000. An assessment of the risk of xenozoonotic disease in pig-to-human xenotransplantation. *Xenotransplantation* 7:143–55

42. Smith DM. 1993. Endogenous retroviruses in xenografts. *N. Engl. J. Med.* 328:142–43

43. Patience C, Takeuchi Y, Weiss RA. 1997. Infection of human cells by an endogenous retrovirus of pigs. *Nat. Med.* 3:282–86

44. Stoye JP, Coffin JM. 1995. The dangers of xenotransplantation. *Nat. Med.* 1:1100

45. Paradis K, Langford G, Long Z, et al. 1999. Search for cross-species transmission of porcine endogenous retrovirus in patients with living pig tissue. *Science* 285:1236–41

46. Chae S, Cooper DKC. 1997. Legal implications of xenotransplantation. *Xenotransplantation* 4:132–39

Annu. Rev. Med. 2002. 53:149–72

IMMUNOLOGIC CONTROL OF HIV-1

Rajesh T. Gandhi and Bruce D. Walker
*Partners AIDS Research Center and Infectious Diseases Division, Massachusetts General
Hospital and Division of AIDS, Harvard Medical School, Boston, Massachusetts 02114;
e-mail: rgandhi@partners.org; bwalker@helix.mgh.harvard.edu*

Key Words human immunodeficiency virus-1 (HIV-1), acquired
  immunodeficiency syndrome (AIDS), immunology, virology, immunotherapy

■ **Abstract** By destroying CD4+ T cells, human immunodeficiency virus-1
(HIV-1) infection results in immunodeficiency and the inability of the immune system
to contain the virus in most individuals. Although treatment of HIV-1 infection with
potent antiretroviral medications has resulted in enormous clinical benefit, there is a
growing recognition of the limitations of this therapy. As a result, novel approaches
to treating HIV-1 infection are being considered. One such strategy is immunotherapy, which seeks to boost immune responses against HIV-1 and control the virus.
This approach is based on studies of other viruses in which a coordinated immune response contains the chronic infection. Recent studies show that CD4+ helper responses,
CD8+ T cell activity, and antibodies may contribute to control of the virus without
antiretroviral therapy in some HIV-positive individuals. Based on this understanding
of the immunologic correlates of control of HIV-1, exciting new immunotherapeutic
strategies for HIV-1 infection are being designed and tested.

INTRODUCTION

Human immunodeficiency virus-1 (HIV-1) infects CD4+ T lymphocytes, resulting in depletion of these cells and progressive immunodeficiency. Combination
antiretroviral therapy (ART) can block replication of HIV-1 and is associated with
an improvement in the ability to resist opportunistic infections. However, because
HIV-1 can establish a latent infection in long-lived memory CD4+ T cells, current
ART cannot eradicate HIV-1 (1; see also 1a, this volume). As a result, life-long
ART is necessary. Such therapy has several limitations, including long-term side
effects and the requirement for strict adherence to the medications to prevent viral
resistance. Thus, new strategies to treat HIV-1 are urgently needed.

Immunotherapy is an exciting new strategy that is being explored for treating
HIV-1. This approach is based on the recognition that the immune system controls
most viral infections, including many that establish a chronic infection of the human host. In contrast, HIV-1 is rarely completely controlled by the immune system.
However, recent evidence suggests that immunologic control of HIV-1 is possible

in some infected patients, and the immunologic correlates of this control are being defined. These new findings form the rationale for innovative immune-based therapies aimed at augmenting immune responses to HIV-1 and achieving long-term control of this infection which, left untreated, is fatal in the vast majority of persons.

THE IMMUNE RESPONSE TO VIRAL INFECTIONS

To understand the basis of immunologic control of HIV-1, it is useful to review how the immune system controls other viral infections. The immune system is often categorized into innate and acquired immunity (2–4). Innate immunity, such as antimicrobial peptides, phagocytes, natural killer cells, and complement, acts rapidly and has an important role in initial control of acute viral infections. For example, humans with a defective natural killer cell response develop recurrent infections by the herpes family of viruses (5). In addition, cells of the innate immune system, such as dendritic cells, are necessary to activate acquired immunity. Acquired immunity consists of humoral (B lymphocyte–mediated) and cellular (T lymphocyte–mediated) responses. Clonal expansion and differentiation of antigen-specific lymphocytes results in the ability to recognize an extremely diverse variety of viral pathogens. In addition, acquired immunity includes memory lymphocytes, which protect against re-exposure to the viral pathogen. Defects in acquired immunity, such as severe combined immunodeficiency and the acquired immunodeficiency syndrome (AIDS), predispose individuals to viral infections.

Each arm of the acquired immune system has an important role in controlling viral infections, but the relative contributions of each vary. Many infections and vaccines trigger protective antibody responses. For example, the presence of antibody responses induced by vaccination with hepatitis B surface antigen correlates with protection from this virus (6). Although congenital defects in antibody production mainly lead to an increased risk of bacterial infections, patients with hypogammaglobulinemia have an increased risk of several viral infections, most notably enteroviruses (7). The mechanism of antibody-mediated immune clearance includes binding to the viral pathogen and removal of the antibody-antigen complex by the reticuloendothelial system. Antibodies can also trigger antibody-dependent complement-mediated virolysis and antibody-dependent cellular cytotoxicity. Finally, antibodies can directly inactivate a virus by preventing attachment to its cellular receptor.

The cellular immune response to viruses consists of both CD8+ cytotoxic T lymphocytes (CTLs) and CD4+ T helper cells. CTLs recognize viral antigens that have been processed intracellularly into peptides. These peptides, typically 8–11 amino acids in length, are then presented on the infected cell in conjunction with a class I major histocompatibility complex (MHC) molecule and $\beta 2$ microglobulin. The T cell receptor of CD8+ T cells recognizes the complex of class I MHC, $\beta 2$ microglobulin, and viral peptide, and this recognition triggers the CTLs to lyse the infected cell (Figure 1a). In addition to their cytolytic function, CD8+ T cells also secrete cytokines that may have an antiviral effect, such as interferon γ (IFNγ)

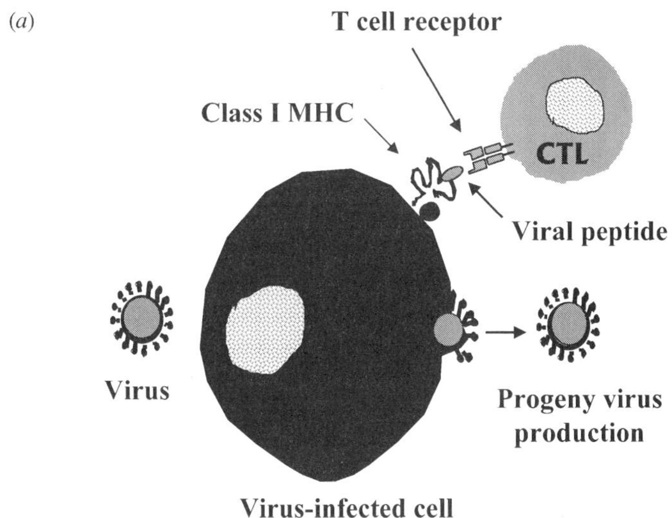

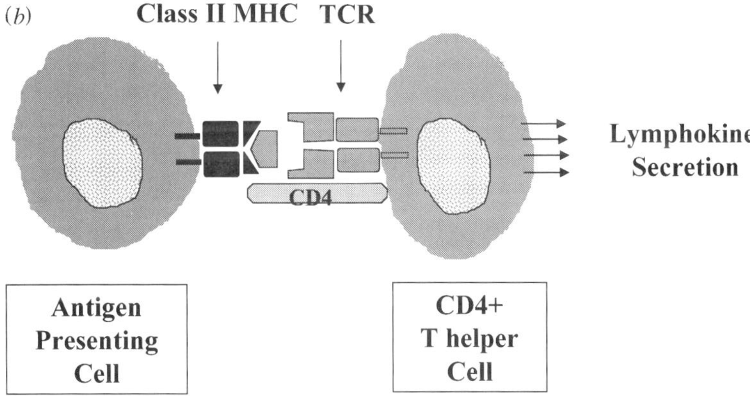

Figure 1   (*a*) Recognition of a viral peptide in conjunction with class I MHC on the surface of an infected cell by a CD8+ cytotoxic T lymphocyte (CTL) leads to lysis of the infected cell. (*b*) A CD4+ T helper cell recognizes viral peptide in conjunction with class II MHC on the surface of an antigen-presenting cell. The helper cell is then activated to secrete lymphokines that coordinate CD8+ T cell and B cell responses. TCR: T cell receptor. (From Reference 7a with permission.)

and tumor necrosis factor α (TNFα). For example, in a transgenic mouse model of hepatitis B virus, CD8+ T cells producing IFNγ and TNFα were critical in clearing hepatocytes of the virus (8, 9). This and other studies indicate that CD8+ T cells are a critical component of the host immune response to viral infections.

In addition to CTLs, acquired immunity involves the generation of virus-specific CD4+ T helper cell responses. The CD4+ T cell response is triggered by exogenous proteins that are endocytosed by antigen-presenting cells and cleaved into peptide antigens. These antigens are presented on the surface of the antigen-presenting cells in conjunction with class II MHC molecules. The peptide–class II MHC complex is recognized by the T cell receptor of CD4+ T cells, and this promotes the activation and differentiation of the CD4+ T cell. These cells can then produce important cytokines that serve as chemical messengers to coordinate the entire immune response to pathogens (Figure 1*b*). For example, activated T helper cells can produce interleukin (IL)-2 and IFNγ (Th1 response), which augment CTL responses. T helper cells also secrete IL-4, IL-5, IL-6, and IL-10, which promote the B cell response to infection (Th2 response). In addition to affecting CTL and B cell responses, T helper cells activate antigen-presenting cells, such as dendritic cells. These antigen-presenting cells are critical in stimulating an effective CTL response. Lack of effective CD4 help may therefore impair antigen presentation and undermine CTL control of a viral infection.

CORRELATES OF IMMUNE CONTROL IN CHRONIC VIRAL INFECTIONS

The innate, humoral, and cellular immune systems all combine to control most viral infections encountered by humans. Before considering why HIV-1 is generally resistant to these immunologic controls, it is useful to examine specifically how the immune system works to contain other viral pathogens.

Lymphocytic Choriomeningitis Virus (LCMV)

The mouse LCMV model has provided some of the most important insights into immunologic control of chronic viral infections. Acute LCMV infection is associated with a massive expansion of virus-specific CD8+ T cells: By eight days, >50% of splenic CD8+ T cells are LCMV-specific (10). Mice that lack CD8+ T cells cannot control acute LCMV, indicating that CTLs are important in immunologic control of this virus (11–13).

The LCMV model also demonstrates that virus-specific CD4+ T cell help is critical in maintaining an effective CTL response. Animals infected with rapidly replicating LCMV variants can clear the infection with CTLs only if CD4 cells are present. If CD4 cells are depleted, there is progressive loss of virus-specific CTL activity and the animals develop lifelong persistence of the infection (14, 15). Lack of CD4 cells may lead to a nonfunctional CD8 T cell response in LCMV (16, 17). This dependence of CTLs on T helper cells for optimal function may also have ramifications for the lack of immunologic control in patients with HIV-1.

Neutralizing antibodies to LCMV may also play a role in control of this virus. Animals that are depleted of CD8+ T cells develop stronger and earlier neutralizing antibody responses after LCMV infection than animals that have CD8+ T cells, perhaps because of the higher titers of LCMV in the CD8-depleted animals. This neutralizing antibody response contributes to transient control of viremia, but containment is eventually lost owing to emergence of neutralizing antibody escape mutations (18). The emergence of neutralization escape mutants is correlated with lack of virus-specific CD4+ helper cells (19), again suggesting that these cells are important in coordinating effective immunologic control of viral infection.

Herpes Viruses

Perhaps the best examples of chronic human viral infections that are controlled by the immune system are in the herpes family of viruses. Herpes simplex virus (HSV), Epstein-Barr virus (EBV), cytomegalovirus (CMV), and varicella zoster virus (VZV) all establish a chronic, latent infection that lasts for the lifetime of the host. The important role of the immune system in controlling these chronic infections is illustrated by the fact that conditions characterized by immunosuppression (such as aging, immunosuppressive medication, cancer, and HIV-1 disease) are associated with an increased risk of reactivation of these viruses. Thus, although the body never eradicates the herpes family of viruses, long-term immunologic control is generally seen.

EPSTEIN-BARR VIRUS   Following acute infection with EBV, there is a massive proliferation of virus-specific CD8 T cells. Thereafter, EBV infection is brought under control, presumably owing to effective CTL control. A congenital condition that impairs the immune response, X-linked lymphoproliferative syndrome, is associated with uncontrolled EBV infection (20). Patients with an acquired defect in cellular immunity, such as after an allogeneic bone marrow transplant, have an increased risk of EBV-induced lymphoproliferative disease. This disease can be prevented by transferring EBV-specific T lymphocytes (21, 22), which underscores the critical role of these cells in the defense against EBV.

HERPES SIMPLEX VIRUS   The critical role of T lymphocytes can also be demonstrated in animal models of HSV infection. Mice lacking CD8+ T cells have delayed clearance of HSV resulting in loss of sensory ganglia. In an in vitro system, CD8 cells present in the sensory ganglia inhibit viral reactivation; removal of these CD8 cells (by a depleting antibody) results in re-emergence of HSV (23). CD4 and B cells also seem to be important in controlling HSV infection (7, 24, 25).

CYTOMEGALOVIRUS   Reactivation of CMV disease after bone marrow transplantation is frequent. In a study of 14 patients undergoing allogeneic bone marrow transplantation who received infusions of CMV-specific CD8+ T cells from the donor, none of the recipients developed CMV viremia or disease (26). This study also suggested that virus-specific CD4+ helper responses might be important in sustaining CD8+ CTL activity, as was indicated by the mouse model of LCMV. In a patient who recovered CMV-specific helper cell activity, there was a sustained

CD8+ T cell response to the virus. In contrast, in patients who did not have helper cells, CMV-specific CTLs generally waned over time.

The above studies of immunologic control of mouse LCMV and herpes viruses suggest that CTLs are critical to containing viral infection. These studies also indicate that CD4 cells may be needed to maintain effective CTL and antibody responses to viruses.

THE IMMUNE RESPONSE TO HIV-1

Following acute HIV-1 infection, a massive viremia triggers an immunologic response. In one cohort of patients with acute HIV-1 infection, the median viral load was approximately 5 million RNA copies/ml of plasma (27). Over the first few months after infection, the viremia declines to a set point, and by one year the average HIV viral load is around 30,000 copies/ml (28). The viral load set point is a strong predictor of how rapidly an individual will develop AIDS (29, 30). Emerging evidence indicates that differences in antiviral immune responses account for the differences in viral load set point and thus in disease progression. There is evidence that antibody, CTL, and CD4 helper responses all play a role in containing HIV-1, so a closer examination of each is important to understanding how immunologic control of HIV-1 is possible.

Antibody

Patients with HIV-1 infection develop a high concentration of antibodies directed at many different viral proteins, generally within one to three months of infection. However, much of the antibody response against HIV-1 may be directed against virion debris (31) and may not have a strong antiviral effect. The first antibodies detected recognize linear determinants in HIV-1 structural proteins, such as p24 and p17 in Gag. Thereafter, antibodies to HIV-1 Env and Pol epitopes appear, and there may also be antibodies to HIV-1 regulatory and accessory proteins, such as Rev, Tat, Vpr, Vpu, Vif, and Nef.

Antibodies that neutralize HIV-1 prior to its entry into cells (neutralizing antibodies) are mainly directed against the HIV-1 envelope (32). These antibodies could theoretically exert an antiviral effect in vivo. Most neutralizing antibodies are directed against a hypervariable region of the gp120 subunit of Env (the V3 loop) as well as against a "neutralization face" on gp120 that overlaps the CD4 binding site and the chemokine receptor binding site (regions necessary for HIV-1 to enter susceptible cells). Neutralizing antibodies against the V3 loop are often more effective against laboratory strains of HIV-1 than against autologous virus or so-called primary HIV-1 isolates, which are derived from infected persons without extensive in vitro passage. This relative resistance of autologous virus and primary isolates to neutralization may limit the in vivo efficacy of these antibodies in controlling HIV-1.

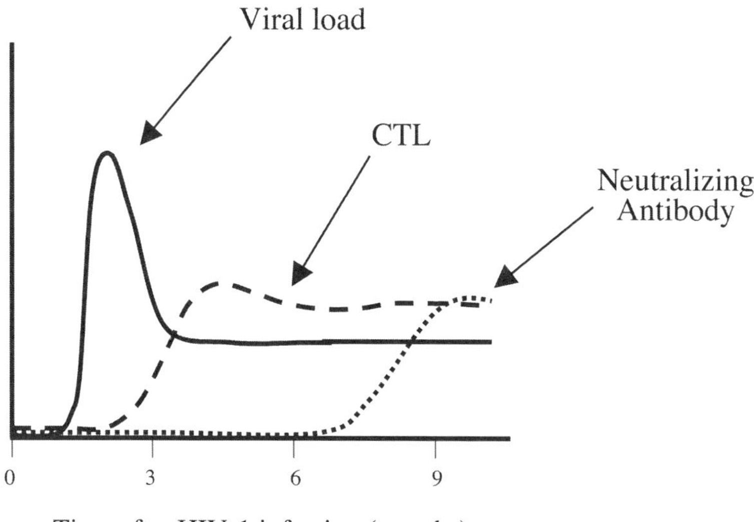

Figure 2   Typical course of HIV-1 viral load and immune response following acute HIV infection.

The precise role of antibodies in controlling HIV-1 in infected individuals remains uncertain. First, patients with acute HIV-1 infection usually have significant decline of the primary viremia before neutralizing antibodies are detectable (Figure 2) (33). Second, although some individuals with long-term control of HIV-1 viremia without ART (called long-term non-progressors or HIV-1 controllers) have strong neutralizing antibody responses, these responses are not present in other patients who control the virus (34). Third, although passive immunization with antibodies can protect monkeys from challenge infections (35, 36), a high concentration of antibodies must be present to protect against infection with primary isolates (isolates obtained from infected persons, as opposed to laboratory isolates that have been adapted to long-term culture).

How does HIV-1 elude the antibody response (32)? First, because of its high mutation rate, HIV-1 may escape antibodies through antigenic variation. For example, even when a laboratory worker was infected with a neutralization-sensitive strain of HIV-1, the virus rapidly developed a neutralization-resistant phenotype in vivo (37), indicative of rapid evolution of the virus to escape immune responses. Second, overlapping hypervariable loops (such as V1 and V2) may restrict accessibility of antibody to those parts of gp120 that are critical for entry of the virus (32). Third, glycosylation of the envelope may mask important epitopes from recognition by antibodies (38, 39). The latter two mechanisms—masking of critical structural determinants by the V1/V2 loop and glycosylation—may lead to neutralization resistance.

Recent evidence suggests that a more effective humoral response to immuno-deficiency viruses can be elicited. Mutations in simian immunodeficiency virus (SIV) envelope glycosylation sites and deletion of the V1/V2 loop were created in an attempt to modify those features of the envelope that contribute to neutralization resistance (39) (R. Desrosiers, personal communication). As compared to infection with unmodified virus, infection of macaques with these mutant viruses generated higher titers of neutralizing antibodies against the parental virus and the mutants. Although the peak viremia after inoculation with the mutant viruses was similar to that seen after parental virus infection, the viral load set point was much lower. This control of viremia may be due to the more effective neutralizing antibody response. Whether these exciting results can be applied in humans remains to be seen.

Cytotoxic T Lymphocytes

Persons with HIV-1 develop strong virus-specific CTL responses against both structural and regulatory genes of HIV-1 (40–42). These responses are sometimes so vigorous that CTL activity can be detected in fresh blood without expansion of CD8+ cells in culture. These CD8+ T cells may control HIV-1 by at least two different mechanisms (43). First, virus-specific CTLs may lyse HIV-infected cells by recognizing viral peptides on the cell surface in conjunction with class I MHC molecules. CTLs can eliminate infected cells before progeny virions are released, demonstrating in vitro that CTLs exhibit potent antiviral activity (44). Second, CD8+ cells may inhibit HIV-1 replication by secreting β chemokines, such as MIP-1α, MIP-1β, and RANTES, which bind HIV-1 coreceptors on the surface of CD4+ T cells and block entry of the virus. These β chemokines are in the same granules that contain cytolytic proteins, and are released in an antigen-specific manner when CTLs encounter their target antigen in the proper HLA context (45). Chemokines may also promote the cytolytic activity of CTLs (46), thereby potentiating control of HIV-1 by CD8+ T cells.

There is substantial evidence that CD8+ T cells have an important role in controlling HIV-1 infection. First, clearance of the primary viremia of acute HIV-1 infection correlates with the appearance of HIV-specific CTLs (Figure 2) (33, 47). Second, CTLs taken from patients with HIV-1 are able to inhibit viral replication in autologous CD4+ T cells in vitro (44). Third, adoptive transfer of virus-specific CTLs into patients with HIV-1 results in homing of the CTLs to areas of HIV infection (48). Finally, the role of CTLs in controlling HIV-1 is strongly supported by studies of rhesus macaques infected with simian immunodeficiency virus (SIV), our best animal model for HIV. Like HIV-1, SIV infection elicits a strong CTL response. Following antibody depletion of macaque CD8+ T cells, SIV viremia increases markedly and is subsequently controlled as the CD8 cells (and CTLs) are restored (49, 50). In animals with persistent CD8 cell depletion, there is a sustained increase in SIV viral load. This series of experiments indicates that CTLs are important in determining the viral load set point at steady state and thus in controlling this immunodeficiency virus. CTLs are likely to play a similar role in containing HIV-1 infection.

New techniques to detect virus-specific CD8+ T cells have greatly expanded our understanding of CTLs in patients with HIV-1. Detection of HIV-specific CTLs originally relied on labeling target cells with radioactive chromium, adding CD8 effector cells, and detecting specific lysis of the targets by measuring the release of chromium. More recently, a technique has been developed to directly visualize epitope-specific CTLs using tetramer staining (51). This technique is based on the fact that a T cell receptor on a CD8+ T cell binds to a specific viral peptide/class I MHC complex. A tetramer complex of MHC class I molecules and viral epitope peptide can be labeled with a fluorescent marker and then used to stain specific T cell receptors on CD8+ cells. Using this method, the frequency of CTLs specific for an individual HIV peptide epitope in chronically infected individuals has been estimated at 0.1%–1%, with some patients having 5% or more of their CD8 cells specific for an HIV-1 epitope.

The tetramer technique has been used to study the relationship between the number of HIV-specific CTLs and the HIV-1 viral load. A cross-sectional study showed an inverse correlation between the number of tetramer-positive CTLs and the viral load; that is, the higher the number of tetramer-positive cells, the lower the HIV-1 viral load (52). This finding suggests that CTLs exert an antiviral effect. However, in patients with low CD4 counts, the inverse correlation between tetramer-positive cells and HIV viral load was not seen (53), perhaps due to nonfunctional CTLs in patients with advanced HIV-1 infection. (see below).

Another new technique to detect HIV-specific CD8 cells measures the ability of CD8+ T cells to produce specific cytokines, such as IFNγ, following recognition of the target epitope. This assay complements the tetramer technique by quantifying cells that are functionally activated in response to antigen (i.e., cells that produce IFNγ). Panels of overlapping peptides that span all the HIV-1 gene products can be used to stimulate CD8+ T cells. Those cells that produce IFNγ (detected by Elispot or intracellular cytokine staining) are thought to be functional epitope-specific CTLs. Use of this technique to detect functional CTLs has suggested that some tetramer-positive CD8 T cells may lack function, especially when CD4 helper cells are not present. For example, CD4 knockout mice infected with LCMV develop a tetramer-positive CTL that does not produce IFNγ or lyse infected cells (16). A nonfunctional CTL response has also been seen in a patient with melanoma (54). In patients with HIV-1, the degree to which tetramer-positive cells lack IFNγ is still under study (53, 55, 56). However, CD8+ T cells in patients with chronic HIV-1 may have other defects, such as lack of perforin and diminished cytolytic activity (56). HIV-specific CD8+ T cells may also exhibit a skewed maturation pattern in infected individuals, which might affect the overall efficacy of these responses in vivo (57).

CD4+ T Cells

The hallmark of HIV-1 infection is progressive depletion of CD4+ T cells. In late-stage AIDS, this CD4 depletion is also associated with a decline in CTL activity. However, even in earlier stages of chronic HIV-1 infection, there is a qualitative defect in CD4+ T cell function (58–60). In fact, the most dramatic hole in the immune repertoire of most infected persons is the selective lack of HIV-specific T helper cells. Since several animal and human studies suggest that helper cell responses are necessary to maintain CTL activity (see above), impairment of these cells in patients with chronic HIV-1 may explain why the immune system cannot control the virus despite the presence of CTLs.

Evidence for the role of CD4+ T cells in control of HIV-1 comes from several studies of infected individuals (61–63). Patients who are long-term nonprogressors (LTNPs) (see below) have strong T cell lymphoproliferative responses to HIV antigen (61, 64). In untreated individuals with chronic HIV-1, an inverse correlation was found between the lymphoproliferative responses to HIV p24 and HIV-1 viral load: Patients with the highest CD4 responses had the lowest viral loads, whereas patients with the lowest CD4 responses had the highest viral loads (Figure 3) (61). In these patients, strong T helper responses were associated with strong CTL responses (62). Thus, CD4 T cells may coordinate the immune response to HIV-1, at least in part by maintaining effective CTL function. Immunologic control of viremia may depend on a strong CD4 helper and CTL response.

These studies measured CD4 helper cell activity by measuring proliferation of CD4+ T cells after stimulation with HIV p24. Using a different technology, Pitcher et al. found that HIV-specific CD4+ T cells, as measured by intracellular IFNγ expression, persisted in patients with chronic HIV-1 infection (65). The frequency

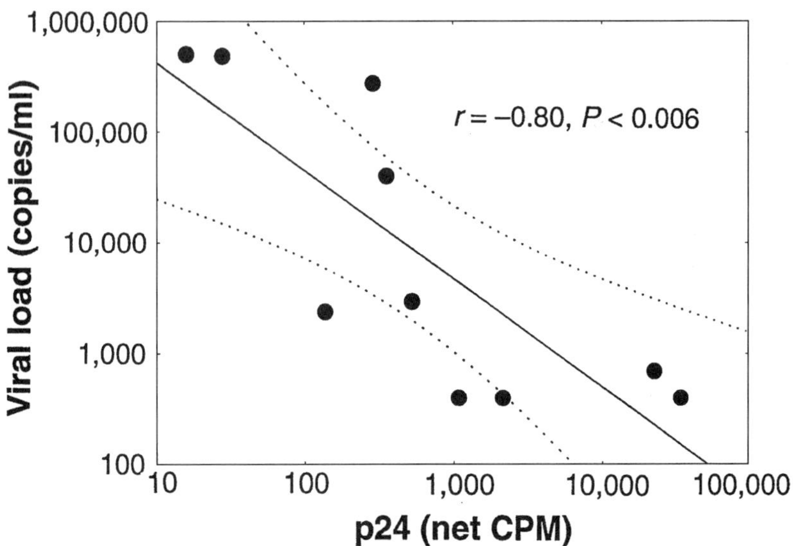

Figure 3 Inverse correlation between HIV viral load and HIV-specific CD4+ T helper response (from Reference 61 with permission).

of HIV-specific CD4+ T cells was lower in patients with chronic HIV-1 than in LTNPs, although there was overlap between the two groups. Also, among patients with chronic HIV-1 infection, the frequency of HIV-specific CD4+ T cells was much lower than the frequency of CMV-specific helper cells. An important goal for future research is to determine whether the IFNγ-positive CD4 cells detected in this study can proliferate and function normally.

Based on studies in HIV-1 and other viral infections, CD4+ T cells seem to play a critical role in maintaining an effective immune response. Loss of immunologic control in patients with HIV-1 may be related to selective destruction of CD4 cell immunity by the virus (see below). Whether this impaired CD4 response is due mainly to a quantitative loss or a functional defect is a topic of great interest. Further elucidation of CD4 cell responses in patients with HIV-1 may have direct relevance for designing immunotherapeutic strategies for this infection.

IMMUNE EVASION

Although HIV-1 can elicit a vigorous immune response, in the vast majority of patients viral replication persists and eventually destroys the immune system. How does HIV-1 persist in the face of this immune response? There are many possible mechanisms by which HIV-1 might elude the immune system (66–68; see also 68a this volume). First, structural features of the HIV-1 envelope may cause resistance to neutralization by antibody responses (as discussed above). Second, because replication of the virus is both error-prone and rapid (69), mutations and antigenic variation occur that allow escape from both humoral and cellular immunity. For example, after acute infection of macaques with SIV, a strong Tat-specific CTL response controls viremia (70), but Tat accumulates mutations that allow the virus to escape from immune control. The remarkable diversity and rapid evolution of HIV-1 make immunologic control particularly challenging. Third, HIV-1 may hide from CTL and natural killer attack by selectively downregulating class I MHC alleles (71–74). Finally, as discussed above, by directly infecting and destroying HIV-specific CD4 cells, the virus may weaken the other arms of the immune response, especially CTLs. If HIV-1 is able to elude the immune response, what are the prospects for immunologic control of this virus?

IMMUNOLOGIC CONTROL OF HIV-1

The evidence that the immune system can control HIV-1 comes from several special circumstances that have provided a great deal of insight into HIV pathogenesis. Both LTNPs and some persons treated with ART during acute seroconversion are able to control HIV-1 viremia. Detailed studies of these two groups of patients suggest that immunologic containment of HIV-1 is possible.

Most patients with HIV-1 infection develop persistent viremia and progressive CD4 cell depletion. However, a small fraction of patients with HIV-1 infection, the LTNPs, maintain low to undetectable viral loads with a stable CD4 count. Over time, some apparent LTNPs develop a rising viral load followed by a decline in their CD4 count. Nevertheless, the long period during which the HIV-1 viral load is kept in check in these individuals suggests that they may offer a unique insight into mechanisms of control of this virus.

Several possible factors may contribute to the control of HIV-1 in these patients. First, certain host factors, such as chemokine receptor genotype, are associated with slow progression of HIV-1 infection to AIDS (75, 76; reviewed in 77). Second, there may be HIV-1 mutations, such as in HIV Nef (78, 79), or other viral polymorphisms (80) that impair viral pathogenicity. Finally, in some LTNPs, the immune system may be responsible for containment of HIV-1.

There is growing evidence for the role of the immune system in patients who control HIV-1. The class I MHC complex, also known as the human leukocyte antigen (HLA) system, coordinates the T cell immune response. Certain HLA types have a strong effect on progression from HIV-1 infection to AIDS. For example, class I MHC homozygosity is associated with more rapid progression of HIV-1 infection to AIDS, perhaps because this homozygosity allows for a less diverse immune response to the virus (81). Particular HLA alleles, such HLA-B35 and Cw4, are also associated with more rapid progression to AIDS (81). Other HLA alleles, such as B57, are associated with slower progression to AIDS (82). Although these studies do not prove that the effect is due to the immune system—the HLA genes may be linked to other unknown genetic factors that influence the course of HIV—they support the hypothesis that control of HIV may be immunologic, and in particular suggest a role for class I restricted CTLs.

In addition to HLA effects on progression, detailed immunologic analyses indicate that some LTNPs have both a strong and diverse CTL response. Some such individuals have little detectable neutralizing antibody, suggesting that the humoral response may not be necessary for control of viremia (34). In contrast to most patients with chronic HIV-1 infection, LTNPs generally have a strong HIV-specific CD4+ T cell response (27, 61, 62) (Figure 4). This preserved CD4+ T cell response may maintain the effectiveness of CD8+ T cells in controlling HIV-1.

If CD4 helper responses are critical in coordinating an effective immune response to HIV-1, why are they lost in most patients with HIV-1? One possibility is preferential infection and destruction of HIV-specific CD4+ T cells by the virus itself. Massive viremia during acute HIV-1 infection may result in widespread activation of the immune system, including HIV-specific CD4+ T cells. Because HIV-1 preferentially infects activated CD4+ T cells, these cells may be deleted during this acute phase of infection. During chronic HIV-1 infection, there may be an inability to regenerate this important immunologic response, even after potent ART controls viremia.

If this model is correct, then early ART during acute HIV-1 infection may preserve the CD4+ helper cell response. And if a strong helper cell response is

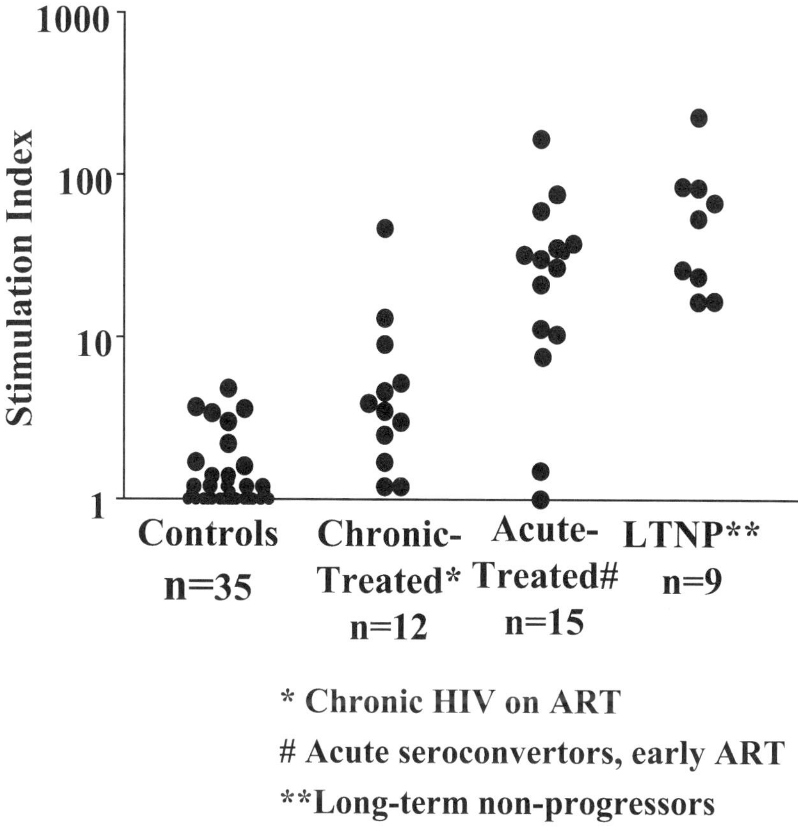

Figure 4   HIV Gag-specific T cell responses (measured by stimulation index) in different groups of individuals with HIV-1 (from Reference 27 with permission).

necessary for immunologic control of HIV-1, patients who retain these cells may be able to effectively control HIV-1 even when ART is stopped.

These hypotheses were tested in a cohort of 16 HIV-positive individuals who were diagnosed during acute HIV-1 seroconversion and started on ART immediately (27). Fifteen patients' viral loads dropped to undetectable levels. Although initially HIV-specific helper cell responses were weak, as viremia was contained all patients developed a strong CD4 T cell response to HIV Gag antigen. The level of CD4 lymphoproliferative response in these patients was comparable to that seen in LTNPs (Figure 4). In addition to this helper cell response, the patients developed CTL responses to HIV-1. However, the CTL responses were lower in magnitude in the patients treated with ART during acute infection than in individuals with chronic HIV-1 (63). In addition, the CD8 response to the virus in patients treated during seroconversion was generally narrow, perhaps owing to the homogeneity of the viral quasispecies during this early stage of infection (63).

To test whether the immune responses generated by early treatment of acute infection could control viremia, eight patients in the cohort had ART discontinued as part of a supervised protocol (27). ART was resumed in patients who had a viral load rebound to $>50,000$ copies/ml on a single occasion or >5000 copies/ml for three consecutive weeks. After a single interruption, three of the eight subjects controlled viremia to <5000 copies/ml. The other five restarted therapy as per the protocol but subsequently underwent a second treatment interruption. During the second interruption, virologic rebound was slower and to a lower peak than after the first interruption. Four of the five patients controlled viremia to <5000 copies/ml after this second treatment interruption; one patient met criteria to restart therapy when his viral load reached 17,100 copies/ml.

The immunologic effects of treatment interruption were striking. The CD8+ CTL response showed a marked increase in magnitude and breadth. Although the CD4 helper response transiently decreased during the viremia after the first treatment interruption, when ART was restarted the helper cell response increased and was maintained during the second treatment interruption.

The results of this pilot study suggest that immunologic control of HIV-1 may be possible, at least transiently, if a strong CD4 helper response can be preserved by early treatment of acute HIV-1. At 30 months after infection, five of eight individuals treated during acute infection had viral loads of <500 copies/ml without ART. In comparison, in a group of historical controls, only 4 of 109 untreated patients with acute HIV-1 had viral loads of <500 copies/ml at a similar time point ($p < 0.001$). This study suggests that immunologic control of HIV-1 is possible, and suggests that a strong HIV-specific CD4 helper response is critical in containing HIV-1.

Studies using the animal models of HIV also support the concept that early treatment can result in subsequent control of immunodeficiency viruses. In an early study, macaques infected with a pathogenic isolate of HIV-2 were treated with d4T monotherapy during acute infection (83). Even after the nucleoside was withdrawn, the treated animals had lower viral loads and higher CD4 counts than untreated animals. In a second study, the majority of macaques who received d4T, ddI, and tenofovir two weeks after infection with SIV had persistent containment of viremia after ART was discontinued, whereas almost all animals that did not receive early treatment failed to control viremia (84). The control of viremia in animals that received early ART correlated with the presence of SIV-specific CD4 helper responses, as seen in the human study discussed above. Finally, a study in which tenofovir alone was given within 1–3 days of SIV infection again demonstrated that animals treated with ART had SIV-specific lymphoproliferative responses and controlled viremia after the drug was discontinued, whereas untreated animals had lower lymphoproliferative responses and did not control viremia (85). These animal studies are compatible with the hypothesis that early treatment of infection results in preservation of critical immunologic responses that can control viremia after withdrawal of ART.

In contrast to the experience in acutely infected patients, individuals with chronic HIV-1 infection do not seem to be able to control viremia when ART is

TABLE 1 Virologic and immunologic differences between acute and chronic HIV-1 infection

Stage of HIV	CD4 response	CD8 response	Viral diversity
Acute	High	Narrow	Narrow
Chronic	Low	Broad	Diverse

stopped (86, 87). With few exceptions, virologic rebound occurs in such patients, usually to a level similar to the baseline viral load (88–90). The explanation for the difference between patients treated during acute versus chronic infection may lie in the function of the virus-specific CD4+ helper response. In patients treated during acute infection, functional CD4+ T cells are preserved, which may maintain an effective CD8+ CTL response against the virus. In contrast, chronically infected individuals treated with HAART (highly active ART) have low numbers of virus-specific CD4+ T cells (27, 63). Thus, when ART is stopped, the immune system is not able to control viremia, perhaps because of an impaired CTL response.

Other immunologic and virologic differences between acute and chronic HIV-1 infection suggest that different immunotherapeutic strategies may be needed (Table 1). In patients who receive effective ART during acute HIV-1 infection, CD4 activity is preserved but CTL response to the virus is narrow (63). The narrow CTL response may be due to the limited viral diversity during early HIV-1 infection (63). Thus, in these individuals, immunotherapy might be aimed at increasing and broadening the CTL response to HIV-1. In contrast, in patients with chronic HIV-1, helper responses are absent and the virus is extremely heterogeneous (63). Therefore, these patients may require enhancement of both CD4 helper responses and CTL activity.

If both CD4+ and CD8+ immune responses were augmented by immunotherapy in patients with HIV-1 on ART, would the immune system be able to control the virus? This question will be addressed by exciting new trials of immunotherapy for HIV-1.

IMMUNOTHERAPY FOR HIV-1

Use of the immune system to control disease is an important concept that has been most fully realized in preventative vaccines for infectious diseases. The data presented above make a compelling case that immunologic control of HIV-1 is possible. The challenge is to boost the immune system in such a way that the experience of the LTNP and the patient with acute HIV-1 who receives early treatment is reproduced in the much larger number of individuals suffering from chronic HIV-1 infection.

Immunotherapy for HIV can be divided into those modalities expected to primarily boost immunity nonspecifically versus those that boost HIV-specific

TABLE 2   Examples of immunotherapeutic approaches for HIV-1 infection

Cytokine-based therapy
    IL-2
    IL-12

Adoptive cell transfers
    CTL
    CD4 T cells

Passive antibody therapy

Therapeutic vaccination
    DNA vaccination
    Viral vectors
        Canarypox
        Modified Vaccinia Ankara
        Venezualan equine encephalitis
        Adenovirus
        Adeno-associated virus
        Vesicular stomatitis virus
        Poliovirus
    Dendritic cells + HIV-1 peptides
    Dendritic cells + viral vectors
    Inactivated HIV-1: Remune
    Combination vaccines

Supervised treatment interruption

Gene therapy

immunity. An example of the former is cytokine therapy, such as with IL-2. An example of the latter is therapeutic vaccination with HIV-1 immunogens. Many different immunotherapeutic strategies are being studied for HIV-1, some of which are listed in Table 2 (see also 90a, this volume).

Interleukin-2

IL-2 was one of the first immune-based therapies for HIV-1, and it continues to generate a great deal of interest. Clinical trials have shown that IL-2 increases CD4 counts in patients with HIV-1 (91, 92). Although prior to HAART this effect was limited to patients with relatively preserved CD4 counts, recent trials suggest that IL-2 also increases CD4 counts in more advanced patients on HAART (92a, 93). The major question is whether this increase will translate into clinical benefit. Given the toxicity of IL-2, the durability of the CD4 response and the quality of life of patients on this medication are also important issues. Two large trials are currently enrolling patients to address these questions.

IL-2 may also be able to boost virus-specific immunity when combined with specific viral antigens. In a recent immunization trial, macaques given a DNA vaccine with IL-2/immunoglobulin (Ig) fusion developed significant CD4 and CD8 immune responses to the viral gene products, unlike animals that received sham vaccination (94). Animals that received DNA vaccine alone developed an intermediate immune response. Although the animals that received DNA vaccine with IL-2/Ig were infected after challenge with an SIV/HIV chimeric virus, they had much lower viral loads than animals that received sham vaccine. Finally, animals that received DNA vaccine + IL-2/Ig did not develop clinical disease, whereas animals that received sham vaccine developed clinical events, including death. Again, the DNA vaccine without IL-2/Ig resulted in an intermediate benefit in terms of viral load reduction and decreased clinical events.

Dendritic Cell Immunization

Dendritic cells are normally present in tissues (including skin) and are specialized to capture antigen (95, 96). After acquiring antigen, they mature and migrate to lymphoid tissue, where they present antigen to T cells. Autologous dendritic cells pulsed with exogenous peptides can elicit strong and durable antigen-specific CD4+ and CD8+ T cell responses (97, 98). Thus, autologous dendritic cells are an attractive adjuvant for HIV-1 immunogens, such as peptides or whole proteins. The precursors of these cells are isolated from the blood, differentiated and expanded in vitro, incubated with immunogen, and then injected subcutaneously. This approach has generated strong influenza peptide-specific CTL response and antigen-specific CD4+ T cell responses (99, 100). A similar strategy is being pursued to boost HIV-specific helper cells and CTLs. If patients with boosted responses can control viremia after withdrawal of ART, then this would shed light on which immune responses are necessary to control HIV-1 and provide proof of concept that immunologic containment is possible in chronic HIV-1.

Viral Vectors

Several viral vectors may be able to boost immunity to HIV-1. One exciting type of vectors are alpha viruses, such as Venezuelan equine encephalitis (VEE), which target dendritic cells (101). Alpha virus vectors have been used successfully to induce protection against a wide variety of pathogens (102, 103). In macaques, immunization with VEE expressing SIV genes can lead to protection from challenge infection (104).

Another promising immunotherapy strategy is to use DNA immunization followed by boosting with an attenuated pox virus called modified vaccinia Ankara (MVA). This strategy has worked well in animal models to protect against malaria (105). Genes from an SIV/HIV chimeric virus have been placed into DNA plasmid constructs and into MVA vectors. Using these constructs, priming with the DNA vaccine and boosting with the MVA vaccine have been able to control viremia in macaques following challenge infection with a related SIV/HIV chimeric virus (106).

Thus, accumulating evidence from animal models suggests that boosting the immune system does allow control of viremia after a challenge infection. Whether the same strategy will work in humans, either for a preventative or a therapeutic vaccine, remains to be demonstrated.

SUMMARY

By depleting CD4+ T cells, HIV-1 infection results in immunodeficiency and the inability of the immune system to control this virus in most individuals. Although potent antiretroviral medications have had enormous clinical benefit in HIV-positive patients, ART has significant limitations, especially since life-long therapy appears to be necessary. Studies of how the immune system controls other chronic viral infections suggest that a coordinated CD4 helper response, CD8+ T cell activity, and antibody response all contribute to immunologic control. These same immune responses seem to be important in containing HIV-1 in recent studies of individuals who control the virus without ART. Based on a growing understanding of the immunologic correlates of control of HIV-1, new immunotherapeutic strategies are being designed. Although there are many challenges, there is genuine excitement and optimism that immunologic control of HIV-1 may be possible. Now we must realize this goal.

Visit the Annual Reviews home page at www.AnnualReviews.org

LITERATURE CITED

1. Finzi D, Blankson J, Siliciano JD, et al. 1999. Latent infection of CD4+ T cells provides a mechanism for lifelong persistence of HIV-1, even in patients on effective combination therapy. *Nat. Med.* 5:512–17

1a. Blankson JN, Persaud D, Siliciano RF. 2002. The challenge of viral reservoirs in HIV-1 infection. *Annu. Rev. Med.* 53:557–93

2. Delves PJ, Roitt IM. 2000. The immune system. First of two parts. *N. Engl. J. Med.* 343:37–49

3. Delves PJ, Roitt IM. 2000. The immune system. Second of two parts. *N. Engl. J. Med.* 343:108–17

4. Medzhitov R, Janeway C Jr. 2000. Innate immunity. *N. Engl. J. Med.* 343:338–44

5. Biron CA, Byron KS, Sullivan JL. 1989. Severe herpesvirus infections in an adolescent without natural killer cells. *N. Engl. J. Med.* 320:1731–35

6. Szmuness W, Stevens CE, Harley EJ, et al. 1982. Hepatitis B vaccine in medical staff of hemodialysis units: efficacy and subtype cross-protection. *N. Engl. J. Med.* 307:1481–86

7. Sanna PP, Burton DR. 2000. Role of antibodies in controlling viral disease: lessons from experiments of nature and gene knockouts. *J. Virol.* 74:9813–17

7a. Cohen DE, Walker BD. 2001. Human immunodeficiency virus pathogenesis and prospects for immune control in patients with established infection. *Clin. Infect. Dis.* 32:1756–68

8. Guidotti LG, Ando K, Hobbs MV, et al. 1994. Cytotoxic T lymphocytes inhibit hepatitis B virus gene expression by a non-cytolytic mechanism in transgenic mice. *Proc. Natl. Acad. Sci. USA* 91:3764–68

9. Guidotti LG, Ishikawa T, Hobbs MV, et al. 1996. Intracellular inactivation of the hepatitis B virus by cytotoxic T lymphocytes. *Immunity* 4:25–36

10. Murali-Krishna K, Altman JD, Suresh M, et al. 1998. Counting antigen-specific CD8 T cells: a reevaluation of bystander activation during viral infection. *Immunity* 8:177–87

11. Lehmann-Grube F, Assmann U, Loliger C, et al. 1985. Mechanism of recovery from acute virus infection. I. Role of T lymphocytes in the clearance of lymphocytic choriomeningitis virus from spleens of mice. *J. Immunol.* 134:608–15

12. Moskophidis D, Cobbold SP, Waldmann H, Lehmann-Grube F. 1987. Mechanism of recovery from acute virus infection: treatment of lymphocytic choriomeningitis virus-infected mice with monoclonal antibodies reveals that Lyt-2+ T lymphocytes mediate clearance of virus and regulate the antiviral antibody response. *J. Virol.* 61:1867–74

13. Quinn DG, Zajac AJ, Frelinger JA. 1995. The cell-mediated immune response against lymphocytic choriomeningitis virus in beta 2-microglobulin deficient mice. *Immunol. Rev.* 148:151–69

14. Matloubian M, Concepcion RJ, Ahmed R. 1994. CD4+ T cells are required to sustain CD8+ cytotoxic T-cell responses during chronic viral infection. *J. Virol.* 6:8056–63

15. Battegay M, Moskophidis D, Rahemtulla A, et al. 1994. Enhanced establishment of a virus carrier state in adult CD4+ T-cell-deficient mice. *J. Virol.* 68:4700–4

16. Zajac AJ, Blattman JN, Murali-Krishna K, et al. 1998. Viral immune evasion due to persistence of activated T cells without effector function. *J. Exp. Med.* 188:2205–13

17. Kalams SA, Walker BD. 1998. The critical need for CD4 help in maintaining effective cytotoxic T lymphocyte responses. *J. Exp. Med.* 188:2199–204

18. Ciurea A, Klenerman P, Hunziker L, et al. 2000. Viral persistence in vivo through selection of neutralizing antibody-escape variants. *Proc. Natl. Acad. Sci. USA* 97:2749–54

19. Ciurea A, Hunziker L, Klenerman P, et al. 2001. Impairment of CD4(+) T cell responses during chronic virus infection prevents neutralizing antibody responses against virus escape mutants. *J. Exp. Med.* 193:297–306

20. Greenberg PD, Riddell SR. 1999. Deficient cellular immunity—finding and fixing the defects. *Science* 285:546–51

21. Heslop HE, Ng CY, Li C, et al. 1996. Long-term restoration of immunity against Epstein-Barr virus infection by adoptive transfer of gene-modified virus-specific T lymphocytes. *Nat. Med.* 2:551–55

22. Rooney CM, Smith CA, Ng CY, et al. 1998. Infusion of cytotoxic T cells for the prevention and treatment of Epstein-Barr virus–induced lymphoma in allogeneic transplant recipients. *Blood* 92:1549–55

23. Liu T, Khanna KM, Chen X, et al. 2000. CD8(+) T cells can block herpes simplex virus type 1 (HSV-1) reactivation from latency in sensory neurons. *J. Exp. Med.* 191:1459–66

24. Nash AA. 2000. T cells and the regulation of herpes simplex virus latency and reactivation. *J. Exp. Med.* 191:1455–58

25. Minagawa H, Yanagi Y. 2000. Latent herpes simplex virus-1 infection in SCID mice transferred with immune CD4+ T cells: a new model for latency. *Arch. Virol.* 145:2259–72

26. Walter EA, Greenberg PD, Gilbert MJ, et al. 1995. Reconstitution of cellular immunity against cytomegalovirus in recipients of allogeneic bone marrow by transfer of T-cell clones from the donor. *N. Engl. J. Med.* 333:1038–44

27. Rosenberg ES, Altfeld M, Poon SH, et al. 2000. Immune control of HIV-1 after early

treatment of acute infection. *Nature* 407: 523–26

28. Lyles RH, Munoz A, Yamashita TE, et al. 2000. Natural history of human immunodeficiency virus type 1 viremia after seroconversion and proximal to AIDS in a large cohort of homosexual men. Multicenter AIDS Cohort Study. *J. Infect. Dis.* 181: 872–80

29. Mellors JW, Kingsley LA, Rinaldo CR Jr., et al. 1995. Quantitation of HIV-1 RNA in plasma predicts outcome after seroconversion. *Ann. Intern. Med.* 122:573–79

30. Mellors JW, Rinaldo CR Jr., Gupta P, et al. 1996. Prognosis in HIV-1 infection predicted by the quantity of virus in plasma. *Science* 272:1167–70

31. Parren PW, Burton DR, Sattentau QJ. 1997. HIV-1 antibody—debris or virion? *Nat. Med.* 3:366–67

32. Parren PW, Moore JP, Burton DR, Sattentau QJ. 1999. The neutralizing antibody response to HIV-1: viral evasion and escape from humoral immunity. *AIDS* 13:S137–62

33. Koup RA, Safrit JT, Cao Y, et al. 1994. Temporal association of cellular immune responses with the initial control of viremia in primary human immunodeficiency virus type 1 syndrome. *J. Virol.* 68:4650–55

34. Harrer T, Harrer E, Kalams SA, et al. 1996. Strong cytotoxic T cell and weak neutralizing antibody responses in a subset of persons with stable nonprogressing HIV type 1 infection. *AIDS Res. Hum. Retroviruses* 12:585–92

35. Mascola JR, Stiegler G, VanCott TC, et al. 2000. Protection of macaques against vaginal transmission of a pathogenic HIV-1/SIV chimeric virus by passive infusion of neutralizing antibodies. *Nat. Med.* 6:207–10

36. Baba TW, Liska V, Hofmann-Lehmann R, et al. 2000. Human neutralizing monoclonal antibodies of the IgG1 subtype protect against mucosal simian-human immunodeficiency virus infection. *Nat. Med.* 6:200–6

37. Beaumont T, van Nuenen A, Broersen S, et al. 2001. Reversal of human immunodeficiency virus type 1 IIIB to a neutralization-resistant phenotype in an accidentally infected laboratory worker with a progressive clinical course. *J. Virol.* 75:2246–52

38. Chackerian B, Rudensey LM, Overbaugh J. 1997. Specific N-linked and O-linked glycosylation modifications in the envelope V1 domain of simian immunodeficiency virus variants that evolve in the host alter recognition by neutralizing antibodies. *J. Virol.* 71:7719–27

39. Reitter JN, Means RE, Desrosiers RC. 1998. A role for carbohydrates in immune evasion in AIDS. *Nat. Med.* 4:679–84

40. Walker BD, Chakrabarti S, Moss B, et al. 1987. HIV-specific cytotoxic T lymphocytes in seropositive individuals. *Nature* 328:345–48

41. Walker BD, Flexner C, Paradis TJ, et al. 1988. HIV-1 reverse transcriptase is a target for cytotoxic T lymphocytes in infected individuals. *Science* 240:64–66

42. Addo MM, Altfeld M, Rosenberg ES, et al. 2001. The HIV-1 regulatory proteins Tat and Rev are frequently targeted by cytotoxic T lymphocytes derived from HIV-1-infected individuals. *Proc. Natl. Acad. Sci. USA* 98:1781–86

43. Yang OO, Walker BD. 1997. CD8+ cells in human immunodeficiency virus type I pathogenesis: cytolytic and noncytolytic inhibition of viral replication. *Adv. Immunol.* 66:273–311

44. Yang OO, Kalams SA, Rosenzweig M, et al. 1996. Efficient lysis of human immunodeficiency virus type 1-infected cells by cytotoxic T lymphocytes. *J. Virol.* 70: 5799–806

45. Wagner L, Yang OO, Garcia-Zepeda EA, et al. 1998. Beta-chemokines are released from HIV-1-specific cytolytic T-cell granules complexed to proteoglycans. *Nature* 391:908–11

46. Hadida F, Vieillard V, Autran B, et al. 1998. HIV-specific T cell cytotoxicity mediated by RANTES via the chemokine receptor CCR3. *J. Exp. Med.* 188:609–14

47. Borrow P, Lewicki H, Hahn BH, et al. 1994. Virus-specific CD8+ cytotoxic T lymphocyte activity associated with control of viremia in primary human immunodeficiency virus type 1 infection. *J. Virol.* 68:6103–10

48. Brodie SJ, Patterson BK, Lewinsohn DA, et al. 2000. HIV-specific cytotoxic T lymphocytes traffic to lymph nodes and localize at sites of HIV replication and cell death. *J. Clin. Invest.* 105:1407–17

49. Schmitz JE, Kuroda MJ, Santra S, et al. 1999. Control of viremia in simian immunodeficiency virus infection by CD8+ lymphocytes. *Science* 283:857–60

50. Jin X, Bauer DE, Tuttleton SE, et al. 1999. Dramatic rise in plasma viremia after CD8(+) T cell depletion in simian immunodeficiency virus-infected macaques. *J. Exp. Med.* 189:991–98

51. Altman JD, Moss PA, Goulder PJ, et al. 1996. Phenotypic analysis of antigen-specific T lymphocytes. *Science* 274:94–96

52. Ogg GS, Jin X, Bonhoeffer S, et al. 1998. Quantitation of HIV-1-specific cytotoxic T lymphocytes and plasma load of viral RNA. *Science* 279:2103–6

53. Kostense S, Ogg GS, Manting EH, et al. 2001. High viral burden in the presence of major HIV-specific CD8(+) T cell expansions: evidence for impaired CTL effector function. *Eur. J. Immunol.* 31:677–86

54. Lee PP, Yee C, Savage PA, et al. 1999. Characterization of circulating T cells specific for tumor-associated antigens in melanoma patients. *Nat. Med.* 5:677–85

55. Goulder PJ, Tang Y, Brander C, et al. 2000. Functionally inert HIV-specific cytotoxic T lymphocytes do not play a major role in chronically infected adults and children. *J. Exp. Med.* 192:1819–32

56. Appay V, Nixon DF, Donahoe SM, et al. 2000. HIV-specific CD8(+) T cells produce antiviral cytokines but are impaired in cytolytic function. *J. Exp. Med.* 192:63–75

57. Champagne P, Ogg GS, King AS, et al. 2001. Skewed maturation of memory HIV-specific CD8 T lymphocytes. *Nature* 410:106–11

58. Lane HC, Depper JM, Greene WC, et al. 1985. Qualitative analysis of immune function in patients with the acquired immunodeficiency syndrome. Evidence for a selective defect in soluble antigen recognition. *N. Engl. J. Med.* 313:79–84

59. Murray HW, Rubin BY, Masur H, Roberts RB. 1984. Impaired production of lymphokines and immune (gamma) interferon in the acquired immunodeficiency syndrome. *N. Engl. J. Med.* 310:883–89

60. Musey LK, Krieger JN, Hughes JP, et al. 1999. Early and persistent human immunodeficiency virus type 1 (HIV-1)-specific T helper dysfunction in blood and lymph nodes following acute HIV-1 infection. *J. Infect. Dis.* 180:278–84

61. Rosenberg ES, Billingsley JM, Caliendo AM, et al. 1997. Vigorous HIV-1-specific CD4+ T cell responses associated with control of viremia. *Science* 278:1447–50

62. Kalams SA, Buchbinder SP, Rosenberg ES, et al. 1999. Association between virus-specific cytotoxic T-lymphocyte and helper responses in human immunodeficiency virus type 1 infection. *J. Virol.* 73:6715–20

63. Altfeld M, Rosenberg ES, Shankarappa R, et al. 2001. Cellular immune responses and viral diversity in individuals treated during acute and early HIV-1 infection. *J. Exp. Med.* 193:169–80

64. Schwartz D, Sharma U, Busch M, et al. 1994. Absence of recoverable infectious virus and unique immune responses in an asymptomatic HIV+ long-term survivor. *AIDS Res. Hum. Retroviruses* 10:1703–11

65. Pitcher CJ, Quittner C, Peterson DM, et al. 1999. HIV-1-specific CD4+ T cells are detectable in most individuals with active HIV-1 infection, but decline with prolonged viral suppression. *Nat. Med.* 5:518–25

66. McMichael AJ, Phillips RE. 1997. Escape of human immunodeficiency virus from immune control. *Annu. Rev. Immunol.* 15:271–96

67. Goulder PJ, Rowland-Jones SL, Mc-Michael AJ, Walker BD. 1999. Anti-HIV cellular immunity: recent advances towards vaccine design. *AIDS* 13:S121–36

68. Brander C, Walker BD. 2000. Modulation of host immune responses by clinically relevant human DNA and RNA viruses. *Curr. Opin. Microbiol.* 3:379–86

68a. Johnson WE, Desrosiers RC. 2002. Viral persistence: HIV's strategies of immune system evasion. *Annu. Rev. Med.* 53:499–518

69. Coffin JM. 1995. HIV population dynamics in vivo: implications for genetic variation, pathogenesis, and therapy. *Science* 267:483–89

70. Allen TM, O'Connor DH, Jing P, et al. 2000. Tat-specific cytotoxic T lymphocytes select for SIV escape variants during resolution of primary viraemia. *Nature* 407:386–90

71. Schwartz O, Marechal V, Le Gall S, et al. 1996. Endocytosis of major histocompatibility complex class I molecules is induced by the HIV-1 Nef protein. *Nat. Med.* 2:338–42

72. Collins KL, Chen BK, Kalams SA, et al. 1998. HIV-1 Nef protein protects infected primary cells against killing by cytotoxic T lymphocytes. *Nature* 391:397–401

73. Le Gall S, Erdtmann L, Benichou S, et al. 1998. Nef interacts with the mu subunit of clathrin adaptor complexes and reveals a cryptic sorting signal in MHC I molecules. *Immunity* 8:483–95

74. Cohen GB, Gandhi RT, Davis DM, et al. 1999. The selective downregulation of class I major histocompatibility complex proteins by HIV-1 protects HIV-infected cells from NK cells. *Immunity* 10:661–71

75. Dean M, Carrington M, Winkler C, et al. 1996. Genetic restriction of HIV-1 infection and progression to AIDS by a deletion allele of the CKR5 structural gene. Hemophilia Growth and Development Study, Multicenter AIDS Cohort Study, Multicenter Hemophilia Cohort Study, San Francisco City Cohort, ALIVE Study. *Science* 273:1856–62

76. Huang Y, Paxton WA, Wolinsky SM, et al. 1996. The role of a mutant CCR5 allele in HIV-1 transmission and disease progression. *Nat. Med.* 2:1240–43

77. Carrington M, Dean M, Martin MP, O'Brien SJ. 1999. Genetics of HIV-1 infection: chemokine receptor CCR5 polymorphism and its consequences. *Hum. Mol. Genet.* 8:1939–45

78. Deacon NJ, Tsykin A, Solomon A, et al. 1995. Genomic structure of an attenuated quasi species of HIV-1 from a blood transfusion donor and recipients. *Science* 270:988–91

79. Kirchhoff F, Greenough TC, Brettler DB, et al. 1995. Brief report: absence of intact nef sequences in a long-term survivor with nonprogressive HIV-1 infection. *N. Engl. J. Med.* 332:228–32

80. Alexander L, Weiskopf E, Greenough TC, et al. 2000. Unusual polymorphisms in human immunodeficiency virus type 1 associated with nonprogressive infection. *J. Virol.* 74:4361–76

81. Carrington M, Nelson GW, Martin MP, et al. 1999. HLA and HIV-1: heterozygote advantage and B*35-Cw*04 disadvantage. *Science* 283:1748–52

82. Migueles SA, Sabbaghian MS, Shupert WL, et al. 2000. HLA B*5701 is highly associated with restriction of virus replication in a subgroup of HIV-infected long term nonprogressors. *Proc. Natl. Acad. Sci. USA* 97:2709–14

83. Watson A, McClure J, Ranchalis J, et al. 1997. Early postinfection antiviral treatment reduces viral load and prevents CD4+ cell decline in HIV type 2-infected macaques. *AIDS Res. Hum. Retroviruses* 13:1375–81

84. Hel Z, Venzon D, Poudyal M, et al. 2000. Viremia control following antiretroviral treatment and therapeutic immunization during primary SIV251 infection of macaques. *Nat. Med.* 6:1140–46

85. Lifson JD, Rossio JL, Arnaout R, et al.

2000. Containment of simian immunodeficiency virus infection: cellular immune responses and protection from rechallenge following transient postinoculation antiretroviral treatment. *J. Virol.* 74:2584–93

86. Davey RT Jr., Bhat N, Yoder C, et al. 1999. HIV-1 and T cell dynamics after interruption of highly active antiretroviral therapy (HAART) in patients with a history of sustained viral suppression. *Proc. Natl. Acad. Sci. USA* 96:15109–14

87. Carcelain G, Tubiana R, Samri A, et al. 2001. Transient mobilization of human immunodeficiency virus (HIV)-specific CD4 T-helper cells fails to control virus rebounds during intermittent antiretroviral therapy in chronic HIV type 1 infection. *J. Virol.* 75:234–41

88. Garcia F, Plana M, Vidal C, et al. 1999. Dynamics of viral load rebound and immunological changes after stopping effective antiretroviral therapy. *AIDS* 13:F79–86

89. Neumann AU, Tubiana R, Calvez V, et al. 1999. HIV-1 rebound during interruption of highly active antiretroviral therapy has no deleterious effect on reinitiated treatment. Comet Study Group. *AIDS* 13:677–83

90. Hatano H, Vogel S, Yoder C, et al. 2000. Pre-HAART HIV burden approximates post-HAART viral levels following interruption of therapy in patients with sustained viral suppression. *AIDS* 14:1357–63

90a. Graham BS. 2002. Clinical trials of HIV vaccines. *Annu. Rev. Med.* 53:207–21

91. Kovacs JA, Baseler M, Dewar RJ, et al. 1995. Increases in CD4 T lymphocytes with intermittent courses of interleukin-2 in patients with human immunodeficiency virus infection. A preliminary study. *N. Engl. J. Med.* 332:567–75

92. Kovacs JA, Vogel S, Albert JM, et al. 1996. Controlled trial of interleukin-2 infusions in patients infected with the human immunodeficiency virus. *N. Engl. J. Med.* 335:1350–56

92a. Mitsuyasu R, Pollard R, Gelman R, Weng D. 2000. *A randomized controlled phase II study of highly active antiretroviral therapy (HAART) with intermittent interleukin-2 (IL-2) by continuous IV (CIV) or subcutaneous (SC) routes in HIV-infected patients with CD4+ counts 50–350 cells/mm³: ACTG 328—results at 60 weeks.* Presented at Int. Congr. Drug Therapy in HIV Infect., 5th, Glasgow, Scotland

93. David D, Nait-Ighil L, Dupont B, et al. 2001. Rapid effect of interleukin-2 therapy in human immunodeficiency virus–infected patients whose CD4 cell counts increase only slightly in response to combined antiretroviral treatment. *J. Infect. Dis.* 183:730–35

94. Barouch DH, Santra S, Schmitz JE, et al. 2000. Control of viremia and prevention of clinical AIDS in rhesus monkeys by cytokine-augmented DNA vaccination. *Science* 290:486–92

95. Banchereau J, Steinman RM. 1998. Dendritic cells and the control of immunity. *Nature* 392:245–52

96. Banchereau J, Briere F, Caux C, et al. 2000. Immunobiology of dendritic cells. *Annu. Rev. Immunol.* 18:767–811

97. Dhodapkar MV, Bhardwaj N. 2000. Active immunization of humans with dendritic cells. *J. Clin. Immunol.* 20:167–74

98. Fong L, Engleman EG. 2000. Dendritic cells in cancer immunotherapy. *Annu. Rev. Immunol.* 18:245–73

99. Dhodapkar MV, Steinman RM, Sapp M, et al. 1999. Rapid generation of broad T-cell immunity in humans after a single injection of mature dendritic cells. *J. Clin. Invest.* 104:173–80

100. Dhodapkar MV, Krasovsky J, Steinman RM, Bhardwaj N. 2000. Mature dendritic cells boost functionally superior CD8(+) T-cell in humans without foreign helper epitopes. *J. Clin. Invest.* 105:R9–R14

101. MacDonald GH, Johnston RE. 2000. Role of dendritic cell targeting in Venezuelan equine encephalitis virus pathogenesis. *J. Virol.* 74:914–22

102. Hevey M, Negley D, Pushko P, et al. 1998. Marburg virus vaccines based upon alphavirus replicons protect guinea pigs and nonhuman primates. *Virology* 251:28–37

103. Davis NL, Brown KW, Johnston RE. 1996. A viral vaccine vector that expresses foreign genes in lymph nodes and protects against mucosal challenge. *J. Virol.* 70:3781–87

104. Davis NL, Caley IJ, Brown KW, et al. 2000. Vaccination of macaques against pathogenic simian immunodeficiency virus with Venezuelan equine encephalitis virus replicon particles. *J. Virol.* 74:371–78

105. Schneider J, Gilbert SC, Blanchard TJ, et al. 1998. Enhanced immunogenicity for CD8+ T cell induction and complete protective efficacy of malaria DNA vaccination by boosting with modified vaccinia virus Ankara. *Nat. Med.* 4:397–402

106. Amara RR, Villinger F, Altman JD, et al. 2001. Control of a mucosal challenge and prevention of AIDS by a multiprotein DNA/MVA vaccine. *Science* 292:69–74

Annu. Rev. Med. 2002. 53:173–88

THE EXPANDING PHARMACOPOEIA FOR BIPOLAR DISORDER

Philip B. Mitchell and Gin S. Malhi

School of Psychiatry, University of New South Wales, Sydney, NSW 2052, Australia; and Mood Disorders Unit, Prince of Wales Hospital, Randwick, NSW 2031, Australia

Key Words   mood stabilizers, carbamazepine, valproate, lamotrigine, olanzapine

■ **Abstract**   Over the past decade, the number of treatments available for bipolar disorder has undergone an extraordinary expansion. In that period, valproate and olanzapine have received regulatory approval in the United States for the acute treatment of mania, and carbamazepine has been indicated for this condition in many other countries. In addition to those agents, a number of other anticonvulsants (in particular lamotrigine, gabapentin, and topiramate) are in trials, as are the atypical antipsychotics clozapine and risperidone, and other novel compounds. This article critically reviews the evidence from controlled trials of these proposed "mood stabilizers," highlighting the strengths and limitations of the data for each compound. A major challenge to the field is the capacity to prove the prophylactic properties of agents for which effectiveness in acute mania and/or bipolar depression has been demonstrated. Finally, as the mechanisms of agents such as lithium are now becoming apparent, and the possibility of understanding the molecular defects underpinning the condition is no longer highly fanciful, the prospect of targeted therapies is considered feasible by both academia and the pharmaceutical industry.

INTRODUCTION

The past decade has witnessed an extraordinary expansion of treatments available for bipolar disorder. Ten years ago, lithium was the only approved agent for this condition. Since that time, valproate and olanzapine have received regulatory approval for the acute treatment of mania in the United States, and carbamazepine has been indicated for the acute treatment of mania and prophylaxis of bipolar disorder in many other countries. Furthermore, it is only in this past decade that the pharmaceutical industry has taken a serious interest in this condition. Large-scale clinical trial programs in bipolar disorder have been undertaken with a number of agents previously marketed for other disorders, in particular some of the anticonvulsants (such as valproate, lamotrigine, gabapentin, and topiramate) and atypical antipsychotics (olanzapine and risperidone). Several of the as-yet-unapproved compounds—particularly lamotrigine, gabapentin, and topiramate—are being widely prescribed off-label in the United States for patients with bipolar

0066-4219/02/0218-0173$14.00   **173**

disorder. Although no novel treatments developed specifically for bipolar disorder have reached the clinical arena, developmental research programs for identifying suitable targets for antibipolar drug action are in progress.

Bipolar disorder is a more common condition than previously thought, with recent community surveys indicating a lifetime prevalence of up to 1.6% (1). The illness comprises periods of mania or hypomania, depression, and "mixed episodes" or "dysphoric mania" (an admixture of manic and depressed symptoms). It is commonly subdivided into Bipolar I Disorder (at least one lifetime manic episode) and Bipolar II Disorder (only periods of hypomania and depression). Most patients experience multiple episodes at an average of 0.4 to 0.7 episodes per year, with each lasting three to six months (2). Illness occurring at a rate of at least four episodes in a 12-month period is termed rapid cycling. This condition remains disabling for the majority of sufferers. For example, Keck et al. (3) investigated the 12-month course of illness of 134 patients following hospitalization for the treatment of a manic or mixed episode. Syndromic recovery occurred in only 48%; even more dramatically, full symptom resolution was found in only 26%, and functional recovery in a mere 24%.

The specific molecular pathology underlying bipolar disorder is not understood; however, dysfunction of various components of intracellular signalling has been proposed (4). Although the condition is strongly genetic, with heritable factors explaining 70% to 80% of the etiological variance, this is a genetically complex trait and no specific genes have yet been identified. This lack of knowledge concerning the precise pathophysiological process places considerable limitations on the development of new therapies specifically tailored for this illness.

MOOD STABILIZERS

The term mood stabilizer has varying definitions. Whereas some authorities would view demonstration of antimanic and antidepressant qualities as sufficient to categorize an agent as a mood stabilizer, others would also expect proven prophylactic capacities (5). This issue has particular pertinence, since several of the new agents discussed in this article are already being described as mood stabilizers. Arguably, only lithium currently fulfils all three criteria (6).

Although globally lithium is still the most widely used agent for bipolar disorder, there has been a clear shift in treatment, with valproate and other new compounds being increasingly prescribed, particularly in U.S. practice. Features that have been found to predict poor response to lithium are dysphoric mania, rapid cycling, depression-mania-interval pattern (the clinical presentation of depressed episodes preceding periods of mania which are then followed by intervals of recovery), multiple episodes of illness, lack of family history, and comorbid medical illness or substance abuse. However, two particular strengths of lithium have emerged in the past few years. First, there is some evidence that lithium may substantially reduce suicide rates—an effect seemingly unrelated to its prophylactic effectiveness (7). Second, preclinical studies indicate that lithium may possess neuroprotective properties (4).

ANTICONVULSANTS

Carbamazepine

The pharmacological actions of carbamazepine include stabilization of sodium and potassium channels, reduction of calcium fluxes, upregulation of $GABA_B$ receptors, and agonism and antagonism of adenosine receptors. The specific mode of mood-stabilizing action, however, remains to be elucidated. The initial report on the efficacy of carbamazepine in bipolar disorder was that of the Japanese psychiatrist Takezaki, who had been prescribing this agent for epilepsy (8). Okuma, also in Japan, subsequently undertook the first controlled studies. However, it was not until Ballenger and Post (9, 10) published the first U.S. studies that widespread international interest in carbamazepine as a mood stabilizer was aroused. Because many of the early studies were of limited methodological rigor, only those reported in peer-reviewed journals are discussed in this review.

ACUTE TREATMENT OF MANIA/MIXED EPISODES   With a few exceptions, the quality of the randomized controlled studies of carbamazepine in acute mania has been surprisingly poor, and relatively few subjects have been involved. There have been only two double-blind placebo-controlled monotherapy trials, involving a total of just 31 subjects (9–11); both found carbamazepine to be effective. The study of Post et al. (10) found responders more likely than nonresponders to be dysphoric or show a rapid-cycling pattern. Supporting those findings, two other double-blind trials found the combination of carbamazepine and a typical antipsychotic more effective than the antipsychotic alone (12, 13).

Three double-blind monotherapy trials have compared the efficacies of carbamazepine and lithium (14–16). Those trials found no overall significant difference between the two agents, though the numbers were small and intention-to-treat analyses were not undertaken. In the Lerer et al. study (14), a measure of overall improvement (the Clinical Global Impression scale) significantly favored lithium, but the other scales did not distinguish between the treatments. Two other studies (17, 18) compared carbamazepine and lithium when added to typical antipsychotic medications, and again found no difference between groups. In a meta-analysis including some of these studies, Emilien et al. (19) concluded that the acute antimanic efficacies of lithium and carbamazepine are the same.

ACUTE TREATMENT OF BIPOLAR DEPRESSION   There have been no placebo-controlled studies of carbamazepine monotherapy in distinct groups with bipolar depression. Although there have been some controlled studies of samples that include both bipolar and unipolar depressed patients (20), it is not possible to distinguish bipolar disorder response rates from those reports. The largest open study found that 63% of patients remitted (21). Post et al. (22) reported that cerebrospinal fluid levels of the active −10,11-epoxide metabolite of carbamazepine correlated with antidepressant efficacy in a mixed bipolar/unipolar group.

PROPHYLAXIS   There has only been one placebo-controlled prophylactic study of carbamazepine (23). This small study of 22 patients over one year failed to demonstrate any significant superiority to placebo, though there was a trend favoring carbamazepine. Only five methodologically acceptable randomized double-blind comparative prophylactic studies against lithium have been reported (15, 24–27), most of which found no difference between the two treatments. A meta-analysis of the first four of these studies, however, found no convincing evidence that carbamazepine had any prophylactic efficacy in bipolar disorder (28). Nevertheless, the recent study by Denicoff et al. (27) is worthy of comment. Fifty-two outpatients with bipolar disorder were randomized in a double-blind fashion to one year of lithium or carbamazepine, with crossover to the opposite drug in the second year and allocation to the combination in the third year. The results indicated that lithium was more effective than carbamazepine in the prophylaxis of mania, but not depression, and that the combination of lithium and carbamazepine was better than either monotherapy. Consistent with this, Greil et al. (29), in an open randomized prospective study of lithium and carbamazepine over 2.5 years, found lithium superior in bipolar I patients, with a lower recurrence rate. However, they found no difference between response rates in bipolar II patients. There have been no head-to-head prophylactic studies comparing lithium and carbamazepine in rapid-cycling patients.

COMBINATION THERAPIES   Substantial evidence suggests enhanced efficacy with the combination of lithium and carbamazepine. Kramlinger & Post reported—for both acute mania (30) and depression (31)—that a significant proportion of nonresponders in double-blind trials of carbamazepine responded to blind addition of lithium. With regard to prophylaxis, Denicoff et al. (27) found the combination more effective than either lithium or carbamazepine monotherapy.

SAFETY ISSUES   There is no indication of differing rates of adverse effects of carbamazepine in bipolar versus epileptic populations. The high risk of spina bifida in fetuses exposed to maternal carbamazepine is a significant issue for females with bipolar disorder, since the illness usually arises in the reproductive years. Carbamazepine appears to be relatively safe during breastfeeding, though no reports are specific to bipolar disorder.

OVERVIEW AS A MOOD STABILIZER   Although studies in acute mania indicate superiority to placebo and comparable efficacy to lithium, the number of subjects involved in most studies has been small. The evidence for prophylaxis is contentious. The single placebo-controlled maintenance study found only a trend favoring carbamazepine (23). Although the overall response rates of carbamazepine and lithium are the same, a meta-analysis (28) reported no convincing evidence of prophylactic benefit. Moreover, the more recent trials of Denicoff et al. (27) and Greil et al. (29) found carbamazepine less effective than lithium, particularly in bipolar I patients. Such studies suggest that carbamazepine is an effective mood stabilizer but probably less potent than lithium, particularly in prophylaxis. There is evidence, though, that the combination of carbamazepine and lithium is more effective than either agent alone (27). With regard to the rapid-cycling and dysphoric-mania subgroups, there is some, albeit slight, evidence of particular efficacy (10), but this should be regarded cautiously in the absence of direct head-to-head comparisons with lithium.

Valproate

Valproate (valproic acid) is usually administered as its sodium salt. Other available forms include valpromide (the amide of valproic acid) and divalproex sodium (a combination of sodium valproate and valproic acid in a 1:1 molar ratio). In this section, the term valproate covers all forms unless specified otherwise. Whereas the antiepileptic effect of valproate is thought to be mediated via the GABAergic system, its mood-stabilizing action is postulated to be on excitatory neurotransmission and excitatory membranes. Like lithium, valproate reduces the activity of the enzymes protein kinase C (PKC) and glycogen synthase kinase 3β (GSK 3β), and levels of the protein MARCKS (myristoylated alanine rich C kinase substrate), which is the most prominent substrate of PKC in the brain (4). The first report of a potential role for valproate in bipolar disorder was that of the French psychiatrist Lambert, who prescribed valpromide for a broad range of psychiatric conditions while he was involved in its initial trials in epileptic patients (8).

ACUTE TREATMENT OF MANIA/MIXED EPISODES   Three studies of valproate in the treatment of mania, involving double-blind comparisons with placebo and/or lithium, have been published in peer-reviewed journals (32–34). The trial of Pope et al. (32), the first of the two double-blind placebo-controlled parallel group studies of divalproex, found that agent significantly more effective than placebo. Freeman et al. (33) undertook the first double-blind active comparator study, comparing sodium valproate and lithium. Most comparisons in that trial demonstrated no differences between these two medications, though several favored lithium. When only subjects with mixed mania were considered, valproate was found to be more effective than lithium. As in the study of Pope et al. (32), however, numbers were relatively small, with less than 20 subjects in each arm.

The study of Bowden et al. (34) represented the pivotal confirmation of the comparative efficacy of valproate against placebo and lithium. The three arms in this double-blind study were divalproex sodium, lithium, and placebo. This study represented the largest-ever parallel group trial in acute mania, with a total of 179 patients. The degree of improvement in the two active drug groups was significantly greater than that observed in the placebo group, but there was no significant difference between divalproex and lithium. Furthermore, there was no difference in response rates between lithium and divalproex in subjects with rapid-cycling illness. Swann et al. (35) later reported that, in this sample, valproate was more effective than lithium in those with dysphoric mania—defined by the presence of two or more depressed symptoms in addition to the manic syndrome—a finding consistent with the previous report of Freeman et al. (33). A further subanalysis by Swann et al. (36) found divalproex more effective than lithium in subjects with more than nine previous episodes, though the finding may have been biased by the inclusion of a high proportion of lithium-refractory patients. A subsequent investigation of the relationship between serum valproate concentrations and response to mania in this trial (37) is the only report of this association. This study found that patients with valproate concentrations of at least 45 μg/ml were more likely than patients with lower levels to show an improvement. It should be noted, though, that there have been no studies of randomly allocated doses or concentration ranges of valproate, for either the acute treatment of mania or its prophylaxis.

A meta-analysis of these controlled valproate studies (19) found no significant difference in effectiveness between lithium and valproate. Consistent with these studies, Mueller-Oerlinghausen et al. (38) recently reported on a randomized double-blind placebo-controlled comparison of sodium valproate as an adjunct to neuroleptic medication. The proportion of responders was significantly higher in the group receiving the combination of valproate and a neuroleptic.

Oral loading of valproate may lead to a more rapid antimanic response. In an open random-assignment comparison with blind evaluators, McElroy et al. (39) found 20 mg/kg divalproex to be as effective as haloperidol in patients with psychotic mania, with both groups demonstrating their greatest rate of improvement in the first three days. A subsequent double-blind study found that oral loading (30 mg/kg for two days, followed by 20 mg/kg) achieved serum concentrations of >50 μg/ml in 84% of patients by day 3, whereas only 30% of the non–loading-dose subjects achieved such levels (40). This loading dosage did not cause a greater incidence of side effects. Unfortunately, the study was insufficiently powered to confirm a more rapid rate of response in the oral loading group. Although the accumulated data indicate a more rapid response with oral loading, a confirmatory double-blind comparison of standard and oral loading doses in a sufficiently large sample has yet to be reported. However, consistent with this suggestion of more rapid response with oral loading, several open studies indicate the benefit of intravenous loading (41).

Only one comparison of sodium valproate and carbamazepine in the acute treatment of mania has been reported. In a randomly allocated open loading-dose comparison with blinded evaluators, Vasudev et al. (42) found that the valproate group experienced significantly more improvement than the carbamazepine group.

ACUTE TREATMENT OF DEPRESSION   There have been no controlled studies of valproate for acute treatment of bipolar depression. Of interest, therefore, is a recent double-blind trial (43) of patients with bipolar depression that found the addition of a second mood stabilizer (lithium or divalproex) to be as effective, though less well-tolerated, as adding the antidepressant paroxetine to the existing mood-stabilizer regimen.

PROPHYLAXIS   There has been only one double-blind trial of the prophylactic value of sodium valproate for bipolar disorder (44). That study of 372 subjects recently recovered from a manic episode compared responses to divalproex, lithium, and placebo over one year. There was no difference in the primary outcome measure—time to the development of any mood disorder—between these three groups. It is possible that the failure to distinguish lithium or divalproex from placebo may have been related to the inclusion of milder or less recurrent forms of bipolar disorder, perhaps due to the requirement that subjects had to have remitted and be randomized to treatment within three months of the onset of a manic episode. The largest open randomized study (45) compared valpromide and lithium in a mixed group of bipolar and recurrent unipolar affective disorder patients over an 18-month period. Patients experienced a reduction in the number of both depressed and manic episodes with both lithium and valpromide, but no breakdown of recurrence rates for the two disorders was reported, nor were detailed statistical analyses provided. There is no detail in the Bowden et al. (44) maintenance trial concerning patients with rapid-cycling illness. Data from open studies of rapid-cycling patients (46) suggest prophylactic antimanic and antimixed effects, but poor antidepressant activity.

COMBINATION THERAPIES   Denicoff et al. (47) reported the outcome of a one-year single-blind study comparing the efficacy of valproate plus lithium in 24 outpatients who had completed a three-year trial comparing lithium, carbamazepine, and their combination. The investigators found that 6 of the 18 evaluable patients had moderate or marked responses to valproate plus lithium, 4 of whom had not responded to any previous treatment.

SAFETY ISSUES   In general, there is no indication of differing rates of adverse effects of valproate in subjects with bipolar disorder versus those with epilepsy. The main area of debate concerns the prevalence of polycystic ovary syndrome. One report has suggested that this syndrome is not seen in women with bipolar disorder (48). Although there have been no specific studies of the safety of valproate in pregnancy in bipolar disorder, there is no reason to consider it other than a markedly teratogenic agent, as has been reported in the epilepsy literature. Reports on breastfeeding mothers with bipolar disorder indicate that infant serum levels of valproate are low, at 1% to 6% of maternal concentrations (49).

OVERVIEW AS A MOOD STABILIZER   Valproate has been confirmed as an effective antimanic agent of comparable efficacy to lithium, and as more effective than lithium in mixed episodes/dysphoric mania. Considerable, though not definitive, data suggest that loading doses may prompt more rapid antimanic response. There is little evidence for a significant antidepressant effect. As yet, there is no controlled support for prophylactic capacity, though this is probably because of methodological difficulties. Furthermore, there are no strong data concerning valproate's effect in rapid-cycling bipolar disorder. Limited evidence suggests that the combination with lithium may be more effective than the respective monotherapies.

Lamotrigine

Lamotrigine was initially developed as an adjunctive therapy for partial and secondary generalized tonic-clonic seizures. Pharmacological actions include the stabilization of neuronal membranes and release of excitatory amino acids (particularly glutamate) by blocking voltage-dependent sodium, calcium, and potassium channels. Mood-elevating effects observed in epileptic patients encouraged clinical application of lamotrigine in mood disorders. The first major open trial found a marked response in 48% of subjects with depressed presentations and in 81% of those with manic, hypomanic, or mixed episodes (50). A later subanalysis of the same study found no substantive differences in response between those with rapid- compared to non-rapid-cycling illness (51).

ACUTE TREATMENT OF MANIA/MIXED EPISODES   No placebo-controlled trials in patients with mania or mixed episodes have been reported. One small randomized comparison of lamotrigine and lithium in acute mania has been published (52). No differences in efficacy were demonstrated, but the trial included only 30 subjects.

ACUTE TREATMENT OF DEPRESSION   A randomized double-blind controlled study compared two doses of lamotrigine (50 mg and 200 mg) with placebo in bipolar I patients in the depressed phase (53). That trial of 195 subjects constituted the largest-ever controlled study of bipolar depression. Lamotrigine was significantly more effective than placebo at a dose of 200 mg daily. The 50 mg dosage showed some antidepressant effect, albeit less robust. Significantly, rates of mania were the same on lamotrigine as on placebo.

PROPHYLAXIS   No controlled prophylactic trials of lamotrigine in non-rapid-cycling bipolar disorder have been published. A potential maintenance role for lamotrigine was indicated in an open trial undertaken through the Stanley Foundation Bipolar Network (54), which found that 65% of patients were very much or much improved. Recently, Calabrese et al. (55) published the outcome of a double-blind placebo-controlled trial of lamotrigine over six months in 182 patients with rapid-cycling illness. There was no significant difference between treatments in the primary outcome measure—time to additional pharmacotherapy for emerging symptoms. Neither the number of episodes nor time to first episode in each treatment group was reported. Some secondary measures, such as survival time in the study and study completion without relapse, favored lamotrigine, particularly for bipolar II patients.

Frye et al. (56) undertook a placebo-controlled randomized crossover trial of lamotrigine and gabapentin in a mixed group of affective-disorder patients, most of whom had refractory bipolar (mainly rapid-cycling) disorder. Lamotrigine was more effective than both gabapentin and placebo in terms of overall global improvement, but unfortunately the findings were not broken down into bipolar and unipolar subgroups. There was no difference between gabapentin and placebo.

SAFETY ISSUES   The major safety issue with lamotrigine in both epilepsy and bipolar disorder populations is the development of serious rash, particularly that related to the potentially fatal Stevens-Johnson syndrome. The risk is minimized by slow dose titration and by reduced dosage when prescribed with valproate.

OVERVIEW AS A MOOD STABILIZER   Currently, the only substantively supported action of lamotrigine in bipolar disorder is in depression (53). This apparent antidepressant effect of lamotrigine, if replicated, would distinguish this putative mood stabilizer from lithium, carbamazepine, and valproate, which do not possess significant antidepressant properties. There is some provisional evidence that lamotrigine may be effective for rapid-cycling illness (55, 56), but the failure of the study of Calabrese et al. (55) to demonstrate an effect on the number of newly emerging episodes indicates that lamotrigine lacks a robust prophylactic effect on that form of the illness. There is no convincing evidence of an antimanic effect, and theoretically, the requirement for slow dose titration makes lamotrigine an unlikely candidate for the management of acute mania, where the clinical imperative is for rapid symptomatic and behavioral control.

Other Anticonvulsants

GABAPENTIN   Gabapentin is a recently developed anticonvulsant that is effective for treatment-refractory partial seizures and secondary generalized tonic-clonic seizures. It was synthesized to be a GABA structural analogue. Several studies noted a possible mood-enhancing effect while gabapentin was in trials as an anticonvulsant. However, only two controlled trials have been published (56, 57). As discussed above, the study of Frye et al. (56) found gabapentin less effective than lamotrigine and no more effective than placebo. Another negative finding—this time in a large placebo-controlled trial of gabapentin as an adjunctive agent in mania—has been reported recently (57). Therefore, on current evidence, it appears that gabapentin does not possess significant mood-stabilizing properties.

TOPIRAMATE   Topiramate, a new antiepileptic drug used as adjunctive therapy for partial-onset seizures, enhances GABA activity and antagonizes glutamate at non-NDMA receptors; however, its antiepileptic mechanism of action is unknown. To date, no double-blind controlled reports of its effectiveness in bipolar disorder have been published. The first published open report was that of Marcotte (58), whose retrospective case review study found that half of his treatment-refractory rapid-cycling bipolar patients had demonstrated a marked or moderate improvement on topiramate. More recently, the Stanley Foundation Bipolar Outcome Network evaluated open-label topiramate in bipolar outpatients (59). The main benefit occurred in those who were manic at the time topiramate treatment commenced. Topiramate was associated with reduction of both appetite and weight, a potentially advantageous clinical effect contrasted with the weight gain commonly observed with other mood-stabilizing agents. It is too early in the research development phase of topiramate to make an informed comment on its mood-stabilizing qualities.

ANTIPSYCHOTICS

From the time of their introduction into clinical practice, typical antipsychotic drugs have been widely used in the treatment of bipolar disorder. In general, though, clinical trials have found their value limited. For example, one meta-analysis of the double-blind randomized studies comparing typical antipsychotics with lithium in the treatment of mania reported the latter to be significantly more effective (60). Despite a lack of controlled studies confirming the efficacy of neuroleptics as maintenance agents, they are commonly used prophylactically in clinical practice, particularly in Europe. The major current interest lies with the atypical antipsychotics clozapine, olanzapine, and risperidone, as increasing evidence suggests that they may possess specific mood-stabilizing properties, rather than merely acting as tranquilizing agents. Also, a few case reports suggest that quetiapine may be effective (61). There have been no studies of other atypical agents such as ziprasidone.

Clozapine

There have been no double-blind controlled trials of clozapine in bipolar disorder. However, several reports of an apparent therapeutic effect began to appear within a few years of its reintroduction to the U.S. market as a treatment for refractory schizophrenia. For example, one prospective open study concluded that clozapine is effective in mania and bipolar-type schizoaffective disorder (62). Other open studies have found clozapine effective in the prophylaxis of bipolar and schizoaffective disorders, either as monotherapy or as an adjunct to other mood stabilizers.

Olanzapine

Potential mood-stabilizing properties of olanzapine were first noted during trials in schizoaffective disorder. There have been two placebo-controlled double-blind trials of olanzapine in the acute treatment of mania (63, 64). Both studies found olanzapine more effective than placebo. In the first study (63), olanzapine produced statistically significant reductions in mania severity scores, and significantly more patients (48.6%) responded to olanzapine than to placebo (24.2%). The second double-blind trial studied the effects of 5–20 mg daily in 55 patients with mania or a mixed state (64). Olanzapine-treated patients demonstrated a statistically significant improvement that was emergent after only one week of treatment. Furthermore, in comparison to placebo-treated patients, a greater proportion responded (65% versus 43%) and returned to euthymia (61% versus 36%), despite a relatively high placebo response. To date, no active comparator trials of olanzapine against typical neuroleptics such as haloperidol, or mood stabilizers such as lithium or valproate, have been published. Although there are promising preliminary reports of the efficacy of olanzapine in major depression, there have been no specific studies in bipolar depressed groups. Similarly, there have been no controlled studies of olanzapine in the prophylaxis of bipolar disorder, with or without a rapid-cycling pattern, though a recent open 12-month continuation phase trial has reported persisting benefit (65). Until such controlled trials are reported, there remains a lingering concern that olanzapine acts no differently in mania than the typical neuroleptics.

Risperidone

No placebo-controlled studies of risperidone in bipolar disorders have been published. There has been, however, one randomized double-blind comparison with haloperidol and lithium in the treatment of mania (66). That study concluded that risperidone's efficacy was equivalent to lithium's, but because of its small number of subjects, its statistical power was insufficient to exclude therapeutic nonequivalence. Most reports concerning risperidone have consisted of single cases or open-label studies, such as the retrospective review (67) which found that manic patients responded to adjunctive risperidone therapy. However, the data are too preliminary as yet to allow definitive comment on any mood-stabilizing properties of risperidone.

OTHER TREATMENTS

The other major class of medications reported to be effective in bipolar disorder is the calcium channel blockers (CCBs). Several double-blind controlled trials (68) have shown that verapamil significantly reduces manic symptoms. The other CCB of note is nimodipine, which has demonstrated efficacy in rapid-cycling bipolar disorder, either as monotherapy (69) or as an adjunct to other mood stabilizers (70). Prophylactic use of CCBs in bipolar disorder has not been investigated. Additionally, several agents hypothesized to act on cellular signal transduction pathways have been studied recently in bipolar disorder, although trials have been few, the number of participants has generally been low, and most trials have employed open designs. One exception, a double-blind placebo-controlled study (71) that examined the prophylactic effect of omega-3 fatty acids, found significant improvement in the short-term course of the illness. (A possible theoretical explanation is the reduction by omega-3 fatty acids of the activity of signal pathways associated with phosphatidylinositol, arachidonic acid, and other systems.) Therapy involving cholinergic systems has also been examined with two different compounds. First, the coadministration of choline and lithium was found to produce a synergistic effect in a small case series (72). Second, donepezil—a reversible acetylcholinesterase inhibitor—was found to be effective for 50% of a treatment-resistant sample (73). Tamoxifen citrate also acts on second messenger pathways by inhibiting PKC and has been shown, in a preliminary single-blind study, to diminish manic symptoms (74).

DISCUSSION

Several themes emerge from the research to date. First, most of the compounds with proven efficacy were originally developed for other conditions, such as epilepsy or schizophrenia, with their effect on mood states being initially observed during clinical trials for those illnesses. Only now, with increasing understanding of some of the mechanisms of agents such as lithium, is the pharmaceutical industry seriously considering the development of novel agents targeted at specific enzymes or receptors. Other approaches to discovering drug targets, such as potential susceptibility genes identified in genetic studies, are also in progress.

Second, it is becoming apparent that whereas it is possible, albeit difficult, to demonstrate acute effects in mania, mixed episodes, and bipolar depression, confirming the prophylactic capacity of a compound is much more complex. There are several reasons for this. Bipolar disorder is by its very nature capricious—it may present in at least three forms (depression, hypomania/mania, or mixed episodes), and these phasic presentations are usually unpredictable and irregular. Furthermore, those patients likely to agree to (or eligible to be ethically considered for) such trials are by necessity those with less severe and less recurrent illness—the very group in which it is difficult to distinguish an active compound from placebo over short periods such as 12 months. This difficulty means that few drugs have confirmed prophylactic capacity—surely the most convincing evidence of an agent being a true mood stabilizer. New methodologies for proving long-term effectiveness are needed. Examples such as those of the Stanley Foundation Network (see 59) and the NIMH-sponsored Systematic Treatment Enhancement Program for Bipolar Disorder (STEP-BD) of Sachs et al. (www.stepbd.org) are worthy of note.

Despite these concerns, it must be acknowledged that major advances have occurred in the recognition and development of effective agents for the treatment of bipolar disorder in the past two decades, with a marked acceleration of progress in the most recent five to ten years. The advent of these new agents means that more patients who were previously refractory to or intolerant of lithium may be successfully treated. The pharmacotherapy of bipolar disorder has been transformed from a field of sterility and stagnation to one of creativity and vigor within this short period. This clinical research area is perhaps on the threshold of comprehending both the molecular pathologies underlying the disorder and the therapeutic mechanisms of these agents. These advances will eventually enable the development of treatments specifically targeted at causative defects—a truly marvelous prospect for those whose lives continue to be devastated by bipolar disorder.

Visit the Annual Reviews home page at www.AnnualReviews.org

LITERATURE CITED

1. Kessler RC, McGonagle KA, Zhao S, et al. 1994. Lifetime and 12-month prevalence of DSM-III-R psychiatric disorders in the United States. *Arch. Gen. Psychiatry* 51:8–19

2. Angst J, Selloro R. 2000. Historical perspectives and natural history of bipolar disorder. *Biol. Psychiatry* 48:445–57

3. Keck PE Jr, McElroy SL, Strakowski SM, et al. 1998. 12-month outcome of patients with bipolar disorder following hospitalisation for a manic or mixed episode. *Am. J. Psychiatry* 155:646–52

4. Manji HK, Moore GJ, Rajkowska G, et al. 2000. Neuroplasticity and cellular resilience in mood disorders. *Mol. Psychiatry* 5:578–93

5. Schou M. 1997. Forty years of lithium treatment. *Arch. Gen. Psychiatry* 54:9–13

6. Potter WZ Ozcan ME. 1998. Methodological considerations for the development of new treatments for bipolar disorder. *Austr. NZ J. Psychiatry* 33:S84–S98

7. Goodwin FK, Ghaemi SN. 1999. The impact of the discovery of lithium on psychiatric thought and practice in the USA and Europe. *Austr. NZ J. Psychiatry* 33:S54–S64

8. Healey D. 2000. *The Psychopharmacologists*, Vol. III. New York: Oxford Univ. Press

9. Ballenger JC, Post RM. 1980. Carbamazepine in manic-depressive illness: a new treatment. *Am. J. Psychiatry* 137:782–90

10. Post RM, Uhde TW, Roy-Byrne PP, et al. 1987. Correlates of antimanic response to carbamazepine. *Psychiatry Res.* 21:71–83

11. Goncalves N, Stoll KD. 1985. Carbamazepine in manic syndromes. A controlled double-blind study. *Nervenarzt* 56:43–47

12. Klein E, Bental E Lerer B, Belmaker RH. 1984. Carbamazepine and haloperidol v placebo and haloperidol in excited psychoses. *Arch. Gen. Psychiatry* 41:165–70

13. Moller HJ, Kissling W, Riehl T, et al. 1989. Doubleblind evaluation of the antimanic properties of carbamazepine as a comedication to haloperidol. *Prog. Neuro-Psychopharm. Biol. Psychiatry* 13:127–36

14. Lerer B, Moore N, Meyendorff E, et al. 1987. Carbamazepine versus lithium in mania: a double-blind study. *J. Clin. Psychiatry* 48:89–93

15. Lusznat RM, Murphy DP, Nunn CMH. 1988. Carbamazepine vs lithium in the treatment and prophylaxis of mania. *Br. J. Psychiatry* 153:198–204

16. Small JG, Klapper MH, Milstein V, et al. 1991. Carbamazepine compared with lithium in the treatment of mania. *Arch. Gen. Psychiatry* 48:915–21

17. Lenzi A, Lazzerini F, Grossi E, et al. 1986. Use of carbamazepine in acute psychosis: a controlled study. *J. Int. Med. Res.* 14:78–84

18. Okuma T, Yamashita I, Takahashi R, et al. 1990. Comparison of the antimanic efficacy of carbamazepine and lithium carbonate by double-blind controlled study. *Pharmacopsychiatry* 23:143–50

19. Emilien G, Maloteaux JM, Seghers A,

et al. 1996. Lithium compared to valproic acid and carbamazepine in the treatment of mania: a statistical meta-analysis. *Eur. Neuropsychopharmacol.* 6:245–52

20. Post RM, Uhde TW, Roy-Byrne P, et al. 1986. Antidepressant effects of carbamazepine. *Am. J. Psychiatry* 143:29–34

21. Dilsaver SC, Swann SC, Chen Y-W, et al. 1996. Treatment of bipolar depression with carbamazepine: results of an open study. *Biol. Psychiatry* 40:935–37

22. Post RM, Uhde TW, Ballenger JC, et al. 1983. Carbamazepine and its −10,11-epoxide metabolite in plasma and CSF. *Arch. Gen. Psychiatry* 40:673–76

23. Okuma T, Inanaga K, Otsuki S, et al. 1981. A preliminary double-blind study on the efficacy of carbamazepine in prophylaxis of manic-depressive illness. *Psychopharmacology* 73:95–96

24. Watkins SE, Callender K, Thomas DR, et al. 1987. The effect of carbamazepine and lithium on remission from affective illness. *Br. J. Psychiatry* 150:180–82

25. Placidi GF, Lenzi A, Lazzerini F, et al. 1986. The comparative efficacy and safety of carbamazepine versus lithium: a randomized, double-blind 3-year trial in 83 patients. *J. Clin. Psychiatry* 47:490–94

26. Coxhead N, Silverstone T, Cookson J. 1992. Carbamazepine versus lithium in the prophylaxis of bipolar affective disorder. *Acta Psychiatr. Scand.* 85:114–18

27. Denicoff KD, Smith-Jackson EE, Disney ER, et al. 1997. Comparative prophylactic efficacy of lithium, carbamazepine, and the combination in bipolar disorder. *J. Clin. Psychiatry* 58:470–78

28. Dardennes R, Even C, Bange F, et al. 1995. Comparison of carbamazepine and lithium in the prophylaxis of bipolar disorders: a meta-analysis. *Br. J. Psychiatry* 166:378–81

29. Greil W, Ludwig-Mayerhofer W, Erazo N, et al. 1997. Lithium versus carbamazepine in the maintenance treatment of bipolar disorders: a randomized study. *J. Affect. Disord.* 43:151–61

30. Kramlinger KG, Post RM. 1989. Adding lithium carbonate to carbamazepine: antimanic efficacy in treatment-resistant mania. *Acta Psychiatr. Scand.* 79:378–85

31. Kramlinger KG, Post RM. 1989. The addition of lithium to carbamazepine. *Arch. Gen. Psychiatry* 46:794–800

32. Pope HG, McElroy SL, Keck PE, et al. 1991. Valproate in the treatment of acute mania: a placebo-controlled study. *Arch. Gen. Psychiatry* 48:62–68

33. Freeman TW, Clothier JL, Pazzaglia P, et al. 1992. A double-blind comparison of valproate and lithium in the treatment of acute mania. *Am. J. Psychiatry* 149:108–11

34. Bowden CL, Brugger AM, Swann AC, et al. 1994. Efficacy of divalproex vs lithium and placebo in the treatment of mania. *JAMA* 271:918–24

35. Swann AC, Bowden CL, Morris D, et al. 1997. Depression during mania: treatment response to lithium or divalproex. *Arch. Gen. Psychiatry* 54:37–42

36. Swann AC, Bowden CL, Calabrese JR, et al. 2000. Mania: differential effects of previous depressive and manic episodes on response to treatment. *Acta Psychiatr. Scand.* 101:444–51

37. Bowden CL, Janicak PG, Orsulak P, et al. 1996. Relation to serum valproate concentration to response in mania. *Am. J. Psychiatry* 153:765–70

38. Mueller-Oerlinghausen B, Retzow A, Henn FA, et al. 2000. Valproate as an adjunct to neuroleptic medication for the treatment of acute episodes of mania: a prospective, randomized, double-blind, placebo-controlled, multicentre study. *J. Clin. Psychopharmacol.* 20:195–203

39. McElroy SL, Keck PE, Stanton SP, et al. 1996. A randomized comparison of divalproex oral loading versus haloperidol in the initial treatment of acute psychotic mania. *J. Clin. Psychiatry* 57:142–46

40. Hirschfeld RMA, Allen MH, McEvoy JP, et al. 1999. Safety and tolerability of oral loading divalproex sodium in acutely

manic bipolar patients. *J. Clin. Psychiatry* 60:815–18

41. Grunze H, Erfurther A, Amann B, et al. 1999. Intravenous valproate loading in acutely manic and depressed bipolar I patients. *J. Clin. Psychopharmacol.* 19:303–9

42. Vasudev K, Goswami U, Kohli K. 2000. Carbamazepine and valproate monotherapy: feasibility, relative safety and efficacy, and therapeutic drug monitoring in manic disorder. *Psychopharmacology* 150:15–23

43. Young LT, Joffe RT, Robb JC, et al. 2000. Double-blind comparison of addition of a second mood stabilizer versus an antidepressant to an initial mood stabilizer for treatment of patients with bipolar depression. *Am. J. Psychiatry* 157:124–26

44. Bowden CL, Calabrese JR, McElroy SL, et al. 2000. A randomized, placebo-controlled 12-month trial of divalproex and lithium in treatment of outpatients with bipolar I disorder. *Arch. Gen. Psychiatry* 57:481–89

45. Lambert PA, Venaud G. 1992. Comparative study of valpromide versus lithium as prophylactic treatment in affective disorders. *Nervure J. Psychiatrie* 7:1–9

46. Calabrese JR, Rapport DJ, Kimmel SE, et al. 1993. Rapid cycling bipolar disorder and its treatment with valproate. *Can. J. Psychiatry* 38:57–60

47. Denicoff KD, Smith-Jackson EE, Bryan AL, et al. 1997. Valproate prophylaxis in a prospective clinical trial of refractory bipolar disorder. *Am. J. Psychiatry* 154:1456–58

48. Rasgon NL, Altshuler LL, Gudeman D, et al. 2000. Medication status and polycystic ovary syndrome in women with bipolar disorder: a preliminary report. *J. Clin. Psychiatry* 61:173–78

49. Piontek CM, Baab S, Peindl KS, et al. 2000. Serum valproate levels in six breast-feeding mother-infant pairs. *J. Clin. Psychiatry* 61:170–72

50. Calabrese JR, Bowden CL, McElroy SL, et al. 1999. Spectrum of activity of lamot-rigine in treatment-refractory bipolar disorder. *Am. J. Psychiatry* 156:1019–23

51. Bowden CL, Calabrese JR, McElroy SL, et al. 1999. The efficacy of lamotrigine in rapid cycling and non–rapid cycling patients with bipolar disorder. *Biol. Psychiatry* 45:953–58

52. Ichim L, Berk M, Brook S. 2000. Lamotrigine compared with lithium in mania: a double-blind randomized controlled trial. *Annals Clin. Psychiatry* 12:5–10

53. Calabrese JR, Bowden CL, Sachs GS, et al. 1999. A double-blind placebo-controlled study of lamotrigine monotherapy in outpatients with bipolar I depression. *J. Clin. Psychiatry* 60:79–88

54. Suppes T, Brown ES, McElroy SL, et al. 1999. Lamotrigine for the treatment of bipolar disorder: a clinical case series. *J. Affect. Disord.* 53:95–98

55. Calabrese JR, Suppes T, Bowden CL, et al. 2000. A double-blind, placebo-controlled, prophylaxis study of lamotrigine in rapid-cycling bipolar disorder. *J. Clin. Psychiatry* 61:841–50

56. Frye MA, Ketter TA, Kimbrell TA, et al. 2000. A placebo-controlled study of lamotrigine and gabapentin monotherapy in refractory mood disorders. *J. Clin. Psychopharmacol* 20:607–14

57. Pande AC, Crockatt JG, Janney CA, et al. 2000. Gabapentin in bipolar disorder: a placebo-controlled trial of adjunctive therapy. *Bipolar Disord.* 2:249–55

58. Marcotte D. 1998. Use of topiramate, a new anti-epileptic as a mood stabilizer. *J. Affect. Disord.* 50:245–51

59. McElroy SL, Suppes T, Keck PE, et al. 2000. Open-label adjunctive topiramate in the treatment of bipolar disorders. *Biol. Psychiatry* 47:1025–33

60. Janicak PG, Newman RH, Davis JM. 1992. Advances in the treatment of manic and related disorders: a reappraisal. *Psychiatr. Ann.* 22:92–103

61. Ghaemi SN, Goodwin FK. 1999. Use of atypical antipsychotic agents in bipolar and schizoaffective disorders: review of the

empirical literature. *J. Clin. Psychopharmacol.* 19:354–61

62. Calabrese JR, Kimmell SE, Woyshville MJ, et al. 1996. Clozapine for treatment of refractory mania. *Am. J. Psychiatry* 153:759–64

63. Tohen M, Sanger TM, McElroy SL, et al. 1999. The Olanzapine HGEH Study Group. Olanzapine versus placebo in the treatment of acute mania. *Am. J. Psychiatry* 156:702–9

64. Tohen M, Jacobs TG, Grundy SL, et al. 2000. Efficacy of olanzapine in acute bipolar mania: a double-blind, placebo-controlled study. *Arch. Gen. Psychiatry* 57:841–49

65. Sanger TM, Grundy SL, Gibson PJ, et al. 2001. Long-term olanzapine therapy in the treatment of bipolar I disorder: an open-label continuation phase study. *J. Clin. Psychiatry* 62:273–81

66. Segal J, Berk M, Brook S. 1998. Risperidone compared with both lithium and haloperidol in mania: a double-blind randomized controlled trial. *Clin. Neuropharmacol.* 21:176–80

67. Keck PE Jr, Wilson DR, Strakowski SM, et al. 1995. Clinical predictors of acute risperidone response in schizophrenia, schizoaffective disorder, and psy-chotic mood disorders. *J. Clin. Psychiatry* 56:466–70

68. Janicak PG, Sharma RP, Pandey G, et al. 1998. Verapamil for the treatment of acute mania: a double-blind, placebo-controlled trial. *Am. J. Psychiatry* 155:972–73

69. Pazzaglia PJ, Post RM, Ketter TA, et al. 1993. Preliminary controlled trial of nimodipine in ultra-rapid cycling affective dysregulation. *Psychiatry Res.* 49:257–72

70. Pazzaglia PJ, Post RM, Ketter TA, et al. 1998. Nimodipine monotherapy and carbamazepine augmentation in patients with refractory recurrent affective illness. *J. Clin. Psychopharmacol.* 18:404–13

71. Stoll AL, Severus E, Freeman MP. 1999. Omega 3 fatty acids in bipolar disorder. *Arch. Gen. Psychiatry* 56:407–12

72. Stoll AL, Sachs GS, Cohen BM, et al. 1996. Choline in the treatment of rapid-cycling bipolar disorder. *Biol. Psychiatry* 40:382–88

73. Burt T, Sachs GS, Demopoulos C. 1998. Donepezil in treatment-resistant bipolar disorder. *Biol. Psychiatry* 45:959–64

74. Bebchuk JM, Arfken CL, Dolan-Manji S, et al. 2000. A preliminary investigation of a protein kinase C inhibitor in the treatment of acute mania. *Arch. Gen. Psychiatry* 57:95–97

Annu. Rev. Med. 2002. 53:189–205

HEART TRANSPLANTATION:
A Thirty-Year Perspective

Douglas N. Miniati and Robert C. Robbins
*Department of Cardiothoracic Surgery, Stanford University School of Medicine, Stanford,
California, 94025; e-mail: dminiati@leland.stanford.edu, robbins@leland.stanford.edu*

Key Words   heart failure, treatment, indications, surgery, immunosuppression

■ **Abstract**   Heart transplantation has evolved over the past 30 years into a mainstay
of therapy for heart failure patients. As the surgical technique and basic immunology
were defined, heart transplantation became a real therapeutic option. Over the next few
decades, thoracic transplant teams at Stanford University and other institutions refined
this mode of therapy. This review addresses the history, current surgical technique,
recipient and donor selection, postoperative care, immunosuppression, short- and long-
term complications, and clinical outcomes associated with this procedure.

INTRODUCTION

Heart transplantation is currently one of the most effective therapies for end-
stage heart disease. Although scientists and physicians have faced many challenges in bringing heart transplantation into the therapeutic realm, the fact that
most of these challenges have been overcome represents a modern example of the
power of medicine. As cardiothoracic surgeons, cardiologists, and basic scientists
have worked side by side over the past 30 years, they have brought the surgical techniques, patient care, and immunology involved in this procedure from
the bedside to the bench and back to the bedside. Accordingly, heart transplantation has continued to improve the quality of life and survival of heart failure
patients.

Recently, the 30-year experience in heart transplantation at Stanford University
was reviewed, demonstrating the refinements and evolution of this program from
a decade of laboratory work into a clinical program of over a thousand heart
transplant recipients (1). From this groundwork sprouted more than 200 heart
transplantation centers throughout the world that have carried the torch of progress
along with Stanford. This review of the world literature describes the historical
aspects of this journey as well as the current state of heart transplantation with
respect to surgical techniques, recipient and donor selection, clinical management,
and potential pitfalls.

HISTORY

Although there are accounts of heart transplantation in ancient civilizations, the development of heart transplantation as a real therapeutic option has occurred only in the past 30 years. After the pioneering work of Carrel & Guthrie (2), who demonstrated the ability of the transplanted heart to survive and resume function, several decades passed before any significant advances were made in this arena. Then, the development of cardiopulmonary bypass in the 1950s made heart transplantation a potential reality. During this decade, several groups around the world attempted to refine the technical aspects of transplanting the heart into the orthotopic (normal anatomic) position (3–8). The landmark paper of Lower et al. (9), which conceptualized and refined the atrial cuff technique of orthotopic heart transplantation in dogs, represented a major step forward. This innovation enabled the transplanted heart to adequately support the circulation and allowed the recipient dogs to survive and exercise normally for up to three weeks. Further experiments by this team using this technique resulted in dogs surviving more than one year (10). Concurrent advances in immunology produced a better understanding of the principles of tissue rejection and the role of the immune system in this process.

The first human-to-human heart transplantation was performed by Christiaan Barnard in Cape Town, South Africa, in December 1967 (11), followed by the first successful cardiac transplantation in the United States by Norman Shumway in January 1968 at Stanford University (12). Thereafter, other leading cardiothoracic surgeons from around the world made a flood of attempts at cardiac transplantation. Because of the lag time in discovering appropriate immunosuppressive agents, however, these investigators were forced to perform a nearly impossible balancing act between infection and rejection. The vast majority of attempts from 1967 to 1971 were unsuccessful, and most surgeons abandoned the procedure.

The teams of Norman Shumway, at Stanford University, and Richard Lower, who had moved to the Medical College of Virginia, worked on the principles of heart transplantation virtually alone through the next decade. During this time, they helped to establish recipient selection criteria (13), the use of the endomyocardial biopsy to diagnose rejection (14), the use of rabbit antithymocyte globulin to treat acute rejection (15), and early and late management principles (16). Thanks to the persistence of these teams, heart transplantation is one of the most effective therapies for end-stage heart disease today, and as of March 2000, over 55,000 heart transplantations have been performed (17).

SURGICAL TECHNIQUE

As the use of heart transplantation spread around the world, a number of investigators began to experiment with variations of the conceptually simple technique described by Lower et al. (9). The "Lower and Shumway" or biatrial method consists of anastomoses of the donor left and right atria to those of the recipient at the midatrial level, allowing short operative time and avoidance of potential complications associated with individual vena caval and pulmonary vein anastomoses (i.e., thrombosis, stenosis) (18, 19). Over time, however, surgeons have found disadvantages of this technique, including enlarged atria with atrioventricular valve insufficiency, impaired atrial contractile function, and associated arrhythmias.

In an attempt to improve function and physiology, surgeons have developed the bicaval and total techniques of heart transplantation. In the bicaval technique (Figure 1), described by Baumgartner et al. (20) and Sievers et al. (21), individual anastomoses of the superior and inferior vena cavae are performed in place of the right atrial cuff anastomosis. The total technique, developed by Yacoub & Banner (22) and Dreyfus et al. (23), includes this modification plus the anastomosis of paired pulmonary veins in place of the left atrial cuff anastomosis. Several studies have compared these methods from both functional and clinical perspectives (see 24 for review). The newer techniques have proven at least as effective as, and in some investigations more effective than, the original biatrial technique with respect to arrhythmia (particularly sinus node dysfunction requiring pacemaker support), valvular function, hemodynamics, exercise capacity, and patient survival. A recent survey of 75% of the world's heart transplantation centers indicated that the bicaval technique is the most frequently used, and the general consensus among heart transplantation surgeons is that ultimately the bicaval technique will be demonstrated to have clinical superiority (25).

RECIPIENT SELECTION

With the success of heart transplantation came the need to establish strict transplantation candidate selection criteria. Such criteria result in the most prudent allocation of scarce donor organs to benefit the largest number of patients. The most common indications for adult heart transplantation are ischemic and idiopathic dilated cardiomyopathies, together comprising almost 90% of all adult indications (Figure 2). In children, the most common indications include congenital anomalies and myopathy, in varying contributions according to age groups (17). The contraindications to heart transplantation vary somewhat from one center to another, but many include irreversible extracardiac end-organ dysfunction (such as cirrhosis), recent cancer with uncertain status, psychiatric illness with poor medical compliance, severe irreversible pulmonary hypertension, and active infection. Other systemic afflictions, such as diabetes mellitus, chronic obstructive pulmonary disease, peripheral vascular disease, and morbid obesity represent relative contraindications.

Determining which heart disease patients should be listed for transplantation should be as objective and judicious as possible. While the number of heart failure patients continually increases, the treatment of heart failure continues to improve. Some patients with severe left ventricular dysfunction remain symptom-free, and

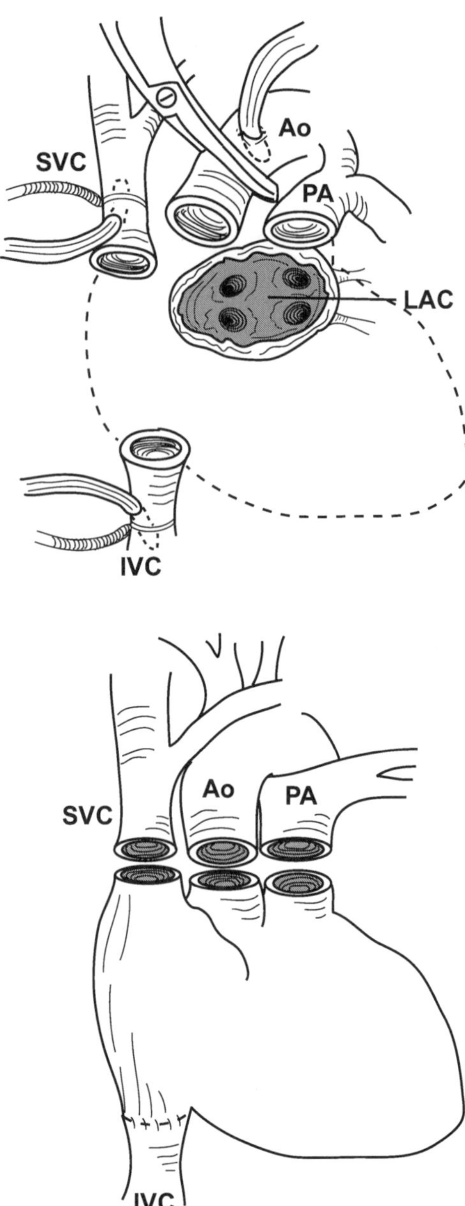

Figure 1 Bicaval orthotopic heart transplantation technique. *Above*, anterior view of the recipient's chest after excision of the native heart. *Below*, anterior view of the transplanted heart partially sewn into place. SVC, superior vena cava; Ao, aorta; PA, pulmonary artery; LAC, left atrial cuff; IVC, inferior vena cava; dotted lines, original position of excised native heart.

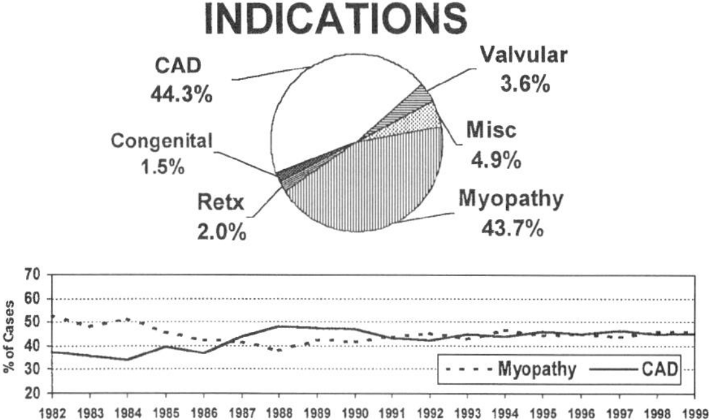

Figure 2   Adult heart transplant indications. CAD, coronary artery disease; Misc, miscellaneous; Retx, retransplantation (reprinted from Reference 17 with permission from Elsevier Science).

some studies indicate that for correctly selected patients, medical management can achieve similar symptomatic and survival outcomes as heart transplantation (26, 27). Therefore, as a general rule, evaluation for potential heart transplantation should be instituted only if a contraindication-free patient continues to suffer severe cardiac disability despite optimal medical management.

One screening method that has been used extensively is the measurement of peak exercise oxygen consumption (VO2). Historically, provided the patient could reach the anaerobic threshold, a peak VO2 of <15 ml/kg/min or <55% of predicted peak VO2 has led to strong consideration for listing for heart transplantation. These set points for listing, however, were derived before beta-blocker therapy was available and may need to be adjusted in the future.

Another important functional parameter to measure is pulmonary vascular resistance (PVR). Patients with severe heart failure often have an increased PVR due to their primary illness, and if this problem cannot be managed medically, a newly transplanted heart could suffer acute right-sided heart failure and cause the patient's immediate demise. Also, increasing PVR has been shown to have a linear impact on one-year and five-year survival rates (17). Optimal PVR for transplantation has been controversial, but most centers accept a value of no greater than 3–4 Wood units with maximal vasodilator therapy, including 100% oxygen, nitroprusside, and inhaled nitric oxide.

Recipient age has been another area of debate among heart transplantation programs. At Stanford, the upper age limit was initially 50 years, and over time this general age limit has been extended to 65 years, although successes have been achieved in carefully selected patients over 70 years old. In addition, the program at the University of California, Los Angeles has instituted an alternative list, including patients up to 75 years old, to receive donor hearts that otherwise might not be used (28). According to the year 2000 Registry of the International Society for Heart and Lung Transplantation (ISHLT), advancing recipient age increases the one-year and five-year post-transplantation mortality risk, with significance beginning at around age 65 (17). Concurrent studies, however, indicate one-year and four-year survival rates similar to younger patients' in carefully selected recipients over age 69 (29).

In the end, the decision to list a patient for heart transplantation must be individualized within a general framework of indications and contraindications. Optimal medical management must be achieved prior to making this decision and must be continued while the patient awaits transplantation. Additional psychological and social factors must also be considered, and the final decision should be made by the transplantation team and the patient together.

DONOR EVALUATION

Like recipient selection, the evaluation of potential donor hearts depends on universally accepted objective criteria that may be modified by the particular circumstances and program-based trends within each case. The most common causes of death of organ donors are intracranial bleed, motor vehicle accident, gunshot wound, and closed head injury. Information obtained at the primary screening, which is generally performed by specialists from organ procurement organizations (see listings at www.aopo.org), includes cause of death, body size, ABO blood type, serologies including HIV and hepatitis B and C status, routine laboratory data, and clinical course. A secondary screen conducted by a transplant cardiologist or cardiac surgeon entails evaluation of relevant (particularly thoracic) injuries, baseline electrocardiogram, chest X-ray, arterial blood gas analysis, and echocardiogram. The final screen is performed by the procuring surgeon, who assesses the donor for any signs of deterioration that may have occurred during the organ allocation process and inspects the physical specimen for signs of contusion or other injuries.

Absolute contraindications for using a potential donor, recommended by the American College of Cardiology 24th Bethesda Conference Report on cardiac transplantation (30), include positive HIV status, carboxyhemoglobin level greater than 20%, intractable ventricular arrhythmia, arterial oxygen saturation less than 80%, previous myocardial infarction, severe echocardiographic ventricular dysfunction (ejection fraction less than 10%), and severe coronary artery disease detected by arteriography. Relative contraindications include, among others, positive hepatitis B or C serology, sepsis, history of metastatic cancer, evidence of cardiac contusion, prolonged hypotension, noncritical coronary artery disease, and history of intravenous drug abuse.

Since heart transplantation has become a viable treatment for heart failure, the scarcity of donor organs has been a major difficulty. A combined consensus conference of the American Society of Transplant Physicians and the American Society of Transplant Surgeons was held in March 2001 in an attempt to establish guidelines for increasing donor organ utilization, and the results of this meeting are to be published in the *American Journal of Transplantation*. One option that has been applied is the use of marginal donors. These hearts generally come from older donors or from young patients with decreased left ventricular function by echocardiogram but with no obvious reason for left ventricular failure. Wheeldon et al. (31) have demonstrated that, in many cases, a donor who is unacceptable by strict physiological criteria can be converted into a satisfactory donor by hormone replacement therapy. The use of this "Papworth protocol" of donor management, with comprehensive monitoring and a cardiac-trained anesthetist on the donor team, has been shown to substantially increase the number of donor hearts without adverse effects on the recipients.

The issue of maximum donor age has been developing over the years. Donors are on average approximately 30 years old, although, in an effort to expand the number of potential donors, many centers will consider donors up to 55 years old. Some studies report the safe and effective use of older donors (32, 33), but the latest ISHLT Registry does cite increasing donor age as a factor that increases the one-year and five-year mortality of transplant recipients in a linear fashion (17). The use of older donors, particularly in teenage pediatric recipients, has been demonstrated to adversely affect long-term outcome (34).

POSTOPERATIVE CARE

The immediate postoperative care of heart transplant recipients is similar to that of other cardiac surgical patients. Extubation and weaning from inotropic support are performed as soon as possible, along with patient mobilization and physical therapy. Occasionally, the recipient's pulmonary vascular resistance is elevated, leading to right-sided failure of the donor heart. This immediate complication has been controlled with inhaled nitric oxide (35, 36), ventricular assist devices (37, 38), and, in extreme cases, extracorporeal membrane oxygenation (39, 40).

Apart from the monitoring and treatment of the patient's cardiopulmonary functional parameters, most attention is focused on the institution and progression of an immunosuppressive protocol. A triple-drug regimen of cyclosporine (CsA) or tacrolimus (FK506), azathioprine (AZA) or mycophenolate mofetil (MMF), and prednisone is typical, starting with higher doses in the immediate postoperative period and weaning to lower doses as tolerated (Table 1). Kobashigawa (41) recently reviewed immunosuppression for heart transplantation and described the mechanisms and major side effects of these drugs along with several agents that may be used clinically in the future. In particular, FK506 (42) and MMF (43) have shown promise as alternatives to CsA and AZA, respectively, and further studies may elucidate additional long-term benefits of these agents (44). Other agents that have had success in solid organ transplantation and will likely be used for heart transplantation in the future include sirolimus (rapamycin) and monoclonal

TABLE 1 Immunosuppression for heart transplantation protocols[a]

Drug	Early	Late
Methylprednisolone	500 mg IV intraoperatively then 125 mg IV q8hr ×3	
OKT3 induction	5 mg IV/d ×7	
Cyclosporine	6–10 mg/kg/d PO[b] or 0.5–2 mg/kg/d IV	3–6 mg/kg/d PO[c]
Or		
Tacrolimus (FK506)	0.15–0.30 mg/kg/d PO	0.15–0.30 mg/kg/d PO[c]
Azathioprine	2 mg/kg/d PO[d]	1–2 mg/kg/d PO
Or		
Mycophenolate mofetil	3000 mg/d PO	3000 mg/d PO
Prednisone	1 mg/kg/d PO tapered to 0.4 mg/kg/d	0.1–0.2 mg/kg/d PO

[a]Reproduced from Reference 68 with permission.

[b]Omit if preoperative serum creatinine level is >1.5 mg/dl and use IV.

[c]Or as modified by blood levels.

[d]Omit if white blood count is <4000/mm^3.

antibody interleukin (IL)-2 receptor antagonists such as dacliximab (daclizumab) and basiliximab.

Many centers perform cytolytic induction therapy with polyclonal or monoclonal antilymphocyte antibodies, usually with a 3- to 10-day course beginning immediately after transplantation. Although the bioactivity of these agents is not fully understood, in general they function by causing the lysis of lymphoid cells. The most commonly used preparations are the equine-derived ATGAM and rabbit-derived RATG (both polyclonal) and the mouse preparation OKT3 (monoclonal). Whereas the polyclonal preparations have pan–T-cell activity (anti-CD2, -CD3, -CD4, -CD8, -CD18, and -HLA-DR), OKT3 is directed specifically against the epsilon chain of the CD3-receptor complex of human T cells. Cytolytic induction clearly benefits some groups of patients, including those at high risk of acute rejection (e.g., females, patients with high panels of reactive antibodies) and patients with renal dysfunction (via avoidance of the nephrotoxic effects of CsA) (45). Disadvantages of antilymphocyte antibody therapy include a slight increase in incidence of cytomegalovirus infection, possible increase in development of post-transplantation lymphoproliferative disorder, sensitization/serum sickness, and the "first-dose effect," which consists of fevers, chills, and mild hypotension (45, 46). In addition, cytolytic induction therapy is more expensive than other modes of induction, although studies have shown that lower doses and shorter courses of administration are as effective as the doses originally used, making this treatment more affordable.

REJECTION SURVEILLANCE

An important aspect of the care of the heart transplant recipient is surveillance for acute rejection. A study by the Cardiac Transplant Research Database Group indicated that the risk for acute rejection normally peaks within the first month after transplantation and then decreases rapidly (47). This report also showed a mean of 1.25 rejection episodes per patient in the first year after transplantation, declining to 0.18, 0.13, and 0.02 in the second, third, and fourth years, respectively. Despite this decline over time, acute rejection continues to cause significant morbidity and mortality in heart transplant recipients, necessitating careful monitoring and prompt treatment.

Because clinical symptoms of rejection are often vague and relatively late in terms of immune cell destruction of myocardial cells, routine testing for rejection in the absence of symptoms is standard procedure. In heart transplants, unlike kidney and liver transplants, there are no reliable serological markers for rejection, although troponin T levels have been suggested as an adjunct (48). In the absence of such a test, the endomyocardial biopsy remains the gold standard method for detecting acute rejection in transplanted hearts. Typically, patients are first biopsied two weeks after the transplantation, then once per week for the next two weeks, once every two weeks for the next eight weeks, once per month for the next three months, and four times per year thereafter. If rejection is detected, patients are treated and then rebiopsied after 10 to 14 days. The uniform criteria established by the ISHLT are described by a scale from 0 to 4 in increasing severity of lymphocyte infiltration and myocyte necrosis (49).

TREATMENT OF ACUTE REJECTION

A standard algorithm for the treatment of acute rejection is shown in Figure 3. Low-grade rejection (ISHLT grade 1A/B or 2) can often be managed with adjustments in the patient's maintenance regimen or with oral steroids, and there is some debate as to whether these grades of rejection should even be treated. In general, intravenous pulse steroids are the initial line of therapy for higher-grade histological rejection (ISHLT grade 3A/B or 4) or for rejection causing significant hemodynamic compromise (necessitating inotropic agents or mechanical ventricular assistance). If the patient does not respond, has demonstrated steroid resistance in the past, and has not been exposed to the anti–T-cell antibodies, OKT3, RATG, or ATGAM can be used (50). Care must be taken when using these agents because patients may develop antibodies against these animal-derived molecules, leading to decreased effectiveness, serum sickness, and possibly acute vascular rejection with graft loss (46, 51). Another alternative for treating recurrent acute rejection consists of conversion from AZA to MMF and/or from CsA to FK506. Occasionally, a patient presents with persistent,

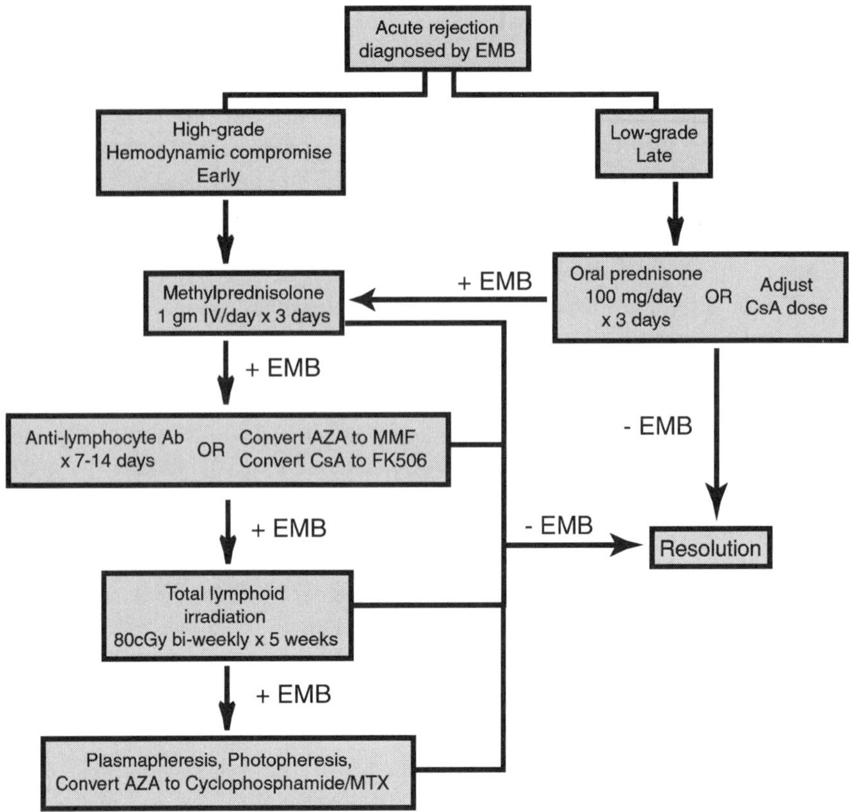

Figure 3   Acute rejection treatment algorithm. EMB, endomyocardial biopsy; CsA, cyclosporine; Ab, antibodies; AZA, azathioprine; MMF, mycophenolate mofetil; FK506, tacrolimus; MTX, methotrexate.

refractory rejection that is resistant to steroids. For these cases, additional strategies for immunosuppression include total lymphoid irradiation, plasmapheresis, photopheresis, and conversion from AZA to cyclophosphamide or methotrexate (50, 52).

As more options for immunosuppression become available, transplant physicians will be able to individualize each patient's induction and maintenance regimen to achieve maximum efficacy with minimum toxicity. A patient's age and gender, renal function, presence or absence of ongoing infection, and predisposition to bone marrow suppression will be important factors to consider. In addition, as the risk factors and pathophysiology of graft coronary artery disease become more apparent, physicians may be able to tailor each patient's immunosuppression to prolong the long-term function of cardiac allografts (53).

GRAFT CORONARY ARTERY DISEASE

Although short-term outcomes continue to improve, the long-term success of heart transplantation is still hindered by graft coronary artery disease (GCAD, also known as cardiac allograft vasculopathy and transplant coronary artery disease). According to the most recent ISHLT Registry, 21.7% of heart transplant recipients are afflicted with GCAD five years post-transplantation, and GCAD represents a significant cause of death (17). This accelerated form of coronary artery disease is characterized by diffuse and heterogeneous narrowing of both large-caliber and small-caliber vessels, and although fibrous neointimal hyperplasia is the predominant underlying pathophysiological process, arteritis and atheromatous changes probably also play a role in this disease (54).

Among the many risk factors postulated, those that appear to have the greatest weight are a recipient's underlying diagnosis of coronary artery disease and increasing donor age, with the five-year odds ratio doubling when donors are 50 years of age or older (17). Other important risks include alloantigen-dependent and alloantigen-independent factors. Alloantigen-dependent factors include donor/recipient histocompatibility (55) and number of acute rejection episodes. Alloantigen-independent factors include donor brain death, recipient cytomegalovirus infection, graft ischemic time, and the myocardial oxidative stress resulting from ischemia and reperfusion of the donor heart. All are believed to play an important role in the development of GCAD (56).

Because of the accelerated nature of this disease process and its associated significant morbidity, early detection is required for any treatment to have a significant response. Because conventional coronary angiography is insufficiently sensitive, intravascular ultrasound (IVUS) has been employed more often for the annual surveillance of heart transplant recipients. IVUS allows for the measurement of intimal area, lumen area, plaque morphology, vessel remodeling, and progression of disease over time (57).

Developing effective therapies for GCAD has been a daunting task. Because of the diffuse nature of the disease, traditional options for coronary artery disease such as bypass grafting and angioplasty have had limited success (58–60). Angioplasty, particularly with stenting (61), can be efficacious for focal lesions, but the restenosis rate may ultimately prove prohibitive. Coronary artery bypass grafting may be performed on carefully selected patients, but perioperative mortality and durability of distal perfusion remain concerns. Retransplantation has also been employed, but GCAD frequently recurs in the retransplanted hearts. In addition, the ethical debate over the appropriateness of allocating a donor heart to an older, previously transplanted patient versus a younger, immunologically naïve patient remains to be resolved.

Ultimately, the key to treating GCAD will probably fall in the realm of prevention. Control or modulation of patient immune responses, environmental influences (lipid profiles, control of diabetes and hypertension, and infections), and donor-specific factors (pretransplantation injury and antigenicity) may be attained with advancements in donor care, organ preservation, new immunosuppressive agents, and the ultimate objective in transplantation, immunological tolerance of the allograft (54). Until these strides are made, the long-term success of heart transplantation will continue to be limited.

COMPLICATIONS

In addition to GCAD, there are several short- and long-term complications associated with heart transplantation. These problems may be broadly categorized into technical complications and complications of immunosuppression.

Adverse events due to technical difficulties related to the transplantation procedure include superior vena caval stenosis and tricuspid regurgitation requiring valve replacement. Although both complications are rare, with reported incidences of 2.4% (62) and 1.8% (63), respectively, they are worth mentioning because of their associated morbidities. Superior vena caval stenosis is usually related to donor-recipient mismatch of caval diameter and can be treated by operative or percutaneous interventional correction. Tricuspid regurgitation can result from chordal disruption by the bioptome during the endomyocardial biopsy procedure and, if severe, may require surgical replacement.

Complications of immunosuppression include drug toxicities, infection, and neoplasms. All immunosuppressive agents have multiple significant toxicities. Corticosteroids, in particular, can take a serious toll on a patient's well-being. If patients require relatively high steroid levels, side effects can include diabetes, hyperlipidemia, osteoporosis, peptic ulcers, weight gain, and psychiatric disorders. Among the other most notable adverse side effects of immunosuppression are nephrotoxicity, which may result from CsA and FK506 therapy; diabetes mellitus, with FK506; bone marrow suppression, with long-term azathioprine administration; and gastrointestinal symptoms, with MMF.

Although immunosuppressive agents have become more specific over the past 30 years, infectious complications persist as a major cause of death, especially within the first year after heart transplantation (17). Within the first month of transplantation, infections are usually of nosocomial bacterial origin, including *Pseudomonas aeruginosa*, *Staphylococcus aureus*, Enterococci, and Enterobacteriaceae. These organisms can cause pneumonia, urinary tract and wound infections, and bacteremia associated with the use of intravascular devices (64). Later infections are commonly caused by viruses and opportunistic fungi (e.g., *Pneumocystis*, *Candida*, and *Aspergillus*).

Cytomegalovirus (CMV) is probably the most frequently encountered infectious organism, and patients may present with pneumonia, gastroenteritis, hepatitis, or retinitis, alone or in combination. Because of the mortality risk, especially with CMV pneumonia, and the association of CMV with the later development of GCAD, prophylaxis against and prompt treatment of CMV infection cannot be overemphasized. In cases of CMV serological mismatch between the donor and the recipient, such prophylaxis includes ganciclovir and hyperimmune globulin for six to eight weeks post-transplantation.

Another clinical problem associated with immunosuppression is the development of neoplasms, the most notable of which is post-transplantation lymphoproliferative disorder (PTLD). Other tumors include malignancies of the skin and lips, non-Hodgkin lymphomas, Kaposi sarcoma, and uterine, cervical, vulval, and perineal neoplasms. Frequencies of common adenocarcinomas such as breast, lung, colon, and prostate do not exceed that in the general population (65). The most common first-line treatment of PTLD consists of drastic reduction of immunosuppressive drug doses, and other options range from conventional chemotherapy to antiviral and immunologically based therapies (66).

SURVIVAL

The overall one-year survival rate of heart transplant recipients, according to the ISHLT database, is currently 81%, with a patient half-life (time to 50% survival) of 9.8 years (17), although many centers report over 90% one-year survival. After the first post-transplantation year, the mortality rate is constant at approximately 4% per year. Patients who have received heart transplants within the past five years have one- and three-year survival rates of 85.6% and 79.5%, respectively. Figure 4, displaying data from the ISHLT database, shows the steady improvement in survival from one era to the next in heart transplantation. Approximately 40% of patients are hospitalized in the first post-transplantation year, for infection, rejection, or other causes, and this value drops to 20% by the third and fifth post-transplantation years. Heart transplant patient physical rehabilitation programs are common and

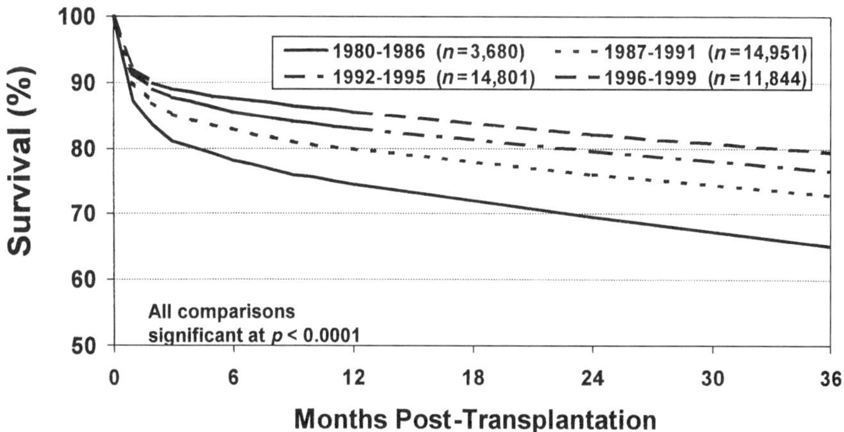

Figure 4   Adult heart transplant actuarial survival by era. (Reprinted from Reference 17 with permission.)

have been shown to increase a patient's capacity for physical work (67). The vast majority of patients report no physical limitations, but less than 40% of heart transplant recipients work full-time. This low value may be explained partly by older recipients having reached retirement age and by the fact that for many heart transplant recipients, gainful employment requires sacrificing disability and insurance benefits, without which they could not afford their maintenance medical therapy.

SUMMARY

The field of cardiac transplantation has steadily evolved into a mainstay of therapy for heart failure patients over the past 30 years. Once the major hurdles of the surgical technique and a basic understanding of immunology were cleared, cardiologists, nurses, infectious disease specialists, social workers, cardiothoracic surgeons, and immunologists continued to refine these aspects of heart transplantation while learning more about long-term obstacles. Acute rejection still occurs, but it does not represent a major difficulty for most patients, who enjoy a quality of life that would not be possible without a heart transplant. The holy grail of tolerance may yet be attained, as knowledge of the immune response and the means to control immunity improve. In the meantime, it is hoped that increasingly individualized immunosuppression will continue to decrease the incidence of infectious complications and may also play a role in preventing graft coronary artery disease.

Unfortunately, the success of heart transplantation has only magnified the shortage of donor organs, which will continue to be a tremendous problem. One positive result from this limitation of heart transplantation has been the intense interest generated in other surgical forms of heart failure treatment, including mechanical support, biventricular pacing, mitral valve repair, coronary artery bypass grafting, the Dor procedure (endoventricular circular patch plasty repair), and cell transplantation. Many of these alternatives, in particular mechanical support systems, probably will progress into long-term destination therapy as alternatives to transplantation. As the population of heart failure patients continues to grow, both heart transplantation and these alternative therapies will become more refined, such that heart transplantation may be reserved for those patients who would benefit most from it. We can expect that as donor utilization improves, so will recipient selection, ultimately resulting in further progress in the survival and quality of life of heart transplant recipients.

Visit the Annual Reviews home page at www.AnnualReviews.org

LITERATURE CITED

1. Robbins RC, Barlow CW, Oyer PE, et al. 1999. Thirty years of cardiac transplantation at Stanford University. *J. Thorac. Cardiovasc. Surg.* 117:939–51

2. Carrel A, Guthrie C. 1905. The transplantation of veins and organs. *Am. J. Med.* 10:1105

3. Webb WR, Howard HS, Neely WA. 1959.

Practical methods of homologous cardiac transplantation. *J. Thorac. Surg.* 37:361–66

4. Cass MH, Brock R. 1959. Heart excision and replacement. *Guy's Hosp. Reps.* 108:285–90

5. Downie HG. 1953. Homotransplantation of the dog heart. *Arch. Surg.* 66:624

6. Sayegh SF, Creech O. 1957. Transplantation of the homologous canine heart. *J. Thorac. Surg.* 34:692

7. Neptune WB, Cookson BA, Bailey CP, et al. 1953. Complete homologous heart transplantation. *Arch. Surg.* 66:174

8. Blanco G, Adam A, Rodriguez-Perez D, Fernandez A. 1958. Complete homotransplantation of canine heart and lungs. *Arch. Surg.* 76:20

9. Lower RR, Stofer RC, Shumway NE. 1961. Homovital transplantation of the heart. *J. Thorac. Cardiovasc. Surg.* 41:196–204

10. Lower RR, Shumway NE. 1960. Studies on orthotopic transplantation of the canine heart. *Surg. Forum* 11:18–20

11. Barnard CN. 1967. The operation. A human cardiac transplant: an interim report of a successful operation performed at Groote Schuur Hospital, Cape Town. *S. Afr. Med. J.* 41:1271–74

12. Shumway NE, Dong E, Stinson EB. 1969. Surgical aspects of cardiac transplantation in man. *Bull. NY Acad. Med.* 45:387–93

13. Griepp RB, Stinson EB, Dong EJ, et al. 1971. Determinants of operative risk in human heart transplantation. *Am. J. Surg.* 122:192–97

14. Caves PK, Billingham ME, Schulz WP, et al. 1973. Transvenous biopsy from canine orthotopic heart allografts. *Am. Heart J.* 85:525–30

15. Bieber CP, Griepp RB, Oyer PE, et al. 1976. Use of rabbit antithymocyte globulin in cardiac transplantation. Relationship of serum clearance rates to clinical outcome. *Transplantation* 22:478–88

16. Baumgartner WA, Reitz BA, Oyer PE, et al. 1979. Cardiac homotransplantation. *Curr. Probl. Surg.* 16:1–61

17. Hosenpud JD, Bennett LE, Keck BM, et al. 2000. The registry of the International Society for Heart and Lung Transplantation: seventeenth official report—2000. *J. Heart Lung Transplant.* 19:909–31

18. Stinson EB, Dong EJ, Iben AB, Shumway NE. 1969. Cardiac transplantation in man. 3. Surgical aspects. *Am. J. Surg.* 118:182–87

19. Barnard CN. 1968. What we have learned about heart transplants. *J. Thorac. Cardiovasc. Surg.* 56:457

20. Baumgartner WA, Traill TA, Cameron DE, et al. 1989. Unique aspects of heart and lung transplantation exhibited in the "domino-donor" operation. *JAMA* 261:3121–25

21. Sievers HH, Weyand M, Kraatz EG, Bernhard A. 1991. An alternative technique for orthotopic cardiac transplantation, with preservation of the normal anatomy of the right atrium. *Thorac. Cardiovasc. Surg.* 39:70–72

22. Yacoub MH, Banner NA. 1989. Recent developments in lung and heart-lung transplantation. In *Transplantation Reviews*, ed. PJ Morris, NE Tilney, 3:1–29. Philadelphia: Saunders

23. Dreyfus G, Jebara V, Mihaileanu S, Carpentier AF. 1991. Total orthotopic heart transplantation: an alternative to the standard technique. *Ann. Thorac. Surg.* 52:1181–84

24. Miniati DN, Robbins RC. 2001. Techniques in orthotopic cardiac transplantation: a review. *Cardiol. Rev.* 9:131–36

25. Aziz TM, Burgess MI, El-Gamel A, et al. 1999. Orthotopic cardiac transplantation technique: a survey of current practice. *Ann. Thorac. Surg.* 68:1242–46

26. Rickenbacher PR, Trindade PT, Haywood GA, et al. 1996. Transplant candidates with severe left ventricular dysfunction managed with medical treatment: characteristics and survival. *J. Am. Coll. Cardiol.* 27:1192–97

27. Levine TB, Levine AB, Goldberg AD, et al. 1996. Clinical status of patients removed from a transplant waiting list rivals

that of transplant recipients at significant cost savings. *Am. Heart J.* 132:1189–94

28. Laks H, Marelli D. 1999. The alternate recipient list for heart transplantation: a model for expansion of the donor pool. *Adv. Cardiovasc. Surg.* 11:233–44

29. Blanche C, Blanche DA, Kearney B, et al. 2001. Heart transplantation in patients seventy years of age and older: a comparative analysis of outcome. *J. Thorac. Cardiovasc. Surg.* 121:532–41

30. Baldwin JC, Anderson JL, Boucek MM, et al. 1993. 24th Bethesda conference: cardiac transplantation. Task Force 2: Donor guidelines. *J. Am. Coll. Cardiol.* 22:15–20

31. Wheeldon DR, Potter CD, Oduro A, et al. 1995. Transforming the "unacceptable" donor: outcomes from the adoption of a standardized donor management technique. *J. Heart Lung Transplant.* 14:734–42

32. Sweeney MS, Lammermeier DE, Frazier OH, et al. 1990. Extension of donor criteria in cardiac transplantation: surgical risk versus supply-side economics. *Ann. Thorac. Surg.* 50:7–10

33. Drinkwater DC, Laks H, Blitz A, et al. 1996. Outcomes of patients undergoing transplantation with older donor hearts. *J. Heart Lung Transplant.* 15:684–91

34. Chin C, Miller J, Robbins R, et al. 1999. The use of advanced-age donor hearts adversely affects survival in pediatric heart transplantation. *Pediatr. Transplant.* 3:309–14

35. Carrier M, Blaise G, Belisle S, et al. 1999. Nitric oxide inhalation in the treatment of primary graft failure following heart transplantation. *J. Heart Lung Transplant.* 18:664–67

36. George SJ, Boscoe MJ. 1997. Inhaled nitric oxide for right ventricular dysfunction following cardiac transplantation. *Br. J. Clin. Pract.* 51:53–55

37. Icenogle TB, Williams RJ, Smith RG, et al. 1989. Extracorporeal pulsatile biventricular support after cardiac transplantation. *Ann. Thorac. Surg.* 47:614–16

38. Esmore DS, Spratt PM, Branch JM, et al. 1990. Right ventricular assist and prostacyclin infusion for allograft failure in the presence of high pulmonary vascular resistance. *J. Heart Transplant.* 9:136–41

39. Whyte RI, Deeb GM, McCurry KR, et al. 1994. Extracorporeal life support after heart or lung transplantation. *Ann. Thorac. Surg.* 58:754–58

40. Barzaghi N, Olivei M, Minzioni G, et al. 1997. ECMO and inhaled nitric oxide for cardiopulmonary failure after heart retransplantation. *Ann. Thorac. Surg.* 63:533–35

41. Kobashigawa JA. 1998. Advances in immunosuppression for heart transplantation. *Adv. Cardiovasc. Surg.* 10:155–74

42. Reichart B, Meiser B, Vigano M, et al. 1998. European Multicenter Tacrolimus (FK506) Heart Pilot Study: one-year results—European Tacrolimus Multicenter Heart Study Group. *J. Heart Lung Transplant.* 17:775–81

43. Kobashigawa J, Miller L, Renlund D, et al. 1998. A randomized active-controlled trial of mycophenolate mofetil in heart transplant recipients. Mycophenolate Mofetil Investigators. *Transplantation* 66:507–15

44. Hunt SA. 2000. New immunosuppressive agents in clinical use: mycophenolate mofetil and tacrolimus. *Cardiol. Rev.* 8:180–84

45. Wahlers T. 1998. Cytolytic induction therapy in heart and lung transplantation: the protagonist opinion. *Transplant Proc.* 30:1100–3

46. Taylor DO, Kfoury AG, Pisani B, et al. 1997. Antilymphocyte-antibody prophylaxis: review of the adult experience in heart transplantation. *Transplant Proc.* 29:13S–15S

47. Kubo SH, Naftel DC, Mills RMJ, et al. 1995. Risk factors for late recurrent rejection after heart transplantation: a multiinstitutional, multivariable analysis. Cardiac Transplant Research Database Group. *J. Heart Lung Transplant.* 14:409–18

48. Dengler TJ, Zimmermann R, Braun K, et al. 1998. Elevated serum concentrations

of cardiac troponin T in acute allograft rejection after human heart transplantation. *J. Am. Coll. Cardiol.* 32:405–12

49. Billingham ME, Cary NR, Hammond ME, et al. 1990. A working formulation for the standardization of nomenclature in the diagnosis of heart and lung rejection: Heart Rejection Study Group. The International Society for Heart Transplantation. *J. Heart Transplant.* 9:587–93

50. Kirklin JK, Bourge RC, McGiffin DC. 1997. Recurrent or persistent cardiac allograft rejection: therapeutic options and recommendations. *Transplant Proc.* 29:40S–44S

51. Ma H, Hammond EH, Taylor DO, et al. 1996. The repetitive histologic pattern of vascular cardiac allograft rejection. Increased incidence associated with longer exposure to prophylactic murine monoclonal anti-CD3 antibody (OKT3). *Transplantation* 62:205–10

52. Koransky ML, Robbins RC. 2001. Additional strategies for immunosuppression. In *Heart and Lung Transplantation*, ed. WA Baumgartner, B Reitz, E Kasper, J Theodore. Philadelphia: Saunders. In press

53. Valantine HA. 1997. Individualizing immunosuppression for heart transplantation: strategies for the next decade. *Transplant Proc.* 29:5S–8S

54. Russell ME. 2000. Cardiac allograft vasculopathy—a changing perspective. *Z. Kardiol.* 89(Suppl. 9):IX/6–10

55. Taylor DO, Yowell RL, Kfoury AG, et al. 2000. Allograft coronary artery disease: clinical correlations with circulating anti-HLA antibodies and the immuno-histopathologic pattern of vascular rejection. *J. Heart Lung Transplant.* 19:518–21

56. Behrendt D, Ganz P, Fang JC. 2000. Cardiac allograft vasculopathy. *Curr. Opin. Cardiol.* 15:422–29

57. Konig A, Theisen K, Klauss V. 2000. Intravascular ultrasound for assessment of coronary allograft vasculopathy. *Z. Kardiol.* 89(Suppl. 9):IX/45–49

58. Patel VS, Radovancevic B, Springer W, et al. 1997. Revascularization procedures in patients with transplant coronary artery disease. *Eur. J. Cardiothorac. Surg.* 11:895–901

59. Musci M, Loebe M, Wellnhofer E, et al. 1998. Coronary angioplasty, bypass surgery, and retransplantation in cardiac transplant patients with graft coronary disease. *Thorac. Cardiovasc. Surg.* 46:268–74

60. Musci M, Pasic M, Meyer R, et al. 1999. Coronary artery bypass grafting after orthotopic heart transplantation. *Eur. J. Cardiothorac. Surg.* 16:163–68

61. Pethig K, Heublein B, Haverich A. 2000. Cardiac allograft vasculopathy—coronary interventions and surgical options. *Z. Kardiol.* 89(Suppl. 9):IX/66–69

62. Sze DY, Robbins RC, Semba CP, et al. 1998. Superior vena cava syndrome after heart transplantation: percutaneous treatment of a complication of bicaval anastomoses. *J. Thorac. Cardiovasc. Surg.* 116:253–61

63. Chan MC, Giannetti N, Kato T, et al. 1999. Severe tricuspid regurgitation after heart transplant. *Circulation* 100:I–163

64. Gentry LO. 1993. Cardiac transplantation and related infections. *Semin. Respir. Infect.* 8:199–206

65. Penn I. 1993. Tumors after renal and cardiac transplantation. *Hematol. Oncol. Clin. N. Am.* 7:431–45

66. Mamzer-Bruneel MF, Bourquelot P, Hermine O, et al. 1997. Treatment and prognosis of post-transplant lymphoproliferative disease. *Ann. Transplant.* 2:42–48

67. Kobashigawa JA, Leaf DA, Lee N, et al. 1999. A controlled trial of exercise rehabilitation after heart transplantation. *N. Engl. J. Med.* 340:272–77; erratum 340(12): 976

68. Miniati DN, Robbins RC, Reitz BA. 2001. Heart and heart-lung transplantation. In *Heart Disease: A Textbook of Cardiovascular Medicine*, ed. E Braunwald, DP Zipes, P Libby, 20:621. Philadelphia: Saunders

Annu. Rev. Med. 2002. 53:207–21

CLINICAL TRIALS OF HIV VACCINES*

Barney S. Graham

Vaccine Research Center, National Institute of Allergy and Infectious Diseases, National Institutes of Health, 40 Convent Drive, Building 40, Room 2502, MSC-3017, Bethesda, Maryland 20892-3017; e-mail: bgraham@nih.gov

Key Words   AIDS, virus, immunity, neutralizing antibody, cytotoxic T lymphocyte

■ **Abstract**   Development of a preventive vaccine for HIV is the best hope of controlling the AIDS pandemic. Evidence from natural history studies and experiments in animal models indicates that immunity against HIV is possible, suggesting that vaccine development is feasible. These studies have shown that sufficient levels of neutralizing antibody against HIV can prevent infection, although the effect is type-specific. In contrast, HIV-specific cytotoxic T lymphocyte (CTL) activity has broad cross-reactivity, and although CTL activity alone cannot prevent HIV infection, it can control the level of viremia at a low level. Evaluation of candidate vaccines in human trials has focused on approaches that can safely elicit HIV-specific antibody and T cell responses. Current strategies have been unable to induce antibody with broad neutralizing activity against primary HIV isolates. However, recombinant poxvirus and DNA vaccines have elicited CTL responses that are broadly cross-reactive against primary HIV isolates from diverse clades. Future advances will require the discovery of new immunogens that can induce neutralizing antibody, as well as efficacy trial evaluation of regimens optimized for CTL induction.

INTRODUCTION

The HIV-1 pandemic has become one of the greatest infectious disease threats to human health and social stability that the world has ever encountered. Nearly 40 million persons are living with HIV-1 infection and more than 21 million have already died from HIV-induced disease. Although effective antiretroviral therapy has slowed the epidemic in some industrialized countries, worldwide there are still an estimated 15,000 new HIV infections occurring daily. In addition to vast personal suffering and the loss of young adult parents, caretakers, and wage-earners, HIV has created an unprecedented strain on the social and economic infrastructure of many developing countries, particularly in sub-Saharan Africa. These facts make it imperative that the epidemic be controlled as rapidly as possible

---

*The US Government has the right to retain a nonexclusive, royalty-free license in and to any copyright covering this paper.

through prevention of new infections. Although education and available public health approaches should be vigorously pursued, development of a preventive vaccine is the best hope of controlling the HIV epidemic.

New molecular tools in virology and immunology, new adjuvants, new gene expression systems, new antigen delivery systems, recent discoveries concerning HIV entry and pathogenesis, evidence that natural immunity is achieved in rare instances, and promising studies of candidate vaccines in animal models have provided reasons to hope for a safe and effective AIDS vaccine. However, some have argued that preventive vaccination for AIDS will not be possible (1), and the complex biology of HIV-1 makes its development a daunting task.

EXPECTATIONS OF A VACCINE AGAINST HIV

Vaccines developed during the last century have provided unprecedented health and freedom from epidemics of many previously common infectious diseases. They have worked by protecting the vaccinated individual from the consequences of infection, but also by reducing the incidence of transmission within the population, diminishing the spread of epidemics. The ultimate goal for HIV vaccine development is to prevent infection in an exposed individual or induce rapid clearance of infected cells to avoid persistent infection. However, no current licensed vaccine for other viral pathogens is known to fully prevent infection, and most are effective because they limit the replication and spread of the pathogen below the threshold for clinical expression of disease. It is unlikely that vaccine-induced immune responses will be able to prevent the establishment of latency. It has been shown that a small proportion of infected CD4+ T cells become quiescent, allowing viral latency to be established in a reservoir of long-lived cells (1a, this volume). Therefore, a more realistic initial goal for HIV vaccine development is to dampen the initial viremia in an infected individual, maintain a low virus load, and prevent progression to AIDS.

Altering the disease course in individuals could potentially have a large impact on the spread of HIV within a population. The determinants of epidemic spread can be expressed as $R_o = \beta \times c \times D$, where R_o is the reproductive rate of the epidemic or a measure of spread; β is the transmission efficiency of the agent; c is the frequency of new partners or new transmission opportunities; and D is the duration of transmissibility. If $R_o > 1$, the epidemic will spread, and if $R_o < 1$ the epidemic will diminish (2). Effective vaccination has the potential to change both β and D, while education, surveillance, and traditional public health approaches can alter c. The significant impact on the incidence of new infections from the use of highly active antiretroviral treatment (HAART), as well as natural history studies, encourage the idea that vaccine-induced immune responses that maintain a low viral load in infected individuals will reduce transmission efficiency in the population (3). Therefore, the initial aim in vaccine development is to identify approaches that will induce immune responses that control infection and prevent disease in individuals, and slow the epidemic spread of HIV within a population.

ASSUMPTIONS RELEVANT TO HIV VACCINE DESIGN

Vaccine-Induced Immunity is Possible

Although many challenges remain, three observations suggest that vaccine development is feasible. First, HIV transmission is relatively inefficient. On average, more than 200 exposures are required to cause one infection in settings of sexual transmission (4) or needle-stick injuries (5). Therefore, modest improvement in antiviral defenses may have a profound impact on the transmissibility of HIV. Furthermore, based on analysis of HIV isolates in acute infection, most individuals are infected with a very small number of infectious particles, in many cases a single virion (6, 7). The small inoculum size improves the chances that vaccine-induced immunity could prevent infection. In addition, these data suggest that transmitted virus may have limited structural and genotypic features, which would further improve the chances for identifying mechanisms of protective immunity. Second, there are examples of natural immunity from studies of highly exposed, uninfected (8, 9), and long-term nonprogressor (10) populations. There is also evidence from western Africa, where there are concurrent epidemics of HIV-1 and HIV-2, that prior infection with the less virulent HIV-2 confers some protection against HIV-1 infection (11). Finally, there are now many examples of passive protection and vaccine-induced immunity in nonhuman primate models of lentivirus infection.

Timing of the HIV-Specific Immune Response is Critical

Several parameters of the vaccine-induced immune response determine its ability to protect the host from infection or disease, including specificity, functional properties, magnitude, and compartmentalization. Another critical factor is timing. The timing of the immune response with respect to initial virus infection and spread is particularly important in the case of HIV-1 infection. One reason is that the longer HIV-1 replicates in the host, the more diverse variants evolve, which may allow escape from subsequent immune responses. In addition, once HIV-1 resides in the extracellular space of lymph node germinal centers and in latently infected cellular reservoirs, or is sequestered in the central nervous system and other sites that are relatively protected from immune responses, it probably cannot be fully eliminated from the host.

After the initial burst of virus replication and high-titer viremia, the titer of virus in plasma is reduced by the initial immune responses and establishes a new plateau about 6 months after infection, referred to as the viral load "set point." The immune response to HIV-1 infection includes potent effector responses that at best achieve a steady state in which virus clearance matches virus production (11a, this volume). The magnitude of the viral load "set point" correlates with the rate of immune system destruction (12). The important advantage of vaccine-induced immune responses is that they are induced prior to infection and can be recalled more rapidly than primary effector mechanisms. Therefore, the success of vaccination may hinge on altering events that occur in the early hours following HIV-1 exposure.

Vaccines Work By Inducing Adaptive Immune Responses

Preventive vaccines work by establishing immunologic memory for antigenic structures presented by the pathogen or by infected cells. Therefore, the immunologic "tool box" accessible for vaccine-induced immunity only includes elements of the adaptive immune response. The basic cellular elements of adaptive immunity include the B and T lymphocytes. The primary effector mechanisms important for protection against viruses are antibodies produced by B cells and cytotoxic activity mediated primarily by CD8+ T cells. In addition, soluble factors produced by activated CD4+ and CD8+ T cells have antiviral activity and can influence the differentiation, expansion, and duration of T cell responses. Elements of the nonadaptive immune system are important during the initial phases of antigen presentation and development of the cytokine microenvironment, mediating many of the activities induced by adjuvants. However, immunity against subsequent infection is determined by adaptive immune responses with memory for key antigens and functional effector activities that can neutralize the pathogen and rapidly eliminate infected cells.

Neutralizing Antibody and Cytotoxic T Cells are the Major Effectors of Antiviral Immunity

The correlates of immunity against HIV-1 have not been defined in an absolute sense, but much is known about HIV-specific immune responses associated with long-term survival and maintenance of low viral loads (11a, this volume). In addition, there is a general understanding about how different elements of the adaptive immune response should work, and these concepts can be tested against observations made in studies of the natural history of HIV infection in humans or experimental data from animal models (13). Alternative vaccine-inducible effector mechanisms mediated by chemokines and other soluble factors produced by T cells may ultimately be shown to have a role in protection (14, 15), but in this review I focus on classical neutralizing antibody and CD8+ cytotoxic T cell activities.

There is debate and speculation about which component of the adaptive immune system is most important for immunity. However, abundant evidence indicates that in HIV and other virus infections, both antibody and CD8+ CTL are important and perform complementary roles in protection from and control of infection. CD4+ T cells are also of obvious importance, especially for influencing differentiation patterns and expansion of selected lymphocyte populations, but their role as a direct effector of virus clearance is less clear. Therefore, another assumption is that CD4+ T cells will be induced in the process of achieving the appropriate antibody and CD8+ CTL responses. CD4+ T cells are not specifically addressed in this paper.

Antibody is the only component of the adaptive immune response that can neutralize a virus particle prior to infection of a cell and is the only immune response associated with protection for any currently licensed vaccines. Antibody titers can be sustained at high levels in serum and in mucosal secretions and be present at the time of infection. T cells, in contrast, recognize virus only in the context of an already infected cell and require a few days for activation and expansion of memory populations to respond. Therefore, an effective neutralizing antibody response is likely to be a critical component of vaccine-induced immunity, because it can prevent infection and thereby reduce inoculum size and establishment of latently infected cells.

Neutralization is defined as the ability to reduce infectivity of cell-free virus, usually measured in susceptible cells in culture. Although this aspect of antibody activity is thought to be the key function associated with protection from infection, there is some debate about its mechanism. The identification of specific neutralizing epitopes suggests that the site of antibody binding is important. However, it has also been suggested that neutralization occurs when a threshold level of the virion surface is covered by antibody that binds the native envelope oligomer regardless of specificity (16). In either case, it is clear that T cell line–adapted viruses are more susceptible to neutralization than primary field isolates, which presents a major obstacle to achieving this immunologic endpoint (17, 18).

T cells recognize virus-infected cells by specific interactions between the T cell receptor and 8–10 amino acid peptides processed from viral antigens and presented in the context of major histocompatibility complex (MHC) molecules. Therefore, T cells can only recognize and clear virus after infection has occurred. The recognition is restricted by the MHC molecule, which means that the particular epitopes recognized by a given individual depend on the set of inherited alleles encoding the MHC molecules. Although each person should have the capacity to recognize multiple epitopes among the antigens included in HIV-1, the hierarchy of recognition or epitope dominance may vary even among individuals who share MHC haplotypes. These issues suggest that the epitope repertoire in an HIV-1 vaccine will need enough breadth to encompass all the relevant MHC haplotypes of potential vaccinees. In addition, it will be important to induce a broad response in each individual against several viral antigens to diminish the possibility of immune escape through genetic variation and to allow for host selection of dominant epitopes.

The need for CD4+ T lymphocytes to initiate the adaptive immune response presents a dilemma, since these cells are the major targets for HIV-1 infection. The challenge is to effectively induce protective immunity against HIV-1 without risking infection of vaccine-induced HIV-specific CD4+ T cells. This emphasizes the need for effective immune responses, preexistent at the time of HIV exposure, so that virus clearance can be accomplished before the burden of infected cells is sufficient to maintain persistent infection. Although CD4+ T cells may have some capacity for lysis of HIV-infected cells (19) and production of antiviral cytokines, their major role is in shaping the immune response by establishing a microenvironment with a particular cytokine composition. For HIV and most other viruses, induction of type 1 cytokines [production of interleukin(IL)-12, IL-2, and interferon (IFN)-γ] is more likely to provide protection than induction of type 2 cytokines (IL-4, IL-5, IL-13). Initial priming with vectors and the use of adjuvants other than alum (which promotes type 2 responses) would provide an advantage.

CD8+ T cells are the principal effector mechanism of the adaptive immune response to clear virus-infected cells. The CD8+ lymphocyte recognizes a virus-infected cell through a cognate interaction between the T cell receptor and a processed peptide epitope presented in the groove of an MHC class I molecule. The lysis of the infected cells occurs through the production and secretion of perforin and granzymes that penetrate the target cell membrane and induce apoptosis. FasL is also upregulated on the activated CD8+ T cell and can bind Fas on the target cell, providing another avenue for inducing apoptosis of the infected target cell. CD8+ T cells also produce cytokines with antiviral properties, such as IFN-γ and tumor necrosis factor (TNF)-α, in addition to other soluble factors that may play a role in virus inhibition. The T cell response causes cytopathology not only of the virus-infected cell but also to some degree in bystander cells. This again points to the importance of clearing virus rapidly to diminish the overall cytopathology and illness associated with the immune response to infection. For a more detailed review of immune control of HIV infection and HIV escape from immunity, see Chapter 9 (11a) and Chapter 28 (19a) in this volume.

DATA FROM STUDIES IN HUMANS AND ANIMALS

Antibody Can Prevent HIV Infection

Passive antibody studies in nonhuman primate models of lentivirus infection have directly proven that sufficient levels of neutralizing antibody can prevent infection. Studies evaluating polyclonal anti-HIV-1 antiserum (20) or monoclonal anti-V3 antibody in HIV-1 infected chimpanzees (20a) or polyclonal serum in SIV-infected macaques (21) have shown that when sufficiently high antibody titers are present prior to intravenous challenge, lentivirus infection can be prevented. Importantly, antibody-mediated protection has also been demonstrated against SHIV (a chimeric virus composed of an HIV envelope and SIV nucleocapsid and replication machinery) with an envelope glycoprotein derived from a dual tropic primary HIV isolate, and the protection could be correlated with in vitro neutralizing activity (22). More recently, passive prophylaxis using HIV immune globulin combined with two monoclonal antibodies has protected macaques from vaginal challenge with SHIV (23), and a mixture of three neutralizing monoclonal IgG1 antibodies given to pregnant macaques has protected their infants from SHIV oral challenge (24).

Definitive evidence of antibody-mediated protection in studies of active immunization has been more difficult to demonstrate, but an example from early studies performed with whole inactivated SIV vaccines is provocative. These studies showed that antibodies to cell constituents incorporated into virions during production of challenge stocks were the best correlate of protection. When the virus used to produce vaccine was grown in human cells, and the virus challenge stock was grown in the same human cells, allogenic responses to the human proteins incorporated by the virus were the dominant mechanism of protection (25–28). Studies done with vaccine produced in monkey cells did not show consistent protection. Even though the antibody response was not specific for virus-encoded antigens, this example of vaccine-induced antibody-mediated protection suggests that protection through induction of virus-specific antibodies may be achievable. When SIV immune globulin was given one day after intravenous challenge with SIV, infection was not prevented, but disease progression was delayed in some animals (29). This again illustrates that the timing of immune responses is critical to the outcome of infection and that preexisting immunity gives the host a distinct advantage.

T Cells Can Control HIV Infection

Control of the initial viremia associated with primary HIV infection temporally correlates with the appearance of CD8+ cytotoxic T lymphocytes (30, 31), and mutations in specific CTL epitopes can be detected in the residual virus population (reviewed in 32). In addition, HIV-specific CD8+ CTL activity has been demonstrated in a small subset of uninfected, seronegative commercial sex workers in the Gambia and in Kenya, which suggests that transient infection may have occurred, inducing protective immunity mediated by CD8+ CTL (8, 9). In persons who remain uninfected despite significant occupational exposure to HIV-1–contaminated material, studies have also focused on HIV-specific T cell responses. Although HIV-specific antibodies cannot be detected, peripheral blood mononuclear cells show lymphoproliferative activity when stimulated with HIV-specific peptides (33). HIV-specific CTL responses have also been seen in this cohort (34), suggesting that transient infection may have occurred and been cleared by natural immune defenses.

Another subset of persons infected with HIV-1 have persistent infection but do not progress to AIDS for >12 years. Some of these individuals are infected with virus isolates that replicate poorly (35, 36). Others, though infected with viruses of normal replication capacity, have maintained a strong and broad set of humoral (36a) and cellular (37, 38) HIV-specific immune responses that may be responsible for their delayed disease progression. This phenomenon has been best associated with HIV-specific CD4+ T cell proliferation (37) and strong CD8+ CTL activity against multiple epitopes (38).

Another clue to the importance of T cell responses in the control of HIV has come from the evaluation of HIV-infected persons treated with HAART soon after primary infection. When these persons undergo structured treatment interruptions, there is a transient rise in the virus load, which results in a boost of functional T cell activity and subsequent control of virus load without HAART (39).

The most compelling evidence for the importance of CD8+ CTL for controlling lentivirus infection comes from studies of pathogenesis and vaccine evaluation in nonhuman primates. The CD8+ CTL response is the best correlate of viremia control after primary SIV infection in macaques (40). Several studies using nucleic acid or other recombinant vector approaches have demonstrated that induction of CD8+ CTL responses with a weak or absent antibody response does not prevent lentivirus infection but reduces viral load and delays disease progression. One of the early demonstrations of this was in macaques immunized with recombinant MVA (modified vaccinia Ankara) prior to challenge with SIV. Vaccination did not prevent infection, and the CTL cell response was associated with delayed disease progression (41). Subsequent studies have shown similar patterns (42–50). As attempts are made to optimize the CD8+ CTL response, such as the addition of an IL-2 adjuvant to a recombinant DNA vaccine regimen (49) or combining modalities of DNA and MVA (50), subsequent SHIV infection can be almost completely controlled. These data are consistent with the premise that vaccines able to establish a preexisting expanded population of HIV-specific CD8+ CTL are likely to delay disease progression in HIV-infected persons.

CLINICAL TRIALS OF CANDIDATE HIV VACCINES

Overview of Concepts Evaluated

Clinical trials have been performed in nearly 10,000 seronegative volunteers to evaluate the safety and immunogenicity of candidate AIDS vaccines. Recombinant envelope products, rgp120 or rgp160, produced in insect, yeast, or mammalian cells formulated with a variety of adjuvants, have been evaluated in clinical trials. Peptides tested to date have been derived from envelope V3 loop or gag sequences of clade B or multiple clades. They have been presented conjugated to an oligolysine backbone, as a lipopeptide conjugate, mixed with adjuvant, or as a fusion protein with the self-assembling yeast protein, Ty, as a particle. They have been administered intramuscularly in the deltoid or anterior thigh (to target lymph nodes that also drain the rectal mucosa), rectally and orally as Ty-gag virus-like particles, and orally encapsulated in polylactide copolymers. Live recombinant vectors including vaccinia, canarypox, and salmonella have been evaluated as well as nucleic acid–based vaccines. These vectors have been delivered by various routes and have been constructed to express either single or multiple HIV-1 antigens from both structural and nonstructural proteins.

New trials utilizing recombinant replication-incompetent adenovirus and MVA are just under way, as is a novel approach in which tat is the vaccine antigen. Tat is secreted from HIV-infected cells and has adverse effects on neighboring cells. It is hypothesized that blocking these effects with vaccine-induced antibody will facilitate virus clearance (51). These and other studies evaluating schedule-of-administration and combination approaches using more than one product in the immunization regimen (52–54) are compiled and updated on the web site of the National Institutes of Health Vaccine Research Center (54). This table also documents studies that have advanced to Phase II and III status, and those that have been performed at sites outside the US. Fortunately, there have been no significant safety concerns other than unacceptable local reactogenicity associated with a few selected adjuvants (55).

Vaccine-Induced Antibody Responses in Clinical Trials

Neutralizing antibody responses have been induced by immunization with recombinant envelope glycoproteins alone or in combination with poxvirus vectors. The antibody response to immunization with rgp120 alone is in general maximal after the third or fourth injection, is dose-dependent, and can be attenuated unless there is a several-month interval between injections. Serum antibody titers have a relatively short half-life, and although they can be boosted, the titers generally achieve their peak level after the third or fourth injections. Repeated boosting does not prolong the half-life significantly. Therefore, it is likely that recombinant envelope glycoprotein products may find their greatest utility in boosting antibody responses in subjects primed with recombinant vector vaccines (56), or other strategies that can induce MHC class I–restricted CTL responses. This combination approach not only adds the CD8+ CTL component to the immune response but also results in a more durable antibody response.

The initial recombinant envelope glycoprotein products were derived from sequences of syncytium-inducing, T cell line–adapted (TCLA), CXCR-4–utilizing X4 viruses from clade B. Newer products, such as the VaxGen B/B product, incorporate sequences from primary isolates that utilize CCR5 (R5), combining the rgp120 from HIV-1$_{MN}$ and the rgp120 from HIV-1$_{GNE8}$ (57). Phase I and II studies have defined how dose, schedule, and formulation affect immunogenicity of purified protein subunit preparations as primary immunogens and as booster immunogens given in combination with other vaccine modalities. The principal findings related to vaccine-induced antibody responses in clinical trials of candidate HIV vaccines are that neutralizing antibody responses against TCLA viruses induced by the most immunogenic formulations are still five- to ten-fold lower than those produced by HIV-1 infection. The responses are type-specific with a relatively short half-life and are unable to neutralize typical primary isolate R5 viruses (54).

Vaccine-Induced CD8+ CTL Responses in Clinical Trials

Induction of HIV-specific CD8+ CTL responses generally requires the delivery of vaccine antigens into the cytoplasmic compartment of an antigen-presenting cell (APC) for display in an MHC class I molecule on the cell surface. Therefore, vector-based approaches or nucleic acid vaccines that rely on antigen production within the target cell are most effective. Delivering vaccine antigens as purified proteins or even whole inactivated virus will primarily access the endocytic pathway for antigen presentation and lead to CD4+ T cell activation. Although this is critical for antibody production and important for supporting CD8+ CTL development, it is not sufficient for inducing CD8+ CTL. In some cases, a novel adjuvant or delivery system is able to provide access for these types of vaccines into the cytoplasmic compartment, but in general vector-based vaccines, including nucleic acids, are more potent methods for inducing CD8+ CTL. One exception is the use of peptides that incorporate a T cell epitope that can bind directly to an MHC class I molecule on the cell surface and induce CD8+ CTL responses.

Vector-based vaccines, beginning with recombinant vaccinia products, were first evaluated in clinical trials in the late 1980s with the expressed purpose of achieving vaccine-induced CD8+ CTL responses. The induction of CD8+ CTL responses has been a primary focus of clinical trials since the mid-1990s. It has been found that recombinant vaccinia expressing envelope glycoprotein only, or multiple antigens, can consistently induce long-lived CD8+ CTL responses in vaccinia-naive subjects (58–61). HIV-specific CD8+ CTL can also be detected in a majority of subjects receiving recombinant canarypoxvirus vectors, and in a subset, CTL activity is detectable for >18 months. The activity is at the threshold of detection in classical ^{51}Cr release assays requiring in vitro stimulation and is detected in only 15%–30% of subjects at any given time (62–66). However, unlike antibody responses, vaccine-induced CTL responses are broadly cross-reactive (67). CTLs induced by recombinant canarypox vectors have been shown to lyse target cells infected with primary R5 HIV-1 isolates from multiple clades (67). CD8+ CTL effectors have also been isolated from rectal mucosa from vaccinees, which suggests that T cells induced by parenteral vaccination may provide some level of protection at mucosal surfaces (M.J. McElrath et al., unpublished observations). Not only is classical MHC class I–restricted cytotoxic activity induced, but vaccine-induced noncytotoxic CD8+-mediated suppression of HIV-1 replication has also been demonstrated in recipients of recombinant canarypox vaccines (68). In summary, vaccine approaches that are currently being evaluated in clinical trials can induce HIV-specific CD8+ CTL activity that is durable and can lyse cells infected with typical primary R5 HIV-1 isolates from multiple clades. A phase III study evaluating the efficacy of combined recombinant canarypox with rgp120 is planned for Thailand, and a decision will be made in 2002 whether to advance this combination to phase III evaluation in the United States.

Recent advances in methods to quantitate T cells and evaluate their function are changing the process of vaccine evaluation. Enumeration of functional T cells by IFN-γ ELIspot or intracellular IFN-γ by FACS analysis, combined with identification of epitope-specific T cells with MHC-peptide tetramers by FACS analysis (69), has improved the ability to detect vaccine-induced responses by improving sensitivity and reproducibility. This allows the use of cryopreserved cells and reduces the number of effector cells needed.

FUTURE SCIENTIFIC CHALLENGES FOR HIV VACCINE DEVELOPMENT

Despite the current optimism, there are still many scientific obstacles to overcome in the development of a vaccine for HIV. Most important is the inability to induce broadly cross-reactive neutralizing antibody against typical primary HIV-1 isolates. This is one of several immune evasion strategies employed by HIV (19a, this volume). Without a high level of neutralizing activity present at the time of infection, it is unlikely that a vaccine-induced immune response can prevent the establishment of latency and infection of immunoprivileged sites. There are also questions involving the importance of HIV genetic variation, mucosal immunity, and duration of vaccine-induced immune responses that will be difficult to address until large-scale efficacy trials are implemented. In addition, many ethical, logistic, and economic challenges lie ahead.

In summary, the ultimate vaccine that can prevent persistent HIV-1 infection will probably require a conceptual breakthrough in the understanding of how to elicit broadly neutralizing antibody against primary R5 HIV-1 isolates. Development of such a vaccine will also involve a number of iterative steps to achieve optimal HIV-specific CD8+ CTL responses. However, a vaccine aimed at controlling viremia, delaying disease progression, and reducing transmission, based on induction of HIV-specific CD8+ CTL, could have a significant impact on the AIDS epidemic and may be within our grasp using currently available technology.

ACKNOWLEDGMENT

I thank R. Stokes Peebles for reviewing the manuscript.

Visit the Annual Reviews home page at www.AnnualReviews.org

LITERATURE CITED

1. Sabin AB. 1992. Improbability of effective vaccination against human immunodeficiency virus because of its intracellular transmission and rectal portal of entry. *Proc. Natl. Acad. Sci. USA* 89:8852–55

1a. Blankson JN, Persaud D, Siliciano RF. The challenge of viral reservoirs in HIV-1 infection. *Annu. Rev. Med.* 53:557–93

2. Holmes KK. 1994. Human ecology and behavior and sexually transmitted bacterial infections. *Proc. Natl. Acad. Sci. USA* 91:2448–55

3. Quinn TC, Wawer MJ, Sewankambo N, et al. 2001. Viral load and heterosexual transmission of human immunodeficiency virus type 1. Rakai Project Study Group. *N. Engl. J. Med.* 342:921–29

4. Gray RH, Wawer MJ, Brookmeyer R, et al. 2001. Probability of HIV-1 transmission per coital act in monogamous, heterosexual, HIV-1-discordant couples in Rakai, Uganda. *Lancet* 357:1149–53

5. Geberding JL. 1994. Incidence and prevalence of human immunodeficiency virus, hepatitis B virus, hepatitis C virus, and cytomegalovirus among health care personnel at risk for blood exposure: final report

from a longitudinal study. *J. Infect. Dis.* 170:1410–17

6. Wolinsky SM, Wike CM, Korber BTM, et al. 1992. Selective transmission of human immunodeficiency virus type-1 variants from mothers to infants. *Science* 255:1134–37

7. Wolfs TF, Zwart G, Bakker M, Goudsmit J. 1992. HIV-1 genomic RNA diversification following sexual and parenteral virus transmission. *Virology* 189:103–10

8. Fowke KR, Nagelkerke NJ, Kimani J, et al. 1996. Resistance to HIV-1 infection among persistently seronegative prostitutes in Nairobi, Kenya. *Lancet* 348: 1347–51

9. Rowland-Jones S, Sutton J, Ariyoshi K, et al. 1995. HIV-specific cytotoxic T-cells in HIV-exposed but uninfected Gambian women. *Nat. Med.* 1:59–64

10. Wagner R, Leschonsky B, Harrer E, et al. 1999. Molecular and functional analysis of a conserved CTL epitope in HIV-1 p24 recognized from a long-term nonprogressor: constraints on immune escape associated with targeting a sequence essential for viral replication. *J. Immunol.* 162:3727–34

11. Kokkotou EG, Sankale JL, Mani I, et al. 2000. In vitro correlates of HIV-2 mediated HIV-1 protection. *Proc. Natl. Acad. Sci. USA* 97:6797–802

11a. Gandhi RT, Walker BD. 2002. Immunologic control of HIV-1. *Annu. Rev. Med.* 53:149–72

12. Mellors JW, Rinaldo CR Jr, Gupta P, et al. 1996. Prognosis in HIV-1 infection predicted by the quantity of virus in plasma. *Science* 272:1167–70

13. Ada GL. 1990. Modern vaccines: the immunological principles of vaccination. *Lancet* 335:523–26

14. Walker CM, Moody DJ, Stites DP, Levy JA. 1986. CD8+ lymphocytes can control HIV infection in vitro by suppressing virus replication. *Science* 234:1563–66

15. Cocchi F, DeVico AL, Garzino-Demo A, et al. 1995. Identification of RANTES, MIP-1 alpha, and MIP-1 beta as the major HIV-suppressive factors produced by CD8+ T cells. *Science* 270:1811–15

16. Parren PW, Burton DR. 2001. The antiviral activity of antibodies in vitro and in vivo. *Adv. Immunol.* 77:195–262

17. Trkola A, Ketas T, Kewalramani VN, et al. 1998. Neutralization sensitivity of human immunodeficiency virus type 1 primary isolates to antibodies and CD4-based reagents is independent of coreceptor usage. *J. Virol.* 72:1876–85

18. Cecilia D, KewalRamani VN, O'Leary J, et al. 1998. Neutralization profiles of primary human immunodeficiency virus type 1 isolates in the context of coreceptor usage. *J. Virol.* 72:698896

19. Siliciano RF, Lawton T, Knall C, Karr RW, Berman P, et al. 1988. Analysis of host-virus interactions in AIDS with anti-gp120 T cell clones: effect of HIV sequence variation and a mechanism for CD4+ cell depletion. *Cell* 54:561–75

19a. Johnson WE, Desrosiers RC. 2002. Viral persistence: HIV's strategies of immune system evasion. *Annu. Rev. Med.* 53:499–518

20. Prince AM, Reesink H, Pascual D, et al. 1991. Prevention of HIV infection by passive immunization with HIV immunoglobulin. *AIDS Res. Hum. Retroviruses* 7:971–73

20a. Emini EA, Schleif WA, Nunberg JH, et al. 1992. Prevention of HIV-1 infection in chimpanzees by gp120 V3 domain-specific monoclonal antibody. *Nature* 355:728–30

21. Putkonen P, Thorstensson R, Ghavamzadeh L, et al. 1991. Prevention of HIV-2 and SIV_{sm} infection by passive immunization in cynomolgus monkeys. *Nature* 352:436–38

22. Shibata R, Igarashi T, Haigwood N, et al. 1999. Neutralizing antibody directed against the HIV-1 envelope glycoprotein can completely block HIV-1/SIV chimeric virus infections of macaque monkeys. *Nat. Med.* 5:204–10

23. Mascola JR, Lewis MG, Stiegler G, et al. 1999. Protection of macaques against pathogenic simian/human immunodeficiency virus 89.6PD by passive transfer of neutralizing antibodies. *J. Virol.* 73:4009–18

24. Baba TW, Liska V, Hofmann-Lehmann R, et al. 2000. Human neutralizing monoclonal antibodies of the IgG1 subtype protect against mucosal simian-human immunodeficiency virus infection. *Nat. Med.* 6:200–6

25. Stott EJ. 1991. Anti-cell antibody in macaques. *Nature* 353:393

26. Stott EJ, Chan WL, Mills KH, et al. 1990. Preliminary report: protection of cynomolgus macaques against simian immunodeficiency virus by fixed infected-cell vaccine. *Lancet* 336:1538–41

27. Langlois AJ, Weinhold KJ, Matthews TJ, et al. 1992. Detection of anti-human cell antibodies in sera from macaques immunized with whole inactivated virus. *AIDS Res. Hum. Retroviruses* 8:1641–52

28. Montefiori DC, Cornell RJ, Zhou JY, et al. 1994. Complement control proteins, CD46, CD55, and CD59, as common surface constituents of human and simian immunodeficiency viruses and possible targets for vaccine protection. *Virology* 205:82–92

29. Haigwood NL, Watson A, Sutton WF, et al. 1996. Passive immune globulin therapy in the SIV/macaque model: early intervention can alter disease profile. *Immunol. Lett.* 51:107–14

30. Koup RA, Safrit JT, Cao YZ, et al. 1994. Temporal association of cellular immune responses with the initial control of viremia in primary human immunodeficiency virus type 1 syndrome. *J. Virol.* 68:4650–55

31. Borrow P, Lewicki H, Hahn BH, et al. 1994. Virus-specific CD8+ cytotoxic T-lymphocyte activity associated with control of viremia in primary human immunodeficiency virus type 1 infection. *J. Virol.* 68:6103–10

32. McMichael AJ, Phillips RE. 1997. Escape of human immunodeficiency virus from immune control. *Annu. Rev. Immunol.* 15:271–96

33. Clerici M, Levin JM, Kessler HA, et al. 1994. HIV-specific T-helper activity in seronegative health care workers exposed to contaminated blood. *JAMA* 271:42–46

34. Pinto LA, Sullivan J, Berzofsky JA, et al. 1995. ENV-specific cytotoxic T lymphocyte responses in HIV seronegative health care workers occupationally exposed to HIV-contaminated body fluids. *J. Clin. Invest.* 96:867–76

35. Deacon NJ, Tsykin A, Soloman A, et al. 1995. Genomic structure of an attenuated quasi species of HIV-1 from blood transfusion donor recipients. *Science* 270:988–91

36. Kirchhoff F, Greenough TC, Brettler DB, et al. 1995. Brief report: absence of intact nef sequences in a long-term survivor with nonprogressive HIV-1 infection. *N. Engl. J. Med.* 332:228–32

36a. Pilgrim AK, Pantaleo G, Cohen OJ, et al. 1997. Neutralizing antibody responses to human immunodeficiency virus type 1 in primary infection and long-term-nonprogressive infection. *J. Infect. Dis.* 176:924–32

37. Rosenberg ES, Billingsley JM, Caliendo AM, et al. 1997. Vigorous HIV-1-specific CD4+ T cell responses associated with control of viremia. *Science* 278:1447–50

38. Ortiz GM, Nixon DF, Trkola A, et al. 1999. HIV-1-specific immune responses in subjects who temporarily contain virus replication after discontinuation of highly active antiretroviral therapy. *J. Clin. Invest.* 104:R13–18

39. Rosenberg ES, Altfeld M, Poon SH, et al. 2000. Immune control of HIV-1 after early treatment of acute infection. *Nature* 407:523–26

40. Reimann KA, Tenner Racz K, Racz P, et al. 1994. Immunopathogenic events in acute infection of rhesus monkeys

with simian immunodeficiency virus of macaques. *J. Virol.* 68:2362–70

41. Hirsch VM, Fuerst TR, Sutter G, et al. 1996. Patterns of viral replication correlate with outcome in simian immunodeficiency virus (SIV)-infected macaques: effect of prior immunization with a trivalent SIV vaccine in modified vaccinia virus Ankara. *J. Virol.* 70:3741–52

42. Ourmanov I, Brown CR, Moss B, et al. 2000. Comparative efficacy of recombinant modified vaccinia virus Ankara expressing simian immunodeficiency virus (SIV) Gag-Pol and/or Env in macaques challenged with pathogenic SIV. *J. Virol.* 74:2740–51

43. Leno M, Kowalski M, Robert-Guroff M. 2000. CD8 T cell anti-HIV activity as a complementary protective mechanism in vaccinated chimpanzees. *AIDS* 14:893–94

44. Allen TM, Vogel TU, Fuller DH, et al. 2000. Introduction of AIDS virus-specific CTL activity in fresh, unstimulated peripheral blood lymphocytes from rhesus macaques vaccinated with a DNA prime/modified vaccinia virus Ankara boost regimen. *J. Immunol.* 164:4968–78

45. Buge SL, Richardson E, Alipanah S, et al. 1997. An adenovirus-simian immunodeficiency virus env vaccine elicits humoral, cellular, and mucosal immune responses in rhesus macaques and decreases viral burden following vaginal challenge. *J. Virol.* 71:8531–41

46. Abimiku AG, Robert-Guroff M, Benson J, et al. 1997. Long-term survival of SIVmac251-infected macaques previously immunized with NYVAC-SIV vaccines. *J. Acq. Immun. Defic. Syndr.* 15:S78–85

47. Davis NL, Caley IJ, Brown KW, et al. 2000. Vaccination of macaques against pathogenic simian immunodeficiency virus with Venezuelan equine encephalitis virus replicon particles. *J. Virol.* 74:371–78

48. Egan MA, Charini WA, Kuroda MJ, et al. 2000. Simian immunodeficiency virus (SIV) gag DNA-vaccinated rhesus monkeys develop secondary cytotoxic T-lymphocyte responses and control viral replication after pathogenic SIV infection. *J. Virol.* 74:7485–95

49. Barouch DH, Santra S, Schmitz JE, et al. 2001. Control of viremia and prevention of clinical AIDS in rhesus monkeys by cytokine-augmented DNA vaccination. *Science* 290:486–92

50. Amara RR, Villinger F, Altman JD, et al. 2001. Control of a mucosal challenge and prevention of AIDS by a multiprotein DNA/MVA vaccine. *Science* 292:69–74

51. Cafaro A, Caputo A, Fracasso C, et al. 1999. Control of SHIV-89.6P-infection of cynomolgus monkeys by HIV-1 Tat protein vaccine. *Nat. Med.* 5:643–50

52. Graham BS, Karzon DT. 1998. AIDS vaccine development. In *Textbook of AIDS Medicine*, ed. TC Merigan, JG Bartlett, D Bolognesi, 42:689–724. Baltimore, MD: Williams & Wilkins. 1063 pp. 2nd ed.

53. Graham BS. 2000. Clinical trials of HIV vaccines. In *HIV Molecular Immunology 2000*, ed. BTM Korber, JP Moore, C Brander, et al., p. I-20–I-38. Los Alamos, NM: Los Alamos Natl. Lab., Theor. Biol. Biophys. http://hiv-web.lanl.gov/immunology

54. Graham BS. 2001. NIH Vaccine Research Center Clinical Studies. http://www.vrc.nih.gov/VRC/clinstudies.htm

55. Keefer MC, Wolff M, Gorse GG, et al. 1997. Safety profile of phase I and II preventive HIV-1 vaccination: experience of the AIDS Vaccine Evaluation Group. *AIDS Res. Hum. Retroviruses* 13:1163–77

56. Graham BS, Matthews TJ, Belshe RB, et al. 1993. Augmentation of human immunodeficiency virus type 1 neutralizing antibody by priming with gp160 recombinant vaccinia and boosting with rgp160 in vaccinia-naive adults. *J. Infect. Dis.* 167:533–37

57. Berman PW, Huang W, Riddle L, et al.

1999. Development of bivalent (B/E) vaccines able to neutralize CCR5-dependent viruses from the United States and Thailand. *Virology* 265:1–9

58. Cooney EL, McElrath MJ, Corey L, et al. 1993. Enhanced immunity to human immunodeficiency virus (HIV) envelope elicited by a combined vaccine regimen consisting of priming with a vaccinia recombinant expressing HIV envelope and boosting with gp160 protein. *Proc. Natl. Acad. Sci. USA* 90:1882–86

59. Corey L, McElrath MJ, Weinhold K, et al. 1998. Cytotoxic T cell and neutralizing antibody responses to HIV-1 envelope with a combination vaccine regimen. *J. Infect. Dis.* 177:301–9

60. Hammond SA, Bollinger RC, Stanhope PE, et al. 1992. Comparative clonal analysis of human immunodeficiency virus type 1 (HIV-1)-specific CD4+ and CD8+ cytolytic T lymphocytes isolated from seronegative humans immunized with candidate HIV-1 vaccines. *J. Exp. Med.* 176:1531–42

61. El-Daher N, Keefer MC, Reichman RC, et al. 1993. Persisting human immunodeficiency virus type 1 gp160-specific human T lymphocyte responses including CD8+ cytotoxic activity after receipt of envelope vaccines. *J. Infect. Dis.* 168:306–13

62. Clements-Mann ML, Matthews TJ, Weinhold K, et al. 1998. HIV-1 immune responses induced by canarypox (ALVAC)-gp160 MN, SF-2 rgp120, or both vaccines in seronegative adults. *J. Infect. Dis.* 177:1230–46

63. Evans TG, Keefer MC, Weinhold KJ, et al. 1999. A canarypox vaccine expressing multiple HIV-1 genes given alone or with rgp120 elicits broad and durable CD8+ CTL responses in seronegative volunteers. *J. Infect. Dis.* 180:290–98

64. Belshe RB, Gorse GJ, Mulligan MJ, et al. 1998. Induction of immune responses to HIV-1 by canarypox virus (ALVAC) HIV-1 and gp120 SF-2 recombinant vaccines in uninfected volunteers. *AIDS* 12:2407–15

65. Salmon-Ceron D, Excler JL, Finkielsztejn L, et al. 1999. Safety and immunogenicity of a live recombinant canarypox virus expressing HIV type 1 gp120 MN tm/gag/protease LAI (ALVAC-HIV, vCP205) followed by a p24E-V3 MN synthetic peptide (CLTB-36) administered in healthy volunteers at low risk for HIV infection. *AIDS Res. Hum. Retroviruses* 15:633–45

66. Belshe RB, Stevens C, Gorse GJ, et al. 2001. Safety and immunogenicity of a canarypox-vectored human immunodeficiency virus type 1 vaccine with or without gp120: a phase 2 study in higher- and lower-risk volunteers. *J. Infect. Dis.* 183:1343–52

67. Ferrari G, Humphrey W, McElrath MJ, et al. 1997. Clade B–based HIV-1 vaccines elicit cross-clade cytotoxic T lymphocyte reactivities in uninfected volunteers. *Proc. Natl. Acad. Sci. USA* 94:1396–401

68. Castillo RC, Arango-Jaramillo S, John R, et al. 2000. Resistance to human immunodeficiency virus type 1 in vitro as a surrogate of vaccine-induced protective immunity. *J. Infect. Dis.* 181:897–903

69. Murali-Krishna K, Altman JD, Suresh M, et al. 1998. Counting antigen-specific CD8 T cells: a reevaluation of bystander activation during viral infection. *Immunity* 8:177–87

Annu. Rev. Med. 2002. 53:223–43

CHEMOPREVENTION OF AERODIGESTIVE TRACT CANCERS

Edward S. Kim, Waun Ki Hong, and Fadlo Raja Khuri
*Thoracic/Head and Neck Medical Oncology, The University of Texas,
M. D. Anderson Cancer Center, 1515 Holcombe Blvd., Houston, Texas 77030;
e-mail: edkim@mdanderson.org; whong@mdanderson.org*

Key Words   head and neck cancer, lung cancer, prevention, retinoids,
biochemoprevention

■ **Abstract**   Epithelial cancers are a major worldwide health problem. Since the
mid-1970s, advances in multidisciplinary cancer therapeutics have only slightly improved the mortality rate from epithelial malignancies. Chemoprevention is the use of
specific natural or synthetic chemical agents to reverse, suppress, or prevent progression
to invasive cancer. Chemopreventive medicine is based on translating basic biologic
research into clinical chemical interventions, thus attempting to impede carcinogenesis. Its principles build on the concepts of field cancerization (diffuse epithelial injury
that results from carcinogen exposure) and multistep carcinogenesis (a stepwise accumulation of cellular and genetic alterations that progress to cancer). Chemoprevention
targets the carcinogenic process at earlier and potentially more reversible stages, focusing on the inhibition of one or many steps in the progression towards cancer. Strategies
of chemoprevention include primary prevention in groups at high risk, reversal of
premalignant lesions, and prevention of second primary tumors.

INTRODUCTION

Epithelial cancers are a major worldwide health problem. Since the mid-1970s,
advances in multidisciplinary cancer therapeutics have only slightly improved the
mortality rate from epithelial malignancies. Although some patients present with
early-stage cancers, a majority present with locally advanced or metastatic disease.
Surgical intervention with adjuvant treatment including radiotherapy and/or concurrent chemoradiation has offered some improvement in long-term survival rates.
However, local recurrence and especially the development of second primary tumors (SPTs) have affected both morbidity and mortality in this patient population.
Thus, novel approaches to epithelial cancers are highly desirable.

Epithelial carcinogenesis is a multistep process in which an accumulation of genetic events leads to a progressively dysplastic cellular appearance, dysregulated
cell growth, and finally frank carcinoma. As the biologic basis for carcinogenesis continues to be elucidated, various strategies for prevention have emerged,

including treatment of premalignant lesions, adjuvant treatment, and prevention of SPTs.

The success of recent clinical trials designed to prevent cancer in patients who are at increased risk for developing it suggests that chemopreventive agents can interrupt the carcinogenic process and that chemoprevention is a rational and appealing treatment strategy.

This review focuses on current chemoprevention approaches, including both laboratory research and clinical trials specifically targeting cancers of the aerodigestive tract, lung, and head and neck. Chemopreventive agents, the mechanism by which they may inhibit abnormal epithelial cell growth and differentiation, and the genetic events associated with epithelial carcinogenesis are also discussed. Furthermore, the utility of intermediate biomarkers as markers of premalignancy is reviewed. Finally, we analyze chemoprevention strategies with reference to specific trials and clinical outcome and propose future directions in chemoprevention based on recently acquired mechanistic insight into carcinogenesis and chemoprevention.

CANCER CHEMOPREVENTION

The term chemoprevention, introduced by Sporn in 1976, can be defined as the use of specific natural or synthetic chemical agents to reverse, suppress, or prevent progression to invasive cancer (1). Early detection techniques tailored to screen for aerodigestive tract cancers included annual chest X-ray and sputum cytology analysis in individuals at high risk for lung cancer. Despite these early efforts, overall mortality and survival did not improve.

The foundation of chemopreventive medicine is the translation of basic biologic research into clinical chemical interventions, thus attempting to halt the process of carcinogenesis. Its principles build on the concepts of field cancerization and multistep carcinogenesis. Field cancerization is the diffuse epithelial injury that results from carcinogen exposure, such as in the aerodigestive tract. Genetic changes, including both premalignant and malignant lesions in one region of the field, translate into an increased risk of cancer development throughout the entire field. Multistep carcinogenesis is a stepwise accumulation of cellular and genetic alterations, both genotypic and phenotypic. Arresting one or several of the steps may impede or delay the development of cancer. This has been described particularly well in studies involving precancerous and cancerous lesions of the head and neck, which focus on oral premalignant lesions (leukoplakia and erythroplakia) and their associated increased risk of progression to cancer.

Field Cancerization

The upper aerodigestive tract (UADT) has become a useful model in studying chemoprevention. Slaughter and colleagues originally described the concept of field cancerization in 1953 (2). Their studies included histologic examination of

783 resected head and neck cancer specimens. Epithelium from sites beyond the original invasive cancer was found to be abnormal in every case; these abnormalities included epithelial hyperplasia and hyperkeratinization, dyskaryosis, and carcinoma in situ. In addition, 88 patients (11.2%) were found to have multiple, distinct invasive cancers within the surgically resected specimen. The authors suggested that oral cavity squamous cell carcinoma originated from epithelium that had been "preconditioned by an as-yet unknown carcinogenic agent," causing an irreversible change that made cancer development inevitable. Thus, a "preconditioned" or "condemned" epithelium could conceivably become activated or break down into cancer at multiple points, producing separate tumors. The interaction of host susceptibility and exposure to carcinogens (e.g., tobacco and/or alcohol) leads to the variation in cancer susceptibility and presentation. The premalignant changes found in areas of carcinogen-exposed epithelium adjacent to tumors, termed field cancerization, suggest that these multiple foci of premalignancy could progress concurrently to form multiple primary cancers or SPTs.

SPTs have become the leading cause of mortality in early-stage treated head and neck cancer and perhaps best illustrate the concept of field cancerization. Multiple genetic abnormalities have been detected in normal and premalignant epithelium of the lung and UADT in high-risk patients. Studies have focused on whether these SPTs are clonally related to the index primary tumor. The field cancerization model raised the issue of whether the areas of abnormality involved separate, independent clones with a unique set of genetic alterations or were genetically related and derived from a single cellular clone. Observations have indicated a common, clonal origin of the histopathologically distinct areas in premalignant lesions. Additional genetic losses were associated with a more malignant phenotype (3). For example, discordant p53 mutations found in multiple tumors in the same field resulted from genetic events such as 3p14 and 9p21 loss preceding p53 mutation (4). Thus, as the clonal population expands, genetic heterogeneity occurs. This may explain the divergent genetic abnormalities found in primary tumors and SPTs. Research analyzing the molecular characteristics of primary and second primary cancers continues in order to distinguish clonal versus multifocal origins.

Multistep Carcinogenesis

The concept of multistep carcinogenesis was derived from pathologic observations in field cancerization. Neoplastic changes evolve over time, progressing from normal tissue to metaplasia, hyperplasia, dysplasia, and finally to malignancy. An understanding of the mechanism of multistep carcinogenesis has awaited the integration of combined molecular biologic techniques with pathologic evaluation of epithelial lesions. This has led to the discovery of genetic abnormalities in premalignant and malignant epithelial cells. Based on animal studies, epithelial carcinogenesis is divided into three phases: initiation, promotion, and progression. DNA damage occurs during initiation, and the mutation becomes clonal after several cellular divisions. Exposure to carcinogens strongly influences this step, since these chemical events occur very rapidly. During promotion, slow phenotypic clonal expansion of the molecularly damaged cell occurs, eventually leading to hyperplasia. Progression is the most complex step because genetic and phenotypic changes occur with rapid cellular expansion (5).

Primary prevention efforts such as avoidance of carcinogens affect the initiation phase. Chemoprevention targets the promotion and progression phases as premalignant lesions evolve during these periods (6). Arresting one or several of the steps may impede the development of cancer. An important goal of clinical and basic research is to establish markers of these carcinogenic steps so as to identify individuals at high risk for UADT cancers. These "intermediate markers" could serve not only as screening devices but also as indicators for early evaluation of chemopreventive agent efficacy (7). The complex fundamental biology of UADT cancer remains poorly understood despite intensive study.

Genetic damage appears to accumulate during neoplastic transformation, and specific genes have been discovered that, when altered, may play a role in epithelial carcinogenesis. These include both tumor suppressor genes and proto-oncogenes, which encode proteins involved in cell-cycle control, signal transduction, and transcriptional regulation. Tumor suppressor genes inhibit clonal expansion by suppressing cell growth and genomic mutability. Some tumor suppressors that have been linked to epithelial carcinogenesis include p53, retinoblastoma (Rb), DCC (deleted in colorectal carcinoma), MCC (mutated in colorectal carcinoma), and APC (adenomatous polyposis coli) genes. Over 500 genes crucial to cell signaling and growth control are altered in cancer cells and, as proto-oncogenes, may be involved in the process of neoplasia. These include ras (H-, N-, and K-ras), myc (C-, N-, and L-myc), and the erbB family [erbB1 (epidermal growth factor receptor), erbB2 (her2/neu), erbB3 (her3), and erbB4/her4]. Chromosomes, also extensively damaged during epithelial carcinogenesis, are detected in the form of nuclear DNA adducts, cytoplasmic DNA fragments, or micronuclei and chromosomal abnormalities, which include aneuploidy as well as intrachromosomal deletions and amplifications. Future studies designed to discover genes disrupted by these chromosomal lesions may reveal both known and novel tumor suppressor genes and oncogenes, which play a role in epithelial carcinogenesis.

THE BIOLOGIC BASIS OF CHEMOPREVENTION

Chemoprevention studies are based on the hypothesis that interruption of the biologic processes involved in carcinogenesis will inhibit it and, in turn, reduce cancer incidence. This hypothesis provides a framework for the design and evaluation of chemoprevention trials, including the rationale for the selection of agents that are likely to inhibit biologic processes and the development of intermediate markers associated with carcinogenesis.

DNA damage and the resulting aberrant epithelial proliferation and differentiation are hallmarks of premalignant and malignant lesions. Treatment approaches include interrupting any of the processes that lead to their development. Discovery and validation of intermediate markers for chemoprevention trials are crucial. Because improvements in cancer incidence are measured directly from treatment, requiring years to evaluate, validated intermediate markers modulated by chemopreventive treatments that correlate with a reduction in cancer incidence would allow more expeditious evaluation of potential chemopreventive agents. Premalignant lesions are a potential source of intermediate markers, and if disappearance of these lesions correlates with a reduction in cancer incidence, then markers of premalignancy may serve as intermediate endpoints for chemoprevention trials. Future studies in chemoprevention will continue to test this hypothesis.

CHEMOPREVENTIVE AGENTS

A long list of potentially effective chemopreventive agents await clinical trials (Table 1), including vitamins, minerals, antioxidants, anti-inflammatory agents, and molecularly targeted agents. As single agents, these compounds will provide material for important clinical trials over the next decade or more.

TABLE 1   Potential chemopreventive agents

Retinoids
    13-cis-retinoic acid, 9-cis-retinoic acid
    4-HPR (N-4-hydroxyphenyl retinamide)
    All-trans retinoic acid (ATRA)
    Bexarotene (Targretin)

Flavonoids

NSAIDs

Curcumin

Polyphenolic compounds
    Tea, green tea, Epigallocatechin (EGCG)

Plant monoterpenes

DFMO combinations (difluoromethylornithine)

Lipoxygenase inhibitors

Cyclooxygenase inhibitors

Farnesyltransferase inhibitors
    R115777, SCH66336

Tyrosine kinase inhibitors
    Epidermal growth factor receptor (ZD1839, OSI-774)

Interferon-α

Protease inhibitors

Selenium

Retinoids have recently undergone extensive development as chemopreventive agents. In addition to 13-cis-retinoic acid (13-cRA), another retinoic acid stereoisomer, 9-cis retinoic acid (9-cRA), has been developed for clinical trials. 9-cRA can bind and activate both RAR and RXR receptor families. Because of its novel nuclear receptor affinities, 9-cRA may have biochemical effects that other retinoic acid stereoisomers lack. In addition there are synthetic retinoids with receptor-specific activity, which may have greater efficacy than natural retinoids if particular receptors are implicated in epithelial carcinogenesis (8–11). One site in which this may prove true is the UADT. RAR-β expression is lower in cancers in this region than in adjacent normal mucosa. In UADT cancer patients, treatment with retinoic acid produces the same chemopreventive response that occurs in those who have undergone resection. The mechanisms by which retinoids induce a chemopreventive effect in the UADT are not fully understood, but in vitro experiments suggest that RAR-β regulates squamous cell growth and differentiation.

Specific gene mutations found in premalignant lesions, such as *ras* and p53 point mutations, may offer additional opportunities for intervention at the molecular level. *Ras* is the most commonly expressed oncogene in human cancer. For example, post-translational farnesylation of mutant *ras* is necessary for activation of its transforming properties. Farnesyltransferase inhibitors (FTIs) block the enzyme farnesyltransferase or its substrate, the lipid moiety, farnesol, from being post-translationally added to *ras* (12). Similarly, in vitro studies suggest that loss or mutation of the p53 gene can be compensated for by ex vivo transfection of multiple copies of the wild-type p53 gene (13, 14). Since p53 is a critical tumor suppressor gene that is lost in $\sim$50% of all cancers, such an approach might be considered to restore p53 tumor suppressor activities within tumor cells.

Combinations of agents that mediate their effects through different pathways might enhance the ultimate chemopreventive effect. For example, agents that decrease the accumulation of intracellular free radicals, such as oltipraz, might be combined with retinoids that activate a separate pathway, that is, the modulation of cell growth and differentiation. Other agents have enhanced the effects of retinoids. In tumor differentiation models, for example, the effects of retinoids are augmented by agents such as phorbol esters or cyclic AMP, which activate protein kinase C (PKC) and protein kinase A, respectively. In a human teratocarcinoma cell line, activation of these kinases enhanced the effects of retinoic acid on RAR-β activation, demonstrating coupling of these kinase pathways with retinoid receptors. In addition to retinoid receptors, another mechanism through which retinoids and kinases might couple is transforming growth factor-β (TGF-β). Intracellular TGF-β production is increased by either retinoic acid treatment or PKC activation. Thus, retinoid and PKC pathways converge on TGF-β. TGF-β has been shown to induce profound growth suppression in many cell types. Studies that illuminate the convergence of different intracellular pathways on molecules that mediate growth suppression, such as retinoid receptors and TGF-β, provide a rationale for combination chemoprevention approaches. This strategy might be used in designing future chemoprevention trials.

Such trials await the development of agents that interact with specific kinase pathways. One possible agent is bryostatin, a PKC activator now entering phase I trials. Other potentially attractive agents for chemoprevention in high-risk patients because of their favorable side-effect profiles include FTIs, tyrosine kinase inhibitors to the epidermal growth factor receptor (EGFR), and inhibitors of the vascular endothelial growth factor (VEGF). Cyclooxygenase (COX-2) inhibitors, lipoxygenase inhibitors, and other nonsteroidal anti-inflammatory drugs (NSAIDs) are promising agents in tumors with high expression. COX-2 inhibitors have already demonstrated efficacy in preventing colon cancer in patients with familial adenomatous polyposis (FAP) (15; 15a, this volume). Immunotherapy with interferon-α combinations has also been studied in high-risk populations, including as bioadjuvant therapy in patients with head and neck cancer at risk for recurrence.

TREATMENT STRATEGIES IN CANCER CHEMOPREVENTION

Current treatment of aerodigestive tract cancers in all stages includes surgery, radiation therapy, and chemotherapy. An estimated 45,000 new cases of head and neck cancer will be diagnosed in 2001 in the United States alone, causing >12,000 deaths (16). The five-year survival rate for head and neck cancer patients in the United States and other developed countries is now 40%, comparable to the five-year survival rate in the 1960s despite advances in detection, surgery, and chemotherapy. Despite significant improvements in diagnosis, local management, and chemotherapy of head and neck cancer, there has been no significant increase in long-term survival over the past 30 years.

Additionally, an estimated 174,600 new cases of lung cancer will be diagnosed in the United States, with 157,400 deaths (16). With new regimens and earlier detection, clinical responses have improved, but the poor five-year survival rate has improved little over the past four decades, from 9% in 1963 to 15.8% in 2000 (17). A better biologic understanding of tumorigenesis may lead to novel approaches to treating aerodigestive tract cancers.

Chemoprevention targets the carcinogenic process at earlier and potentially more reversible stages, focusing on the inhibition of one or many steps in the progression toward cancer. As a cell's exposure to carcinogens increases, genetic mutations and other processes eventually lead to excessive proliferation of genetically altered cells and ultimately cancer. Strategies of chemoprevention include primary prevention in groups at high risk, reversal of premalignant lesions, and prevention of SPTs.

Primary Prevention

Clinical trials examining the prevention of primary lung tumors have been disappointing. These chemoprevention efforts have involved current smokers and have shown little efficacy. Strikingly, 50% of new lung cancer cases are among former smokers (17a,b,c), a population of roughly 46 million people in the United States. Early detection methods are now of great interest in lung cancer treatment. Screening techniques analyzing sputum cytology, chest X-rays, and spiral computed tomography (CT) scans have been evaluated. Recent studies have specifically tested the efficacy of screening individuals at high risk with spiral CT scanning (18–20). The results, though promising, are not yet definitive, and debate continues as to whether they are sufficient to mandate broad lung cancer screening programs. Thus, smoking cessation and primary prevention of smoking remain the best-established measures to prevent primary lung cancer.

Reversal of Premalignant Lesions

Early detection of lung cancer by chest X-ray has not yet significantly changed the outcome for patients with lung cancer. However, premalignant markers detected by sputum cytology studies or found in bronchial metaplasia have been investigated as early predictors of lung cancer. Reversal of these premalignant lesions may prevent progression to lung cancer.

Studies have included various agents to treat sputum atypia (21) or bronchial squamous metaplasia (22–25). One study remarkably showed improvement of bronchial epithelium metaplasia in smokers taking folate and vitamin B_{12} (26). However, because of problems with the consistency of the endpoints, these positive results must be viewed cautiously. Larger trials of biologic endpoints are needed to confirm the efficacy of these agents. Reversal of premalignant head and neck lesions using retinoids has met with some success. However, lessons from UADT chemoprevention trials have not yet been proven applicable to lung cancer. A maintenance regimen of low-dose 13-cRA was shown to decrease oral premalignancy (27). These studies have led to translational lung cancer trials based on the biologic activity of 13-cRA in the aerodigestive tract. Trials targeting intermediate biologic markers, including molecular indicators of genetic damage, may well hold the greatest promise for cancer chemoprevention.

ORAL PREMALIGNANCY AND UADT TRIALS

The UADT has been a good model for chemoprevention and its utility. Retinoids, β-carotene, vitamin E, and selenium have all shown activity in the reversal of oral premalignancy, but only retinoids have demonstrated positive results in randomized trials.

Leukoplakia and erythroplakia are the predominant premalignant lesions in oral cancer (28–30). Leukoplakia, a white patch that cannot be scraped off, is clearly associated with oral cancer development (31). Erythroplakia, a red, velvety lesion in the oral mucosa, is more often associated with in situ or invasive carcinoma (32). Both lesions harbor histologic abnormality, including both hyperplasia and dysplasia, and in the United States are found predominantly in tobacco users. Standard therapy for these lesions is surgical removal or laser excision. Leukoplakia and erythroplakia have a propensity for relapse or development of new lesions despite surgical intervention, most commonly in patients with tobacco, cigarette, and alcohol histories (33). Spontaneous regression occurs in 10%–20% of lesions.

In the largest U.S. series, Silverman et al. followed 257 leukoplakia patients for 7.2 years (34). Malignant transformation occurred in 45 of these patients (17.5%), all of whom developed squamous cell carcinoma of the oral cavity. Cancer development was fourfold higher in patients with erythroplakia than in those with leukoplakia, and marginal improvement of both kinds of lesions occurred with smoking cessation. These facts support the notion of field cancerization, that oral leukoplakia is a marker of this damage, and that systemic treatment is required. Because these lesions are accessible and can be monitored safely, they serve as an excellent model for chemoprevention and biomarker studies.

Vitamin A, because of its effects on epithelial differentiation, has been studied as both a topical and systemic treatment for oral leukoplakia. These trials, initiated in the 1950s, demonstrated regression of oral leukoplakia and also documented the toxic effects of vitamin A (35–38). As studies continued, a balance between toxicity and efficacy of other natural and synthetic vitamin A agents was critical for the development of chemoprevention trials in oral cancer. Stich et al. reported a 57% complete clinical response rate using vitamin A to reverse leukoplakia (39) and pioneered a series of trials testing β-carotene in high-risk groups, namely betel-nut and snuff users (40). Micronucleated buccal mucosa cells were studied, introducing the concept of intermediate endpoints as markers of activity. These investigators studied 130 patients who received placebo, β-carotene alone, or β-carotene plus retinol. They found that the combination of β-carotene plus retinol was twice as active as β-carotene alone in inducing remission in leukoplakia (41). Subsequent single-arm trials of β-carotene reported decreasing response rates with increasing doses, but these studies were not randomized and their responses were not histologically documented (42–44). However, these trials have been extremely important in developing potentially useful chemopreventive regimens against carcinogenesis. Other agents studied in the model of human oral leukoplakia include α-tocopherol (vitamin E) and selenium. A nonrandomized trial in oral leukoplakia using selenium (45) produced a 33% response rate. A trial of α-tocopherol (46) produced a 46% response rate. Continued studies will help devise combination regimens, which may be more efficacious than single agents. Following successful treatment of leukoplakia lesions with vitamin A treatment, other retinoids have been studied, including all-trans retinoic acid, etretinate, 13-cRA, and N-4-(hydroxycarbophenyl) retinamide. Clinical responses have been reported with all these agents (35, 47–53).

In 1986, a landmark trial by Hong et al. reported several important aspects of retinoid treatment in oral premalignancy (54). In this pioneering double-blind trial, 44 patients were randomized to either high-dose 13-cRA (2 mg/kg per day) or placebo for 3 months and then followed for 6 months. Complete or partial clinical responses were observed in 67% of those treated with the high-dose retinoid and in 10% of those given placebo ($p = 0.0002$). Histologic responses, including reversal of dysplasia, occurred in 54% of retinoid-treated patients and in 10% of patients given placebo ($p = 0.01$). Several important facts arose from this short high-dose retinoid regimen. First, toxicity was dose-related and was reversible with drug cessation. Among patients receiving 2 mg/kg, 88% experienced moderate to severe cheilitis, dry skin, and peeling, and 76% had conjunctivitis. Dose reduction to 1 mg/kg was necessary in 47% of patients, and many still experienced mild skin toxicities. This group also had significantly lower response rates than did the 2-mg/kg-per-day dose group. Second, remission was short-lived after therapy was stopped; >50% of participants relapsed within 3 months after drug cessation. These findings suggested long-term administration of chemopreventive drugs is needed to confer protection from cancer development.

A second trial examined the effects of low-dose maintenance isotretinoin (0.5 mg/kg per day) or β-carotene (30 mg per day) for 9 months following 3 months of high-dose induction therapy with isotretinoin (1.5 mg/kg per day) (27). Sixty-six patients completed the first phase of the study. The premalignant disease progression rates were 8% in patients who received low-dose isotretinoin and 55% in patients who received β-carotene ($p < 0.001$). The percentage of patients whose lesions decreased in size was 33% among those treated with isotretinoin and 10% among those treated with β-carotene. Carcinoma developed in seven patients who received β-carotene and only one who received isotretinoin. This study not only confirmed the activity of isotretinoin demonstrated in the first study but also showed that isotretinoin is superior to β-carotene in this setting and revealed that low-dose maintenance therapy with isotretinoin may yield better long-term effects than a short course of high-dose therapy. However, a 10-year update of the study revealed no differences in cancer rates between the two groups (55). Nevertheless, these studies established the rationale for the treatment of premalignant disease with chemopreventive agents.

The above results led to a currently ongoing randomized trial in oral premalignancy. This study compares low-dose 13-cRA (0.5 mg/kg per day) for 1 year, and then 0.25 mg/kg per day for the next 2 years, versus a combination of β-carotene (50 mg per day) and retinyl palmitate (25,000 I.U. per day) for a total of 3 years. This study will attempt to identify an appropriate maintenance dose, maximizing efficacy while minimizing toxicity. Intermediate markers will also be assessed. However, the β-carotene dose was removed after results from the Alpha Tocopherol, Beta Carotene (ATBC) Cancer Prevention study (56) and the β-Carotene and Retinol Efficacy Trial (CARET) (57) reported adverse outcomes with β-carotene supplementation in smokers and the Physicians' Health Study (58) reported its lack of efficacy.

LUNG CANCER PREMALIGNANCY

Because of the overall poor prognosis associated with lung cancer, chemoprevention strategies in high-risk patients are being studied. However, most studies performed in premalignant lung lesions have shown no benefit to retinoid chemoprevention. Most notable were randomized trials of 13-cRA and 4-HPR versus placebo in active and current smokers with a minimum 15- to 20-pack-year smoking history (22, 59). In these studies, retinoids showed no benefit in the reversal of premalignant lesions of the airways in active smokers. However, one of them (59) demonstrated that 13-cRA was more effective than placebo, both in reversing metaplasia and in upregulating RAR-β in the airways of former smokers. Other studies of retinoids in lung cancer premalignancy have failed to show a benefit in active smokers (21, 60, 61).

The Lung Cancer Biomarker Chemoprevention Consortium is planning a multi-institutional trial studying the effects of oral biologic compounds, ZD1839 (IRESSA), a tyrosine kinase inhibitor to epidermal growth factor receptor, and R115777, a farnesyl transferase inhibitor, on the reversal of premalignant lesions in the lung. Patients will have a previous definitively treated cancer of the head and neck or lung, evidence of sputum cytology, and at least a 30-pack-year history of smoking. Serial bronchoscopies will assess histologic changes. Patients will take one drug for 6 months and be followed subsequently. The primary endpoint will be histologic improvement. These trials, to begin in late 2001, are the first randomized trials to directly test the chemopreventive potential of these novel molecularly targeted agents.

Prevention of Lung Cancer

The rationale for lung cancer prevention is similar to that for head and neck cancer prevention. In both diseases, chronic exposure to tobacco is the major risk factor and dysplastic epithelial lesions are thought to represent a premalignant stage. Preclinical data indicate that retinoids reverse dysplastic bronchial epithelial lesions; however, placebo-controlled, randomized trials in smokers have revealed that retinoid treatment adds no significant benefit to the effects of smoking cessation and reversal of bronchial metaplasia. Research is under way to identify intermediate markers that predict retinoid chemopreventive effects on bronchial epithelial cells.

Trials in lung cancer chemoprevention have demonstrated the importance of smoking status when testing these agents. The ATBC Cancer Prevention study was a randomized, double-blind, placebo-controlled primary-prevention trial in which 29,133 Finnish male smokers received either α-tocopherol alone at 50 mg per day, β-carotene alone at 20 mg per day, both α-tocopherol and β-carotene, or placebo. These men were 50–69 years of age and all smoked 5 or more cigarettes per day. Patients were followed for 5–8 years. Lung cancer incidence, the primary endpoint, did not change with the addition of α-tocopherol alone, nor did overall mortality. However, both groups who received β-carotene supplementation (alone or with α-tocopherol) had an 18% increase in the incidence of lung cancer. There appeared to be a stronger adverse effect from β-carotene in those men who smoked >20 cigarettes a day. This trial raised the serious issue that pharmacologic doses of β-carotene could potentially be harmful in active smokers (56).

CARET confirmed the results of the Finnish trial. This randomized, double-blind, placebo-controlled trial tested the combination of 30 mg β-carotene and 25,000 I.U. retinyl palmitate against placebo in 18,314 men and women aged 50–69 years at high risk for lung cancer. 14,254 had at least a 20-pack-year smoking history and were either current smokers or recent former smokers. 4060 men had extensive occupational exposure to asbestos. This trial was stopped after 21 months because no benefit and even possible harm was found. Lung cancer incidence, the primary endpoint, increased 28% in the active intervention group. Overall mortality also increased 17% in this group (57). Given these results, as well as those of the ATBC trial, high-dose β-carotene is not recommended for high-risk patients who continue to smoke.

The Physicians Health Study, a randomized, double blind, placebo-controlled trial, studied 22,071 healthy male physicians, of whom 11,036 received 50 mg β-carotene on alternate days and 11,035 received placebo. The use of supplemental β-carotene showed virtually no adverse or beneficial effects on cancer incidence or overall mortality during a 12-year follow-up (58).

In China, a study evaluating β-carotene, α-tocopherol, and selenium in the prevention of gastric and esophageal cancer showed a nonsignificant decrease in the risk of lung cancer in a small cohort of patients (61a).

Subgroup analysis of the above studies, especially ATBC and CARET, has provided few explanations for the increase in lung cancer incidence. Apparently, β-carotene is harmful only to high-risk heavy smokers or those with previous exposure to asbestos. It is currently recommended that these people avoid supplemental β-carotene in large doses (62).

Prevention of Second Primary Tumors

Head and neck cancer patients who have been successfully treated remain at a significantly increased risk for developing additional neoplasms within the UADT and lungs (63–69). The concept of multistep field cancerization explains the development of multiple independent tumor sites within the aerodigestive tract. In fact, although SPTs occur in all treatment stages of head and neck cancer, they have the greatest impact on patients treated for early-stage disease (stage I or II), which is usually curative (70, 71). The lifetime risk of developing an SPT in head and neck squamous cell cancer is 20% and the annual rate is 4%–6%. One study in oral cancer reported a rate of 3.6% per year (72). SPTs are the major cause of death after curative surgery in head and neck cancer and are the leading cause of death in early-stage disease, causing more deaths than recurrence (70–75). Retinoids have been proven active in oral premalignancy. These facts are the basis for chemoprevention trials in head and neck cancer evaluating SPTs and the impact of smoking.

Variations in reported occurrence rates depend on the population studied and the methods used for diagnosing an SPT. Currently, the Warren-Gates criteria (76), published in the 1930s, are used to diagnose an SPT. The definition of SPT is as follows:

1. It is a new cancer of a different histologic type.

2. It is a cancer, regardless of site, that occurs after >3 years.

3. In the head and neck, the lesion is separated from the initial primary tumor by >2 cm of clinically normal epithelium.

4. In the lung, the cancer presents as a solitary mass, is of squamous cell histologic type, develops within 3 years, and occurs in the absence of local or regional disease accompanied by evidence of dysplasia or carcinoma in situ within the bronchial epithelium.

Using these criteria, the risk of local recurrence seems to decline over time, whereas the risk of SPT is constant for the first 8 years following initial head and neck cancer (75).

Because of the morbidity associated with the development of SPTs in head and neck cancer, Hong et al. performed the first phase III adjuvant chemoprevention trial in 1990 (77). This randomized, placebo-controlled, double-blind study followed 103 patients with stage I through IV (M0) head and neck cancer who were randomized to receive high-dose 13-cRA (100 mg/m^2 per day) or placebo for 1 year after definitive local therapy. The dosage of 13-cRA was reduced to 50 mg/m^2 per day after 13 of the first 44 patients experienced intolerable side effects. The primary endpoints were primary recurrence and SPT development. The two treatment arms showed no difference in local recurrence or distant metastases. However, the patients treated with 13-cRA had a dramatically lower incidence of SPTs. Among the 103 patients followed for a median of 42 months, SPTs developed in 6% (3 of 49) of those in the 13-cRA arm whereas 28% (14 of 51) developed SPTs in the placebo arm.

After 54.5 months of follow-up, there was still no difference in the rates of recurrence between the isotretinoin-treated group and the placebo group (78). However, there remained a statistically significant reduction of SPTs in the isotretinoin-treated group versus placebo group (14% vs. 31%). Consistent with field carcinogenesis, in the placebo group, 14 of 17 SPTs developed in the UADT, esophagus, and lung and were histologically squamous cell type. Additionally, none of the patients receiving 13-cRA developed an SPT during the year of active treatment. Although only 47% of patients in the 13-cRA treatment arm completed the therapy as prescribed, the reduction in SPT development was still significant.

Based on the important findings of the this study, a chemoprevention trial in head and neck squamous cell cancer (HNSCC) designed to prevent SPT development was instituted in 1991 through the University of Texas M. D. Anderson Cancer Center and its affiliated Community Clinical Oncology Program (CCOP), along with the Radiation Therapy Oncology Group (RTOG) (79, 80). This randomized, double-blind trial studied the ability of low-dose 13-cRA to prevent SPTs in patients definitively treated for stage I or II squamous cell carcinoma for up to 3 years before participation (T1N0M0 or T2N0M0). Patients received 30 mg per day of 13-cRA or placebo for 3 years and were followed for an additional 4 years. This study recently completed accrual with 1190 randomized and 1384 registered patients. SPT incidence has been reported according to prior tumor stage, as well as related to smoking status (current, former, never). The annual primary tumor recurrence rate was 2.8% and annual SPT occurrence rate was 5.1%. Stage II HNSCC had a higher rate of SPT development than did stage I. Additionally, active smokers had a significantly higher recurrence rate than former and never smokers (4.3% vs. 3.3% vs. 1.9%). This prospective study demonstrated for the first time the impact of active smoking status on SPT development. The SPT rate was significantly higher in active smokers than in the other groups ($p = 0.018$) and the difference was marginally significant between former and never smokers ($p = 0.11$). The site of the SPT differed depending on the site of the primary index tumor. Patients with primary laryngeal cancers were most likely to develop an SPT in either the lung or larynx whereas patients with oral cavity primaries were most likely to develop SPTs in either the oral cavity or the lung. Finally, patients with an index primary tumor of the pharynx developed SPTs in the lung, oral cavity, pharynx, or esophagus. Compared with previous trials, SPTs occurred more frequently than expected at the index primary sites of the oral UADT. The lower dose of 13-cRA was also well tolerated with few grade 3 toxicities. This trial is scheduled to be unblinded in 2002 (81–83).

In resected non–small cell lung cancer (NSCLC) patients, SPTs occur at the rate of 2%–4% per year. Similar to its effects in head and neck cancer patients, retinoid treatment reduces the incidence of SPTs in lung cancer patients who have undergone resection. In a randomized study, 307 patients whose stage I NSCLCs were completely resected received either 12 months of treatment with retinol palmitate (300,000 I.U. a day) or no treatment. At a median of 46 months follow-up, patients who received retinol palmitate had a 35% lower incidence of SPTs than the control group (3.1% vs. 4.8%) (60). As in studies of head and neck cancer patients, retinoid treatment had no observed effect on survival duration or the rate of primary disease recurrence. These trials in NSCLC patients point out the need to further investigate the effects of different retinoids in this setting and to extend these trials to include patients cured of small cell lung cancer, whose SPT rate is double that of patients treated for early-stage head and neck cancer.

Other recently reported major phase III studies include EUROSCAN and the US-Intergroup NCI 91-0001 trial. EUROSCAN, a randomized adjuvant chemo-prevention study of the European Organization for Research and Treatment of Cancer (EORTC) Head/Neck and Lung Cancer Groups, studied the effects of vitamin A (retinyl palmitate) and N-acetylcysteine in patients with early-stage head and neck and lung cancer. In the trials, 2592 patients with cancers of the larynx (Tis–T3, N0–N1), oral cavity (Tis–T2, N0–N1), and NSCLC (T1–T2, N0–N1) received retinyl palmitate (300,000 I.U. per day in year 1; 150,000 I.U. per day in year 2), N-acetylcysteine (600 mg per day for 2 years), both drugs, or placebo. There were no endpoint differences between the three active treatment arms and the placebo group in terms of lung cancer incidence, occurrence of second primary cancer, or survival. There was a statistically significant difference in time to development of SPTs within the carcinogen-exposed field ($p = 0.045$) in favor of the retinoid-treated group. The majority (93%) of the patient population were considered regular smokers, of whom at least half had >43 pack-years of tobacco exposure. Problems with the study included differences in medication adherence across the three treatment groups and the testing of N-acetylcysteine, a drug with little established efficacy in chemoprevention, in 1300 patients at risk (84).

US-Intergroup NCI 91-0001 was a randomized, double-blind study using low-dose 13-cRA after complete resection of stage I NSCLC; 1304 patients were randomized to receive either 13-cRA or placebo. The study objectives were to evaluate the efficacy of 13-cRA in reducing the incidence of SPTs after complete resection of stage I NSCLC, to look at the qualitative and quantitative toxicity of daily low-dose 13-cRA, and to compare the overall survival rates of the two groups. All patients had undergone complete resection of primary stage I NSCLC (postoperative T1 or T2, N0) 6 weeks to 3 years prior to registering. After a median follow-up of 3.5 years, there were no statistically significant differences between the placebo and isotretinoin arms with respect to the time to SPTs, recurrences, or mortality, nor did isotretinoin improve the overall rates of SPTs, recurrences, or mortality in stage I NSCLC. Secondary multivariate and subset analyses suggested that isotretinoin was harmful in current smokers and beneficial in never smokers (61).

Large trials such as the Euroscan and US-Intergroup studies help define new avenues for future chemopreventive treatment. Currently, an Eastern Cooperative Oncology Group trial is studying the effect of daily selenium supplementation on patients with stage I lung cancer.

Other SPT prevention trials are ongoing. A randomized, double-blind, placebo-controlled trial at Yale University is evaluating the efficacy of β-carotene (50 mg per day) in reducing local recurrence and SPTs in head and neck cancer (85). Patients are being recruited from the state tumor registry, a procedure that may eventually serve as a model for future chemoprevention studies.

Biochemoprevention

Biochemoprevention is currently being studied as another method to prevent treatment failure. A prospective trial evaluated 36 patients with advanced premalignant lesions of the UADT (86). Patients were treated with isotretinoin at 100 mg/m^2 per day, α-tocopherol at 1200 I.U./day, and interferon-α 3 μ/m^2 twice weekly for 12 months. Laryngeal lesions favored response at 6 and 12 months (47% and 50%) versus oral lesions (9% and 0%).

A phase II study using 13-cRA (50 mg/m^2 per day), interferon-α (3 million units/m^2 three times weekly), and α-tocopherol (1200 I.U./day) for 12 months in patients with stage III and IV head and neck cancer after definitive therapy was reported recently (87). Thirty-eight of 44 patients completed the 12-month treatment plan. With a median follow-up of 24 months, 4 patients (9%) had local/regional recurrence and 2 patients (5%) had local/regional recurrence and distant metastases. The median 2-year rate of overall survival was 91% and of disease-free survival was 84%. The results suggest a role for biologic adjuvant therapy in high-risk patients to prevent disease recurrence and SPTs, and perhaps that more aggressive therapies for prevention are warranted. A phase III randomized study to confirm these phase II results is under way, and its results may potentially influence treatment of late-stage head and neck cancers.

CONCLUSIONS AND FUTURE DIRECTIONS

The future of lung cancer chemoprevention remains open to innovation. While new regimens combining chemotherapy, radiation therapy, and surgery for the treatment of aerodigestive tract cancers continue to proliferate, the mechanisms underlying tumor biology are becoming better understood. Thus, new chemopreventive agents will be tested in an attempt to reduce the aerodigestive cancer mortality rate. Obviously, smoking cessation campaigns need to continue because tobacco use is still the most important cause of lung cancer. Furthermore, dissuading people from starting tobacco use is of great importance, as statistics have shown an increased risk of lung cancer even after smokers quit.

Chemopreventive agents appear thus far to have efficacy, and we hope to define their future role in treating and, more importantly, preventing head and neck cancers in high-risk individuals. SPTs have emerged as an increasingly important problem, despite curative local therapy, underscoring the principle of field cancerization. Chemopreventive agents have affected this arena as well, and as further studies are performed, their role in prevention of SPTs will be further defined. Combination regimens targeting specific molecular defects show early promise. Development of a risk model will be important to help guide and tailor therapy for patients with various risk profiles. A multidisciplinary approach involving clinicians and basic researchers is needed to study the biology of aerodigestive tract cancers before chemoprevention can be incorporated into a societal standard of care.

Visit the Annual Reviews home page at www.AnnualReviews.org

LITERATURE CITED

1. Sporn MB. 1976. Approaches to prevention of epithelial cancer during the preneoplastic period. *Cancer Res.* 36:2699–702
2. Slaughter DP, Southwick HW, Smejkal W. 1953. Field cancerization in oral stratified squamous epithelium. *Cancer* 6(5):963–68
3. Califano J, van der Riet P, Westra W, et al. 1996. A genetic progression model for head and neck cancer; implications for field cancerization. *Cancer Res.* 56:2488–92

4. Chung KY, Mukhopadhyay T, Kim J, et al. 1993. Discordant p53 mutations in primary head and neck cancer and corresponding second primary cancers of the upper aerodigestive tract. *Cancer Res.* 53:1676–83
5. Meyskens FL Jr. 1997. Micronutrients. In *Cancer: Principles and Practice of Oncology*, ed. VT DeVita, S Hellman, SA Rosenberg, 3:573–84. Philadelphia: Lippincott-Raven
6. Clayman GL, Lippman SM, Laramore

GE, Hong WK. 1997. Head and neck cancer. In *Cancer Medicine*, ed. JF Holland, RC Bast, DL Morton, et al., 1:1645–1710. Baltimore: Williams & Wilkins

7. Lippman SM, Lee JS, Lotan R, et al. 1990. Biomarkers as intermediate endpoints in chemoprevention trials. *J. Natl. Cancer Inst.* 82(7):555–60

8. Wolbach SB, Howe PR. 1925. Tissue changes following deprivation of fat soluble A vitamin. *J. Exp. Med.* 42:753

9. Whelan P. 1999. Retinoids in chemoprevention. *Eur. Urol.* 35:424–28

10. Xu XC, Lee JS, Lee JJ, et al. 1999. Nuclear retinoid acid receptor beta in bronchial epithelium of smokers before and during chemoprevention. *J. Natl. Cancer Inst.* 91(15):1317–21

11. Xu XC, Sozzi G, Lee JS, et al. 1997. Suppression of retinoic acid receptor β in non–small-cell lung cancer *in vivo*: implications for lung cancer development. *J. Natl. Cancer Inst.* 89(9):624–29

12. Sepp-Lorenzino L, Ma Z, Rands E, et al. 1995. A peptidomimetic inhibitor of farnesylprotein transferase blocks the anchorage-dependent and -independent growth of human tumor cell lines. *Cancer Res.* 55(22):5302–9

13. Hollstein M, Sidransky D, Vogelstein B, Harris CC. 1991. p53 mutations in human cancers. *Science* 253:49–53

14. Clayman GL, El-Nagger AK, Roth JA, et al. 1995. *In vivo* therapy with p53 adenovirus for microscopic residual head and neck squamous carcinoma. *Cancer Res.* 55:1–6

15. Steinbach G, Lynch PM, Phillips RK, et al. 2000. The effect of celecoxib, a cyclooxygenase-2 inhibitor, in familial adenomatous polyposis. *N. Engl. J. Med.* 342(26):1946–52

15a. Turini ME, DuBois RN. 2002. Cyclooxygenase-2: a new therapeutic target. *Annu. Rev. Med.* 53:35–57

16. Greenlee RT, Hill-Harmon MB, Murray T, Thun M. 2001. Cancer statistics, 2001. *CA Cancer J. Clin.* 51:15–36

17. Ries L, Eisner M, Kosary C, et al. 2000. *SEER Cancer Statistics Review, 1973–1997*. Bethesda, MD: Natl. Cancer Inst.

17a. Lubin JH, Blot WJ. 1993. Lung cancer and smoking cessation: patterns of risk. *J. Natl. Cancer Inst.* 85:422–23

17b. Tong L, Spitz MR, Fueger JJ, Amos CA. 1996. Lung carcinoma in former smokers. *Cancer* 78:1004–10

17c. Lee JJ, Liu D, Lee JS, et al. 2001. Long-term impact of smoking on lung epithelial proliferation in current and former smokers. *J. Natl. Cancer Inst.* 93:1081–88

18. Fontana RS, Sanderson DR, Taylor WF, et al. 1984. Early lung cancer detection: results of the initial (prevalence) radiologic and cytologic screening in the Mayo Clinic Study. *Am. Rev. Respir. Dis.* 130:561–65

19. Fontana RS, Sanderson DR, Woolner LB, et al. 1991. Screening for lung cancer. A critique of the Mayo Lung Project. *Cancer* 67:1155–64

20. Henschke CI, McCauley DI, Yankelevitz DF, et al. 1999. Early lung cancer action project: overall design and findings from baseline screening. *Lancet* 354:99–105

21. Arnold AM, Browman GP, Levine MN, et al. 1992. The effect of the synthetic retinoid etretinate on sputum cytology: results from a randomised trial. *Br. J. Cancer* 65:737–43

22. Gouveia J, Hercend T, Lemaigre G, et al. 1982. Degree of bronchial metaplasia in heavy smokers and its regression after treatment with a retinoid. *Lancet* 1:710–12

23. Lee JS, Lippman SM, Benner SE, et al. 1994. A randomized placebo-controlled trial of isotretinoin in chemoprevention of bronchial squamous metaplasia. *J. Clin. Oncol.* 12:937–45

24. Mathe G, Gouveia J, Hercend R, et al. 1982. Correlation between precancerous bronchial metaplasia and cigarette consumption, and preliminary results of retinoid treatment. *Cancer Detect. Prev.* 5:461–66

25. Misset JL, Santelli G, Homasson JP, et al. 1986. Regression of bronchial epidermoid metaplasia in heavy smokers with etretinate treatment. *Cancer Detect. Prev.* 9:167–70

26. Heimburger DC, Alexander CB, Birch R, et al. 1988. Improvement in bronchial squamous metaplasia in smokers treated with folate and vitamin B12: report of a preliminary randomized double-blind intervention trial. *JAMA* 259:1525–30

27. Lippman SM, Batsakis JG, Toth BB, et al. 1993. Comparison of low-dose isotretinoin with beta carotene to prevent oral carcinogenesis. *N. Engl. J. Med.* 328:15–20

28. Shklar G. 1986. Oral leukoplakia. *N. Engl. J. Med.* 315:1544–45

29. Mashberg A, Samit AM. 1989. Early detection, diagnosis, and management of oral and oropharyngeal cancer. *Cancer* 39:67–88

30. Waldron CA, Shafer WG. 1975. Leukoplakia revisited: a clinicopathologic study of 3256 oral leukoplakias. *Cancer* 36:1386–92

31. WHO Collaborating Centre for Oral Precancerous Lesions. 1978. Definition of leukoplakia and related lesions: an aid to studies on oral precancer. *Oral Surg. Oral Med. Oral Pathol.* 46:518–39

32. Silverman S, Shillitoe EJ. 1990. Etiology and predisposing factors. In *Oral Cancer*, ed. S Silverman, 3:7–39. Atlanta, GA: Am. Cancer Soc.

33. Chiesa F, Tradati N, Marazza M, et al. 1992. Prevention of local relapses and new localizations of oral leukoplakias with synthetic retinoid fenretinide (4-HPR): preliminary results. *Eur. J. Cancer B Oral Oncol.* 28B:97–102

34. Silverman S, Gorsky M, Lozada F. 1984. Oral leukoplakia and malignant transformation: a follow-up study of 257 patients. *Cancer* 53:563–68

35. Koch HF. 1981. Effect of retinoids on precancerous lesions of oral mucosa. In *Retinoids, Advances in Basic Research and Therapy*, ed. CE Orfanos, O Braun-Falco, EM Farber, 3:307–12. Berlin: Springer-Verlag

36. Wulf K. 1957. Zur vitamin A behandlung der leukoplkien. *Arch. Klin. Exp. Dermatol.* 206:495–98

37. Silverman S, Renstrup G, Pindborg JJ. 1963. Studies in oral leukoplakias: III. Effects of vitamin A comparing clinical, histopathologic, cytologic, and hematologic responses. *Acta Odont. Scand.* 21:271–92

38. Silverman S, Eisenberg E, Restrup G. 1965. A study of the effects of high doses of vitamin A on oral leukoplakia (hyperkeratosis), including toxicity, liver function, and skeletal metabolism. *J. Oral Ther. Pharmacol.* 2:9–23

39. Stich HF, Hornby AP, Mathew B, et al. 1988. Response of oral leukoplakias to the administration of vitamin A. *Cancer Lett.* 40:93–101

40. Stich HF, Rosin MP, Vallejera MO. 1984. Reduction with vitamin A and beta-carotene administration of the proportion of micronucleated buccal cells in Asian betel nut and tobacco chewers. *Lancet* 1:1204–6

41. Stich HF, Rosin MP, Hornby AP, et al. 1988. Remission of oral leukoplakias and micronuclei in tobacco/betel quid chewers treated with beta-carotene and with beta-carotene plus vitamin A. *Int. J. Cancer* 42:195–99

42. Garewal HS, Meyskens FL, Killen D, et al. 1990. Response of oral leukoplakia to beta-carotene. *J. Clin. Oncol.* 8:1715–20

43. Malaker K, Anderson BJ, Beecroft WA, Hodson DI. 1991. Management of oral mucosal dysplasia with beta-carotene retinoic acid: a pilot cross-over study. *Cancer Detect. Prev.* 15:335–40

44. Toma S, Benso S, Albanese E, et al. 1992. Treatment of oral leukoplakia with beta-carotene. *Oncology* 42:77–81

45. Toma S, Coialbu T, Collecchi P, et al. 1990. Aspetti biologici e prospettive

applicative della chemioprevenzione nel cancro delle vie aerodigestive superiori. *Acta Otorhinolaryngol. Ital.* 10:41–54

46. Benner SE, Winn RJ, Lippman SM, et al. 1993. Regression of oral leukoplakia with alpha-tocopherol: a Community Clinical Oncology Program (CCOP) chemoprevention study. *J. Natl. Cancer Inst.* 85:44–47

47. Ryssel HJ, Brunner KW, Bollag W. 1971. Die perorale Anwedung von Vitamin-A-Saure bie Leukoplakien, Hyperkeratosen und Plattenepithelkarzinomen: Ergebnisse und Vertaglichkeit. *Schweiz. Med. Wochenschr.* 101:1027–30

48. Stuttgen G. 1975. Oral vitamin A acid therapy. *Acta Dermatol. Venereol.* 74 (Suppl.):174–79

49. Raque CJ, Biondo RV, Keeran MG, et al. 1975. Snuff dippers keratosis (snuff-induced leukoplakia). *South. Med. J.* 68:565–68

50. Koch HF. 1978. Biochemical treatment of precancerous oral lesions: the effectiveness of various analogues of retinoic acid. *J. Oral Maxillofac. Surg.* 6:59–63

51. Cordero AA, Allevato MAJ, Barclay CA. 1981. Treatment of lichen planus and leukoplakia with the oral retinoid RO 10–9359. In *Retinoids, Advances in Basic Research and Therapy*, ed. CE Orfanos, O Braun-Falco, EM Farber, 3:273–78. Berlin: Springer-Verlag

52. Shah JP, Strong EW, DeCosse JJ, et al. 1983. Effect of retinoids on oral leukoplakia. *Am. J. Surg.* 146:466–70

53. Han J, Jiao L, Lu Y, et al. 1990. Evaluation of N-4-(hydroxycarbophenyl)retinamide as a cancer agent. *In Vivo* 4:153–60

54. Hong WK, Endicott J, Itri LM, et al. 1986. 13-cis-retinoic acid in the treatment of oral leukoplakia. *N. Engl. J. Med.* 315:1501–5

55. Papadimitrakopoulou VA, Hong WK, Lee JS, et al. 1997. Low-dose isotretinoin versus beta-carotene to prevent oral carcinogenesis: long-term follow-up. *J. Natl. Cancer Inst.* 89(3):257–58

56. The Alpha-Tocopherol, Beta-Carotene Cancer Prevention Study Group. 1994. The effect of Vitamin E and beta carotene on the incidence of lung cancer and other cancers in male smokers. *N. Engl. J. Med.* 330:1029–35

57. Omenn GS, Goodman GE, Thornquist MD, et al. 1996. Effects of a combination of beta carotene and vitamin A on lung cancer and cardiovascular disease. *N. Engl. J. Med.* 334:1150–55

58. Hennekans CH, Buring JE, Manson JE, et al. 1996. Lack of effect of long-term supplementation with beta-carotene on the incidence of malignant neoplasms and cardiovascular disease. *N. Engl. J. Med.* 334:1145–49

59. Kurie JM, Lee JS, Khuri FR, et al. 2000. N-(4-hydroxyphenyl) retinamide in the chemoprevention of squamous metaplasia and dysplasia of the bronchial epithelium. *Clin. Cancer Res.* 8:2973–79

60. Pastorino U, Infante M, Maioli M, et al. 1993. Adjuvant treatment of stage I lung cancer with high-dose vitamin A. *J. Clin. Oncol.* 11(7):1216–22

61. Lippman SM, Lee JJ, Karp DD, et al. 2001. Randomized phase III intergroup trial of isotretinoin to prevent second primary tumors in stage I non–small-cell lung cancer. *J. Natl. Cancer Inst.* 93(8):605–18

61a. Wang GQ, Dawsey SM, Li JY, et al. 1994. Effects of vitamin/mineral supplementation on the prevalence of histological dysplasia and early cancer of the esophagus and stomach: results from the General Population Trial in Linxian, China. *Cancer Epidemiol. Biomarkers Prev.* 3:161–66

62. Goodman M, Morgan RW, Ray R, et al. 1999. Cancer in asbestos-exposed occupational cohorts: a meta-analysis. *Cancer Causes Control* 10(5):453–65

63. Boice JD, Fraumeni JF. 1985. Second cancer following cancer of the respiratory

system in Connecticut, 1935–1982. *Natl. Cancer Inst. Monogr.* 68:83–98

64. Gluckman JL, Crissman JD. 1983. Survival rates in 548 patients with multiple neoplasms of the upper aerodigestive tract. *Laryngoscope* 93:71–74

65. Cooper JS, Pajak TK, Rubin P, et al. 1989. Second malignancies in patients who have head and neck cancer: incidence, effect on survival and implications based on the RTOG experience. *Int. J. Radiat. Oncol. Biol. Phys.* 17:449–56

66. De Vries N, Snow GB. 1986. Multiple primary tumours in laryngeal cancer. *J. Laryngol. Otol.* 100:915–18

67. Yellin A, Hill LR, Benfield JR. 1986. Bronchogenic carcinoma associated with upper aerodigestive cancers. *J. Thorac. Cardiovasc. Surg.* 91:674–83

68. Vokes EE, Weichselbaum RR, Lippman SM, Hong WK. 1993. Head and neck cancer. *N. Engl. J. Med.* 328:184–93

69. Lippman SM, Hong WK. 1993. Not yet standard: retinoids versus second primary tumors. *J. Clin. Oncol.* 11:1204–7

70. Lippman SM, Hong WK. 1989. Second malignant tumors in head and neck squamous cell carcinoma: the overshadowing threat for patients with early stage disease. *Int. J. Radiat. Oncol. Biol. Phys.* 17:691–94

71. Larson JT, Adams GL, Fattah HA. 1990. Survival statistics for multiple primaries in head and neck cancer. *Otolaryngol. Head Neck Surg.* 103:14–24

72. Tepperman BS, Fitzpatrick PJ. 1981. Second respiratory and upper digestive tract cancers after oral cancer. *Lancet* 9:547–49

73. McDonald S, Haie C, Rubin P, et al. 1989. Second malignant tumors in patients with laryngeal carcinoma: diagnosis, treatment and prevention. *Int. J. Radiat. Oncol. Biol. Phys.* 17:457–65

74. Licciardello JT, Spitz MR, Hong WK. 1989. Multiple primary cancers in patients with cancer of the head and neck: second cancer of the head and neck, esophagus

and lung. *Int. J. Radiat. Oncol. Biol. Phys.* 17:467–76

75. Vikram B. 1984. Changing patterns of failure in advanced head and neck cancer. *Arch. Otolaryngol.* 110:564–65

76. Warren S, Gates O. 1932. Multiple primary malignant tumors: a survey of the literature and statistical study. *Am. J. Cancer* 16(4):1358–403

77. Hong WK, Lippman SM, Itri LM, et al. 1990. Prevention of second primary tumors with isotretinoin in squamous-cell carcinoma of the head and neck. *N. Engl. J. Med.* 323:795–801

78. Benner SE, Pajak TF, Lippman SM, et al. 1994. Prevention of second primary tumors with isotretinoin in patients with squamous cell carcinoma of the head and neck: long-term follow-up. *J. Natl. Cancer Inst.* 86(2):140–41

79. Benner SE, Lippman SM, Hong WK. 1992. Current status of chemoprevention of head and neck cancer. *Oncology* 6:61–66

80. Benner SE, Pajak TF, Stetz J, et al. 1994. Toxicity of isotretinoin in a chemoprevention trial to prevent second primary tumors following head and neck cancer. *J. Natl. Cancer Inst.* 86:1799–801

81. Khuri FR, Lee JJ, Winn RJ, et al. 1999. Interim analysis of randomized chemoprevention trial of HNSCC. *Proc. Am. Soc. Clin. Oncol.* 18:1503 (Abstr.)

82. Kim ES, Khuri FR, Lee JJ, et al. 2000. Second primary tumor incidence related to primary index tumor and smoking status in a randomized chemoprevention study of head and neck squamous cell cancer. *Proc. Am. Soc. Clin. Oncol.* 19:1642 (Abstr.)

83. Khuri FR, Kim ES, Lee JJ, et al. 2001. The impact of smoking status, disease stage, and index tumor site on second primary tumor incidence and tumor recurrence in the head and neck retinoid chemoprevention trial. *Cancer Epid. Biomarkers Prev.* 10:823–29

84. van Zandwijk N, Dalesio O, Pastorino U,

et al. 2000. EUROSCAN, a randomized trial of vitamin A and N-acetylcysteine in patients with head and neck cancer or lung cancer. For the European Organization for Research and Treatment of Cancer Head and Neck and Lung Cancer Cooperative Groups. *J. Natl. Cancer Inst.* 92(12):977–86

85. Mayne ST, Zheng T, Janerich DT, et al. 1992. A population based trial of β-carotene chemoprevention of head and neck cancer. *Adv. Exp. Med. Biol.* 320:119–27

86. Papadimitrakopoulou VA, Clayman GL, Shin DM, et al. 1999. Biochemoprevention for dysplastic lesions of the upper aerodigestive tract. *Arch. Otolaryngol. Head Neck Surg.* 125(10):1083–89

87. Shin DM, Khuri FR, Murphy B, et al. 2001. Combined interferon-alfa, 13-cis-retinoic acid, and alpha-tocopherol in locally advanced head and neck squamous cell carcinoma: novel bioadjuvant phase II trial. *J. Clin. Oncol.* 19(12):3010–17

Annu. Rev. Med. 2002. 53:245–67

DIABETES AND CARDIOVASCULAR DISEASE

Helaine E. Resnick and Barbara V. Howard
MedStar Research Institute, 108 Irving Street NW, Washington, DC 20010;
e-mail: helaine.e.resnick@medstar.net, barbara.v.howard@medstar.net

Key Words epidemiology, insulin resistance, sex, inflammation, glycosylation
end products

■ **Abstract** This review focuses on several topics related to the epidemiology of diabetes and cardiovascular disease (CVD). These include the CVD risk factors common
in the metabolic syndrome, behavioral risk factors and diabetes, gender differences in
the association between diabetes and CVD risk, and how the clinical definition of
diabetes influences the association of diabetes and CVD. Nontraditional risk factors
potentially linking diabetes and CVD are also discussed, including chronic inflammation, advanced glycation endpoints, autonomic neuropathy, sleep-disordered breathing,
and genetic susceptibility to diabetes-associated CVD risk.

INTRODUCTION

Diabetes mellitus and cardiovascular disease (CVD) share several important characteristics. The occurrence of both conditions increases with age; both are associated with an adverse lipid profile, obesity, and a sedentary lifestyle; and the
risk of both can be reduced by lifestyle modifications of common risk factors
(1). Diabetes is a potent, independent risk factor for CVD. Coronary heart disease (CHD) is the most common and costly vascular complication of diabetes
(2).

Cross-sectional epidemiologic studies have consistently shown an association between diabetes and prevalence of CVD in the U.S. population and in
community-based studies in the United States and abroad (3–8). Diabetes is associated with an unfavorable distribution of CVD risk factors among people with
existing diabetes, and unfavorable CVD risk factors are also present prior to diagnosis of diabetes (9–11). Prospective epidemiologic studies of individuals at
risk for CVD yield consistent temporal relationships between diabetes and both
incident CVD and mortality (12–21). Results from epidemiologic studies linking diabetes to CVD are consistent in the United States and abroad, in younger
and older individuals, among both men and women, and across race/ethnicity
(3, 22).

0066-4219/02/0218-0245$14.00

This paper reviews the relationship between diabetes and CVD with an emphasis on findings from epidemiologic studies. Rather than providing an exhaustive summary of the existing literature on diabetes and its relationship to cardiovascular complications, this review highlights several key points related to the epidemiology of diabetes and CVD. These include a discussion of the "metabolic syndrome" that often characterizes diabetes, the differential effect of diabetes on CVD risk in men and women, and how the definition of diabetes influences not only population estimates of diabetes but also the association of diabetes with CVD. This report also explores the new focus on measurement of "nontraditional" risk factors, such as markers of inflammation, advanced glycosylation end products (AGEs), cardiac autonomic neuropathy, sleep-disordered breathing, and polymorphic genes, which may provide novel insights into mechanisms linking diabetes and CVD.

THE METABOLIC SYNDROME

People with type 2 diabetes often have distinct physical and metabolic profiles. Diabetic individuals are considerably heavier than their nondiabetic counterparts, and weight differences between the groups persist even into old age (9, 23). In epidemiologic studies, the body mass index (BMI) is the most common measure of body size. Nonwhite women have higher BMIs than nonwhite men or white women, a phenomenon that is directly related to the high prevalence of diabetes in minority women (9, 23). Apart from elevated BMI, diabetic individuals tend to have an android fat distribution pattern, with accumulation of fat in the abdomen. It has been postulated that abdominal visceral fat is involved in glucose dysregulation and plays a much greater role in the development of diabetes than subcutaneous fat (24–26). In epidemiologic studies, however, it is not possible to distinguish these two fat compartments by using conventional abdominal girth measures such as waist circumferences. Despite this limitation, circumference measures have been consistently associated with diabetes in a number of epidemiologic studies (27–30).

In addition to overall and abdominal obesity, people with diabetes exhibit a pattern of dyslipidemia characterized by elevated triglycerides, low levels of high-density lipoprotein (HDL) cholesterol and small, dense low-density lipoprotein (LDL) particles (9, 23). In contrast, levels of LDL cholesterol do not consistently differ between diabetic and non-diabetic people (i.e., diabetic patients may present with normal or below-normal LDL levels). Appearing prior to frank diabetes, this constellation of physical and metabolic characteristics (sometimes accompanied by hypertension, hyperuricemia, and abnormalities in hemostatic factors) has been termed the metabolic syndrome, although these features persist following diagnosis of diabetes. A recent study showed an association between the metabolic syndrome and ischemic heart disease, further highlighting the importance of this set of metabolic disorders in risk of CVD (31).

BEHAVIORAL RISK FACTORS AND CVD AMONG DIABETIC INDIVIDUALS

Smoking, Exercise, and Diet

Several behavioral risk factors increase the risk of adverse health events among diabetic individuals, although the effects of these risk factors are not limited to people with diabetes. Smoking has repeatedly been associated with development of diabetic complications and with increased mortality risk among people with diabetes (32–36). It is for this reason that the American Diabetes Association (ADA) recommends prevention and cessation of smoking among individuals with diabetes (37). Diabetic individuals are less likely to participate in regular physical activity than nondiabetic individuals (38). Lack of physical activity, in turn, is associated with mortality among people with diabetes (33, 39). Although sustained physical activity is generally beneficial to health, diabetic individuals should be evaluated by a physician before beginning an exercise program (40). Factors such as ischemic changes in the foot, loss of protective sensation, risk of vitreous hemorrhage, resting tachycardia, and orthostasis are associated with specific diabetic vascular complications. These factors must be considered in the design and implementation of exercise programs in order to ensure patient safety.

Studies of the role of diet in development of diabetes have yielded varied results regarding the risk associated with specific nutrients (41). However, it is clear that a diet high in saturated fat is associated with an adverse CVD risk factor profile both in the presence and absence of diabetes. The ADA does not recommend a single "diabetic diet" but rather one that is based on detailed patient assessment and treatment goals (42).

GENDER DIFFERENCES: PREVALENCE OF DIABETES AND DIFFERENTIAL EFFECTS OF DIABETES ON CVD RISK

When evaluating the effect of gender on the occurrence of diabetes and the association of diabetes with CVD, it is critical to consider other CVD risk factors to determine if gender plays an independent role in the development of either condition. When the gender distribution of key diabetes risk factors, such as obesity, is considered, there is no consistent difference in the occurrence of diabetes between men and women, nor does gender appear to influence the progression of glucose disorders (43, 44). The lack of risk-factor-adjusted differences in diabetes between men and women suggests that intrinsic characteristics distinguishing men from women do not play a role in the pathway from normoglycemia to a state of abnormal glucose metabolism leading to diabetes.

Although risk-factor-adjusted rates of diabetes do not consistently differ by gender, it is important to stress that the public health burden of diabetes is quite dissimilar in men and women. This is partly because key diabetes risk factors such as obesity are more prevalent in women, as are other factors potentially related to maintenance of normal glucose metabolism in the presence of obesity (45). In the United States, black, Hispanic, and American Indian women are considerably more obese than men of the same ethnicity (9), and these women experience higher rates of diabetes than their male counterparts (46, 47).

Women have lower unadjusted risk of CHD than men. In many studies, rates of CVD in women with diabetes equal or exceed those in men (5, 10, 14, 48–53), although not all studies have demonstrated this relationship (16, 54). A number of mechanisms have been proposed to explain the excess CVD risk among diabetic women.

Estrogen is generally associated with an antiatherogenic CVD risk factor profile, including higher HDL, lower LDL, and lower blood pressure, as well as a peripheral rather than central distribution of fat. The favorable effect of estrogen on these factors may therefore protect premenopausal women from CVD in comparison to men of similar age. At menopause, cessation of ovarian function leads to a reduction in estrogen levels and to elevated LDL and blood pressure, reduced HDL, and changes in body composition that favor deposition of fat in the abdomen. All of these phenomena also accompany chronological aging and are risk factors for CVD. Thus, after menopause and with aging, the favorable CVD risk factor profile commonly observed during women's reproductive years is reduced or eliminated compared to men of similar age, i.e., women's CVD risk may rise more steeply than men's as they age. However, changes in CVD risk factors at menopause do not fully explain the association between diabetes and CVD in women.

What, then, is the link between diabetes and CVD among diabetic women? Insulin resistance may be one answer. A period of insulin resistance often precedes the appearance of frank diabetes, and this period may last for years. During this time, peripheral tissues do not respond normally to the biological effects of insulin. Tissue resistance to insulin results in increased pancreatic beta cell activity, ultimately leading to a state of compensatory hyperinsulinemia that helps maintain euglycemia. At some point, a relative decrease in insulin production results in hyperglycemia because the compensatory hyperinsulinemia common in insulin resistance is no longer sufficient to maintain euglycemia. Paradoxically, diagnosis of diabetes is often accompanied by supranormal levels of insulin despite the high glucose levels.

The hyperinsulinemia of insulin resistance and diabetes is important in understanding the link between female gender and risk of CVD. Insulin resistance is associated with lower estrogen and higher androgen levels. Thus, even premenopausal women who are insulin-resistant or diabetic often have relatively low estrogen and higher androgen levels, characteristics associated with an unfavorable distribution of CVD risk factors. Premenopausal women with insulin resistance or diabetes do not benefit from the protective effects of estrogen experienced by women without these conditions. Although CVD events are relatively rare in the premenopausal years, the adverse effects of unfavorable CVD risk factor levels occurring before menopause may accumulate over time and only become apparent in the postmenopausal years. Thus, the estrogen deficiency characterizing menopause may be an especially potent CVD risk factor among women who were insulin-resistant earlier in life. Their late-life CVD risk may be a function not only of the unfavorable changes in CVD risk factors that often accompany menopause but also of the cumulative effects of unfavorable CVD risk factors that characterized their reproductive years.

Although estrogen may play a role in reducing CVD risk among diabetic women, secondary trials of postmenopausal women taking exogenous estrogen have not shown a reduction in CVD risk, and hyperestrogenemia has been linked to heart disease in men (55, 56). Studies of the effect of estrogen on CVD risk in both diabetic and nondiabetic women are needed to clarify this relationship.

Other pathways may link diabetes to higher CVD risk in women than in men. For example, although it is known that LDL is a risk factor for CVD, LDL levels are similar in people with and without diabetes (9, 57). However, one study showed not only that the composition of LDL differed between diabetic and nondiabetic individuals, with both diabetic men and women having smaller LDL particle size, but also that after adjustment for other CHD risk factors including lipids, no differences in LDL size remained in diabetic men whereas unfavorable differences persisted in diabetic women (58). Because small, dense LDL may enhance the atherosclerotic process (59), results from this cross-sectional study suggest an additional mechanism by which diabetes may increase CVD risk more in women than in men. This study also highlights the fact that LDL characteristics may play an important role in the vascular disease of diabetes, even at levels similar to those in nondiabetic people.

Another study of diabetic men and women showed that diabetes has a greater adverse effect on multiple CVD risk factors among women than among men (10). This study examined diabetes × gender interactions and found significant effects for waist-hip ratio, LDL cholesterol, HDL cholesterol, LDL size, apoB, and apoA1, findings that suggest a stronger effect of diabetes on CVD risk in women than in men. Differences in levels of these risk factors may be responsible for the observation of increased CVD risk in diabetic women compared with diabetic men.

EFFECT OF DEFINITION OF DIABETES
ON DIABETES PREVALENCE

A key requirement in interpreting epidemiologic research relating diabetes to CVD is the ability to compare results across studies. To achieve this, standardized methods for ascertaining and classifying abnormalities of glucose metabolism are necessary. Similarly, standardized criteria for defining CVD are important. For many years there was no set of standard diagnostic criteria for either type 1 or type 2 diabetes. This resulted in inconsistent practices in both clinical and research settings and in difficulty interpreting research findings across studies (60, 61). In response, the National Diabetes Data group and the World Health Organization

(WHO) proposed criteria for classification and diagnosis of diabetes based on either a fasting glucose of ≥ 140 mg/dL or a two-hour post-challenge glucose of ≥ 200 mg/dL following an oral glucose tolerance test (OGTT) using a standard 75-g carbohydrate challenge (62, 63). These criteria became known as the WHO criteria, and for more than 10 years, epidemiologic studies that collected both fasting and post-challenge glucose often used an "either-or" approach to define prevalence and incidence of diabetes—that is, diabetes was defined as an abnormality of *either* screening test. Diabetic individuals (people with an abnormality of either fasting or post-challenge glucose) were then studied in relation to prevalence and incidence of CHD and other diabetic complications (4–8, 18).

As the dust was settling after publication of the WHO criteria, in 1997 the ADA proposed changing the diagnostic criteria. Two principal features distinguish the ADA criteria from the WHO criteria: (*a*) a reduction in the fasting glucose threshold that is diagnostic of diabetes from 140 mg/dL to 126 mg/dL; (*b*) a recommendation against use of the OGTT for diagnosing or classifying diabetes, with a specific recommendation against use of the OGTT in epidemiologic studies (64). Following publication of the ADA criteria, a flurry of papers and editorials addressed not only comparisons in diabetes prevalence and incidence between the 1997 ADA and 1985 WHO criteria but also the relationship between the two definitions of diabetes and outcomes such as CVD and mortality, as well as principles of diabetes screening in general (57, 65–74).

Although one study showed a slight increase in the prevalence of diabetes under the ADA criteria (71), another showed few differences in the prevalence of diabetes under the two sets of criteria but hinted that differences increased with age (65). The latter findings are supported by another report showing that the ADA criteria under-ascertained diabetes by $\sim 50\%$ in older adults (75) and by results from a representative sample of U.S. adults in which an age-associated bias in ADA-defined diabetes diagnosis was demonstrated with increasing age, with proportionally fewer cases of diabetes identified as age increased (57). These results were due to the "missed" cases of diabetes that would have been identified by the OGTT had this test result been included in the ADA definition of diabetes. Consistent with known age-associated decrements in the OGTT with increasing age (76), individuals with post-challenge glucose ≥ 200 mg/dL often do not have a fasting glucose that is diagnostic of diabetes under the ADA criteria (57, 75, 77, 78). This has direct implications for the ADA criteria, which rely on fasting glucose alone to ascertain diabetes.

Whether the prevalence of diabetes was higher, lower, or about the same under the two sets of criteria, most investigators agreed that the lack of concordance of individuals defined as diabetic under the two sets of criteria was a matter of concern. This issue raised questions about which screening tool is appropriate for identifying diabetes in epidemiologic studies, and how these considerations should apply in a clinical setting. The matter of greatest clinical importance, however, is how the choice of tool to identify people with "diabetes" influences the association of abnormal glucose metabolism with adverse health outcomes.

The most obvious question was whether cases of diabetes that were "missed" under the ADA criteria were clinically relevant. Did people with isolated post-challenge hyperglycemia (IPH—those with fasting glucose <126 mg/dL and an OGTT ≥200 mg/dL) have worse CVD risk factor profiles than "nondiabetic" people (those with fasting glucose <126 mg/dL and an OGTT <200 mg/dL), and did they experience higher rates of CVD or other adverse health events that clearly distinguished them from people with OGTT <200 mg/dL? These questions were addressed by several studies examining CVD risk factors in groups of individuals in various glucose tolerance categories, as well as the relative strength of fasting versus post-challenge glucose in prediction of CVD and mortality. In most (69, 77–79) but not all (80) studies, the data suggested that after fasting glucose was considered, elevated post-challenge glucose was associated with additional risk of adverse health events, including CVD.

Questions concerning the magnitude of association between diabetes and CVD are complicated by studies in which only one of the two glucose measures was collected and by those in which diabetes is defined by self report, without blood chemistry data. Some investigators hold that diabetes should be defined based on a glycemic threshold that could conclusively be linked with diabetes-associated vascular damage, rather than a cut-point that maximizes concordance between fasting and post-challenge glucose (64). Others propose that diabetes should be diagnosed only when there is clear evidence of glycation, a mechanism by which high blood glucose is thought to be causally linked with vascular damage (81).

Whatever the ultimate conclusion to the controversy over the diagnosis and classification of diabetes, both in clinical and epidemiologic settings, researchers will need to address the belief of some investigators that the OGTT provides information on the risk of CVD that is distinct from that yielded by measuring fasting glucose (82). These considerations must be weighed against the fact that in the United States, the OGTT is not routinely performed in clinical practice, making the clinical application of findings from epidemiologic studies in which OGTTs have been collected and studied somewhat limited. However, use of glycated hemoglobin, in conjunction with fasting glucose, may help identify individuals with normal fasting glucose who show evidence of glycation.

THE FUTURE OF DIABETES-CVD RESEARCH: MEASUREMENT AND EVALUATION OF NONTRADITIONAL RISK FACTORS

Chronic Inflammation

Much attention has been focused recently on how inflammation may contribute to the development of CVD and on the possible role of diabetes in this pathway. It has been proposed that markers of inflammation are part of a complex clustering of pro-CVD risk factors characterizing the insulin resistance syndrome and that these markers contribute to CVD risk independently of established metabolic abnormalities commonly observed in insulin resistance (83–85).

The inflammatory response involves a complex cascade of events involving many cell types that have interrelated functions. Considerable redundancy is built into this system, a feature that makes specific disease-outcome attributions of inflammatory markers difficult. Studies of diabetes and CVD focusing on inflammation are limited by the nonspecific nature of existing markers, lack of definition of clinically meaningful levels of these markers, and inability of epidemiologic studies to sufficiently distinguish acute inflammation from chronic, low-grade inflammation. Despite these limitations, there is remarkable consistency in findings from a number of studies on the relationship between markers of inflammation, abnormalities of glucose metabolism, and CVD endpoints.

Interleukin 6 (IL-6) regulates the expression of C-reactive protein (CRP). Data from a small, clinic-based study showed that adipose tissue was associated with increased production of IL-6 and CRP, and that these two inflammatory markers were related to insulin resistance (86). These data suggested that low-level, chronic inflammation was associated with endothelial dysfunction, a pathway potentially linking obesity and insulin resistance to CVD. Results from this study are supported by a larger cross-sectional study that found elevated levels of CRP associated with obesity. This report showed elevated CRP in obese individuals as young at 17 years. Compared to their nonobese counterparts, obese men in this study were 2.13 times as likely to have elevated CRP, but women were 6.21 as likely to have elevated CRP (87). If markers of inflammation such as CRP are shown to be causally related to CVD risk, the gender difference in risk of elevated CRP at similar levels of obesity hints at another explanation for differences in CVD risk between men and women with similar CVD risk factor profiles. A study exploring the role of diabetes in relation to obesity and CRP, conducted in the same sample, showed that within levels of BMI, individuals with abnormalities of glucose metabolism had higher levels of CRP than normoglycemic people (88). These findings suggested that the association between diabetes and inflammation does not operate solely through the increased obesity that is common in diabetic individuals. However, it should be noted that data from this sample showed no association between CRP and self-reported angina pectoris but did show an association between CRP and self-reported stroke (89, 90). The inconsistency of these findings may be due to differences in detecting associations between "soft" outcome measures such as angina and "hard" outcomes such as stroke. Findings from these cross-sectional studies have been supported by prospective studies, which can show true CVD risk associated with inflammation.

IL-6 has been shown to predict mortality in women with CVD but not in those without CVD (91), suggesting that the mortality risk associated with this inflammatory marker may be primarily attributable to prevalent CVD. In a prospective study of older adults, markers of inflammation predicted clinically meaningful increases in fasting glucose levels (92). In this study, baseline levels of inflammatory markers predicted changes in ADA-defined categories of glucose regulation from nondiabetic to impaired fasting glucose, and from impaired fasting glucose to diabetes. Another study of middle-aged adults showed that elevated white-cell count and fibrinogen predicted a new diagnosis of diabetes (93). Although these studies suggest a role for inflammation in the development of glucose abnormalities, others support the temporal relationship between markers of inflammation and occurrence and progression of CVD and CVD mortality (94–97). Two recent studies showed that higher levels of CRP predicted both CVD and long-term mortality in unstable CHD (98, 99) and raised questions about whether a broad recommendation to measure these markers would help reduce CVD-associated morbidity and mortality.

Despite the growing body of evidence linking markers of inflammation to CVD, it is important to stress that these observations may be nonspecific. That is, elevated levels of inflammatory markers are observed in several conditions that are common in old age and may be indicators of the development and/or progression of these conditions (100). Data relating these markers to specific outcomes should therefore be interpreted with caution. The evolving literature on the role of inflammation in risk of CVD seems to indicate that diabetes plays a role, but the complex links between elevated inflammatory markers, impaired glucose regulation, and the occurrence of CVD have not yet been fully described.

Advanced Glycosylation End Products in Vascular Complications of Diabetes

A central pathologic feature of diabetic vascular complications may be the formation of advanced glycosylation end products (AGEs) in the tissues of diabetic individuals, a process that is accelerated in the presence of hyperglycemia (101, 102). Glucose forms early glycosylation products with proteins at a rate proportional to glucose concentrations. Because the amount of these products is reversible depending on the concentration of glucose and does not accumulate in stable tissue proteins, they are not consistently correlated with diabetic complications (103). However, over time, some of the early products undergo further changes and form bonds with other proteins. Levels of AGEs do not return to normal when hyperglycemia is eliminated; they continue to accumulate on wall proteins of both large and small vessels (104). Through several mechanisms, the accumulation of AGEs in tissue is thought to result in increased vascular permeability and thickened, inelastic vessel walls. In contrast to the lack of association between early glycosylation products and diabetic complications, AGEs are related to diabetic vascular disease (105). Numerous AGEs have been characterized (106, 107) but the relative importance of specific AGEs in diabetes-associated vascular damage is still unknown, as are the potentially differential effects of specific AGEs in different tissues.

One way in which AGEs may accelerate the development of macrovascular disease is by linking plasma lipoproteins with matrix proteins, a process that slows the efflux of lipoproteins from the tissues. This process has been demonstrated in vitro (108). Another mechanism potentially linking diabetes with CVD via AGEs is the induction of endothelial cell surface adhesion molecules resulting from the interaction of AGEs with their receptors (RAGE) (109, 110), a phenomenon that may be a marker for amount and progression of vascular disease in diabetes (111). One study suggested that blocking the activity of RAGE inhibits the accelerated atherosclerosis characterizing the diabetic state and may be a future target for new therapies (112).

Yet another mechanism potentially linking AGEs with vessel disease involves the inflammatory processes described above. Several studies have suggested that binding of AGEs induces release of inflammatory cytokines (113, 114). It is possible that sustained interaction between the stable AGEs and RAGE in tissues of diabetic individuals may result in a long-term proinflammatory environment that increases risk of CVD. The potential role of AGEs as a "fuel" for a pro-CVD inflammatory process may therefore be an important piece of the diabetes-CVD puzzle.

Despite promising data linking AGEs and diabetes-associated vascular damage, measurement and reporting of AGEs in epidemiologic studies have been limited. Although methods for standardization have been proposed (115), use of AGEs in epidemiologic studies has been sparse owing to lack of standardized measurements and the continuing evolution of knowledge about which AGEs are involved in the vascular damage observed in diabetes. In addition, although several studies have shown accumulation of AGEs in tissues of diabetic individuals, it will be important to validate serum measures of AGEs against tissue AGEs, because it is postulated that AGE-associated damage to vessels is more closely related to CVD than circulating AGEs are. However, because tissue samples are rarely available in epidemiologic studies, this type of validation may be difficult.

Chemical characterization of AGEs shows the existence of multiple products, each of which may be differentially related to diabetes and specific vascular complications. However, existing assays for polyclonal anti-AGE antibodies do not distinguish between individual AGEs, a key weakness in efforts to link specific products with vascular damage. Despite these limitations in the application of AGEs in epidemiologic studies, small clinic-based reports have shown that serum levels of AGEs are elevated in children with type I diabetes even before vascular complications appear (116). Such findings suggest important future opportunities for epidemiologic studies of AGEs and CVD.

Cigarette smoke is also a source of AGEs (117, 118), which may be one mechanism linking smoking with increased occurrence of CVD in both the presence and absence of diabetes. This is important because it is known that smoking increases the risk of peripheral arterial disease (PAD) among diabetic individuals, who are already at increased PAD risk, and that smoking can influence relationships between risk factors and the development of PAD.

Diabetes, Sleep-Disordered Breathing, and Cardiovascular Disease

Snoring is the most common symptom of sleep-disordered breathing (SDB) and has been suggested as a risk factor for CVD (119–121). Adverse CVD events attributable to snoring may be related to the occurrence of sleep apnea among people who snore. SDB is common in people with hypertension, overweight individuals, and older adults (121–123).

Hypertension, obesity, and older age are also well-established characteristics of people with diabetes. The substantial overlap between risk factors for SDB and those for diabetes raises questions about the potential relationship between diabetes and SDB, and how this relationship may be associated with the development of CVD. It is not clear if a potential SDB-CVD association is modified by diabetes or if this relationship is partly or entirely attributable to diabetic complications or metabolic abnormalities characterizing diabetes.

Severity of diabetes is associated with sleep disruption (124), which may result from the activation of metabolic processes involving insulin action or glucose regulation, although these potential pathways are not well-described (125). One mechanism through which diabetes may be involved in the SDB-CVD relationship is through the effects of diabetic cardiovascular autonomic neuropathy (CAN) on CVD risk.

A growing body of literature describes the contribution of CAN to increased CVD risk among diabetic individuals (126, 127). Although impairment of CAN-associated CVD reflexes, such as heart rate variability, may be associated with increased risk of CVD, other mechanisms may link diabetes to CVD via CAN. A recent study showed that one in four diabetic individuals with CAN had obstructive sleep apnea, a proportion significantly greater than in diabetic individuals without CAN (128). The relatively high prevalence of sleep disturbance in the presence of diabetic neuropathy raises the possibility that impairments in CAN-associated central control of respiration may link diabetes and SDB by enhancing the occurrence or consequences of sleep disorders on CVD (129). Reports of increased prevalence of sleep apnea and nocturnal oxygen desaturation in diabetic patients with CAN support a diabetes-SDB link (130–132). However, diabetes and SDB may also be related in the opposite direction, with SBD leading to decrements in glucose metabolism. A recent study showed a reduction in glucose tolerance following sleep deprivation and raised the possibility that disrupted sleep has deleterious effects on endocrine function (133). However, in such small cross-sectional studies, statistical power is often limited, and it is difficult to determine the direction of diabetes and SDB factors and to infer their independent effects because of confounding by obesity. Additionally, clinic-based studies of severe sleep deprivation do not mirror the experience of most people in the community. In cross-sectional studies, individuals with a history of CVD may adopt lifestyle modifications that further hinder interpretation of data related to diabetes and SDB.

Existing prospective studies of SDB and CVD are limited and do not provide the full complement of CVD risk factor data, including diabetes status. However, a large community-based prospective study of SDB and CVD is ongoing (134). Data from this study will begin to address deficiencies in previous studies by allowing improved examination not only of SDB's contribution to CVD but also the role of diabetes in this relationship.

Genetic Susceptibility to Diabetes-Associated Vascular Damage

Genetics may play a key role in determining the severity of vascular complications a diabetic individual is likely to experience. In the future, identification of "susceptibility genes" among diabetic individuals may become an important tool for clinicians as they tailor treatment plans for "susceptible" or "protected" patients. Although no clinical practice guidelines currently exist for genetic screening of diabetic patients for susceptibility to complications, intriguing new data suggest the existence of genes that confer differential susceptibility.

One such gene encodes haptoglobin (Hp), a hemoglobin-binding protein that protects against oxidative stress. Oxidative stress has been implicated as an important mediator of numerous pathophysiological processes, including diabetic vascular complications. The two common Hp alleles yield three phenotypes that appear to differ in their ability to function as antioxidants because of their different biochemical and biophysical properties. Three recent studies examining the Hp gene in relation to diabetic retinopathy, diabetic nephropathy, and coronary restenosis showed that individuals who are homozygous for the Hp 1 allele (1-1) appear to be protected against the development of these diabetic complications (135–137). As the field of genetics continues to develop, new strategies for risk stratification of diabetic patients may be tailored to their genetic profiles.

Risk Factors for Cardiovascular Disease in Diabetes: Possible Interventions

LIPIDS   Individuals with type 2 (non-insulin-dependent) diabetes have dyslipidemia characterized by high triglyceride levels, low levels of HDL, and small, dense LDL particles. This pattern results from both hyperglycemia per se and the insulin resistance syndrome that accompanies diabetes (138). Subgroup analyses of several major trials provide evidence that aggressive lipid lowering can be highly effective in reducing CVD risk in diabetic individuals. For primary prevention, the Helsinki Heart Study showed a 60% reduction (NS) in CVD events in a subgroup of 155 diabetic patients treated with gemfibrozil (139), and the Air Force/Texas Coronary Atherosclerosis Prevention Study (AFCAPS/TEXCAPS) showed a 30% (NS) reduction in CVD events in a subgroup of 264 diabetic patients treated with Lovastatin (140). For secondary prevention, the Cholesterol And Recurrent Events (CARE) Study showed a 25% reduction ($p < 0.02$) of CVD in a subgroup analysis of 586 diabetic individuals (141), and the Scandinavian Simvastatin Survival Study (4S) showed a 50% reduction of CVD in 202 diabetic individuals treated with simvastatin (142). The DAIS Study, the first lipid-lowering study to be completed solely in diabetic patients, showed reduced progression of atherosclerosis with fenofibrate therapy (143).

There is considerable debate concerning appropriate targets for LDL lowering among diabetic (and also nondiabetic) patients. Except for the CARE Study, all intervention studies show consistent risk reduction across the range of LDL levels; i.e, there is little evidence for a threshold below which LDL reduction does not mitigate CVD risk. Currently, the National Cholesterol Education Program (NCEP) ATP III guidelines indicate a goal of 100 mg/dL for individuals with diabetes (144). The American Diabetes Association (ADA) recommends a target of 100 mg/dL for all such individuals because of their known high risk for CVD and tendency to have multiple risk factors. High LDL levels in diabetic patients are thought to be particularly atherogenic because of altered composition, glycation, and susceptibility to oxidation.

In the above trials, LDL goals were between 100 and 130 mg/dL. However, it has often been suggested that therapeutic goals could be lower. In the Post Coronary Artery Bypass Graft (Post CABG) Trial, the role of aggressive (goal LDL 85 mg/dL) versus moderate (goal LDL 130–140 mg/dL) cholesterol reduction was evaluated in 1351 patients with prior saphenous vein CABG and baseline LDL levels of 130–175 mg/dL using lovastatin (40–80 mg) $\pm$ cholestyramine (2.5–5 mg/d). The aggressive therapy arm produced a 31% relative reduction in the progression of atherosclerosis in the grafts and 29% relative reduction in revascularization procedures compared with moderate therapy (145). In a more recent evaluation of aggressive lipid management in asymptomatic to moderately symptomatic individuals with known CVD, the AVERT Trial revealed that aggressive lipid lowering to 77 mg/dL utilizing 80 mg of atorvastatin daily (with baseline LDL levels $\geq$115 mg/dL) reduced the 18-month ischemic event rate by an absolute 8% (NS, a relative reduction of 36%) compared with those treated with angioplasty, and significantly increased the time to the first ischemic event (146). Because the risk of initial CVD events in diabetic patients appears at least as great as the risk for recurrent events in those with proven CVD (147), it appears that the benefits of the aggressive interventions evidenced in secondary prevention would be applicable to those with diabetes.

BLOOD PRESSURE   Hypertension in the setting of type 2 diabetes is frequently associated with both CVD and progressive renal insufficiency. Intensive blood pressure (BP) control in patients with type 2 diabetes is associated with a substantial reduction in CVD risk. This has been well described in a number of pivotal trials, including a subgroup analysis of 1501 patients in the Hypertension Optimal Treatment (HOT) Trial ($N = 1501$) (148) and the Israeli Multicenter Study ($N = 94$) (149). Two studies, however, have clearly defined the importance of more rigorous BP control in type 2 diabtes: the United Kingdom Prospective Diabetes Study (UKPDS) (150) and the Heart Outcomes Prevention Evaluation (HOPE) Trial (151). In the UKPDS study, more than 1000 hypertensive diabetic subjects were randomized to either tight (144/82 mmHg) or less tight BP control (154/87 mmHg). The 10/5 mmHg difference in BP was associated with a 15% decrease in CVD, a 32% decrease in death due to diabetes, and a 44% reduction in the incidence of CVA. The HOPE Trial extended these observations in 3577 hypertensive diabetic individuals by demonstrating that the addition of 10 mg ramipril for patients who already had "well-controlled" BP (139/79 mmHg) further reduced CVD death by 37% and all forms of microvascular complications. Other clinical trials, such as the ABCD Study (152), the CAPPP Trial (153), and the FACET Trial (154), have similarly demonstrated the survival advantage of more rigorous BP control with ACE inhibitors plus other drugs.

Although the optimum target BP for hypertensives with diabetes has not yet been determined with certainty, completed trials indicate that reducing systolic BP to at least 130 mmHg provides substantial reduction in both macro- and microvascular disease progression. Moreover, these benefits can be demonstrated without increasing the risk for adverse events or myocardial infarction, as some have previously suggested (J-curve effect) (33). Adler et al. carefully assessed the risk of diabetic complications associated with systolic BP in the UKPDS and demonstrated that, with increasing systolic BP, there was a continuous and linear risk of progressive development of both macrovascular and microvascular events (155). Clinical trials have also demonstrated that treatment of BP even in the so-called normotensive range of type 2 diabetes is associated with prevention of BP elevation and increasing urinary protein excretion, and would likely reduce the risk of CVD and the progression of renal disease (156–158). Viberti et al. randomized both type 1 and type 2 diabetic subjects with microalbuminuria to treatment with either an ACE inhibitor or a placebo even though their BP prior to therapy was 124/77 mmHg. This study demonstrated that this intervention, despite minimal BP reduction (4/2 mmHg), was associated with a significant reduction in the risk for progression from microalbuminuria to macroalbuminuria (156). Likewise, Ravid et al. demonstrated in a five-year prospective randomized controlled trial that an ACE inhibitor was capable of preventing BP elevation and increasing proteinuria in type 2 diabetics with a BP of 130/80 mmHg and only 130 mg protein in the urine per 24 h (157, 158). Moreover, within five years, differences in the rate of loss of renal function over time, favoring therapy with the ACE inhibitor, were demonstrated.

These studies in diabetics indicate that early treatment of BP even in the normotensive range may forestall the development of progressive nephropathy. A recent pooled analysis of 11 large randomized controlled trials demonstrated that the optimal systolic BP for preventing progression of nondiabetic renal disease is approximately 110 mmHg (159). Thus, these data show that earlier and more rigorous BP control, particularly with ACE inhibitors, prevents progression of renal disease, and strongly suggest that CVD will also be reduced.

SUMMARY

Diabetes remains a growing public health problem. The aging of the population, along with increasing obesity and decreasing physical activity, will ensure that the number of diabetic individuals will continue to grow. The most effective strategy for preventing diabetes-associated CVD is prevention of diabetes. Among people with diabetes, aggressive modification of conventional CVD risk factors remains a cornerstone of risk reduction. As clinical applications of modern genetics and molecular biology continue to develop, new therapies will likely focus on novel targets in the multiple pathways between hyperglycemia and CVD.

Visit the Annual Reviews home page at www.AnnualReviews.org

LITERATURE CITED

1. Pyorala K, Laakso M, Uusitupa M. 1987. Diabetes and atherosclerosis: an epidemologic view. *Diab. Met. Rev.* 3:463–524

2. American Diabetes Association. 1998. Economic consequences of diabetes mellitus in the U.S. in 1997. *Diab. Care* 21:296–309

3. Wingard DL, Barrett-Connor E. 1995. Heart disease and diabetes. In *Diabetes in America*, pp. 429–34. Natl. Inst. Health, Natl. Inst. Diab. and Digestive and Kidney Dis. NIH Pub. No. 95-1468. 2nd ed.

4. Scheidt-Nave C, Barrett-Connor E, Wingard DL. 1990. Resting electrocardiographic abnormalities suggestive of asymptomatic ischemic heart disease associated with non-insulin-dependent diabetes mellitus in a defined population. *Circulation* 81:899–906

5. Rewers M, Shetterly SM, Baxter J, et al. 1992. Prevalence of coronary heart disease in subject with normal and impaired glucose tolerance and non-insulin-dependent diabetes mellitus in a biethnic Colorado population. The San Luis Valley Diabetes Study. *Am. J. Epidemiol.* 12:1321–30

6. Mitchell BD, Hazuda HP, Haffner SM, et al. 1991. Myocardial infarction in Mexican-Americans and non-Hispanic whites: the San Antonio Heart Study. *Circulation* 83:45–51

7. Fujimoto WY, Leonetti DL, Kinyoun JL, Shuman WP, et al. 1987. Prevalence of complications among second generation Japanese-American men with diabetes, impaired glucose tolerance, or normal glucose tolerance. *Diabetes* 36:730–39

8. Fujimoto WY, Leonetti DK, Bergstrom RW, et al. 1991. Glucose intolerance and diabetic complications among Japanese-American women. *Diab. Res. Clin. Prac.* 13:119–29

9. Cowie CC, Harris MI. 1995. Physical and metabolic characteristics of persons with diabetes. See Ref. 3, pp. 117–32

10. Howard BV, Cowan LD, Go O, et al. 1998. Adverse effects of diabetes on multiple cardiovascular disease risk factors in women. *Diab. Care* 21:1258–65

11. McPhillips JB, Barrett-Connor E, Wingard D. 1990. Cardiovascular disease risk factors prior to the diagnosis of impaired glucose tolerance and non-insulin-dependent diabetes mellitus in a community of older adults. *Am. J. Epidemiol.* 131:443–53

12. Wilson PW, Cupples AD, Kannel WB. 1991. Is hyperglycemia associated with cardiovascular disease? The Framingham Study. *Am. Heart J.* 121:(2 Pt. 1):586–90

13. Manson JE, Colditz GA, Stampfer MJ, et al. 1991. A prospective study of maturity-onset diabetes mellitus and risk of coronary heart disease and stroke in women. *Arch. Int. Med.* 151:1141–47

14. Barrett-Connor E, Cohn BA, Wingard DL, Edelstein SL. 1991. Why is diabetes mellitus a stronger risk factor for fatal ischemic heart disease in women than in men? The Rancho Bernardo Study. *JAMA* 265:627–31

15. Seeman T, Mendes de Leon C, Berkman L, Ostfeld A. 1993. Risk factors for coronary heart disease among older men and women: a prospective study of community-dwelling elderly. *Am. J. Epidemiol.* 138:1037–49

16. Kleinman JC, Donohue RP, Harris MI, et al. 1988. Mortality among diabetics in a national sample. *Am. J. Epidemiol.* 128:389–401

17. Howard BV, Robbins DC, Sievers ML, et al. 2000. LDL cholesterol as a strong predictor of coronary heart disease in diabetic individuals with insulin resistance

and low LDL: the Strong Heart Study. *Arterioscler. Thromb. Vasc. Biol.* 20:830–35

18. Howard BV, Lee ET, Cowan LD, et al. 1999. Rising tide of cardiovascular disease in American Indians: the Strong Heart Study. *Circulation* 99:2389–95

19. Garcia MJ, McNamara PM, Gordon T, Kannell WB. 1974. Morbidity and mortality in diabetics in the Framingham population. Sixteen-year follow-up study. *Diabetes* 23:105–11

20. Standl E, Balletshofer B, Dahl B, et al. 1996. Predictors of 10-year macrovascular and overall mortality in patients with NIDDM: the Munich General Practitioner Project. *Diabetologia* 39:1540–45

21. Haffner SM, Lehto S, Ronnemaa T, et al. 1998. Mortality from coronary heart disease in subjects with type 2 diabetes and in nondiabetic subjects with and without prior myocardial infarction. *New Engl. J. Med.* 339:229–34

22. Nathan DM, Meigs J, Singer DE. 1997. The epidemiology of cardiovascular disease in type 2 diabetes mellitus: How sweet it is . . . or is it? *Lancet* 350(Suppl. 1):S14–S19

23. Resnick HE, Shorr RI, Kuller L, et al. 2001. Prevalence and clinical implications of American Diabetes Association–defined diabetes and other categories of glucose dysregulation in older adults: the Health, Aging, and Body Composition Study. *J. Clin. Epidemiol.* In press

24. Abate N. 1996. Insulin resistance and obesity: the role of fat distribution pattern. *Diab. Care* 19:292–94

25. Stern MP, Haffner SM. 1986. Body fat distribution and hyperinsulinemia as risk factors for diabetes and cardiovascular disease. *Arteriosclerosis* 6:123–130

26. Despres JP, Nadeau A, Tremblay A, et al. 1989. Role of deep abdominal fat in the association between regional adipose tissue distribution and glucose tolerance in obese women. *Diabetes* 38:304–9

27. Cassano PA, Rosner B, Vokonas PS, Weiss ST. 1992. Obesity and body fat distribution in relation to the incidence of non-insulin dependent diabetes mellitus. *Am. J. Epidemiol.* 136:1474–86

28. Karter AJ, Mayer-Davis EJ, Selby JV, et al. 1996. Insulin sensitivity and abdominal obesity in African-American, Hispanic and non-Hispanic white men and women: the Insulin Resistance and Atherosclerosis Study. *Diabetes* 45:1547–55

29. Haffner SM, Stern MP, Hazuda HP, et al. 1987. Do upper-body and centralized adiposity measure different aspects of regional body-fat distribution? *Diabetes* 36:43–51

30. Okosun IS, Cooper RS, Rotimi CN, et al. 1998. Association of waist circumference with risk of hypertension and type 2 diabetes in Nigerians, Jamaicans, and African-Americans. *Diab. Care* 21:1836–42

31. Lindblad U, Langer RD, Wingard DL, et al. 2001. Metabolic syndrome and ischemic heart disease in elderly men and women. *Am. J. Epidemiol.* 153:481–89

32. Haire-Joshu D, Glasgow RE, Tibbs TL. 1999. Smoking and diabetes. *Diab. Care* 22:1887–98

33. Ford ES, DeStefano F. 1991. Risk factors for mortality from all causes and from coronary heart disease among persons with diabetes: findings from the National Health and Nutrition Examination Survey I Epidemiologic Follow-up Study. *Am. J. Epidemiol.* 133:1220–30

34. Nielsen MM, Hjollund E. 1978. Smoking and diabetic microangiopathy. *Lancet* 2:533–34

35. Stegmayr BG. 1990. A study of patients with diabetes mellitus (type 1) and end-stage renal failure: tobacco usage may increase risk of nephropathy and death. *J. Intern. Med.* 228:121–24

36. Hamman RF, Mayer EJ, Moo-Young GA, et al. 1989. Prevalence and risk factors of diabetic retinopathy in non-Hispanic whites and Hispanics with NIDDM. San

Luis Valley Diabetes Study. *Diabetes* 38:1231–37

37. American Diabetes Association: smoking and diabetes. 2001. *Diab. Care* 24(Suppl. 1):S64–S65

38. Ford ES, Herman WH. 1995. Leisure-time physical activity patterns in the U. S. diabetic population. Findings from the 1990 National Health Interview Survey— Health Promotion and Disease Prevention Supplement. *Diab. Care* 18:27–33

39. Kohl HW, Gordon NF, Villegas JA, Blair SN. 1992. Cardiorespiratory fitness, glycemic status, and mortality risk in men. *Diab. Care* 15:184–92

40. American Diabetes Association. 2001. Diabetes mellitus and exercise. *Diab. Care* 24(Suppl. 1):S51–S55

41. Rewers M, Hamman RF. 1995. Risk factors for non-insulin dependent diabetes. See Ref. 3 pp. 179–220

42. American Diabetes Association. 2001. Nutrition recommendations and principles for people with diabetes mellitus. *Diab. Care* 24(Suppl. 1):S44–S47

43. King H, Rewers M. 1993. Global estimates for prevalence of diabetes mellitus and impaired glucose tolerance in adults. *Diab. Care* 16:157–77

44. Edelstein SL, Knowler WC, Bain RP, et al. 1997. Predictors of progression from impaired glucose tolerance to NIDDM. An analysis of six prospective studies. *Diabetes* 46:701–10

45. Sumner AE, Kushner H, Sherif KD, et al. 1999. Sex differences in African-Americans regarding sensitivity to insulin's glucoregulatory and antilipolytic actions. *Diab. Care* 22:71–77

46. Harris MI. 1991. Epidemiological correlates of NIDDM in Hispanics, whites and blacks in the U.S. population. *Diab. Care* 14(Suppl. 3):639–48

47. Resnick HE, Valsania P, Halter JB, Lin X. 1998. Differential effects of BMI on diabetes risk among black and white Americans. *Diab. Care* 21:1828–35

48. Kannel WB, McGee DL. 1979. Diabetes and glucose tolerance as risk factors for cardiovascular disease: the Framingham Study. *Diab. Care* 2:120–26

49. Kannel WB, Wilson PW. 1995. Risk factors that attenuate the female coronary disease advantage. *Arch. Intern. Med.* 155:57–61

50. Heyden S, Heiss G, Bartel AG, Hames CG. 1980. Sex differences in coronary mortality among diabetics in Evans County, Georgia. *J. Chron. Dis.* 33:265–73

51. Pan WH, Cedres LB, Liu K, et al. 1986. Relationship of clinical diabetes and asymptomatic hyperglycemia to risk of coronary heart disease mortality in men and women. *Am. J. Epidemiol.* 123:504–16

52. DeStefano F, Ford ES, Newman J, et al. 1993. Risk factors for coronary heart disease mortality among persons with diabetes. *Ann. Epidemiol.* 3:27–34

53. Sprafka JM, Pankow J, McGovern PG, French LR. 1993. Mortality among type 2 diabetic individuals and associated risk factors: the Three City Study. *Diab. Med.* 10:627–32

54. Head J, Fuller JH. 1990. International variation in mortality among diabetic patients: the WHO Multinational Study of Vascular Disease in Diabetics. *Diabetologia* 33:477–81

55. Wilson PW, Garrison RJ, Castelli WP. 1985. Postmenopausal estrogen use, cigarette smoking, and cardiovascular morbidity in women over 50. The Framingham Study. *N. Engl. J. Med.* 313:38–1043

56. Phillips GB, Castelli WP, Abbott RD, McNamara PM. 1983. Association of hyperestrogenemia and coronary heart disease in men in the Framingham cohort. *Am. J. Med.* 74:863–69

57. Resnick HE, Harris MI, Brock DB, Harris TB. 2000. American Diabetes Association diabetes diagnostic criteria, advancing age, and cardiovascular disease risk factor profiles: results from the Third

National Health and Nutrition Examination Survey. *Diab. Care* 23:176–80

58. Haffner SM, Mykkanen L, Stern MP, Paidi M, Howard BV. 1994. Greater effect of diabetes on LDL size in women than in men. *Diab. Care* 17:1164–71

59. Tribble DL, Holl LG, Wood PD, Krauss RM. 1992. Variations in oxidative susceptibility among six low density lipoprotein subfractions of differing density and particle size. *Atherosclerosis* 93:189–99

60. West KM. 1975. Substantial differences in the diagnostic criteria used by diabetes experts. *Diabetes* 24:641–44

61. West KM. 1979. Standardization of definition, classification, and reporting in diabetes-related epidemiologic studies. *Diab. Care* 2:65–76

62. National Diabetes Data Group. 1979. Classification and diagnosis of diabetes mellitus and other categories of glucose intolerance. *Diab.* 28:1039–57

63. World Health Organization. 1985. *Diabetes mellitus, report of a study group.* WHO Tech. Rep. Ser. No. 727, Geneva, Switzerland

64. The Expert Committee on the Diagnosis and Classification of Diabetes Mellitus. 1997. Report of the Expert Committee on the Diagnosis and Classification of Diabetes Mellitus. *Diab. Care* 20:1183–97

65. Lee ET, Howard BV, Go O, et al. 2000. Prevalence of undiagnosed diabetes in three American Indian populations. A comparison of the 1997 American Diabetes Association diagnostic criteria and the 1985 World Health Organization diagnostic criteria: the Strong Heart Study. *Diab. Care* 23:181–86

66. Vinicor F. 1999. When is diabetes diabetes? *JAMA* 281:1222–24

67. Resnick HE, Harris TB. 1999. New diabetes diagnostic criteria result in fewer cases in older adults. *BMJ* 318:531

68. Balkau B. 1999. New diabetes diagnostic criteria for diabetes and mortality in older adults. DECODE Study Group. European Diabetes Epidemiology Group. *Lancet* 353:68–69

69. Gabir MM, Hanson RL, Dabelea D, et al. 2000. Plasma glucose and prediction of microvascular disease and mortality: evaluation of 1997 American Diabetes Association and 1999 World Health Organization criteria for diagnosis of diabetes. *Diab. Care* 23:1113–18

70. Mannucci E, Bardini G, Ognibene A, Rotella CM. 1999. Comparison of ADA and WHO screening methods for diabetes mellitus in obese patients. *Diab. Med.* 16:579–85

71. Unwin N, Alberti KGMM, Bhopal R, et al. 1998. Comparison of the current WHO and new ADA criteria for the diagnosis of diabetes mellitus in three ethnic groups in the UK. *Diab. Med.* 15:554–57

72. Alberti KGGM, Zimmet PZ. 1998. New diagnostic criteria and classification of diabetes—again? *Diab. Med.* 15:535–36

73. Goyder E, Irwig L. 1998. Screening for diabetes: What are we really doing? *BMJ* 317:1644–46

74. de Vegt F, Dekker JM, Stehouwer CDA, et al. 1998. The 1997 American Diabetes Association criteria versus the 1985 World Health Organization criteria for the diagnosis of abnormal glucose tolerance: poor agreement in the Hoorn Study. *Diab. Care* 21:1686–90

75. Wahl PW, Savage PJ, Psaty BM, et al. 1998. Diabetes in older adults: comparison of 1997 American Diabetes Association classification of diabetes mellitus with 1985 WHO classification. *Lancet* 352:1012–15

76. Andres R. 1971. Aging and diabetes. *Med. Clin. N. Am.* 55:835–46

77. Shaw JE, Hodge AM, de Courten M, et al. 1999. Isolated post-challenge hyperglycaemia confirmed as a risk factor for mortality. *Diabetologia* 42:1050–54

78. Barrett-Connor E, Ferrara A. 1998. Isolated postchallenge hyperglycemia and the risk of fatal cardiovascular disease

in older women and men: the Rancho Bernardo Study. *Diab. Care* 21:1236–39

79. Barzilay JI, Spiekerman CF, Wahl PW, et al. 1999. Cardiovascular disease in older adults with glucose disorders: comparison of American Diabetes Association criteria for diabetes mellitus with WHO criteria. *Lancet* 354:622–25

80. Hu D, Zhang Y, Yeh F, et al. 2000. Comparison of ADA and WHO diagnostic criteria for predicting CHD risk: the Strong Heart Study. *Diabetes* 49:A186–A187 (Abstract)

81. Davidson MB, Schriger DL, Peters AL, Lorber B. 1999. Relationship between fasting plasma glucose and glycosylated hemoglobin. Potential for false-positive diagnosis of type 2 diabetes using new diagnostic criteria. *JAMA* 281:1203–10

82. Hanefeld M, Temelkova-Kurktschiev T. 1997. The postprandial state and the risk of atherosclerosis. *Diab. Med.* 14(Suppl. 3):S6–S11

83. Sakkinen PA, Wahl P, Cushman M, et al. 2000. Clustering of procoagulation, inflammation and fibrinolysis variables with metabolic factors in insulin resistance syndrome. *Am. J. Epidemiol.* 152:897–907

84. Pickup JC, Mattock MB, Chusney GD, Burt D. 1997. NIDDM as a disease of the innate immune system: association of acute-phase reactants and interleukin-6 with metabolic syndrome X. *Diabetologia* 40:1286–92

85. Mendall MA, Patel P, Asante M, et al. 1997. Relation of serum cytokine concentrations to cardiovascular risk factors and coronary heart disease. *Heart* 78:273–77

86. Yudkin JS, Stehouwer CDA, Emeis JJ, Coppack SW. 1999. C-reactive protein in healthy subjects—association with obesity, insulin resistance and endothelial dysfunction. *Arterioscler. Thromb. Vasc. Biol.* 19:972–78

87. Visser M, Bouter LM, McQuillan GM, et al. 1999. Elevated C-reactive protein levels in overweight and obese adults. *JAMA* 282:2131–35

88. Ford ES. 1999. Body mass index, diabetes, and C-reactive protein among U. S. adults. *Diab. Care* 22:1971–77

89. Ford ES, Giles WH. 2000. Serum C-reactive protein and fibrinogen concentrations and self-reported angina pectoris and myocardial infarction: findings from National Health and Examination Survey III. *J. Clin. Epidemiol.* 53:95–102

90. Ford ES, Giles WH. 2000. Serum C-reactive protein and self-reported stroke: findings from the Third National Health and Nutrition Examination Survey. *Arteriscler. Thromb. Vasc. Biol.* 20:1052–56

91. Volpato S, Guralnik JM, Ferrucci L, et al. 2001. Cardiovascular disease, interleukin-6 and risk of mortality in older women: the Women's Health and Aging Study. *Circulation* 103:947–53.

92. Barzilay JI, Abraham L, Heckbert SR, et al. 2001. The relation of markers of inflammation to the development of glucose disorders in the elderly: the Cardiovascular Health Study. *Diabetes* 50:2384–89

93. Schmidt MI, Duncan BB, Sharrett AR, et al. 1999. Markers of inflammation and prediction of diabetes mellitus in adults (Atherosclerosis Risk in Communities study): a cohort study. *Lancet* 353:1649–52

94. Ridker PM, Cushman M, Stampfer MJ, et al. 1997. Inflammation, aspirin and the risk of cardiovascular disease in apparently healthy men. *N. Engl. J. Med.* 336:973–79

95. Jager A, van Hinsbergh VW, Kostense PJ, et al. 1999. von Willebrand factor, C-reactive protein, and 5-year mortality in diabetic and nondiabetic subjects: the Hoorn Study. *Arterioscler. Thromb. Vasc. Biol.* 19:3071–78

96. Gussekloo J, Schapp MC, Frolich M, et al. 2000. C-reactive protein is a strong but nonspecific risk factor of fatal stroke in elderly persons. *Arterioscler. Thromb. Vasc. Biol.* 20:1047–51

97. Kuller LH, Tracy RP, Shaten J, Meilahn EN. 1996. Relation of C-reactive protein and coronary heart disease in the MR-FIT nested case-control study. Multiple Risk Factor Intervention Trial. *Am. J. Epidemiol.* 144:537–47

98. Ridker PM, Hennekens CH, Buring JE, Rifai N. 2000. C-reactive protein and other markers of inflammation in the prediction of cardiovascular disease in women. *N. Engl. J. Med.* 342:836–43

99. Lindahl B, Toss H, Siegbahn A, et al. 2000. Markers of myocardial damage and inflammation in relation to long-term mortality in unstable coronary artery disease. FRISC Study Group. Fragmin during instability in coronary artery disease. *N. Engl. J. Med.* 343:1139–47

100. Papanicolaou DA, Wilder RL, Manolagas SC, Chrousos GP. 1998. The pathophysiologic roles of interleukin-6 in human disease. *Ann. Intern. Med.* 128:127–37

101. Brownlee M, Cerami A, Vlassara H. 1988. Advanced glycosylation end products in tissue and the biochemical basis of diabetic complications. *N. Engl. J. Med.* 318:1315–21

102. Vlassara H. 1996. Advanced glycation end-products and atherosclerosis. *Ann. Med.* 28:419–26

103. Vishwanath V, Frank KE, Elmets CA, et al. 1986. Glycation of skin collagen in type I diabetes mellitus. Correlation with long-term complications. *Diabetes* 35:916–21

104. Brownlee M, Vlassara H, Cerami A. 1984. Nonenzymatic glycosylation and the pathogenesis of diabetic complications. *Ann. Intern. Med.* 101:527–37

105. Monnier VM, Vishwanath V, Frank KE, et al. 1986. Relation between complications of type I diabetes mellitus and collagen-linked fluorescence. *N. Engl. J. Med.* 314:403–8

106. Ling X, Sakashita N, Takeya M, et al. 1998. Immunohistochemical distribution and subcellular localization of three distinct specific molecular structures of advanced glycation end products in human tissues. *Lab. Invest.* 78:1591–1606

107. Sakata N, Imanaga Y, Meng J, et al. 1998. Immunohistochemical localization of different epitopes of advanced glycation end products in human athersclerotic lesions. *Atherosclerosis* 141:61–75

108. Brownlee M, Vlassara H, Cerami A. 1985. Nonenzymatic glycosylation products on collagen covalently trip low-density lipoprotein. *Diabetes* 34:938–41

109. Schmidt AM, Hori O, Chen JX, et al. 1995. Advanced glycation endproducts interacting with their endothelial receptor induce expression of vascular cell adhesion molecule-1 (VCAM-1) in cultured human endothelial cells and in mice. A potential mechanism for the accelerated vasculopathy of diabetes. *J. Clin. Invest.* 96:1395–1403

110. Yan SD, Stern D, Schmidt AM. 1997. What's the RAGE? The receptor for advanced glycation end products (RAGE) and the dark side of glucose. *Eur. J. Clin. Invest.* 27:179–81

111. Schmidt AM, Crandall J, Hori O, et al. 1996. Elevated plasma levels of vascular cell adhesion molecule-1 (VCAM-1) in diabetic patients with microalbuminuria: a marker of vascular dysfunction and progressive vascular disease. *Br. J. Haematol.* 92:747–50

112. Park L, Raman KG, Lee KJ, et al. 1998. Suppression of accelerated diabetic atherosclerosis by the soluble receptor for advanced glycation endproducts. *Nat. Med.* 4:1025–31

113. Vlassara H, Brownlee M, Manogue KR, et al. 1988. Cachectin/TNF and IL-1 induced by glucose-modified proteins: role in normal tissue remodeling. *Science* 240:1546–48

114. Morohoshi M, Fujisawa K, Uchimura I, Numano F. 1995. The effect of glucose and advanced glycosylation end products on IL-6 production by human monocytes. *Ann. NY Acad. Sci.* 748:562–70

115. Mitsuhashi T, Vlassara H, Founds HW, Li YM. 1997. Standardizing the immunological measurement of advanced glycation endproducts using normal human serum. *J. Immunol. Methods* 207:79–88

116. Berg TJ, Dahl-Jorgensen K, Torjesen PA, Hanssen KF. 1997. Increased serum levels of advanced glycation end products (AGEs) in children and adolescents with IDDM. *Diab. Care* 20:1006–8

117. Cerami C, Founds H, Nicholl I, et al. 1997. Tobacco smoke is a source of toxic reactive glycation products. *Proc. Natl. Acad. Sci. USA* 94:13915–20

118. Nicholl ID, Bucala R. 1998. Advanced glycation endproducts and cigarette smoking. *Cell. Mol. Biol.* 44:1025–33

119. Partinen M, Palomaki H. 1985. Snoring and cerebral infarction. *Lancet* 14:1325–26

120. Koskenvuo M, Kaprio J, Partinen M, et al. 1985. Snoring as a risk factor for hypertension and angina pectoris. *Lancet* 1:893–96

121. Nieto FJ, Young TB, Lind BK, et al. 2000. Association of sleep disordered breathing, sleep apnea, and hypertension in a large community-based study. Sleep Heart Health Study. *JAMA* 283:1829–36

122. Kiely JL, McNicholas WT. 2000. Cardiovascular risk factors in patients with obstructive sleep apnoea syndrome. *Eur. Respir. J.* 16:128–33

123. Foley DJ, Monjan AA, Masaki KH, et al. 1999. Associations of symptoms of sleep apnea with cardiovascular disease, cognitive impairment, and mortality among older Japanese-American men. *J. Am. Geriatr. Soc.* 47:524–28

124. Lamond N, Tiggemann M, Dawson D. 2000. Factors predicting sleep disruption in Type II diabetes. *Sleep* 23:415–16

125. Strohl KP. 1996. Diabetes and sleep apnea. *Sleep* 19(10 Suppl.):S225–S228

126. Ziegler D. 1999. Cardiovascular autonomic neuropathy: clinical manifestations and measurement. *Diab. Rev.* 7:342–57

127. Rathmann W, Ziegler D, Jahnke M, et al. 1993. Mortality in diabetic patients with cardiovascular autonomic neuropathy. *Diab. Med.* 10:820–24

128. Ficker JH, Dertinger SH, Siegfried W, et al. 1998. Obstructive sleep apnoea and diabetes mellitus: the role of cardiovascular autonomic neuropathy. *Eur. Respir. J.* 11:14–19

129. Page MM, Watkins PJ. 1978. Cardiorespiratory arrest and diabetic autonomic neuropathy. *Lancet* 1:14–16

130. Rees PJ, Prior JG, Cochrane GM, Clark TJ. 1981. Sleep apnoea in diabetic patients with autonomic neuropathy. *J. R. Soc. Med.* 74:192–95

131. Neumann C, Martinez D, Schmid H. 1995. Nocturnal oxygen desaturation in diabetic patients with severe autonomic neuropathy. *Diab. Res. Clin. Pract.* 28:97–102

132. Sobotka PA, Liss HP, Vinik AI. 1986. Impaired hypoxic ventilatory drive in diabetic patients with autonomic neuropathy. *J. Clin. Endocrinol. Metab.* 62:658–63

133. Spiegel K, Leproult R, Van Cauter E. 1999. Impact of sleep debt on metabolic and endocrine function. *Lancet* 354:1435–39

134. Quan SF, Howard BV, Iber C, et al. 1997. The Sleep Heart Health Study: design rationale and methods. *Sleep* 20:1077–85

135. Levy AP, Roguin A, Hochberg I, et al. 2000. Haptoglobin phenotype and vascular complications in patients with diabetes. *N. Engl. J. Med.* 343:969–70

136. Nakhoul FM, Marsh S, Hochberg I, et al. 2000. Haptoglobin genotype as a risk factor for diabetic retinopathy. *JAMA* 284:1244–45

137. Nakhoul FM, Zoabi R, Kanter Y, et al. 2001. Haptoglobin phenotype and diabetic nephropathy. *Diabetologia* 44:602–4

138. Howard BV. 1995. Epidemiology of the pleurimetabolic syndrome. In *Atherosclerosis X*, ed. FP Woodford, J Davignon, A Sniderman, pp. 516–19. Int. Congr. Ser. 1066. New York: Elsevier

139. Koskinen P, Manttari M, Manninen V, et al. 1992. Coronary heart disease incidence in NIDDM patients in the Helsinki Heart Study. *Diab. Care* 15:820–25

140. Downs JR, Clearfield M, Weis S, et al. 1998. Primary prevention of acute coronary events with lovastatin in men and women with average cholesterol levels: results of AFCAPS/ TexCAPS. Air Force/Texas Coronary Atherosclerosis Prevention Study. *JAMA* 279(20):1615–22

141. Goldberg RB, Mellies MJ, Sacks FM, et al. 1998. Cardiovascular events and their reduction with pravastatin in diabetic and glucose-intolerant myocardial infarction survivors with average cholesterol levels. Subgroup analyses in the cholesterol and recurrent events (CARE) trial. *Circulation* 98:2513–19

142. Pyorala K, Pedersen TR, Kjekshus J, et al. 1997. Cholesterol lowering with simvastatin improves prognosis of diabetic patients with coronary heart disease. A subgroup analysis of the Scandinavian Simvastatin Survival Study (4S). *Diab. Care* 20:614–20

143. Diabetes Atherosclerosis Intervention Study Investigators. 2001. Effect of fenofibrate on progression of coronary-artery disease in type 2 diabetes: The Diabetes Atherosclerosis Intervention Study, a randomised study. *Lancet* 357:905–10

144. Expert Panel on Detection, Evaluation, and Treatment of High Blood Cholesterol in Adults. 2001. Executive summary of the Third Report of the National Cholesterol Program (NCEP) Expert Panel on Detection, Evaluation, and Treatment of High Blood Cholesterol in Adults (Adult Treatment Panel III). *JAMA* 285:2486–97

145. Post Coronary Artery Bypass Graft Trial Investigators. 1997. The effect of aggressive lowering of low-density lipoprotein cholesterol levels and low-dose anticoagulation on obstructive changes in saphenous-vein coronary-artery bypass grafts. *N. Engl. J. Med.* 336:153–62

146. Pitt B, Waters D, Brown WV, et al. 1999. Aggressive lipid-lowering therapy compared with angioplasty in stable coronary artery disease. Atorvastatin versus Revascularization Treatment Investigators. *N. Engl. J. Med.* 341:70–76

147. Haffner SM, Lehto S, Ronnemaa T, et al. 1998. Mortality from coronary heart disease in subjects with type 2 diabetes and in nondiabetic subjects with and without prior myocardial infarction. *N. Engl. J. Med.* 339:229–34

148. Hansson L, Zanchetti A, Carruthers SG, et al., for the HOT Study Group. 1998. Effects of intensive blood pressure lowering and low-dose aspirin in patients with hypertension: principal results of the Hypertension Optimal Treatment (HOT) randomized trial. *Lancet* 351:1755–62

149. Sive PH, Medalie JH, Kahn HA, et al. 1971. Distribution and multiple regression analysis of blood pressure in 10,000 Israeli men. *Am. J. Epidemiol.* 93:317–27

150. UK Prospective Diabetes Study (UKPDS) Group. 1998. Intensive blood-glucose control with sulphonylureas or insulin compared with conventional treatment and risk of complications in patients with type 2 diabetes (UKPDS 33). *Lancet* 352:837–52

151. Heart Outcomes Prevention Evaluation (HOPE) Study Investigators. 2000. Effects of ramipril on cardiovascular and microvascular outcomes in people with diabetes mellitus: results of the HOPE study and Micro-HOPE substudy. *Lancet* 355:253–59

152. Estacio RO, Jeffers BW, Hiatt WR, et al. 1998. The effect of nisoldipine as compared with analapril on cardiovascular outcomes in patients with non–insulin dependent diabetes and hypertension. *N. Engl. J. Med.* 338:645–52

153. Hansson L, Lindholm LH, Niskanen L, et al. 1999. Effect of angiotensin-converting enzyme inhibition compared with conventional therapy on cardiovascular

morbidity and mortality in hypertension: The Captopril Prevention Project (CAPP) randomized trial. *Lancet* 353:611–15

154. Tatti P, Pahor M, Byington RP, et al. 1998. Outcome results of the Fosinopril versus Amlodipine Cardiovascular Events Trial (FACET) in patients with hypertension and NIDDM. *Diab. Care* 21:597–603

155. Adler A, Statton I, McElroh H, et al. Risk of macrovascular and microvascular complications of diabetes at different levels of blood pressure—observations from the UKPDS. 59th Annu. Sci. Sess. of ADA Abstr. 0064

156. Viberti GC, Mogensen CE, Groop LC, Pauls JF, for the European Microalbuminuria Captopril Study Group. 1994. Effect of captopril on progression to clinical proteinuria in patients with insulin-dependent diabetes mellitus and microalbuminuria. *JAMA* 271:275–79

157. Ravid M, Savin H, Jutrin I, et al. 1993. Long-term stabilizing effect of angiotensin-converting enzyme inhibition on plasma creatinine and on proteinuria in normotensive type II diabetic patients. *Ann. Intern. Med.* 118:577–81

158. Ravid M, Lang R, Rachmani R, Lishner M. 1996. Long-term renoprotective effect of angiotensin-converting enzyme inhibition in non–insulin-dependent diabetes mellitus. A 7-year follow-up study. *Arch. Intern. Med.* 156:286–89

159. Jafar TH, Schmid CH, Stark PC, et al. 2000. The optimal level of blood pressure and urine protein excretion for the prevention of progression of chronic renal disease. *J. Am. Soc. Nephrol.* 11:63A (Abstr.)

Annu. Rev. Med. 2002. 53:269–84

IMMUNE RECONSTITUTION IN PATIENTS WITH HIV INFECTION

Gregory D. Sempowski[1] and Barton F. Haynes[1,2]

Departments of [1]Medicine and [2]Immunology, and the Center For AIDS Research and Human Vaccine Institute, Duke University Medical Center, Durham, North Carolina 27710; e-mail: hayne002@mc.duke.edu; gsem@acpub.duke.edu

Key Words   AIDS, thymus, immune reconstitution, thymus atrophy

■ **Abstract**   The peripheral T cell pool is damaged by HIV-1 infection and can be regenerated by production of new T lymphocytes either from the thymus or from proliferation of post-thymic T cells. A critical question for AIDS patients is whether treatment with antiretroviral drugs can restore the capability to produce new T lymphocytes. The development of a new assay of thymus function in adults (the measurement of T cell receptor excision circles, TRECs), and studies of thymus biopsies in untreated and treated HIV-1-infected patients, have suggested that in select patients the thymus can regenerate on antiretroviral therapy. New strategies to overcome the thymic atrophy of aging are needed to improve thymic function in the majority of AIDS patients.

INTRODUCTION

HIV-1 infection results in progressive loss of peripheral CD4$^+$ T cells and leads to immune deficiency and opportunistic infections. With the development of successful treatment regimens to reduce viral load in HIV-1-infected individuals, the current challenge is to develop strategies to optimize regeneration of the peripheral T cell pool in these individuals and reestablish a functional immune system. Recently, there have been advances in understanding human postnatal thymic function throughout aging and new insights into homeostasis of the adult peripheral T cell pool. In addition, several reports have explored the effects of HIV infection and highly active antiretroviral therapy (HAART) on both the thymus and the peripheral T cell pool. Together, these observations have significantly contributed to the prospect of successful immune reconstitution in patients infected with HIV-1. This chapter reviews these recent studies and discusses the current status of thymus transplantation as a possible immune reconstitution strategy for patients infected with HIV-1.

THYMOPOIESIS

Thymus Function During Aging

The human peripheral T cell pool is established early in fetal development by education of bone marrow–derived T cell progenitors in the thymic microenvironment and subsequent emigration of mature thymocytes into peripheral sites (e.g., lymph node and spleen) (1). This process of thymopoiesis is essential for establishing the peripheral T cell pool in early life, and it has recently been shown to continue throughout life, with thymic output occurring well into the fourth and fifth decades (2–4).

Recent data have also demonstrated an age-dependent decline in thymus function in normal adults (2). Whereas children rapidly reconstitute their peripheral CD4 T cell compartment after cytotoxic chemotherapy, regeneration of the T cell pool after chemotherapy in individuals >20 years old is prolonged and occurs primarily by expansion of peripheral post-thymic T cells (5, 6). Thus, the impact of aging on both thymopoiesis and peripheral T cell homeostasis must be considered in a discussion of immune reconstitution in adults.

The 1985, Steinmann et al. were the first to report a study of thymus morphology that demonstrated thymopoiesis began to decrease shortly after birth (7, 8). This was in contrast to the erroneous dogma that thymopoiesis ceased at puberty. In addition, Steinmann et al. identified two components of the human thymus: the true thymic epithelial space, the site of thymopoiesis, and the nonepithelial, nonthymopoietic perivascular space (7–9) (Figure 1, see color insert).

A recent breakthrough for the study of thymopoiesis and naive peripheral T cells in humans was the development of the T cell receptor excision circle (TREC) assay for the study of thymic function in vivo (10). Kong et al. showed in chickens that excised T cell receptor DNA circles were present in recently produced T cells (11). These extrachromosomal DNA circles are the byproduct of T cell receptor (TCR) gene rearrangement, are not replicated, and are therefore diluted by T cell proliferation. Douek et al. developed a real-time polymerase chain reaction (PCR) assay for the quantitation of these signal joint T cell receptor excision circles (sjTRECs) and reported that they localize in naive human T cells and that they decline in peripheral blood CD4 and CD8 T cells throughout life (10, 12). Thus, measurement of sjTRECs has provided an invaluable assay for the assessment of thymic function and the status of T cell immune reconstitution in humans (Figure 2) (10).

Using sjTREC (3) or TCR ligation-mediated PCR (LM-PCR) (4) analysis, Jamieson et al. and Flores et al. demonstrated that the thymopoietic activity per 100,000 thymocytes remains constant until at least age ~50 years. However, work from Steinmann et al. (7, 8), Flores et al. (4), and Sempowski et al. (2) has shown that the thymic epithelial space shrinks to <10% of the total thymus tissue by age 70, and that sjTRECs decline with aging when analyzed per wet weight of thymus tissue. Thus, the perivascular space (adipocytes, peripheral lymphocytes, stroma) expand with age, resulting in a shift in the ratio of true

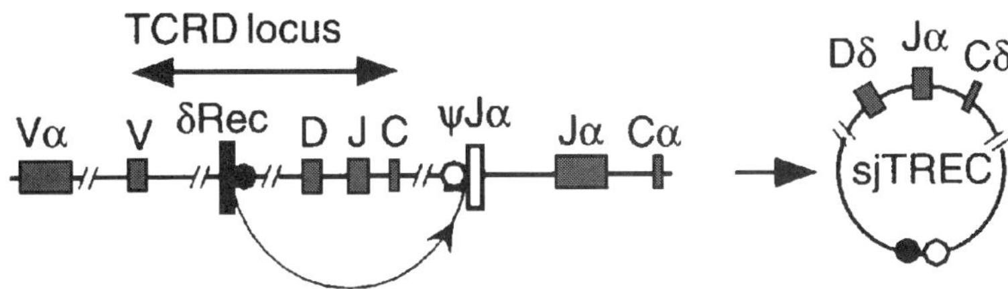

Figure 2   Generation of signal joint (sj) TRECs during *TCRA* rearrangement. The figure shows a simplified representation of the *TCRD* locus flanked by portions of the *TCRA* locus. Rearrangement of the *TCRA* gene forms a single TREC containing a unique sj sequence that is ampified by real-time PCR for quantitation of sjTRECs. Adapted and reprinted with permission from Reference 10.

thymic epithelial space to perivascular space. Overall, the capacity of the thymus to export new T lymphocytes to the periphery begins decreasing at age one year and steadily decreases throughout life, owing to the atrophy of thymopoietic tissue (Figure 1).

Thymus Cytokine Expression During Aging

Several hypotheses have been suggested to explain the progressive atrophy of the thymus during aging. It has been attributed to blocks in TCR rearrangements (13), loss of self-peptides in thymic epithelial major histocompatibility complex (MHC) molecules (14), aging of thymic stroma with loss of trophic cytokines (15–17), and aging of the stem cell populations (18, 19). However, none of these theories has been proven.

Analysis of hematopoietic cytokine expression (mRNA and protein) by thymic epithelial cells or whole thymus tissue has shed new light on possible regulatory mechanisms of thymopoiesis and thymic involution. Thymic epithelial cells produce hematopoietic cytokines, such as G-CSF, GM-CSF, IL-1, IL-3, IL-6, IL-7, M-CSF, oncostatin M (OSM), and leukemia inhibitory factor (LIF) (2, 20–23). Given the pleiotropic effects of cytokines, Sempowski et al. studied steady-state mRNA levels of a large panel of cytokines in normal human thymuses, ranging in age from 3 days to 78 years, and identified changes in cytokine mRNA steady-state levels during aging (2). We identified a group of cytokines whose expression fell (IL-2, IL-9, IL-10, IL-13, IL-14), as well as a group whose expression levels did not change (IL-7, IL-15, G-CSF). We found that mRNA levels of stem cell factor (SCF), M-CSF, and members of the IL-6 family (IL-6, OSM, and LIF) rose during aging and correlated with a concomitant drop in numbers of molecules of sjTREC per milligram of thymus tissue. We then showed that LIF, OSM, IL-6, and M-CSF were produced by adipocytes in addition to thymic epithelial cells (2).

To explore the hypothesis that LIF, OSM IL-6, and SCF and/or M-CSF may actively drive inhibition of thymopoiesis, we administered each of these cytokines to mice and evaluated their thymus 3 days later. LIF, OSM, IL-6, and SCF each induced acute thymic atrophy; LIF and OSM were the most potent followed by IL-6 and then SCF (2).

Two additional cytokines evaluated for thymosuppressive effects are ciliary neurotropic factor (CNTF, another member of the IL-6 cytokine family) and TGF-β (2). Similar to IL-6, LIF, and OSM, intraperitoneal injection of CNTF in Balb/C mice induced acute thymic atrophy (25% reduction in thymus weight compared with saline controls) (A.F. Wells, G.D. Sempowski, M. Alam, B.F. Haynes, manuscript in preparation). Analysis by RNase protection assay of thymus tissue from 10 normal (age 3 days to 78 years) subjects revealed detectable levels of the TGF-β1 isoform, as well as a significant correlation between increasing TGF-β1 mRNA levels in thymus and increasing age ($p < 0.04$) (2).

IL-7 is an important thymic epithelial cell–produced cytokine that drives thymopoiesis in young subjects. One hypothesis for thymic aging is that the thymus ceases to produce IL-7 over time. However, surprisingly, we found that IL-7 mRNA production by the thymic microenvironment was maintained throughout life (2).

Taken together, these data suggest that during aging, overproduction of thymosuppressive cytokines by cells of the expanding thymic perivascular space or by thymic epithelial cells themselves may actively induce thymic atrophy. Thus, it may be important that future therapeutic strategies to augment thymopoiesis and T cell immune reconstitution involve both addition of thymopoietic cytokines and inhibition of thymosuppressive cytokines.

PERIPHERAL T CELL POOL

Peripheral Naive and Memory T Cells

There is emerging evidence in mice that the naive and memory CD8$^+$ T cell pools are independently regulated, with each pool of T cells having its own niche. Both naive and memory CD8$^+$ T cells require MHC class I expression on antigen-presenting cells to survive (25). However, naive T cells survive by not dividing, whereas memory T cells survive by proliferating upon engagement of TCRs with antigen-presenting-cell MHC I and MHC II molecules (25). Data from animal models indicate that the rate of thymic emigrant production is fixed and is not responsive to T cell levels in the periphery (26, 27). If so, the existence of separate niches for naive and memory T cells is critical to ensure the presence of naive T cells for the maximal period of time, particularly if thymic export dwindles (25, 28–30).

Thus, when thymus production of naive T cell emigrants is high, naive T cell turnover in the periphery is high, in order to "make room" for new thymic emigrants. The immune system must also retain its memory pool for T cell immunity to be robust (25, 28). As thymus output gradually dwindles with age, the half-life of naive T cells increases, which assures the organism of a reservoir of naive T cells in the absence of thymic output (25). These notions can explain the persistence of

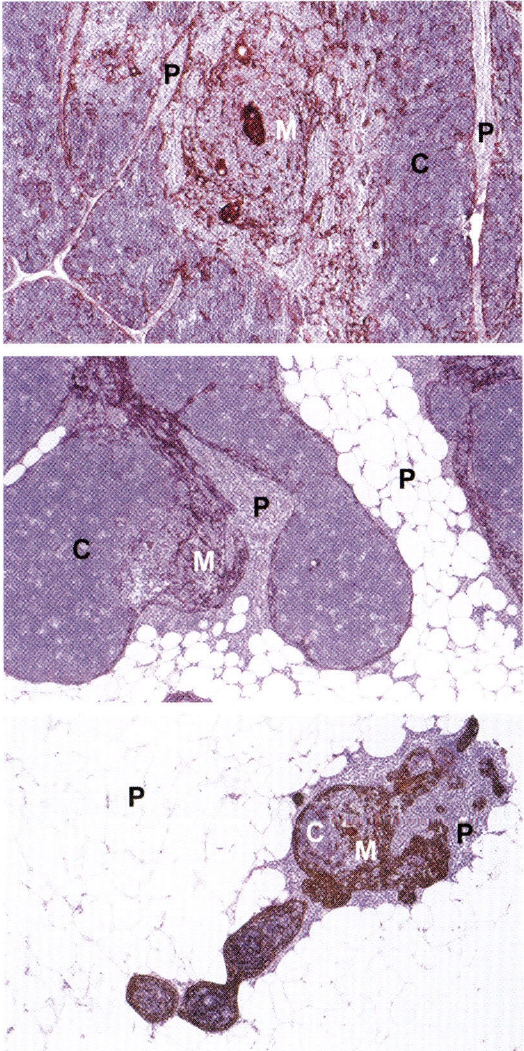

Figure 1 The human thymus during normal aging. All panels are hematoxylin- and eosin-stained sections of human thymus counterstained with an antibody against keratin (*brown areas*). *Top*, thymus of a 2-month-old male with cortex (C) and medulla (M) of the true thymic epithelial space and narrow perivascular spaces (P) indicated. Dark central area is a Hassall's body. *Center,* thymus of a 36-year-old female with well-defined cortex (C) and medulla (M). The perivascular space (P) is enlarged with both lymphoid cells (*blue P areas*) and adipose tissue (*white P areas*). *Bottom,* thymus of a 60-year-old male having very small areas of normal cortex (C) and medulla (M), with perivascular space (P) adipose tissue (*white P area*) predominating and a small amount of lymphoid tissue in the perivascular space around thymic epithelium (*blue P area*). All panels ×10. Reprinted with permission from Reference 9.

peripheral blood T cells with very low but measurable sjTREC levels in humans many years after thymectomy (10). These findings may also explain why peripheral memory T cell expansion in the absence of thymopoiesis may be inefficient in filling the peripheral T cell pool. In this scenario, proliferation of peripheral memory T cells would fill the memory T cell niche but not the naive T cell niche.

Peripheral T Cell Pool Regeneration

Throughout adult life, the peripheral T cell pool is maintained by a dynamic interplay between thymopoiesis and post-thymic expansion of peripheral T cells (28, 31) (Figure 3). Thymic function is greatest during fetal and neonatal development. At this time, the peripheral T cell pool is predominately sjTREC$^+$ and the T cells express a naive cell-surface marker (CD45RA$^+$, CD62L$^+$) phenotype (10). In contrast, thymic atrophy is profound at the end of life, resulting in decreased thymic output (32). Therefore, the level of peripheral T cells in elderly individuals is maintained primarily by proliferation of the post-thymic peripheral T cells (Figure 1). In aged individuals, the frequency of naive peripheral blood T cells is substantially reduced; sjTREC levels are also significantly lower in peripheral T cell subsets, due to peripheral T cell expansion and decreased thymopoiesis (10).

Thus, a working hypothesis is that thymopoiesis contributes more to the peripheral T cell pool in normal subjects at younger ages, and proliferation of post-thymic peripheral T cells contributes more at older ages (Figure 3). The relative contributions of the thymus and proliferating T cell pool at any given time depend on a variety of factors, including the size of the thymopoietic thymic epithelial space of the thymus (32), the degree of peripheral T cell recirculation back to the perivascular space of the thymus to provide feedback on the size of the peripheral T cell pool (33), and the size of the peripheral T cell pool itself (28).

A fundamental question regarding any setting of T cell immune reconstitution is whether the restoration of T cell function at any given time is via the thymus or via peripheral expansion. Immune reconstitution via the thymus generates sjTREC$^+$ naive T cells. The T cell repertoire generated from thymopoiesis is polyclonal and thus is capable of mediating T cell responses to neoantigens. In contrast, immune

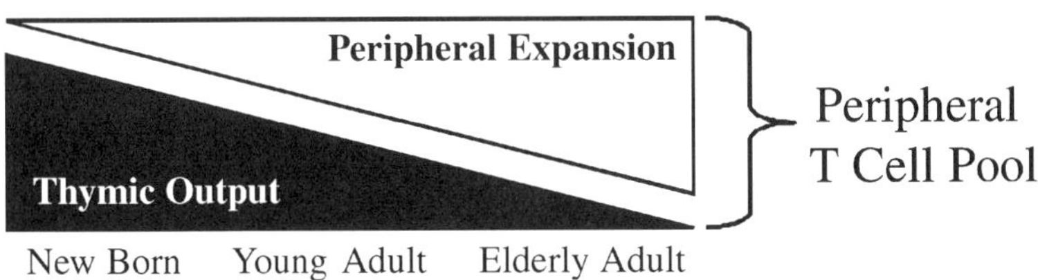

Figure 3 Composition of peripheral T cell pool. Schematic representation of the relative contributions of thymopoiesis versus proliferation of post-thymic T cells for maintainence of the peripheral T cell pool. Adapted and reprinted with permission from Reference 31.

reconstitution via peripheral expansion of existing T cells may limit the T cell repertoire to preexisting memory T cells, with reduced capacity to respond to new antigens (6, 34, 35). In general, thymopoiesis is more efficient in restoring peripheral T cell levels than is peripheral expansion of T cells. Mackall and Gress have demonstrated that in the presence of a functioning thymus, peripheral T cell expansion may be suppressed; this suppression is reversed by eliminating thymic-derived progeny (5, 36). In the absence of active thymopoiesis, peripheral expansion of T cells is enhanced (5, 36), although peripheral expansion may not fully restore peripheral T cell levels or function (5, 6, 34–36).

The phenotype of peripheral blood T cells can be helpful in evaluating the mode of T cell reconstitution. T cell reconstitution via thymopoiesis is associated with the presence of CD45RA$^+$ and CD62L$^+$ T cells and high sjTREC levels, whereas T cell regeneration via peripheral expansion is associated with CD45RO$^+$ T cells and low sjTREC levels (5, 6, 12, 34–36). Thus, the status of thymic output and the peripheral T cell pool significantly influence the degree and mechanism of immune reconstitution in adults.

HIV INFECTION AND CENTRAL AND PERIPHERAL T CELL PRODUCTION

Effect of HIV Infection on the Thymus

HIV-1 RNA-expressing cells are found both in the thymic perivascular space and within the true thymic epithelial space during early and late HIV-1 infection (37). To more fully understand the impact of HIV-1 infection on thymus tissue, it is important to compare the thymus in early and late stages of HIV-1 infection with age-matched control subjects (32, 37). Early HIV-1 infection of the thymus is associated with increased lymphoid infiltrate of the thymic perivascular space, relative to normal thymus tissue, and with the presence of germinal centers in the thymic perivascular space (32, 37–39). These changes are very similar to those seen in the hyperplastic thymus associated with the autoimmune disease myasthenia gravis (40). High endothelial venules, characterized by MECA-1$^+$ immunostaining, are found in peripheral lymph nodes and are induced in the thymic perivascular space of both HIV-1-infected and myasthenia gravis thymus tissues (32, 40). In late HIV-1 infection, the changes in the thymus resemble, but are more exaggerated than, the atrophy associated with normal aging (32, 37, 41). Thymus tissue from a 30-year-old subject with late-stage AIDS can resemble the normally atrophic thymus of a 60-year-old uninfected subject (Figure 4) (32). In addition to thymic atrophy, the HIV-1-infected thymus tissue has islands of thymic epithelium devoid of lymphocytes that are surrounded by a dense lymphoid infiltrate of CD8$^+$ cytotoxic T lymphocytes (CTLs), monocytes, and B cells (32, 37, 38). CD8$^+$ T cells that are present in the perivascular space of the HIV-1-infected thymus express the CTL and natural killer cell (NK) granule antigen TIA-1, suggesting mature "killer" effector cell function. This is similar to the CTL infiltrate seen in

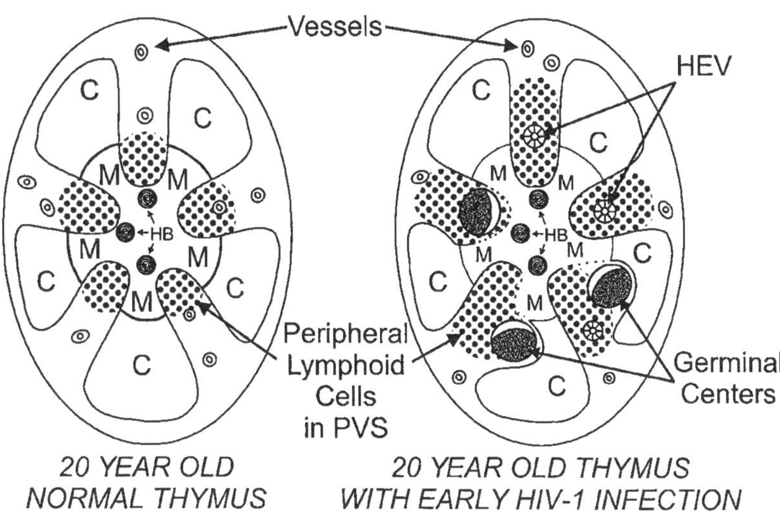

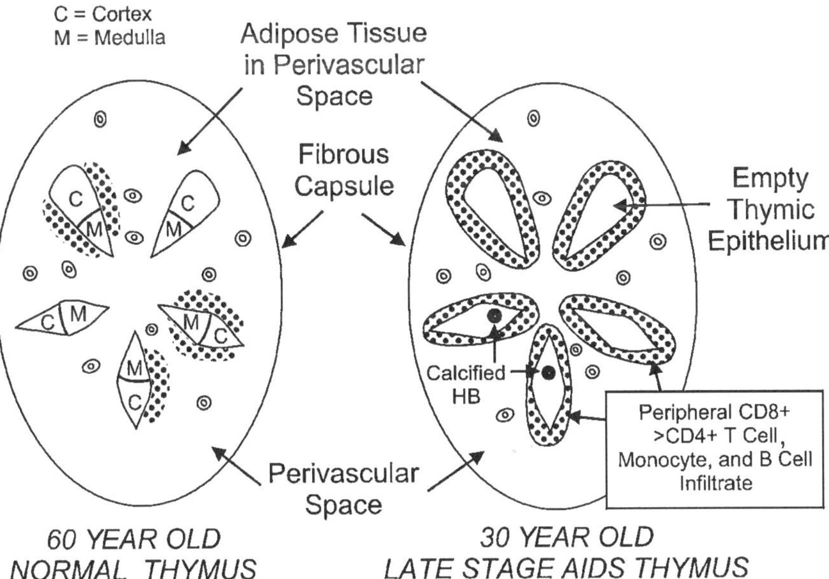

Figure 4 Schematic representations of the morphology of the human thymus in (*top*) early and (*bottom*) late stages of HIV-1 infection. Adapted and reprinted with permission from Reference 32.

HIV-1$^+$ peripheral lymph nodes (37). However, it is important to note that even patients with profound lymphopenia in late-stage AIDS may retain small islands of thymus with active thymopoiesis (37).

Douek et al. reported a decrease of sjTREC levels in the peripheral T cells of untreated HIV-1-infected patients, which suggests a suppressive effect of HIV viremia on sjTREC$^+$ T cell production in the thymus (10). HIV-1 may directly kill thymocytes (42–44), may kill thymic dendritic cells required for normal thymocyte development (45), may damage thymic epithelial cells required for normal thymopoiesis (42), or may inhibit thymocyte signaling.

Experimental models using simian immunodeficiency virus (SIV) have provided hints into thymus function during HIV-1 infection (46). An early stage of suppressed thymopoiesis, evidenced by a decrease in thymocyte numbers due to increased thymocyte apoptosis, decreases peripheral CD4$^+$ T cell levels. Approximately two months after infection, a rebound in thymic function occurs with increased thymocyte production, which is independent of viral load in SIV-infected monkeys. Since thymic rebound preceded any evidence of peripheral lymphopenia, it may be a response to thymic injury rather than to feedback signals from the peripheral T cell pool (46).

In contrast, others (47–50) have reported that lymphopenia in bone marrow transplantation or AIDS is associated with high IL-7 levels, which suggests a possible feedback loop between T cell lymphopenia and IL-7 production. Since IL-7 stimulates both thymopoiesis and peripheral T cell proliferation, elevated IL-7 may act either on peripheral T cells or on the thymus.

With respect to HIV-1 infection, thymic size has been documented using computerized tomogram (CT) scans in 20–40-year-old HIV-1-infected patients (51, 52). McCune and colleagues observed abundant thymus tissue in 50% of HIV-1-infected subjects studied, and the size of thymus shadow on CT correlated with rises in naive (CD4$^+$, CD45RA$^+$) peripheral T cell levels. To directly address the issue of thymic contribution to rises in peripheral T cell levels, Douek et al. used sjTREC analysis to show that HAART induced increases in peripheral CD4$^+$ T cell counts and sjTREC levels in younger HIV-1-infected patients (10), although some of the early rises in CD4$^+$ T cells were probably due to redistribution of CD4$^+$ T cells into the peripheral blood after treatment.

The use of HAART in HIV-1-infected patients has led to suppression of plasma HIV RNA, improvement in peripheral blood CD4$^+$ T cell counts, and in some cases thymic enlargement (51–54). Increased thymus size on HAART has been hypothesized to result from increased thymopoiesis. However, it could also result from infiltration of peripheral lymphocytes into the thymic perivascular space, particularly in untreated HIV patients (37). This distinction is important for HIV-1-infected patients. If the increase in thymic size indicates thymopoiesis, one might conclude that the accompanying increase in CD4$^+$ T cells represents an improvement in T cell receptor repertoire and the ability to respond to neoantigens. However, if the increase in thymus size represents the migration of peripheral lymphocytes to the thymic perivascular space, with resulting thymus "inflammation" and suppression of thymopoiesis, then any accompanying increase in peripheral

CD4$^+$ T cells probably represents proliferation of existing peripheral naive and memory T cells without new expansion of the T cell receptor repertoire.

Markert et al. have directly addressed this question by studying the thymus and peripheral blood T cells of two HIV-seropositive patients with CD4$^+$ T lymphopenia who were treated with HAART, had control of plasma viral RNA, and then developed thymic enlargement (55). With HAART, peripheral blood CD4$^+$ T cell counts increased from $\sim$60/mm^3 to 552/mm^3 and 750/mm^3 for patients 1 and 2, respectively. Thymic biopsies from both patients showed normal thymus histology with active thymopoiesis. Percentages of peripheral blood naive CD4$^+$ T cells and sjTREC levels also reflected active thymopoiesis in both patients. In HIV-1-infected adults after HAART, thymic enlargement can represent active thymopoiesis. Renewed thymopoiesis in select treated adult AIDS patients may contribute to immune reconstitution even after prolonged CD4$^+$ T lymphopenia. In contrast, enlarged thymus tissue in untreated AIDS patients may represent thymus inflammation and not thymopoiesis.

In summary, the morphologic changes observed in the thymus during HIV-1 infection include increased perivascular-space infiltrates of CTLs and condensation of thymic epithelium with large areas devoid of thymopoiesis. These changes are either identical to or exaggerated versions of the thymic atrophy seen in older uninfected patients and in myasthenia gravis thymus tissues. Thus, it appears that untreated HIV-1 infection suppresses thymopoiesis, with associated perivascular-space B and T cell infiltrates similar to those seen in lymph nodes. HAART can, in select patients, allow the thymus to "heal," as has been reported for peripheral lymph nodes in HAART-treated patients (56). Therefore, if HIV virus burden can be suppressed or eliminated with effective treatment, thymic function can be restored to some degree in a subset of patients.

Effect of HIV Infection on the Peripheral T Cell Pool

Studies of patients on and off HAART have been extremely useful in understanding the effect of HIV-1 infection and HAART on peripheral T cell dynamics. Two studies investigating the effect of HAART on peripheral T cells have suggested high levels of CD4$^+$ T cell turnover per day with a concomitantly high number of new T cells generated to replace those lost to turnover (57, 58). As Mackall et al. have clearly shown in humans, there are two distinct pathways for the generation of TCR$\alpha\beta$ T cells in humans: thymopoiesis and expansion of peripheral T cells (59). Recent studies demonstrated that the major components of early rises of CD4$^+$ T cells in peripheral blood during HAART are the decrease in the activation state of T cells sequestered in lymphoid tissues and the redistribution of T cells from tissue to the peripheral blood circulation, rather than thymopoiesis (58, 60, 61). This phenomenon was clearly seen in the study of HAART-treated HIV-1-infected patients previously thymectomized for myasthenia gravis (37). In a patient who had been totally thymectomized eight years prior to onset of HAART for HIV-1 infection, the initial rise of CD4$^+$ T cells comprised increases in existing naive T cells as well as memory T cells (37). At the time of naive T cell increases, peripheral sjTREC levels were very low, proving that these naive CD4$^+$ T cell increases resulted from peripheral expansion, redistribution of naive cells, or redistribution of revertants from the memory T cell pool (37). After the initial CD4$^+$ T cell rise over the first three months, this subject's naive T cell levels stabilized, and all subsequent rises in CD4$^+$ T cell count were sjTREC-negative and of the memory T cell phenotype, owing to peripheral T cell expansion (37).

By using a novel deuterium-labeled glucose technique for assessing in vivo cellular turnover in humans, Hellerstein et al. demonstrated that total T cell (CD4 and CD8) half-life in HIV-1 infection is shortened from 82 days in uninfected controls to 23 days in HIV-1-infected patients (62). CTL (CD8$^+$) production in HIV-1-infected patients increased approximately fourfold over uninfected control subjects, whereas CD4$^+$ T cell production was unchanged. Interestingly, the half-life of T cells decreased after 12 weeks of HAART, with increased absolute production rates of CD4$^+$ and CD8$^+$ T cells (62). Together, these and other studies demonstrated that the CD4$^+$ T cell lymphopenia in HIV-1 infection is due to both shortened CD4$^+$ T cell survival time and a failure to increase production of new T cells (63, 64).

It has been estimated that the peripheral T cell pool is reduced by ~50% in lymphopenic patients with AIDS (63). We know from the studies by Mackall and Gress that peripheral expansion of post-thymic T cells neither efficiently reconstitutes the peripheral T cell pool nor regenerates a complete T cell repertoire (34–36, 59). Thus, untreated adult HIV-1-infected patients frequently have oligoclonal T cell repertoires, which with prolonged HAART can become more polyclonal (53, 65). This trend toward a polyclonal repertoire is presumably due to the addition of new T cells (sjTREC$^+$) from the thymus to the peripheral T cell pools.

It has been conclusively demonstrated that the postnatal thymus is functional to some degree in HIV-1-infected adults (9, 37, 55). However, the key question remains, "how much does the thymus contribute to the peripheral T cell pool in HIV-1 infection, both before and after HAART?" Zhang et al. demonstrated normal thymus function in many HIV-1-infected patients, as well as HAART-induced rises in *TCRA* TRECs in a subset of infected patients with low pretreatment TRECs (66). They suggest that in spite of documented thymus function in adults, the quantity of new T cells after HAART is not sufficient to fully explain the post-HAART increase in peripheral T cells (66). Thus, both peripheral T cell expansion and continued thymus production of new T cells are probably critical to reconstitute the peripheral T cell pool in HIV-1 infection (Figure 3).

IMMUNE RECONSTITUTION IN HIV PATIENTS

Effect of HAART

HAART has led to significant decreases in AIDS-associated morbidity and mortality. The growing body of published evidence suggests clinically significant immune recovery in a sizable fraction of HIV-infected patients treated with HAART.

Gea-Banacloche & Lane have comprehensively reviewed the clinical evidence for immune recovery in HIV patients from a number of clinical reports and summarized the outstanding attributes into four categories (66a):

1. Emergence of effective immune responses to infections that were previously refractory to treatment (e.g., oral candidiasis, molluscum, contagiosum, cryptosporidiosi/microsporidiosis, mycobacterium avium complex bacterium) and regression of Kaposi's sarcoma lesions and lymphoma.

2. A fast temporal course of opportunistic infections. Patients feel better within days instead of weeks.

3. Anomalous increased immune responses such as cytomegalovirus-induced uveitis or shingles.

4. Restoration of general immune competence. After CD4 cell count increases there are infrequent opportunistic infections.

Despite these highly promising improvements in immune function, these reports also demonstrated that very few patients regained immune function equivalent to preinfection. For example, some opportunistic infections still occurred during the first 2–3 months after initiation of therapy. Moreover, others have reported partial reconstitution of T cell function in HIV-1-infected patients receiving HAART. In a study of 20 patients with fewer than 250 CD4$^+$ T cells/mm^3 prior to protease inhibitor treatment, half the patients developed proliferative responses to the T cell recall antigens cytomegalovirus (CMV) and tuberculin, and half were nonresponders (67). Other studies reported similar increased CMV and tuberculin T cell proliferative responses in HIV-1-infected patients after treatment with HAART for six months (53, 68). Alternatively, a study of 44 patients during 12 weeks of HAART found no significant increase above baseline in T cell proliferative response to tetanus toxoid and streptokinase (69). These patients have done reasonably well clinically; however, the concern remains that a number of patients on HAART fail to generate a broad proliferative response to T cell recall antigens.

It is interesting to compare aspects of immune reconstitution in thymectomized subjects during HAART (37) with thymectomized patients given bone marrow transplants (BMT) (70). After HAART, peripheral blood naive CD4$^+$ T cells were present in the thymectomized HIV-1-infected patient, whereas after BMT, naive peripheral blood T cells were absent in the thymectomized recipient. It is important to note that the thymectomized patient received preconditioning irradiation prior to BMT, and after BMT received cyclosporine A. Thus, any existing CD4$^+$ naive T cells were probably reduced prior to transplant, leaving no naive peripheral CD4$^+$ T cells to expand after BMT. In contrast, the HAART-treated thymectomized patient had no irradiation preconditioning, and the naive CD4$^+$ T cells that increased after HAART were negative for sjTRECs and therefore were the result of post-thymic peripheral T cell expansion. Thus, the early rise of naive T cells in the peripheral blood following HAART can be attributed to redistribution of T cells from tissues to peripheral blood.

Thymus Transplantation

One possible reason that complete immune reconstitution (response to recall and neoantigens) does not occur in some HIV-1-infected patients on HAART is that age and viral injury of the thymus have severely compromised the ability of the thymic microenvironment to produce new T cells. In an attempt to remedy this problem, thymic transplantation has been attempted in untreated HIV-1-infected patients (71–73). Unfortunately, in these trials, thymic grafts were rejected and/or infected with HIV-1. Markert et al. have been successful in restoring normal immune function to infants with complete DiGeorge syndrome by transplanting allogeneic cultured postnatal thymus tissue (74). T cell proliferative responses to mitogens developed in four out of five patients. Biopsies of thymus transplants showed active thymopoiesis that correlated with rises in naive peripheral T cells and increases in peripheral blood sjTREC levels, and there was no evidence of graft-versus-host disease (74).

Markert et al. recently investigated whether this method of thymus transplantation in conjunction with HAART would augment T cell immune reconstitution in HIV-1-infected patients (75). Six treatment-naive HIV-1-infected patients with $CD4^+$ T cell counts of 200–500 mm^3 were treated with HAART and four of the six received HLA-unmatched cultured thymus tissue without immunosuppression. In each case, the thymus graft was rejected by host $CD8^+$ T cells (75).

CONCLUSION

To date, the best hope of improving immune reconstitution in HIV infection is combining new and less toxic forms of HAART with strategies to reverse the thymic atrophy of aging and increase thymopoiesis in the HIV-1-infected adult. Evidence that some patients with AIDS can augment thymopoiesis on HAART provides hope that ultimately new thymopoietic regimens may increase thymic output, so that patients can live with HIV infection without clinical immunodeficiency.

ACKNOWLEDGMENTS

The authors acknowledge M. Louise Markert, John Bartlett, Nathan Thielman, Dhaval Patel, Laura Hale, and Africa Alvarez-McLeod for collaborations, and our patients for allowing us to study them.

Visit the Annual Reviews home page at www.AnnualReviews.org

LITERATURE CITED

1. Haynes BF, Denning SM, Le PT, Singer KH. 1990. Human intrathymic T cell differentiation. *Semin. Immunol.* 2:67–77

2. Sempowski GD, Hale LP, Sundy JS, et al. 2000. Leukemia inhibitory factor, oncostatin M, IL-6, and stem cell factor

mRNA expression in human thymus increases with age and is associated with thymic atrophy. *J. Immunol.* 164:2180–87

3. Jamieson BD, Douek DC, Killian S, et al. 1999. Generation of functional thymocytes in the human adult. *Immunity* 10:569–75

4. Flores KG, Li J, Sempowski GD, et al. 1999. Analysis of the human thymic perivascular space during aging. *J. Clin. Invest.* 104:1031–39

5. Mackall CL, Fleisher TA, Brown MR, et al. 1995. Age, thymopoiesis, and CD4+ T-lymphocyte regeneration after intensive chemotherapy. *N. Engl. J. Med.* 332:143–49

6. Mackall CL, Hakim FT, Gress RE. 1997. T-cell regeneration: all repertoires are not created equal. *Immunol. Today* 18:245–51

7. Steinmann GG. 1986. Changes in the human thymus during aging. *Curr. Topics Pathol.* 75:43–88

8. Steinmann GG, Klaus B, Muller-Hermelink HK. 1985. The involution of the ageing human thymic epithelium is independent of puberty. A morphometric study. *Scand. J. Immunol.* 22:563–75

9. Haynes BF, Markert ML, Sempowski GD, et al. 2000. The role of the thymus in immune reconstitution in aging, bone marrow transplantation, and HIV-1 infection. *Annu. Rev. Immunol.* 18:529–60

10. Douek DC, McFarland RD, Keiser PH, et al. 1998. Changes in thymic function with age and during the treatment of HIV infection. *Nature* 396:690–95

11. Kong F, Chen CH, Cooper MD. 1998. Thymic function can be accurately monitored by the level of recent T cell emigrants in the circulation. *Immunity* 8:97–104

12. Douek DC, Vescio RA, Betts MR, et al. 2000. Assessment of thymic output in adults after haematopoietic stem-cell transplantation and prediction of T-cell reconstitution. *Lancet* 355:1875–81

13. Aspinall R. 1997. Age-associated thymic atrophy in the mouse is due to a deficiency affecting rearrangement of the TCR during intrathymic T cell development. *J. Immunol.* 158:3037–45

14. Hartwig M, Steinmann G. 1994. On a causal mechanism of chronic thymic involution in man. *Mech. Ageing Dev.* 75:151–56

15. Hirokawa K, Sato K, Makinodan T. 1982. Influence of age of thymic grafts on the differentiation of T cells in nude mice. *Clin. Immunol. Immunopathol.* 24:251–62

16. Leiner H, Greinert U, Scheiwe W, et al. 1984. Repopulation of lymph nodes and spleen in thymus chimeras after lethal irradiation and bone marrow transplantation: dependence on the age of the thymus. *Immunobiology* 167:345–58

17. Utsuyama M, Kasai M, Kurashima C, Hirokawa K. 1991. Age influence on the thymic capacity to promote differentiation of T cells: induction of different composition of T cell subsets by aging thymus. *Mech. Ageing Dev.* 58:267–77

18. Tyan ML. 1977. Age-related decrease in mouse T cell progenitors. *J. Immunol.* 118:846–51

19. Kadish JL, Basch RS. 1976. Hematopoietic thymocyte precursors. I. Assay and kinetics of the appearance of progeny. *J. Exp. Med.* 143:1082–99

20. Le PT, Lazorick S, Whichard LP, et al. 1990. Human thymic epithelial cells produce IL-6, granulocyte-monocyte-CSF, and leukemia inhibitory factor. *J. Immunol.* 145:3310–15

21. Le PT, Tuck DT, Dinarello CA, et al. 1987. Human thymic epithelial cells produce interleukin 1. *J. Immunol.* 138:2520–26

22. Le PT, Kurtzberg J, Brandt SJ, et al. 1988. Human thymic epithelial cells produce granulocyte and macrophage colony-stimulating factors. *J. Immunol.* 141:1211–17

23. Galy AH, de Waal Malefyt R, Barcena A, et al. 1993. Untransfected and SV40-transfected fetal and postnatal human thymic stromal cells. Analysis of phenotype,

cytokine gene expression and cytokine production. *Thymus* 22:13–33

24. Deleted in proof

25. Tanchot C, Fernandes HV, Rocha B. 2000. The organization of mature T-cell pools. *Phil. Trans. R. Soc. London Ser. B* 355:323–28

26. Gabor MJ, Scollay R, Godfrey DI. 1997. Thymic T cell export is not influenced by the peripheral T cell pool. *Eur. J. Immunol.* 27:2986–93

27. Ramanathan S, Norwich K, Poussier P. 1998. Antigen activation rescues recent thymic emigrants from programmed cell death in the BB rat. *J. Immunol.* 160:5757–64

28. Tanchot C, Rocha B. 1995. The peripheral T cell repertoire: independent homeostatic regulation of virgin and activated $CD8^+$ T cell pools. *Eur. J. Immunol.* 25: 2127–36

29. DeKoning J, DiMolfetto L, Reilly C, et al. 1997. Thymic cortical epithelium is sufficient for the development of mature T cells in relB-deficient mice. *J. Immunol.* 158:2558–66

30. Laufer TM, DeKoning J, Markowitz JS, et al. 1996. Unopposed positive selection and autoreactivity in mice expressing class II MHC only on thymic cortex. *Nature* 383:81–85

31. Haynes BF. 1999. HIV infection and the dynamic interplay between the thymus and the peripheral T cell pool. *Clin. Immunol.* 92:3–5

32. Haynes BF, Hale LP. 1998. The human thymus. A chimeric organ comprised of central and peripheral lymphoid components. *Immunol. Res.* 18:175–92

33. Mehr R, Perelson AS, Fridkis-Hareli M, Globerson A. 1996. Feedback regulation of T cell development: manifestations in aging. *Mech. Ageing Dev.* 91:195–210

34. Mackall CL, Fleisher TA, Brown MR, et al. 1997. Distinctions between CD8+ and CD4+ T-cell regenerative pathways result in prolonged T-cell subset imbalance after intensive chemotherapy. *Blood* 89:3700–7

35. Mackall CL, Bare CV, Granger LA, et al. 1996. Thymic-independent T cell regeneration occurs via antigen-driven expansion of peripheral T cells resulting in a repertoire that is limited in diversity and prone to skewing. *J. Immunol.* 156:4609–16

36. Mackall CL, Granger L, Sheard MA, et al. 1993. T-cell regeneration after bone marrow transplantation: differential CD45 isoform expression on thymic-derived versus thymic-independent progeny. *Blood* 82:2585–94

37. Haynes BF, Hale LP, Weinhold KJ, et al. 1999. Analysis of the adult thymus in reconstitution of T lymphocytes in HIV-1 infection. *J. Clin. Invest.* 103:453–60

38. Burke AP, Anderson D, Benson W, et al. 1995. Localization of human immunodeficiency virus 1 RNA in thymic tissues from asymptomatic drug addicts. *Arch. Pathol. Lab. Med.* 119:36–41

39. Prevot S, Audouin J, Andre-Bougaran J, et al. 1992. Thymic pseudotumorous enlargement due to follicular hyperplasia in a human immunodeficiency virus seropositive patient. Immunohistochemical and molecular biological study of viral infected cells. *Am. J. Clin. Pathol.* 97: 420–25

40. Bofill M, Janossy G, Willcox N, et al. 1985. Microenvironments in the normal thymus and the thymus in myasthenia gravis. *Am. J. Pathol.* 119:462–73

41. Schuurman HJ, Krone WJ, Broekhuizen R, et al. 1989. The thymus in acquired immune deficiency syndrome. Comparison with other types of immunodeficiency diseases, and presence of components of human immunodeficiency virus type 1 *Am. J. Pathol.* 134:1329–38

42. Stanley SK, McCune JM, Kaneshima H, et al. 1993. Human immunodeficiency virus infection of the human thymus and disruption of the thymic microenvironment

in the SCID-hu mouse. *J. Exp. Med.* 178: 1151–63

43. Bonyhadi ML, Rabin L, Salimi S, et al. 1993. HIV induces thymus depletion in vivo. *Nature* 363:728–32

44. Kourtis AP, Ibegbu C, Nahmias AJ, et al. 1996. Early progression of disease in HIV-infected infants with thymus dysfunction. *N. Engl. J. Med.* 335:1431–36; erratum 336:595

45. Valentin H, Nugeyre MT, Vuillier F, et al. 1994. Two subpopulations of human triple-negative thymic cells are susceptible to infection by human immunodeficiency virus type 1 in vitro. *J. Virol.* 68:3041–50

46. Wykrzykowska JJ, Rosenzweig M, Veazey RS, et al. 1998. Early regeneration of thymic progenitors in rhesus macaques infected with simian immunodeficiency virus. *J. Exp. Med.* 187:1767–78

47. Bolotin E, Annett G, Parkman R, Weinberg K. 1999. Serum levels of IL-7 in bone marrow transplant recipients: relationship to clinical characteristics and lymphocyte count. *Bone Marrow Transplant.* 23:783–88

48. Fry TJ, Christensen BL, Komschlies KL, et al. 2001. Interleukin-7 restores immunity in athymic T-cell-depleted hosts. *Blood* 97:1525–33

49. Fry TJ, Connick E, Falloon J, et al. 2001. A potential role for interleukin-7 in T-cell homeostasis. *Blood* 97:2983–90

50. Napolitano LA, Grant RM, Deeks SG, et al. 2001. Increased production of IL-7 accompanies HIV-1-mediated T-cell depletion: implications for T-cell homeostasis. *Nat. Med.* 7:73–79

51. McCune MM, Loftus R, Schmidt DK, et al. 1998. High prevalence of thymic tissue in adults with human immunodefiency virus-1 injection. *J. Clin. Invest.* 101:2301–8

52. Smith KY, Valdez H, Landay A, et al. 2000. Thymic size and lymphocyte restoration in patients with human immunodeficiency virus infection after 48 weeks of zidovudine, lamivudine, and ritonavir therapy. *J. Infect. Dis.* 181:41–47

53. Autran B, Carcelain G, Li TS, et al. 1997. Positive effects of combined antiretroviral therapy on CD4+ T cell homeostasis and function in advanced HIV disease. *Science* 277:112–16

54. Connors M, Kovacs JA, Krevat S, et al. 1997. HIV infection induces changes in CD4+ T-cell phenotype and depletions within the CD4+ T-cell repertoire that are not immediately restored by antiviral or immune-based therapies. *Nat. Med.* 3:533–40

55. Markert ML, Alvarez-McLeod AP, Sempowski G, et al. 2001. Thymopoiesis in HIV-infected adults after highly active antiretroviral therapy. *AIDS Res. Hum. Retroviruses.* In press

56. Zhang ZQ, Notermans DW, Sedgewick G, et al. 1998. Kinetics of CD4+ T cell repopulation of lymphoid tissues after treatment of HIV-1 infection. *Proc. Natl. Acad. Sci. USA* 95:1154–59

57. Wei X, Ghosh SK, Taylor ME, et al. 1995. Viral dynamics in human immunodeficiency virus type 1 infection. *Nature* 373:117–22

58. Pakker NG, Notermans DW, de Boer RJ, et al. 1998. Biphasic kinetics of peripheral blood T cells after triple combination therapy in HIV-1 infection: a composite of redistribution and proliferation. *Nat. Med.* 4:208–14

59. Mackall CL, Hakim FT, Gress RE. 1997. Restoration of T-cell homeostasis after T-cell depletion. *Semin. Immunol.* 9:339–46

60. Bucy RP, Hockett RD, Derdeyn CA, et al. 1999. Initial increase in blood CD4$^+$ lymphocytes after HIV antiretroviral therapy reflects redistribution from lymphoid tissues. *J. Clin. Invest.* 103:1391–98

61. Wolthers KC, Bea G, Wisman A, et al. 1996. T cell telomere length in HIV-1 infection: no evidence for increased CD4+ T cell turnover. *Science* 274:1543–47

62. Hellerstein M, Hanley MB, Cesar D, et al.

1999. Directly measured kinetics of circulating T lymphocytes in normal and HIV-1-infected humans. *Nat. Med.* 5:83–89

63. Haase AT. 1999. Population biology of HIV-1 infection: viral and CD4+ T cell demographics and dynamics in lymphatic tissues. *Annu. Rev. Immunol.* 17:625–56

64. Rowland-Jones S. 1999. HIV infection: Where have all the T cells gone? *Lancet* 354:5–7

65. Gorochov G, Neumann AU, Kereveur A, et al. 1998. Perturbation of CD4+ and CD8+ T-cell repertoires during progression to AIDS and regulation of the CD4+ repertoire during antiviral therapy. *Nat. Med.* 4:215–21

66. Zhang L, Lewin SR, Markowitz M, et al. 1999. Measuring recent thymic emigrants in blood of normal and HIV-1-infected individuals before and after effective therapy. *J. Exp. Med.* 190:725–32

66a. Gea-Banacloche JC, Lane HC. 1999. Immune reconstitution in HIV infection. *AIDS* 13(Suppl. A):S25–S38

67. Li TS, Tubiana R, Katlama C, et al. 1998. Long-lasting recovery in CD4 T-cell function and viral-load reduction after highly active antiretroviral therapy in advanced HIV-1 disease. *Lancet* 351:1682–86

68. Kelleher AD, Carr A, Zaunders J, Cooper DA. 1996. Alterations in the immune response of human immunodeficiency virus (HIV)-infected subjects treated with an HIV-specific protease inhibitor, ritonavir. *J. Infect. Dis.* 173:321–29

69. Lederman MM, Connick E, Landay A, et al. 1998. Immunologic responses associated with 12 weeks of combination antiretroviral therapy consisting of zidovudine, lamivudine, and ritonavir: results of AIDS Clinical Trials Group Protocol 315. *J. Infect. Dis.* 178:70–79

70. Heitger A, Neu N, Kern H, et al. 1997. Essential role of the thymus to reconstitute naive (CD45RA+) T-helper cells after human allogeneic bone marrow transplantation. *Blood* 90:850–57

71. Dwyer JM, Wood CC, McNamara J, Kinder B. 1987. Transplantation of thymic tissue into patients with AIDS. An attempt to reconstitute the immune system. *Arch. Intern. Med.* 147:513–17

72. Dupuy JM, Gilmore N, Goldman H, et al. 1991. Thymic epithelial cell transplantation in patients with acquired immunodeficiency syndrome. Evidence for infection by HIV-1 of newly differentiated T cells at the site of transplantation. *Thymus* 17:205–18

73. Danner SA, Schuurman HJ, Lange JM, et al. 1986. Implantation of cultured thymic fragments in patients with acquired immunodeficiency syndrome. *Arch. Intern. Med.* 146:1133–36

74. Markert ML, Boeck A, Hale LP, et al. 1999. Transplantation of thymus tissue in complete DiGeorge syndrome. *N. Engl. J. Med.* 341:1180–89

75. Markert ML, Hicks CB, Bartlett JA, et al. 2000. Effect of highly active antiretroviral therapy and thymic transplantation on immunoreconstitution in HIV infection. *AIDS Res. Hum. Retroviruses* 16:403–13

Annu. Rev. Med. 2002. 53:285–302

MULTIPLE SCLEROSIS

B. Mark Keegan and John H. Noseworthy

*Department of Neurology, Mayo Clinic and Mayo Foundation, 200 First Street SW,
Rochester, Minnesota 55905; e-mail: noseworthy.john@mayo.edu*

Key Words   interferon beta, glatiramer acetate, genetics, pathogenesis, pathology

■ **Abstract**   Multiple sclerosis (MS) is a common inflammatory disease of the central nervous system (CNS). Diagnosis rests upon identifying typical clinical symptoms and interpreting supportive laboratory and radiological investigations. The etiology is unknown; however, strong evidence suggests that MS is an autoimmune disease directed against CNS myelin or oligodendrocytes. Genetic factors are important in the development of MS. Contributing environmental determinants (possibly including infectious agents) appear important but remain unidentified. Both cell-mediated and humorally mediated immune mechanisms contribute to pathological injury. Axonal damage occurs in addition to demyelination and may be the cause of later permanent disability. Distinct pathological subtypes may differentiate among patients with MS. Treatment is directed at acute attacks (with corticosteroids) and reduction of attack frequency (primarily with type-1 β interferons and glatiramer acetate). Research into the causes and treatments of MS has expanded our knowledge of this disease and promises improved care for MS patients in the future.

BACKGROUND

Multiple sclerosis (MS) is the most common inflammatory demyelinating disease of the central nervous system (CNS). It affects between 250,000 and 350,000 people in the United States (1). It remains a major cause of disability in both young and older populations (2). Although MS has been studied for centuries (3), its etiologies have remained elusive. Until recently, no definitive therapies aimed at reducing attacks and slowing the disease process were available. Much progress has been made over the past decade in elucidating the causes of MS and directing therapies toward improving patient outcomes (4). This paper reviews the diagnosis of MS, its disease course and prognosis, current studies investigating its genetic basis and suspected pathogenesis, and recent therapeutic trials.

Diagnosis

Multiple sclerosis continues to be diagnosed on a clinical basis, although this is facilitated by supportive laboratory and radiological investigations. The classical

Poser diagnostic criteria (5) have recently been revised by an international panel of MS experts in order to acknowledge the contribution of magnetic resonance imaging (MRI) and to include progressive forms of the disease (5a). A purely clinical diagnosis of MS is made upon the occurrence of two or more distinct attacks *and* objective clinical evidence of two or more lesions in separate locations within the myelinated regions of the CNS (i.e., cerebral white matter, brain stem, cerebellar tracts, optic nerves, spinal cord). A diagnosis of MS is also made if a single clinical attack is accompanied by additional lesions discovered by paraclinical evidence [e.g., MRI abnormalities, cerebrospinal fluid (CSF) changes, abnormal evoked potentials (see below)]. Again, the lesions must be clearly disseminated in time and location within the CNS. Paraclinical criteria become more stringent if the clinical presentation is less definite, as in patients with a single demyelinating event or insidious progressive disease. Besides meeting these criteria, a diagnosis of MS requires that no better explanation can be found for the clinical presentation and paraclinical abnormalities.

Typical of a demyelinating etiology, "attacks" or "relapses" of neurological dysfunction commonly arise subacutely over hours to days, then plateau and improve (sometimes incompletely) over days to weeks, either spontaneously or with corticosteroid treatment. The neurological symptoms reflect the location of the lesion within the CNS; for example, visual loss reflects a lesion of the optic nerve; hemi-, para-, or quadriparesis, with or without bowel/bladder dysfunction, reflects a lesion of the spinal cord; vertigo or diplopia, a lesion of the brain stem; and ataxia, a lesion of the cerebellum. However, many lesions are clinically silent. Other symptoms, such as debilitating fatigue, paresthesias on neck flexion (Lhermitte's symptom), and heat-exacerbated symptomatic worsening (e.g., Uhthoff's symptom), may be present. Occasionally, severe attacks occur with multifocal neurological involvement. Although MS is common, other causes for this symptom complex must be considered. The full differential diagnosis of focal or multifocal CNS disease consistent with MS is broad and is covered comprehensively in other articles (6).

CSF analysis, evoked potentials, and especially MRI of the brain and spinal cord often support a clinical diagnosis of MS. CSF parameters are abnormal in the majority of patients at some time during the disease course and underscore the presumed inflammatory and immune-mediated etiology of MS. Abnormalities may include mildly elevated CSF white blood cell count (typically ≤ 50 lymphocytes), elevated immunoglobulin G within CSF compared to serum (IgG index), and identification of two or more unique oligoclonal bands (OCBs) by CSF protein electrophoresis. Although found in 90%–95% of MS patients later in the disease process, OCBs are not consistently present in MS patients early in the course of the disease. Once present, however, they persist throughout the disease course. OCBs may be present in other conditions [e.g., acute disseminated encephalomyelitis (ADEM), subacute sclerosing panencephalitis, Behçet's disease, systemic lupus erythematosus, and sarcoidosis (7)], and therefore are characteristic of but not entirely specific for MS.

Evoked potentials measure conduction along afferent CNS pathways following stimulation of a sensory receptor. Conduction along visual, somatosensory (upper and lower extremity), and brain-stem auditory pathways may be determined. Abnormal conduction may identify a clinically occult demyelinated lesion fulfilling the criterion of separation of distinct events in time and location within the CNS (8).

MRI of the brain and spinal cord is the most sensitive investigational technique aiding the diagnosis of MS (9). Different MR sequences detect various aspects of the disease process. Typical MR sequences include T1-weighted (T1) with and without gadolinium administration, T2-weighted (T2), proton-density (PD), and fluid-attenuated inversion recovery (FLAIR). T1 images demonstrate CNS anatomy to advantage and identify cerebral, corpus callosal, and spinal cord atrophy that may occur as MS progresses. T1 does not demonstrate most routine demyelinated lesions, but chronic, nonenhancing hypointense areas ("T1 black holes") appear to reflect lesions of more severe tissue damage (10). Acute and actively demyelinating lesions enhance after the administration of intravenous gadolinium, reflecting a breach in the normal blood-brain barrier. T2, PD, and FLAIR sequences demonstrate most demyelinated lesions very well; however, they do not clearly distinguish new, actively demyelinating lesions from older lesions. T2 and PD reveal posterior fossa (i.e., brain stem and cerebellum) lesions better than FLAIR. FLAIR imaging reduces artifact from the CSF signal and is therefore superior in identifying periventricular and juxtacortical lesions.

Specific criteria discriminate MRI lesions both typical of and predictive for the development of MS (11, 12). Although there is heterogeneity in the appearance of demyelinating lesions, typical features on T2, PD, or FLAIR are ovoid shape, size >5 mm, and location in the periventricular, corpus callosal, and posterior fossa white matter. An "open ring" of gadolinium enhancement directed toward the cortex may be a helpful sign in determining a demyelinating etiology of typical and atypical lesions (13, 14). Monophasic illnesses where all lesions enhance simultaneously lend support to a diagnosis of ADEM rather than MS where both enhancing (acute) and nonenhancing (older) lesions are seen. Rarely, demyelinating lesions are large and demonstrate mass effect that simulates a neoplasm (known as tumefactive MS or Marburg variant MS) or have large concentric rings of demyelination (Balo's concentric sclerosis).

Given the availability of partially effective therapy, there is greater interest in making a diagnosis of MS prior to the appearance of the classically required two distinct clinical attacks. MRI is of benefit in identifying risk of progression to clinically definite MS (defined by the occurrence of a second clinical attack) in patients with a single demyelinating episode. Monosymptomatic patients who present with one or no brain MRI lesions are at a low risk (15%–20%) of developing a second clinical attack in the subsequent decade. Patients with two or more cerebral MRI lesions are at high risk (~85%) for a second attack over the same period (15). MS appears to be a more continuously active disease when monitored by MRI, since new lesions appear to occur seven to ten times more frequently than clinical attacks (16). The correlation between T2 lesions and disability in MS, however, is poor. This may relate to concomitant disease in the spinal cord, where small lesions may cause significant disability regardless of the number of brain lesions. Whether the number of T2 lesions is a helpful guideline in deciding when to administer immunomodulatory therapy is unknown.

Cerebral and spinal cord atrophy progressively occurs in MS and is detected by MRI (17, 18). The degree of atrophy in the cerebrum, corpus callosum, and spinal cord, as well as third ventricular size, correlate directly with severity of disability. The exact etiology of this atrophy is uncertain; however, it may be related to progressive axonal loss. Progressive impairment in the absence of clinical relapses or new MRI lesions may also be due to continuing loss of axons not associated with a predominant inflammatory component.

Clinical Course and Prognosis

Current diagnostic categories provide a clinical description of the disease course of MS. Most patients (~85%) initially have a relapsing-remitting form of MS (RRMS), which is characterized by discrete clinical "attacks" or "relapses" followed by subsequent improvement. RRMS is the most typical presentation in younger patients. Many years after onset, a majority of RRMS patients will develop a slow, insidiously progressive, neurological deterioration (usually progressive gait impairment) over many years with or without clinical attacks superimposed. This is termed secondary progressive MS (SPMS). A minority of patients (~15%) have primary progressive MS (PPMS) characterized by a progressive course from onset, an absence of clinically evident relapses, and less conspicuous inflammation on MRI (19). Progressive relapsing MS (PRMS) (20) involves a progressive course from onset with occasional relapses later in the disease. This category may be of less prognostic significance, however, as occasional relapses occurring in the context of a predominantly progressive course do not appear to significantly alter long-term outcome (21, 22).

The prognosis of MS is widely variable. Natural history studies prior to the use of current immunomodulatory treatment showed that, on average, patients achieved an Expanded Disability Status Scale (EDSS) score of 6 (requires unilateral assistance with ambulation) at a median of 15 years following diagnosis (23). At the same time point following diagnosis, ~10%–15% required the use of a wheelchair, but 20%–25% remained unrestricted in their ambulation (EDSS ≤ 3.0, a condition termed "benign MS"). The factors responsible for this observed variation are unclear and it therefore remains difficult to estimate prognosis in individual patients at the time of diagnosis. Clinical indicators of a relatively good prognosis are female gender, younger age of onset, optic neuritis, sensory attacks, complete recovery from attacks, few attacks, and long interattack interval (24). Relatively poor prognostic factors include male gender, predominant cerebellar and motor involvement, incomplete resolution of attacks, progressive course from onset, frequent early attacks, and short interattack interval.

PATHOGENESIS

Epidemiology/Genetics

The precise etiology of MS remains unknown. Populations vary in their susceptibility to MS. A clear gender difference, females being more susceptible than males (~1.6:1), is evident in RRMS but not PPMS. The incidence of MS is greatest at the extremes of latitude in both the northern and southern hemispheres. The cause of this association remains in question (25); a genetic predisposition has been postulated, since these are sites of migration of people of Northern European descent, who have a high prevalence of MS (26). Also, there exist relatively "resistant" populations within areas of otherwise very high prevalence rate [e.g., Maoris in New Zealand (27), Hutterites and Natives in western Canada (28)]. Others believe the latitudinal effect to be caused by an infectious agent (possibly viral) that may be endemic in temperate areas (29).

It is clear that genetic factors play a prominent role in susceptibility to MS. The disease appears to conform to the inheritance pattern of a polygenic disease (30). Confirmation of a genetic predisposition comes primarily from twin and sibling studies. The concordance rate for MS in monozygotic twins is 25%–30%, in contrast to 3%–5% concordance between dizygotic twins and non-twin siblings and a population risk of 0.1%–0.4% (31). Genetically unrelated family members living with an index case are at no higher risk of MS than the background population (32). Independent whole-genome screens, searching for a uniting genetic locus or loci for MS (33, 34), confirmed previous reports demonstrating linkage to the human leukocyte antigen (HLA) DR2 locus. Genetic factors, however, must explain only part of the susceptibility to MS, since monozygotic twins remain 70%–75% discordant for MS despite identical genetic background.

Investigations are ongoing to identify further genetic loci associated with susceptibility to MS and the severity of its disease course, as well as loci associated with atypical presentations of inflammatory demyelinating diseases. A point mutation in a gene coding for the expression of isoforms of CD 45 on immune cells is reportedly associated with a familial type of MS in Germans (35). Specific polymorphisms in the glutathione-S-transferase gene superfamily that appear to regulate response to free radical scavenging have been associated with a more severe disease course (36). Inheritance of the apolipoprotein E ε-4 allele may be associated with a more rapid progression of disability (37). A Japanese demyelinating disease involving exclusively the optic nerves and spinal cord, closely resembling Devic's neuromyelitis optica (38), is linked to HLA loci (DPA1 *0202 and DPB1 *0501) distinct from those associated with typical MS (39). Genetic studies need to be reproduced in differing populations of patients before firm conclusions can be made as to particular genes' contributions to the demyelinating diseases (40).

Infectious Agents

The list of infectious agents reportedly associated with MS, either serologically or pathologically, is extensive (41), but none of the associations are conclusive, and separate laboratories have not always replicated earlier preliminary results. Infectious agents are known to cause demyelinating diseases in animals [e.g., visna, Theiler's murine encephalomyelitis virus (TMEV)], as well as in humans (e.g., JC virus causes progressive multifocal leukoencephalopathy). Exposure to an infectious agent in a genetically susceptible individual or within a critical time in development is proposed to cause MS, with acute attacks possibly relating to reactivation of a latent infection. Genetic determinants of susceptibility and severity of disease are evident in TMEV (42). Exposure to foreign agents that are antigenically similar to normal tissue may lead to autoimmune attack against self-antigens [i.e., molecular mimicry (43)]. Damage to normal tissue may expose novel antigens to the immune system that would otherwise not be contacted and further direct attack against nearby self-antigens (i.e., epitope spreading).

Infectious agents undergoing current investigation as to their relationship to MS include Epstein-Barr virus (EBV), human herpesvirus 6 (HHV-6), and *Chlamydia pneumoniae* (44). EBV is a lymphotropic herpes virus. Prior exposure to EBV as determined by seropositivity for IgG antibodies is reported in close to 100% of MS patients, compared with only 90% IgG and 4% IgM of seropositivity in normal controls (45). Investigators argue that prior exposure to EBV is necessary, although obviously not sufficient, for the development of MS. Reactivation as evidenced by EBV DNA within blood appeared to correspond to acute relapses of MS in one report (45).

HHV-6 is a beta–herpes virus that is both lymphotropic and neurotropic. Some investigators have found HHV-6 DNA directly within actively demyelinating plaques (46). HHV-6 DNA and high levels of IgM antibodies to HHV-6 antigen are found serologically in RRMS (47). Other investigators, however, have not found a similar association between HHV-6 and MS (48).

Chlamydia pneumoniae, a gram-negative intracellular organism, is a common respiratory pathogen. In one study, investigators cultured *C. pneumoniae* from the CSF in 64% of MS patients but only 11% of controls (49). The investigators found evidence of *C. pneumoniae* protein within the CSF by polymerase chain reaction (PCR) assay and elevated immunoglobulins specific for *C. pneumoniae* antigens within the CSF. Again, these results have not invariably been confirmed by other laboratories (50).

It is unclear whether these ubiquitous organisms are pathogenic or are merely revealed because the patients have a damaged CNS and an ongoing autoimmune disease. More studies are needed, ideally with replication in different laboratories using standardized techniques, to identify the organisms and clearly delineate the mechanisms of these agents in the pathogenesis or maintenance of demyelinating disease. Currently, it is probably premature to test individual patients or initiate treatment aimed at eradicating suspected pathogenic organisms outside of an investigational setting

Cell-Mediated Autoimmunity

Autoreactive T lymphocytes appear crucial in the development of demyelinating lesions. Their contribution has been studied extensively with the experimental allergic encephalomyelitis (EAE) animal model of demyelinating disease. EAE is an inflammatory demyelinating disease induced by the subcutaneous administration of myelin peptide antigens [e.g., myelin basic protein (MBP), proteolipid protein] with Freund's adjuvant (51). T cells within the CNS have a predominant role in demyelination and subsequent disability in EAE. Their importance is also demonstrated by the induction of EAE in previously unaffected animals by passive transfer of autoreactive T lymphocytes (52).

Autoreactive T lymphocytes are present in patients with MS (53). T cells within the peripheral circulation are activated by an unknown mechanism. Once activated, these T cells easily cross the blood-brain barrier from the systemic circulation into the CNS aided by upregulation of adhesion molecules [e.g., intercellular adhesion molecule 1 (ICAM-1), vascular-cell adhesion molecule 1 (VCAM-1), E-selectin] on endothelial cells (54). Penetration of the T cells into the brain parenchyma from the circulation is enhanced by increased activity of endogenous matrix metalloproteinases responsible for the breakdown of extracellular matrix material.

Within the CNS, the T cells are specifically activated by binding of the T cell receptor with the class II major histocompatibility complex (MHC) and antigen (trimolecular complex) on the surface of an antigen-presenting cell (astrocyte, microglia, or macrophage) in association with appropriate costimulatory factors. The CD4+ (T4, T helper) T lymphocytes proliferate and secrete either a relatively proinflammatory cytokine repertoire known as Th1 type [secrete tumor necrosis factor (TNF)-α, interferon (INF)-γ, interleukin (IL)-12] or a relatively anti-inflammatory cytokine repertoire known as Th2 type [secrete transforming growth factor (TGF)-β, IL-4, IL-10]. The Th1 cytokines enhance macrophage and microglial activity that may injure either the myelin processes or the oligodendroglial cells. Cytotoxic (CD8+) T cells may directly damage the oligodendrocytes and myelin as well. Final pathways of cell death are unclear but may involve upregulation of apoptosis mediators such as Fas and Fas ligand (55) and TNF receptors.

Humoral and Antibody-Mediated Contribution

Unlike activated T cells, B cells do not appear to cross the blood-brain barrier. Disruption of the blood-brain barrier that occurs in MS however, will allow the entry of B cells, antibodies, and the complement factors into the CNS. Within the CNS,

B cells may be activated by T cells in association with antigen (T-cell-dependent B cell activation). Following activation, they differentiate into antibody-secreting plasma cells. Antibody-mediated effector mechanisms may cause damage by opsonization of an autoimmune target, which aids macrophage-mediated phagocytosis, and by activation of the complement membrane attack complex, which may open pores in myelin membranes (56).

Autoantibodies against several myelin components are present in normal controls and in patients with inflammatory neurological diseases as well as in those with MS (57). The pathological significance of these antibodies is unclear. Antibodies against myelin oligodendrocyte glycoprotein (MOG) may have pathogenic importance. MOG is found exclusively in CNS myelin and, although it is only a minor component of myelin, it has an extracellular domain that is similar to the immunoglobulin superfamily, which may make it susceptible to autoimmune attack. Murine and mammalian (marmoset) EAE is worsened in the presence of MOG antibodies (58). Antibodies to MOG have been demonstrated to occur within human MS lesions (59).

Pathological Heterogeneity

Recent evidence suggests that distinct pathological subtypes may exist in MS (60). These subtypes are characterized by the degree of humoral contribution to the lesion, the suspected target of immune-mediated attack (i.e., oligodendrocyte versus myelin components), and the apparent potential for remyelination. The pathological subtype appears to remain consistent in separate plaques within an individual but appears heterogenous between patients. Lucchinetti and colleagues have described four distinct pathological subtypes based on their large series of biopsy and autopsy specimens (61). Pattern 1 is characterized by predominant T lymphocyte infiltration and macrophage-mediated demyelination. Pattern 2 resembles pattern 1 with T lymphocyte and macrophage infiltration but is distinguished by a prominent humoral component with deposition of complement and IgG. In both patterns 1 and 2, demyelination surrounds small venules, and lesions appear to have high potential for remyelination as evidenced by the presence of thinly remyelinated old lesions ("shadow plaques"). Pattern 3 is characterized by the conservation of a rim of myelin surrounding the small venules, a severe loss of oligodendrocytes by apoptosis, and a selective loss of myelin-associated glycoprotein (MAG) with preservation of other myelin proteins. Pattern 4 demonstrates nonapoptotic oligodendroglial death without selective MAG loss. Both patterns 3 and 4 lack shadow plaques, perhaps indicating poor potential for remyelination. Studies are ongoing to determine if these subtypes have prognostic or therapeutic implications.

Axonal Pathology and Remyelination

Although MS predominantly affects the CNS myelin, attention has refocused on axonal pathology (62). Axonal loss may be the major determinant of long-term (permanent) disability in MS. Confocal microscopic techniques demonstrated transection of axons within early demyelinating lesions (63). Decreased N-acetyl aspartate (NAA) peaks on brain and spinal cord magnetic resonance spectroscopy (MRS) and abnormalities seen on magnetic transfer imaging (MTI) indicate axonal pathology. A reduction in NAA appears an appropriate marker of axonal loss, since the vast majority of NAA lies within neurons (64). MTI demonstrates the capacity of molecules within brain tissue to exchange magnetization with water molecules, and reduction in this capacity reflects damage to myelin or axonal membranes (65). Abnormalities on MRS and MTI exist both within inflammatory demyelinating lesions and in "normal-appearing white matter" (NAWM). This seems to indicate that diffuse axonal loss may occur separately from the discrete pathological lesions.

Axons are at least partially remyelinated, especially early in the disease course (66). Both pooled human intravenous IgG (IVIg) and human monoclonal antibodies enhance remyelination in the TMEV animal model of demyelination (67). This finding holds potential for future treatments directed at enhancing the natural remyelination process or inhibiting factors that impede this process.

THERAPY

Therapies in MS (Table 1) are directed at resolving acute attacks, reducing the number of exacerbations, treating the sequelae of previous attacks, and preventing progression of disability. Symptomatic treatments focus on pharmacological and nonpharmacological methods to protect function and improve quality of life despite the sequelae of MS. These include problems with ambulation, spasticity, fatigue, neurogenic sphincter dysfunction, and cognitive and affective disorders. The diverse symptomatic treatment strategies are beyond the scope of this paper but have been reviewed elsewhere (68).

Relapsing-Remitting Multiple Sclerosis

ACUTE RELAPSES   Precipitating factors of acute attacks of MS are unknown; however, some occur in association with acute viral infections (69). Treatment of acute attacks of MS depends on the degree of associated functional impairment. Mild attacks causing little or no functional impairment may require no treatment other than rest and often resolve spontaneously. Relapses causing functional impairment (e.g., visual loss, weakness, significant gait impairment) are typically treated with corticosteroids. Treatment regimens vary; 1 g methylprednisolone intravenously once daily for 3–5 days, with or without a brief oral corticosteroid taper, is typical. The goal of treatment is to expedite recovery (70). Rarely, acute, severe attacks do not respond adequately to corticosteroids and a severe deficit remains. A recent masked, sham-controlled, randomized study showed a functional improvement in ~40% of corticosteroid-unresponsive patients treated with therapeutic plasma

TABLE 1 Treatments of multiple sclerosis

Indication	Drug and dosage	Lab prior to therapy	Lab during therapy	Common side effects	Contraindication
Acute relapse	Methylprednisolone 1g IV qd for 3–5 days ± prednisone po up to 12 days	CBC, urinalysis/ culture, serum sodium, potassium	None	Insomnia, irritability, increased appetite, rare avascular hip necrosis	Systemic infections, known hypersensitivity
Acute, severe relapse unresponsive to corticosteroids	Plasma exchange 7 exchanges qod over 14 days	CBC	CBC qod during treatment; heparin/platelet factor 4 antibodies if HATS suspected	Central line insertion (50%), anemia, hypotension, HATS, HIT	Hemodynamically unstable patient
RRMS	Interferon β1-a (Avonex®) 30 μg IM weekly or (Rebif®)[a] 22 or 44 μg SC 3×/week	CBC, liver enzymes, TSH at 6 mos.	CBC, liver enzymes 1st week, at 1 month, then q 3 mos.	Fever, myalgia, chills, asthenia, depression, injection site reaction	Hypersensitivity to interferon β1-a or human albumin, pregnancy
RRMS, possibly SPMS	Interferon β1-b (Betaseron®) 8 MIU SC qod	CBC, liver enzymes, TSH at 6 mos.	CBC, liver enzymes 1st week, at 1 month, then q 3 mos.	Injection site reaction 85%, site necrosis 5%, fever, myalgia, chills, menstrual irregularities, depression	Hypersensitivity to interferon β1-b or human albumin, pregnancy
RRMS	Glatiramer acetate (Copaxone®)[a] 20 mg SC daily	None	None	Injection site reaction, flushing, transient chest pain and dyspnea, eosinophilia	Hypersensitivity to glatiramer acetate or mannitol, pregnancy
RRMS/SPMS	Mitoxantrone 5 or 12 mg/m^2 IV q 3 mos. Maximum lifetime cumulative dose 100 mg/m^2	CBC, liver enzymes, creatinine, ECG, transthoracic echocardiogram	CBC (hold if neutrophil count <1500/mm^3), liver enzymes, creatinine q weekly for 1 month following each dose, ECG and echocardiogram evaluating ejection fraction q 3 mos., D/C if ejection fraction <50%	Myelosuppression, nausea, alopecia, secondary amenorrhea, cardiotoxicity	Cardiac disease or significant cardiac risk factors, previous anthracycline use, prior mediastinal irradiation, pregnancy

Abbreviations: q, once every; qd, once daily; qod, every other day; mos., months; IV, intravenous; IM, intramuscular; SC, subcutaneous; po, by mouth; D/C, discontinue; CBC, complete blood count; ECG, electrocardiogram; TSH, thyroid-stimulating hormone; MIU, million international units; HATS, heparin-associated thrombocytopenia syndrome; HIT, heparin-induced thrombocytopenia.

[a]At the time of this review, Rebif® is not available in the United States and Copaxone® is not available in the United Kingdom.

exchange (71). Therapeutic plasma exchange is not indicated for progressive types of MS or for mild deficits following acute attacks.

DEFINITIVE TREATMENT OF RELAPSING-REMITTING MULTIPLE SCLEROSIS   Immuno-modulatory therapies approved for RRMS include the type-1 beta interferons [interferon β1-b (Betaseron®), interferon β1-a (Avonex®, Rebif®) and glatiramer acetate (Copaxone®)]. The type-1 interferons are naturally occurring cytokines. Their predominant mechanism of action is unknown, but they have been found to suppress T cell proliferation, reduce T cell migration from the systemic circulation into the CNS, and alter the T cell cytokine secretion repertoire from relatively proinflammatory Th1 to relatively anti-inflammatory Th2 response (72). Glatiramer acetate is a random polymer of four amino acids (L-glutamic acid, L-lysine, L-alanine, and L-tyrosine) that compose myelin basic protein (MBP). Its mechanism of action is also unclear, but evidence points to induction of tolerance to MBP-specific T cells as well as alteration of the immune response from Th1 to Th2 predominance (73).

The pivotal studies of the beta interferons demonstrated efficacy to decrease relapse rate by $\sim$30% in studies of 18–36 months' duration (74), and a reduction in the number of MRI lesions occurred as well (75). These early findings have been confirmed by further studies investigating differing preparations and doses (76–78). Glatiramer acetate has also been demonstrated to reduce attacks by $\sim$30% in mildly affected patients (79). Its efficacy has been confirmed by longer-term follow-up studies (80) and reduction of enhancing lesions on MRI scans over a short duration (81). There is evidence that these agents may delay disability progression in the short term (less than five years), but evidence of long-term benefits and the magnitude of this desired effect remain controversial. There are currently no accepted guidelines to assist in the selection of these agents. MS specialists disagree as to which agent is most effective and the sequence in which they should be tried in given clinical situations.

Treatment of patients with a single demyelinating event and a "high-risk" MRI (two or more cerebral lesions) remains controversial. These patients are at an elevated risk to develop MS (as determined by the occurrence of a second clinical attack). A recent study demonstrated that weekly intramuscular interferon β1-a reduced the proportion experiencing a second clinical attack over a three-year follow-up (cumulative probability of second clinical attack: 50% with placebo versus 35% with treatment) (82). In monosymptomatic patients, however, the effect of early initiation of treatment on long-term outcome and disability remains uncertain and therefore therapeutic practices differ.

Intravenous immunoglobulin (IVIg) administered monthly or every second month has been shown to decrease relapses (83). These studies have not significantly influenced treatment decisions in North America, and IVIg is not currently approved for use in RRMS in the United States or Canada. The cost, recent shortage of IVIg and potential risk of exposure to infectious agents may also limit the widespread use of this treatment.

Mitoxantrone has recently been approved for RRMS as well as SPMS based on positive outcomes from European studies (84, 85), despite equivocal previous trials (86). Mitoxantrone is an anthracycline-based chemotherapeutic agent used primarily in the treatment of acute myelogenous leukemia. Significant side effects include leukopenia, infections, amenorrhea, and cardiotoxicity; however, it appears to be safely administered at lifetime cumulative doses up to 100–140 mg/m^2 (87). It is not clear which patients will most benefit from mitoxantrone. We have used mitoxantrone in patients who have failed traditional immunomodulatory agents and continue to have inflammation as evidenced by clinical relapses and active MRI scans.

Secondary Progressive Multiple Sclerosis

One trial has reported slowing the progression of disability in SPMS with the use of interferon β1-b subcutaneously every other day (88). This trial entered patients who continued to have clinical attacks within two years prior to enrollment. Active treatment appeared to delay progression by 9–12 months. A systematic review of MRI scans from patients in this study showed significant reduction in new lesion formation (89). A similar North American study reported in abstract form did not confirm the beneficial results of interferon in SPMS (90). These results suggest that SPMS patients with continued relapses or evidence of inflammatory activity on MRI may be more likely to experience a mild benefit from interferon treatment. Final results from these and other studies will help to guide treatment decisions for the majority of SPMS patients who do not experience continuing clinical attacks.

Primary Progressive Multiple Sclerosis

The currently available immunomodulatory medications have not been adequately evaluated in patients with PPMS. These patients have no discrete attacks, and less inflammation is noted by T2-weighted and gadolinium-enhanced lesions on MRI scans (19). Because the main effect of current treatments may be suppression of inflammation, response is not likely to be as pronounced. These patients should mainly be treated symptomatically. If available, enrollment in controlled clinical trials is warranted (studies are in progress with glatiramer acetate and the type-1 interferons). Some PPMS patients with recent apparent clinical progression may transiently benefit from a short course of high-dose corticosteroids. If there is a dramatic response (regrettably, a small minority of cases), steroid administration may be repeated at monthly or quarterly intervals provided the benefit is prolonged and the treatment well-tolerated.

Negative Trial Results

Some recent clinical trials leading from basic science work have yielded disappointing results. TNF neutralization and administration of altered peptide ligands are beneficial in murine EAE, but in clinical trials, TNF neutralization with lenercept increased the number of attacks and enhancing lesions on MRI (91). Two separate phase II studies of altered peptide ligands of MBP were halted because they were encephalitogenic and poorly tolerated (92, 93). IVIg has been shown to increase remyelination in TMEV (94), but it did not produce clinically important improvement in fixed deficits of strength and optic nerve function (95). Although the therapeutic outcomes are disappointing, they have contributed to further understanding of the disease process and will guide future trials.

FUTURE DIRECTIONS

Active research in MS continues in both basic science laboratories and large, multicenter clinical trials. Mechanisms of autoimmunity, inflammation, remyelination, and axonal injury continue to be elucidated and are likely to form the basis of future therapies for MS. The currently available treatments are being studied aggressively to determine guidelines for therapeutic decision making. There is reason for optimism as treatments for MS are investigated in increasingly well-designed clinical trials.

ACKNOWLEDGMENT

We wish to thank Ms. Mary Bennett for her assistance with the typing of the manuscript.

Visit the Annual Reviews home page at www.AnnualReviews.org

LITERATURE CITED

1. Anderson DW, Ellenberg JH, Leventhal CM, et al. 1992. Revised estimate of the prevalence of multiple sclerosis in the United States. *Ann. Neurol.* 31:333–36
2. Rodriguez M, Siva A, Ward J, et al. 1994. Impairment, disability, and handicap in multiple sclerosis: a population-based study in Olmsted County, Minnesota. *Neurology* 44:28–33
3. Charcot JM. 1868. Histologie de la sclérose en plaques. *Gaz. Hop. civils et militaires* 140,141,143:554–55,7–8,66
4. Noseworthy J. 1999. Progress in determining the causes and treatment of multiple sclerosis. *Nature* 399(Suppl.):A40–A47
5. Poser CM, Paty DW, Scheinberg L, et al. 1983. New diagnostic criteria for multiple sclerosis: guidelines for research protocols. *Ann. Neurol.* 13:227–31
5a. McDonald WI, Compston A, Edan G, et al. 2001. Recommended diagnostic criteria for multiple sclerosis: guidelines from the International Panel on the Diagnosis of Multiple Sclerosis. *Ann. Neurol.* 50(1):121–27
6. Weinshenker B, Lucchinetti C. 1998. Acute leukoencephalopathies: differential diagnosis and investigation. *Neurologist* 4:148–66
7. McLean BN, Miller D, Thompson EJ. 1995. Oligoclonal banding of IgG in CSF, blood-brain barrier function, and MRI findings in patients with sarcoidosis, systemic lupus erythematosus, and Behcet's disease

involving the nervous system. *J. Neurol. Neurosurg. Psychiatry* 58:548–54

8. Gronseth G, Ashman E. 2000. Practice parameter: the usefulness of evoked potentials in identifying clinically silent lesions in patients with suspected multiple sclerosis (an evidence-based review). Report of the Quality Standards Subcommittee of the American Academy of Neurology. *Neurology* 54:1720–25

9. Fazekas F, Barkhof F, Filippi M, et al. 1999. The contribution of magnetic resonance imaging to the diagnosis of multiple sclerosis. *Neurology* 53:448–56

10. van Walderveen MA, Kamphorst W, Scheltens P, et al. 1998. Histopathologic correlate of hypointense lesions on T1-weighted spin-echo MRI in multiple sclerosis. *Neurology* 50:1282–88

11. Fazekas F, Offenbacher H, Fuchs S, et al. 1988. Criteria for an increased specificity of MRI interpretation in elderly subjects with suspected multiple sclerosis. *Neurology* 38:1822–25

12. Barkhof F, Filippi M, Miller DH, et al. 1997. Comparison of MRI criteria at first presentation to predict conversion to clinically definite multiple sclerosis. *Brain* 120:2059–69

13. Masdeu JC, Moreira J, et al. 1996. The open ring. A new imaging sign in demyelinating disease. *J. Neuroimaging* 6:104–7

14. Masdeu JC, Quinto C, Olivera C, et al. 2000. Open-ring imaging sign: highly specific for atypical brain demyelination. *Neurology* 54:1427–33

15. O'Riordan JI, Thompson AJ, Kingsley DP, et al. 1998. The prognostic value of brain MRI in clinically isolated syndromes of the CNS. A 10-year follow-up. *Brain* 121:495–503

16. Miller DH, Albert PS, Barkhof F, et al. 1996. Guidelines for the use of magnetic resonance techniques in monitoring the treatment of multiple sclerosis. *Ann. Neurol.* 39:6–16

17. Simon JH, Jacobs LD, Campion MK, et al. 1999. A longitudinal study of brain atrophy in relapsing multiple sclerosis. *Neurology* 53:139–48

18. Losseff N, Webb S, O'Riordan J, et al. 1996. Spinal cord atrophy and disability in multiple sclerosis. A new reproducible and sensitive MRI method with potential to monitor disease progression. *Brain* 119:701–8

19. Thompson A, Polman C, Miller D, et al. 1997. Primary progressive multiple sclerosis. *Brain* 120:1085–96

20. Lublin FD, Reingold SC. 1996. Defining the clinical course of multiple sclerosis: results of an international survey. *Neurology* 46:907–11

21. Kremenchutzky M, Cottrell D, Rice G, et al. 1999. The natural history of multiple sclerosis: a geographically based study 7. Progressive-relapsing and relapsing-progressive multiple sclerosis: a re-evaluation. *Brain* 122:1941–49

22. Confavreux C, Vukusic S, Moreau T, Adeleine P. 2000. Relapses and progression of disability in multiple sclerosis. *N. Engl. J. Med.* 343:1430–38

23. Weinshenker BG. 1995. The natural history of multiple sclerosis. *Neurol. Clin.* 13:119–46

24. Weinshenker BG, Rice GPA, Noseworthy JH, et al. 1991. The natural history of multiple sclerosis: a geographically based study. III. Multivariate analysis of predictive factors and models of outcome. *Brain* 114:1045–56

25. Compston A. 1990. Risk factors for multiple sclerosis: race or place? *J. Neurol. Neurosurg. Psychiatry* 53:821–23

26. Bulman D, Ebers G. 1992. The geography of multiple sclerosis reflects genetic susceptibility. *J. Trop. Geogr. Neurol.* 2:66–72

27. Skegg DC, Corwin PA, Craven RS, et al. 1987. Occurrence of multiple sclerosis in the north and south of New Zealand. *J. Neurol. Neurosurg. Psychiatry* 50:134–39

28. McFarlin DE, Lachmann PJ. 1989. Multiple sclerosis: hopeful genes and immunology. *Nature* 341:693–94

29. Miller DH, Hammond SR, McLeod JG,

et al. 1990. Multiple sclerosis in Australia and New Zealand: Are the determinants genetic or environmental? *J. Neurol. Neurosurg. Psychiatry* 53:903–5

30. Oksenberg JR, Baranzini SE, Barcellos LF, Hauser SL. 2001. Multiple sclerosis: genomic rewards. *J. Neuroimmunol.* 113: 171–84

31. Sadovnick A, Ebers G, Dyment D, Risch N, and Canadian Collaborative Study Group. 1996. Evidence for genetic basis of multiple sclerosis. *Lancet* 347:1728–30

32. Ebers G, Sadovnick A, Risch N, Canadian Collaborative Study Group. 1995. A genetic basis for familial aggregation in multiple sclerosis. *Nature* 377:150–51

33. Ebers G, Kukay K, Bulman D, et al. 1996. A full genome search in multiple sclerosis. *Nat. Genet.* 13:472–76

34. Sawcer S, Jones H, Feakes R, et al. 1996. A genome screen in multiple sclerosis reveals susceptibility loci on chromosome 6p21 and 17q22. *Nat. Genet.* 13:464–68

35. Jacobsen M, Schweer D, Ziegler A, et al. 2000. A point mutation in PTPRC is associated with the development of multiple sclerosis. *Nat. Genet.* 26:495–99

36. Mann C, Davies M, Boggild M, et al. 2000. Glutathione S-transferase polymorphisms in multiple sclerosis: their relationship to disability. *Neurology* 5:552–57

37. Chapman J, Vinokurov S, Achiron A, et al. 2001. APOE genotype is a major predictor of long-term progression of disability in MS. *Neurology* 56:312–16

38. Wingerchuk DM, Hogancamp WF, O'Brien PC, Weinshenker BG. 1999. The clinical course of neuromyelitis optica (Devic's syndrome). *Neurology* 53:1107–14

39. Ito H, Yamasaki K, Kawano Y, et al. 1998. HLA-DP-associated susceptibility to the optico-spinal form of multiple sclerosis in the Japanese. *Tissue Antigens* 52:179–82

40. Weinshenker B, Kantarci O. 2000. Seeking genes for MS: big risks for big gains. *Neurology* 545:542–44

41. Dalgleish AG. 1997. Viruses and multiple sclerosis. *Acta Neurol. Scand. Suppl.* 169:8–15

42. Rivera-Quinones C, McGavern D, Schmelzer J, et al. 1998. Absence of neurological deficits following extensive demyelination in a class 1–deficient murine model of multiple sclerosis. *Nat. Med.* 4:187–93

43. Albert LJ, Inman RD. 1999. Molecular mimicry and autoimmunity. *N. Engl. J. Med.* 341:2068–74

44. Hunter SF, Hafler DA. 2000. Ubiquitous pathogens—links between infection and autoimmunity in MS? *Neurology* 55:164–65

45. Wandinger KP, Jabs W, Siekhaus A, et al. 2000. Association between clinical disease activity and Epstein-Barr virus reactivation in MS. *Neurology* 55:178–84

46. Challoner P, Smith K, Parker J, et al. 1995. Plaque-associated expression of human herpesvirus 6 in multiple sclerosis. *Proc. Natl. Acad. Sci. USA* 92:7440–44

47. Soldan S, Berti R, Secchiero P, et al. 1997. Association of human herpes virus 6 (HHV-6) with multiple sclerosis: increased IgM response to HHV-6 early antigen and detection of serum HHV-6 DNA. *Nat. Med.* 3:1394–97

48. Mayne M, Krishnan J, Metz L, et al. 1998. Infrequent detection of human herpesvirus 6 DNA in peripheral blood mononuclear cells from multiple sclerosis patients. *Ann. Neurol.* 44:391–94

49. Sriram S, Stratton C, Yao S, et al. 1999. *Chlamydia pneumoniae* infection of the central nervous system in multiple sclerosis. *Ann. Neurol.* 46:6–14

50. Boman J, Roblin P, Sundstrom P, et al. 2000. Failure to detect *Chlamydia pneumoniae* in the central nervous system of patients with MS. *Neurology* 54:265

51. Dal Canto M, Melvolv R, Kim B, Miller S. 1995. Two models of multiple sclerosis: experimental allergic encephalomyelitis (EAE) and Theiler's murine encephalomyelitis virus (TMEV) infection. A pathological and immunological comparison. *Micro. Res. Tech.* 32:215–29

52. McCarron R, McFarlin DE. 1988. Adoptively transferred experimental autoimmune encephalomyelitis in SJL/J, PL/J, and (SJL/J × PL/J)F1 mice. Influence of I-A haplotype on encephalitogenic epitope of myelin basic protein. *J. Immunol.* 141:1143–49

53. Zhang J, Markovic-Plese S, Lacet B, et al. 1994. Increased frequency of interleukin 2-responsive T cells specific for myelin basic protein and proteolipid protein in peripheral blood and cerebrospinal fluid of patients with multiple sclerosis. *J. Exp. Med.* 179:973–84

54. Archelos J, Hartung H-P. 1999. Adhesion molecules in multiple sclerosis: a review. In *Frontiers in Multiple Sclerosis*, ed. A Siva, J Kesselring, A Thompson, pp. 85–116. London: Martin Dunitz

55. D'Souza SD, Bonetti B, Balasingam V, et al. 1996. Multiple sclerosis: Fas signaling in oligodendrocyte cell death. *J. Exp. Med.* 184:2361–70

56. Archelos JJ, Storch MK, Hartung HP. 2000. The role of B cells and autoantibodies in multiple sclerosis. *Ann. Neurol.* 47:694–706

57. Reindl M, Linington C, Brehm U, et al. 1999. Antibodies against the myelin oligodendrocyte glycoprotein and the myelin basic protein in multiple sclerosis and other neurological diseases: a comparative study. *Brain* 122:2047–56

58. Raine C, Cannella B, Hauser S, Genain C. 1999. Demyelination in primate autoimmune encephalomyelitis and acute multiple sclerosis lesions: a case for antigen-specific antibody mediation. *Ann. Neurol.* 46:144–60

59. Genain CP, Cannella B, Hauser SL, Raine CS. 1999. Identification of autoantibodies associated with myelin damage in multiple sclerosis. *Nat. Med.* 5:170–75

60. Lucchinetti CF, Bruck W, Rodriguez M, Lassmann H. 1998. Multiple sclerosis: lessons from neuropathology. *Sem. Neurol.* 18:337–49

61. Lucchinetti CF, Bruck W, Parisi J, et al. 2000. Heterogeneity of multiple sclerosis lesions: implications for the pathogenesis of demyelination. *Ann. Neurol.* 47:707–17

62. Ferguson B, Matyszak MK, Esiri MM, Petty VH. 1997. Axonal damage in acute multiple sclerosis lesions. *Brain* 120:393–99

63. Trapp BD, Peterson J, Ransohoff RM, et al. 1998. Axonal transection in the lesions of multiple sclerosis. *N. Engl. J. Med.* 338:278–85

64. Arnold DL. 1999. Magnetic resonance spectroscopy: imaging axonal damage in MS. *J. Neuroimmunol.* 98:2–6

65. Filippi M, Rovaris M. 2000. Magnetization transfer imaging in multiple sclerosis. *J. Neurovirol.* 6:S115–S20

66. Prineas JW, Barnard RO, Kwon EE, et al. 1993. Multiple sclerosis: remyelination of nascent lesions. *Ann. Neurol.* 33:137–51

67. Warrington AE, Asakura K, Bieber AJ, et al. 2000. Human monoclonal antibodies reactive to oligodendrocytes promote remyelination in a model of multiple sclerosis. *Proc. Natl. Acad. Sci. USA* 97:6820–25

68. Metz L. 1998. Multiple sclerosis: symptomatic therapies. *Semin. Neurol.* 18:389–95

69. Sibley WA, Bamford CR, Clark K. 1985. Clinical viral infections and multiple sclerosis. *Lancet* 1:1313–15

70. Beck RW, Cleary PA, Anderson MM Jr, et al. 1992. A randomized, controlled trial of corticosteroids in the treatment of acute optic neuritis. The Optic Neuritis Study Group. *N. Engl. J. Med.* 326:581–88

71. Weinshenker B, O'Brien P, Petterson T, et al. 1999. A randomized trial of plasma exchange in acute central nervous system inflammatory demyelinating disease. *Ann. Neurol.* 46:878–86

72. Yong VW, Chabot S, Stuve O, Williams G. 1998. Interferon beta in the treatment of multiple sclerosis: mechanisms of action. *Neurology* 51:682–89

73. Neuhaus O, Farina C, Wekerle H, Hohlfeld R. 2001. Mechanisms of action of glatiramer acetate in multiple sclerosis. *Neurology* 56:702–8

74. The IFNB Multiple Sclerosis Study Group. 1993. Interferon beta-1b is effective in relapsing-remitting multiple sclerosis. I. Clinical results of a multicenter, randomized, double-blind, placebo-controlled trial. *Neurology* 43:655–61

75. Paty DW, Li DKB, the UBC MS/MRI Study Group and the IFNB Multiple Sclerosis Study Group. 1993. Interferon beta-1b is effective in relapsing-remitting multiple sclerosis. II. MRI analysis results of a multicenter, randomized, double-blind, placebo-controlled trial. *Neurology* 43:662–67

76. Jacobs LD, Cookfair DL, Rudick RA, et al. 1996. Intramuscular interferon beta-1a for disease progression in relapsing multiple sclerosis. The Multiple Sclerosis Collaborative Research Group (MSCRG). *Ann. Neurol.* 39:285–94

77. PRISMS (Prevention of Relapses and Disability by Interferon beta-1a Subcutaneously in Multiple Sclerosis) Study Group. 1998. Randomized double-blind, placebo-controlled study of interferon beta-1a in relapsing-remitting multiple sclerosis. *Lancet* 352:1498–504

78. Simon JH, Jacobs LD, Campion M, et al. 1998. Magnetic resonance studies of intramuscular interferon β-1a for relapsing multiple sclerosis. *Ann. Neurol.* 43:79–87

79. Johnson KP, Brooks BR, Cohen JA, et al. 1995. Copolymer 1 reduces relapse rate and improves disability in relapsing-remitting multiple sclerosis: results of a phase III multicenter, double-blind placebo-controlled trial. The Copolymer 1 Multiple Sclerosis Study Group. *Neurology* 45:1268–76

80. Johnson KP, Brooks BR, Ford CC, et al. 2000. Sustained clinical benefits of glatiramer acetate in relapsing multiple sclerosis patients observed for 6 years. *Multiple Scler.* 6:255–66

81. Comi G, Filippi M, Wolinsky JS. 2001. European/Canadian multicenter, double-blind, randomized, placebo-controlled study of the effects of glatiramer acetate on magnetic resonance imaging–measured disease activity and burden in patients with relapsing multiple sclerosis. *Ann. Neurol.* 49:290–97

82. Jacobs LD, Beck RW, Simon JH, et al. 2000. Intramuscular interferon beta-1a therapy initiated during a first demyelinating event in multiple sclerosis. *N. Engl. J. Med.* 343:898–904

83. Fazekas F, Deisenhammer F, Strasser-Fuchsy S, et al. 1997. Randomized placebo-controlled trial of monthly intravenous immunoglobulin therapy in relapsing-remitting multiple sclerosis. *Lancet* 349:589–93

84. Krapf H, Morrissey S, Zenker O, et al. 1999. Mitoxantrone in progressive multiple sclerosis: MRI results of the European Phase III Trial. *Neurology* 52:A495

85. Mauch E, Eisenmann S, Hahn A. 1999. *Mitoxantrone in the treatment of patients with multiple sclerosis (MS): a large single-center experience.* Presented at ECTRIMS/ACTRIS, Basel, Switzerland September, 1999

86. Noseworthy JH, Hopkins MB, Vandervoort MK, et al. 1993. An open-trial evaluation of mitoxantrone in the treatment of progressive MS. *Neurology* 43:1401–6

87. Crossley RJ. 1984. Clinical safety and tolerance of mitoxantrone. *Semin. Oncol.* 11:54–58

88. Kappos L, European Study Group on Interferon beta-1b in Secondary-Progressive MS. 1998. Placebo-controlled multicentre randomised trial of interferon beta-1b in treatment of secondary progressive multiple sclerosis. *Lancet* 352:1491–97

89. Miller D, Molyneux P, Barker G, et al. 1999. Effect of interferon β-1b on magnetic resonance imaging outcomes in secondary progressive multiple sclerosis: results of a European multicenter, randomized, double-blind, placebo-controlled trial. *Ann. Neurol.* 46:850–59

90. Goodkin DE, North American Study Group on Interferon β-1b in Secondary Prevention MS. 2000. Interferon beta 1-b in secondary progressive MS: clinical and MRI results of a 3-year randomized controlled trial. *Neurology* 54(Suppl.):2352 (Abstr.)

91. Arnason BGW, Jacobs G, Hanlon M, et al. 1999. TNF neutralization in MS—results of a randomized, placebo-controlled multicenter study. *Neurology* 53:457–65

92. Bielekova B, Goodwin B, Richert N, et al. 2000. Encephalitogenic potential of the myelin basic protein peptide (amino acids 83–99) in multiple sclerosis: results of a phase II clinical trial with an altered peptide ligand. *Nat. Med.* 6:1167–75

93. Kappos L, Comi G, Panitch H, et al. 2000. Induction of a non-encephalitogenic type 2 T helper-cell autoimmune response in multiple sclerosis after administration of an altered peptide ligand in a placebo-controlled, randomized phase II trial. *Nat. Med.* 6:1176–82

94. Rodriguez M, Lennon VA. 1990. Immunoglobulins promote remyelination in the central nervous system. *Ann. Neurol.* 27:12–17

95. Noseworthy J, O'Brien P, Weinshenker B, et al. 2000. IVIg does not reverse established weakness in MS: a double-blind, placebo-controlled trial. *Neurology* 55:1135–43

Annu. Rev. Med. 2002. 53:303–18

GENE EXPRESSION PROFILING
OF LYMPHOID MALIGNANCIES*

Louis M. Staudt

Metabolism Branch, Center for Cancer Research, National Cancer Institute, 9000 Rockville Pike, Bethesda, Maryland 20892; e-mail: lstaudt@mail.nih.gov

Key Words   genomics, microarray, lymphoma, leukemia, BCL-6

■ **Abstract**   Comprehensive gene expression profiling using DNA microarrays is providing a molecular classification of cancer into disease categories that are homogeneous with respect to pathogenesis and clinical behavior. Gene expression profiling revealed that diffuse large B cell lymphoma (DLBCL) consists of at least two molecularly distinct diseases that are derived from distinct stages of B cell differentiation and have strikingly different clinical outcomes. By contrast, chronic lymphocytic leukemia (CLL) was found to be a single disease defined by a characteristic gene expression signature. Nonetheless, gene expression profiling distinguished two clinically divergent CLL subtypes and provided evidence that signaling through the B cell antigen receptor may play a role in the clinically aggressive subtype. Gene expression analysis also illuminated the mechanism of lymphomagenesis caused by BCL-6 translocations and provided evidence that the NF-κB signaling pathway is a new molecular therapeutic target in DLBCL.

INTRODUCTION

The diagnosis of cancers is currently based largely on morphological examination of tumor cells coupled with clinical data. The inadequacy of the current diagnostic methods is evident in the heterogeneous treatment responses of cancer patients within a diagnostic category. The importance of establishing a new molecular diagnosis of cancer is twofold. First, the assignment of cancer patients to molecularly defined diagnostic categories will often provide prognostic information that can guide patients to the most appropriate treatments. Second, a molecular diagnosis of cancer provides a detailed blueprint of the abnormal molecular circuitry of the cancer cell, which will lead to the development of molecularly targeted therapies that have specificity and potency for defined cancer types.

Recently, new genomics-based technologies have enabled a more comprehensive approach to the molecular diagnosis of cancer (1–4). In particular, DNA

---

*The US Government has the right to retain a nonexclusive, royalty-free license in and to any copyright covering this paper.

microarray technology has been used to analyze the expression of thousands of genes in parallel in normal and malignant lymphoid cells. Several versions of this technology are widely used, each based on an ordered array of DNA fragments on a solid support that represent distinct genes.

One form of microarray relies on robotic spotting of cDNAs for defined genes in an ordered microscopic array on a glass slide (5, 6). Fluorescently labeled cDNA probes are prepared from total cellular mRNA derived from the cell of interest and hybridized at high concentration to this microarray. The extent of hybridization of the probes to each cDNA on the microarray is then quantitated using a modified confocal microscope. It is possible to compare two cell types on the same microarray by labeling the cDNA from each cell with a different fluorochrome. The method is sensitive over three logs of gene expression and gives quantitative results that mesh well with parallel analysis of gene expression using Northern blots or quantitative RT-PCR (reverse transcription–polymerase chain reaction). Both known genes and anonymously cloned cDNAs can be arrayed for analysis, thus allowing insight into defined cellular pathways as well as allowing the discovery of novel genes that influence the biology of the cell. Using microarrays, a cancer biopsy sample can be described with unprecedented molecular detail based on its mRNA expression profile. However, this technology produces an avalanche of data that must be crafted into a biologically coherent and clinically useful molecular diagnosis of cancer.

Much of this review focuses on how comprehensive molecular technologies will rewrite disease definitions in the medical textbooks of the future. How should we judge whether we have arrived at a molecular definition of a homogeneous disease? A first requirement might be that all cases assigned to a given diagnostic category share a common pathogenetic basis. In cancer, the nature of the normal cell from which the cancer cell arises is a critical component of its pathogenesis. As discussed below, much of the gene expression of a cancer cell is "inherited" from its normal cellular counterpart. The second component of pathogenesis in cancer is the molecular mechanism of malignant transformation. Oncogene expression and tumor suppressor loss can impart a characteristic gene expression signature to the cancer cell that distinguishes it from its normal cellular counterpart. However, clinically apparent cancers often result from multiple progression events that each confer a growth or survival advantage to the cell. We may therefore need to define molecular subtypes of a given molecular cancer diagnosis based on these progression events.

Currently, the clinical courses of patients given the same cancer diagnosis can be highly variable, and this undoubtedly stems, in part, from an underlying molecular heterogeneity among their tumors. Therefore, a second requirement for a molecular definition of cancer types is that cases within a particular type should be clinically homogeneous. Indeed, if this is not the case, a search for further molecular heterogeneity within the cancer cells should be undertaken. There are, however, host factors that contribute to a patient's clinical course, such as the metabolism of cancer therapeutic drugs, an issue currently being addressed by the field of pharmacogenomics (7). Additionally, the patient's immune competence

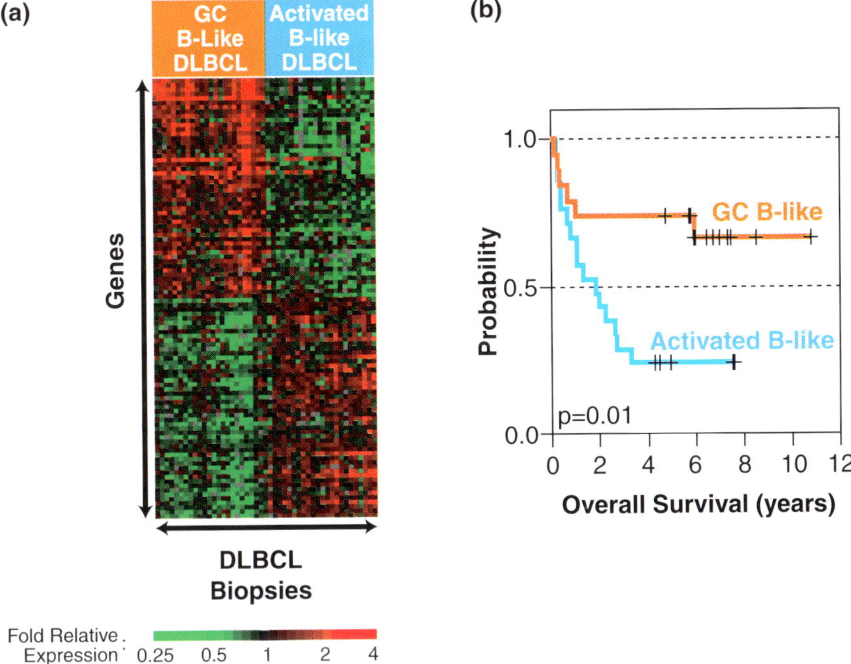

Figure 1 Diffuse large B cell lymphoma (DLBCL) comprises at least two distinct diseases. (*a*) Gene expression differences between germinal center B-like DLBCL and activated B-like DLBCL. Relative expression of ~100 genes that discriminate most significantly between the two DLBCL types is depicted over a 16-fold range using the graded color scale shown at the bottom. Shades of red indicate higher expression and shades of green indicate lower expression of a particular gene (*row*) in a particular DLBCL lymph node biopsy (*column*). (*b*) Kaplan-Meyer plot of overall patient survival following multiagent, anthracycline-based chemotherapy. Gene expression profiles of tumor biopsy samples can stratify DLBCL patients into prognostically distinct groups.

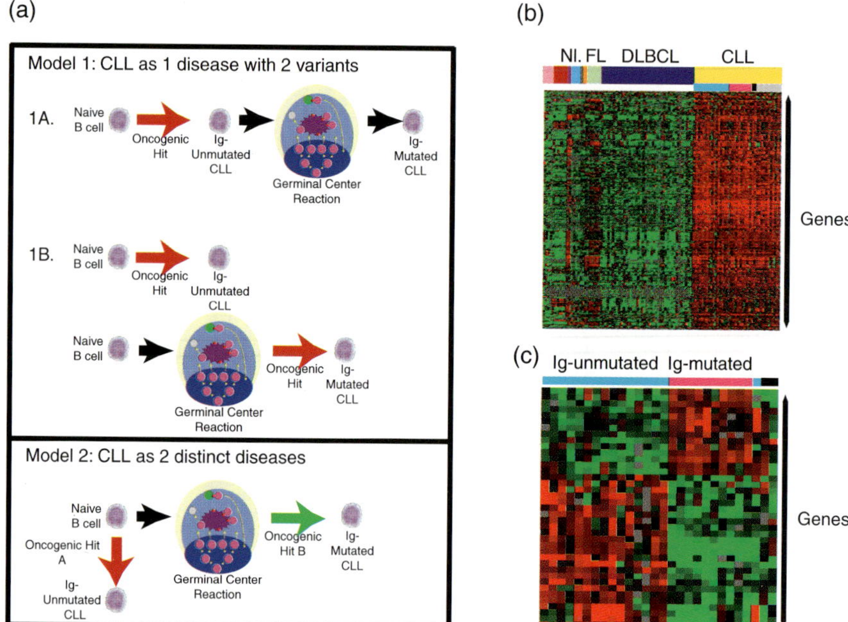

Figure 2 Chronic lymphocytic leukemia (CLL) is one disease with two common variants. (*a*) Models to explain the observation that leukemia cells of some CLL patients have unmutated immunoglobulin (Ig) genes, whereas others have mutated Ig genes. In model 1A, all cases of CLL arise from a naïve B cell with unmutated Ig genes by a common mechanism of malignant transformation. In some instances, this transformed B cell may be driven through a germinal center reaction and mutate its Ig genes. In model 1B, a single mechanism of oncogenic transformation is responsible for CLL, but Ig-unmutated CLL arises from a naïve, pre-germinal center B cell and Ig-mutated CLL arises from a post-germinal center B cell. Both model 1A and model 1B predict that all CLL cases should share a common gene expression signature due to a common cell of origin and/or a common mechanism of malignant transformation. In model 2, Ig-unmutated and Ig-mutated CLL arise from different stages of B cell differentiation by distinct mechanisms of malignant transformation. This model predicts that there should not be a common gene expression signature shared by all CLL cases. (*b*) More than 200 genes are characteristically expressed in CLL but not DLBCL, follicular lymphoma (FL), or in most normal lymphocyte subpopulations (Nl). These CLL signature genes are expressed equivalently in Ig-unmutated and Ig-mutated CLL, consistent with models 1A and 1B in Figure 2*a*. Data are depicted as described in the legend to Figure 1. (*c*) Ig-unmutated and Ig-mutated CLL can be readily distinguished by gene expression analysis. These genes are different from the CLL signature genes represented in Figure 2*b*.

and other less well-defined biological factors such as age and tumor burden may influence the disease course. The immune response to a tumor can be visualized by microarray analysis of gene expression and thus could be incorporated into the molecular definition of a cancer.

The final, and most important, test of a molecular cancer diagnosis is its utility. A useful diagnostic category should allow the physician to choose the optimal therapy based on the molecular characteristics of the patient's tumor. As more molecularly targeted therapies become available, the gene expression profile of a tumor cell could be used to identify whether the target of a given drug is active in the tumor cell.

Equally important will be the use of gene expression profiles to identify new targets for therapeutic development in the future. Individual signaling pathways can produce characteristic gene expression signatures when they are active in a cell. The detection of such a pathway-specific gene expression signature in a cancer cell can prompt investigation into whether the signaling pathway is pro-proliferative or antiapoptotic for the cancer cell. The long-term benefit of a genomic approach to cancer diagnosis is its ability to discover previously unsuspected molecular etiologies.

GENE EXPRESSION PROFILING USING THE LYMPHOCHIP DNA MICROARRAY

To study gene expression in lymphoid malignancies comprehensively, we created a specialized DNA microarray, termed the Lymphochip, that is enriched in genes that are selectively expressed in lymphocytes and in genes that regulate lymphocyte function (8). The Lymphochip currently contains over 18,500 cDNAs, many of which were derived from a normalized cDNA library generated from germinal center B lymphocytes. The rationale underlying this focus on the germinal center B cell was based on the hypothesis that many non-Hodgkin's lymphomas originate from mature B cells that have participated in a germinal center reaction. The germinal center is a novel microenvironment that is formed by antigen-specific B cells and T cells in response to antigenic challenge. During the course of this reaction, which occurs histologically in the follicular regions of secondary lymphoid organs, the B cells proliferate very rapidly and differentiate. As part of this differentiation process, the B cells activate a specialized mutational machinery, termed somatic hypermutation, that dramatically alters the rearranged immunoglobulin (Ig) gene sequences. Mutations are found in the Ig genes of many types of non-Hodgkin's lymphomas, including diffuse large B cell lymphoma (DLBCL), follicular lymphoma, Burkitt's lymphoma, and a variety of less common entities. Thus, the B cell that gives rise to these malignancies is likely to have participated in a germinal center reaction at some point in its history.

The germinal center B cell cDNA library was subjected to high-throughput expressed sequence tag (EST) sequencing as part of the Cancer Genome Anatomy Project (CGAP) (9). This library was sequenced deeply (>59,000 clones) based on a bioinformatics analysis of its EST sequences that revealed a high frequency of potentially novel genes (8). Subsequently, we used the same analytical tools to discover novel genes in CGAP cDNA libraries that were derived from lymphoid malignancies, including DLBCL, follicular lymphoma, mantle cell lymphoma, and chronic lymphocytic leukemia (CLL) (8). In all, the Lymphochip includes ~15,000 cDNA clones from these libraries. Additionally, a set of 3500 cDNA clones were curated that represent "named" human genes known to function in the immune system or in oncogenesis. Thus, the Lymphochip has two components that contribute to its effectiveness in defining subtypes of human lymphoid malignancies. First, the novel genes on the Lymphochip, though currently of unknown function, are often variably expressed in normal and malignant lymphoid cells and thus provide pattern recognition power. Second, the named-gene component of the Lymphochip provides immediate biological insight into the malignancies under study.

DIFFUSE LARGE B CELL LYMPHOMA IS AT LEAST TWO DISTINCT DISEASES

The lymphoid malignancies provide a wonderful test case for a new molecularly based paradigm of cancer diagnosis. Despite the concerted efforts of pathologists and clinicians over the past two decades, certain categories of non-Hodgkin's lymphomas have resisted consistent classification. In particular, DLBCL has alternately been split into multiple subcategories on morphological grounds or lumped into a single category, as it is in the current WHO (World Health Organization) classification (10). Indeed, it was conclusively demonstrated that pathologists could not reliably distinguish subtypes of DLBCL on morphological grounds alone (11). Nonetheless, since the advent of multi-agent chemotherapy for DLBCL in the 1970s, it has been clear that ~40% of DLBCL patients can be cured by these regimens, whereas the remainder eventually succumb to this disease (12, 13). No change in this outcome ratio has occurred in the intervening years, despite numerous attempts to devise alternative chemotherapeutic combinations (14).

These considerations suggested that the clinical heterogeneity of DLBCL patients might be explained by an underlying molecular heterogeneity in their tumor cells, and this hypothesis was directly tested by Lymphochip microarray analysis of gene expression in DLBCL (1). A critical component of this study was the comparative analysis of gene expression in DLBCL, in other lymphoid malignancies, and in a variety of normal lymphocyte subsets. An important concept that emerged from this systematic approach was that complex gene expression profiles can be broken down into component gene expression signatures. A gene expression signature can be defined as a group of genes that is characteristically expressed in a particular cell type or during a particular biological response. These signatures can be found using mathematical algorithms, such as hierarchical clustering, that identify patterns within large datasets (15). Cell type gene expression signatures can be broadly specific for a lineage (e.g., a pan–B cell signature) or specific for a discrete stage of differentiation (e.g., the germinal center B cell signature). A prominent example of a gene expression signature tied to biological function was the proliferation signature, a group of hundreds of genes that are more highly expressed in cycling cells than in cells in a quiescent, G0 stage. The gene expression signatures detected in a complex clinical sample can thus provide an "executive summary" that describes the relationship of the tumor cells to a particular stage of normal differentiation, quantifies the extent of tumor cell proliferation, and measures the quantity and quality of the host immune response to the tumor.

The challenge in the analysis of DBLCL was to identify which genes would best subdivide the DLBCLs into clinically and biologically meaningful subgroups. Indeed, the germinal center B cell, T cell, and proliferation gene expression signatures were independently variable features of these tumors, any of which could have been used to categorize the DLBCL cases. Initially, the germinal center signature genes were chosen, based on the assumption that a tumor cell "inherits" a broad gene expression program from its normal cellular precursor and that this inherited gene expression profile could significantly influence the clinical behavior of the tumor. Indeed, germinal center B cells differ in the expression of hundreds of genes from both resting and mitogenically activated blood B cells (16). DLBCLs were subdivided using the hierarchical clustering algorithm based on expression of roughly 100 germinal center signature genes, leading to the definition of two DLBCL subgroups. One subgroup, termed germinal center B–like DLBCL, closely resembled normal germinal center B cells in gene expression. The other subgroup, termed activated B–like DLBCL, lacked expression of the germinal center B cell genes and instead expressed genes that are characteristic of mitogenically activated blood B cells. Once these two DLBCL subtypes were defined by their expression of germinal center genes, many hundreds of other genes were found to be differentially expressed between the subtypes. Indeed, as many or more genes distinguished the two DLBCL subtypes as distinguished acute lymphoblastic leukemia and acute myelogenous leukemia (http://llmpp.nih.gov/lymphoma/images/sfigure1.html) (3).

Activated B–like DLBCL may be derived from a post–germinal center B cell, based on analysis of somatic mutation of the Ig genes in these two DLBCL subtypes (17). Germinal center B–like DLBCLs had mutant Ig genes that showed evidence of ongoing mutations within the malignant clone. By contrast, although activated B–like DLBCLs had mutated Ig genes, no variation in Ig sequences was found within a given case. This finding demonstrates that germinal center B–like DLBCL not only retains the gene expression signature of normal germinal center B cells but also maintains the somatic hypermutation machinery that distinguishes this differentiation stage. In this respect, germinal center B–like DLBCL resembles follicular lymphoma, which was also found to closely resemble normal germinal center B cells in gene expression (1) and had previously been shown to have ongoing somatic hypermutation (18). Activated B–like DLBCLs share gene expression with a rare germinal center subset that lacks expression of BCL-6 and expresses IRF-4/MUM1 and blimp-1 (19, 20). It has been suggested that these cells are at the transition between germinal center B cells and plasma cells, given that

IRF-4/MUM1 and blimp-1 are both expressed in plasma cells. Taken together, these observations suggest that activated B–like DLBCL may arise in some cases by malignant transformation of a post–germinal center transitional B cell. Recently, however, a subpopulation of normal B cells has been defined in which somatic Ig mutations apparently accumulate in the absence of germinal centers (21, 22). These Ig-mutated peripheral B cells express IgM, IgD, and CD27 and are also candidate precursor cells for activated B–like DLBCL.

Patients with these two types of DLBCL had strikingly different responses to chemotherapy (1). Patients with germinal center B–like DLBCL had a favorable prognosis: 75% of these patients were cured by anthracycline-based, multiagent chemotherapy. Patients with activated B–like DLBCL had a poor outcome following chemotherapy, less than one quarter achieving a long-term remission. A previously defined clinical prognostic indicator, the International Prognostic Index (IPI), amalgamates several clinical parameters and can be used to assign patients to prognostic groups (12). DLBCL patients in a low-clinical-risk group (IPI 0–2) could still be separated into two distinct prognostic subgroups based on gene expression: patients in this favorable IPI subset with the activated B–like DLBCL gene expression profile had a markedly inferior overall survival rate. Thus, gene expression profiling appears to provide prognostic information that is independent of the IPI.

These results show that the diagnosis of DLBCL lumps together two distinct diseases that have different cells of origin and strikingly different clinical courses. This demonstrates that genomic-scale gene expression analysis can define clinically important subtypes of human cancer.

An important point, however, is that residual heterogeneity was evident within these DLBCL subtypes, both molecularly and clinically. The proliferation, T cell, and lymph node gene expression signatures were all variable phenotypes among the DLBCL samples that varied independently of one another and of the germinal center B cell signature. In the first analysis, the expression of these other signatures did not correlate with clinical overall survival, but the potential role of these and other gene expression signatures will need to be reevaluated using a much larger cohort of DLBCL patients. Clinically, each DLBCL subtype was distinct, but neither subtype was homogeneous in clinical behavior: Some patients with the prognostically favorable germinal center B–like phenotype died within the first few years of therapy, whereas some patients with the prognostically poor activated B–like subtype were long-term survivors (Figure 1*b*, see color insert). Two broad hypotheses can be advanced to explain this clinical heterogeneity. First, minor DLBCL subtypes may exist that can only be discerned by analysis of larger numbers of DLBCL samples. Second, individual genes or signaling pathways may be differentially active within tumors assigned overall to the same DLBCL subtype. The testing of these and other hypotheses will be enabled by a large international consortium, the Lymphoma/Leukemia Molecular Profiling Project, that is currently profiling gene expression in hundreds of DLBCLs and other lymphoid malignancies (http://llmpp.nih.gov).

CHRONIC LYMPHOCYTIC LEUKEMIA: ONE DISEASE WITH TWO MOLECULARLY AND CLINICALLY DISTINCT VARIANTS

B cell chronic lymphocytic leukemia (CLL) is the most common human leukemia, comprising 25%–30% of all leukemia cases. Despite the prevalence of CLL, little is understood regarding its molecular pathogenesis, in part because CLL is not characterized by the recurrent translocations that have been pivotal in the analysis of other lymphoid malignancies. A few discrete chromosomal abnormalities are common in CLL, namely trisomy 12 and deletion of a presumptive tumor suppressor gene on 13q14, but the role of these genomic changes in the biology of CLL remains to be elucidated. CLL also presents a clinical challenge. Although it is a chemotherapy-responsive tumor, fludarabine, the most effective drug, produces only a 20% complete response rate (23), and there are no proven cures. Thus, advancing our understanding of the molecular biology of CLL may have important ramifications for developing new and more effective therapies and understanding the molecular basis for fludarabine resistance.

Recently, sequence analysis of the Ig genes in CLL has led to the proposal that CLL encompasses more than one disease (24–26). The leukemic cells in ~50% of CLL patients have rearranged Ig genes with extensive somatic mutations, whereas the other ~50% have leukemic cells in which the Ig genes are germ-line in sequence. Given the critical role of the germinal center microenvironment in the process of somatic hypermutation of Ig genes, these findings suggested that one subtype of CLL (Ig-unmutated CLL) may be derived from naive pre–germinal center B cells and the other subtype (Ig-mutated CLL) may be derived from a germinal center or post–germinal center B cell. The two types of CLL defined in this manner had different clinical courses: Ig-unmutated CLL patients had progressive disease requiring early treatment, whereas Ig-mutated CLL patients had relatively stable disease requiring either late or no treatment (24, 25). Based on this evidence, it was possible that CLL, like DLBCL, comprises two distinct diseases derived by distinct oncogenic mechanisms, one from a pre–germinal center B cell and the other from a post–germinal center B cell (Figure 2a, model 2; see color insert). In this model, as in DLBCL, the gene expression profiles of Ig-unmutated and Ig-mutated CLL should be largely distinct. Alternatively, CLL could have a common cell of origin (Figure 2a, model 1A) or a common mechanism of malignant transformation (Figure 2a, model 1B). These models predict that all CLL cases should share a common gene expression signature reflecting a common normal cellular counterpart and/or oncogenic mechanism.

To test the hypothesis that CLL is more than one disease, the gene expression profiles of CLL cells were related to their Ig mutational status and to other types of normal and malignant B cells (27). More than 200 genes were identified as being highly expressed in CLL in comparison with DLBCL (Figure 2b, see color insert). Importantly, these genes were expressed equivalently in all CLL samples, regardless of Ig mutational status. Many of these genes constituted a CLL-specific gene expression signature in that they were not expressed highly in normal resting or activated blood B cells or in germinal center B cells. Additional genes were identified that were expressed in both CLL cells and resting blood B cells but not in mitogenically activated blood B cells, germinal center B cells, or DLBCL. The CLL-specific gene expression signature suggested that all CLL cases have a common cellular origin and/or mechanism of malignant transformation. From this perspective, Ig-unmutated and Ig-mutated CLL should be considered variants of the same disease.

Despite the existence of a CLL-specific gene expression profile, the two CLL subtypes were distinguished from each other by the expression of $\sim$177 human genes with high statistical significance ($p < 0.001$) (Figure 2b, see color insert). We next developed a statistical algorithm to predict the CLL Ig mutational subtype based on gene expression alone. The subtype predictor assigned 27 out of 28 cases to the correct mutational subtype, including 9 out of 10 new CLL cases that were not used to form the predictor. In fact, we found that we could reduce the number of genes in the predictor to 3 and achieve 100% predictive accuracy. Conceivably, this small group of genes could form the basis of a clinical test for the CLL subtype distinction that would be easier to implement in routine diagnosis than DNA sequencing of Ig variable regions.

Finally, the set of CLL subtype distinction genes showed enhanced expression of genes related to B cell activation through the B cell antigen receptor (BCR). Specifically, genes that are upregulated during BCR stimulation were more highly expressed in Ig-unmutated CLL, and genes that are downregulated during BCR stimulation were expressed at lower levels in Ig-unmutated CLL. This finding suggests that stimulation through the BCR may play a role in the pathogenesis of CLL. Support for this notion comes from previous analyses of Ig variable region usage in CLL. The repertoire of Ig variable regions in CLL is a nonrandom selection of the total repertoire, and each Ig mutational subtype of CLL preferentially rearranges different variable genes (24–26). The Ig D_H and J_H segment utilization in CLL Ig rearrangements is also nonrandom, suggesting that the CLL variable regions are selected for antigen-binding properties (24–26, 28, 29). Indeed, the CLL Igs are often autoantibodies (30–32). Further, it has previously been noted that CLL cells from patients with progressive disease (e.g., Ig-unmutated CLL) can be stimulated through the BCR, whereas CLL cells from patients with stable disease cannot (33). These various lines of evidence support the hypothesis that Ig-unmutated CLL cells receive ongoing stimulation through the BCR, giving rise to the gene expression profile that we found to distinguish the two Ig mutational subtypes. Despite these considerations, it is also possible that the expression of the B cell activation genes in Ig-unmutated CLL reflects the stimulation of these cells by another mitogenic mechanism.

In summary, CLL gene profiling studies support the view that CLL is a single disease with a common cell of origin and/or mechanism of transformation. However, the heterogeneity in the clinical courses of CLL patients can be traced to a gene expression profile that distinguishes two CLL subtypes. The CLL subtype distinction genes further suggest that ongoing BCR stimulation in the Ig-unmutated CLL subtype contributes to the more progressive clinical course of these patients.

GENE EXPRESSION PROFILING REVEALS MECHANISMS OF MALIGNANT TRANSFORMATION

The power of DNA microarrays to view gene expression across the genome has the potential to reveal the regulatory logic of normal and malignant cells. The complex interplay of transcription factors and signaling proteins can be daunting when approached in a conventional fashion in which each protein-protein and protein-DNA interaction is detailed. DNA microarrays can reveal the gene expression consequences of inhibiting or overexpressing a regulatory factor, without requiring full knowledge of each intermediate step involved in altering the gene expression profile. Oncogenic transformation often involves translocation and/or amplification of genes encoding regulatory factors or loss of these genes by chromosomal deletion. These oncogenic events can be modeled experimentally, and DNA microarrays can be used to understand the regulatory consequences for the cell.

Mechanism of BCL-6 Lymphomagenesis

BCL-6 is the most frequently translocated gene in DLBCL, and approximately one sixth of all non-Hodgkin's lymphoma patients have tumors with BCL-6 translocations (34). BCL-6 protein is selectively expressed at high levels in germinal center B lymphocytes and in a variety of B cell lymphomas that are putatively derived from germinal center B cells (35–37). Disruption of the BCL-6 gene in the mouse germ line results in failure of B cells to differentiate to the germinal center stage (38–40). These observations point to an intimate link between the role of BCL-6 in normal B cell differentiation and its role in causing lymphoma.

BCL-6 encodes a zinc finger DNA binding protein that can potently repress the transcription of promoters containing its binding site (41–43). This observation suggested that BCL-6 normally functions by repressing the expression of genomic target genes that encode key regulators of B cell differentiation and immune responses. To identify these target genes, Lymphochip DNA microarrays were used to measure gene expression in biological systems in which BCL-6 function can be manipulated (44). Wild-type BCL-6 was expressed in cell types that normally lack BCL-6 expression, or dominant negative forms of BCL-6 were expressed in cells that express the endogenous BCL-6 gene. Lymphochip microarray analysis revealed 14 putative BCL-6 target genes that could be grouped into four broad functional categories: genes regulated during B cell activation, genes encoding inflammatory chemokines, genes regulating cellular proliferation, and genes regulating terminal differentiation of B cells.

The B cell activation genes repressed by BCL-6 were all induced by stimulation of B cells through the B cell antigen receptor (BCR), suggesting a model (44) in which BCL-6 blocks one of two developmental fates available to an antigen-stimulated mature B cell (45, 46). On one hand, antigen-stimulated B cells can migrate into the follicular area and form germinal centers. Alternatively, antigen-stimulated B cells can differentiate into plasma cells within the T cell–rich periarteriolar sheath, and these cells are responsible for the majority of antibody production within the first week following immunization. Plasmacytic differentiation in this pathway is preceded by a stage of B cell activation in which many BCL-6 target genes are expressed. This is understandable, since most antigen-stimulated B cells do not express BCL-6. However, some antigen-stimulated B cells do express BCL-6 within two days of antigenic stimulation (39). This model proposes that BCL-6 expression in these cells blocks rapid plasmacytic differentiation and promotes the alternative cell fate, germinal center B cell differentiation.

Support for this model comes from another BCL-6 target gene that regulates this developmental decision point: blimp-1. Blimp-1 is a transcriptional repressor that is sufficient for terminal differentiation of B cells into plasma cells (47). Thus, by repressing blimp-1, BCL-6 would be expected to block plasmacytic differentiation. Expression of BCL-6 mRNA and protein is extinguished during plasmacytic differentiation (39), and this downregulation of BCL-6 would allow expression of blimp-1. Therefore, BCL-6 has emerged from these studies as a key upstream regulator of terminal B cell differentiation. Recent in situ immunohistochemical staining for BCL-6 and blimp-1 supports this model (20). Although a majority of germinal center B cells express BCL-6 and not blimp-1, a minority lose BCL-6 expression and gain blimp-1 expression. These cells also express the B cell activation gene, IRF-4, and are presumed to be transitional cells poised between the germinal center and plasma cell stages (19). The importance of BCL-6 in regulating plasmacytic differentiation was directly supported by experiments in which dominant negative BCL-6 evoked partial plasmacytic differentiation in a Burkitt's lymphoma cell line (44). Subsequently, the finding that BCL-6 represses blimp-1 and blocks plasmacytic differentiation was confirmed in a mouse model of plasmacytic differentiation (48).

The regulation of plasmacytic differentiation by BCL-6 suggests a plausible mechanism by which translocation of BCL-6 generates non-Hodgkin's lymphomas. BCL-6 translocations substitute the BCL-6 promoter with a variety of cellular promoters that are constitutively active in mature B cells. Thus, BCL-6 translocations prevent the normal physiological downregulation of BCL-6 transcription that occurs during plasmacytic differentiation. In this way, BCL-6 translocations prevent blimp-1 expression and trap the cell in a perpetual germinal center state of differentiation. A second important BCL-6 target gene that may play a role in lymphomagenesis is p27kip1, an inhibitor of the cyclin-dependent kinases that blocks the cell cycle when expressed highly (49, 50). The repression of p27kip1 expression by BCL-6 may contribute to the rapid proliferation of normal germinal center B cells as well as lymphoma cells in which BCL-6 is highly expressed.

BCL-6 translocations may therefore promote lymphomagenesis by simultaneously blocking differentiation and promoting proliferation (44). Increasingly, the germinal center B cell is being viewed as a mutagenic cellular milieu, given the recent demonstration that somatic hypermutation introduces double-stranded breaks into genomic DNA (51, 52), as does Ig heavy-chain class switching. Our model of BCL-6 lymphomagenesis therefore proposes that BCL-6 translocations prolong the exposure of a B cell to this mutagenic environment, allowing secondary oncogenic hits to accumulate.

New Therapeutic Targets in Lymphoma Revealed by Gene Expression Profiling

Genomic-scale gene expression analysis of cancer has the potential to uncover the aberrant signaling pathways that tumor cells use to proliferate, survive, and evade immune detection. The challenge is to develop a comprehensive understanding of gene expression "physiology" that allows us to "read" the gene expression profiles of cancers (53). In other words, a signaling pathway will evoke characteristic gene expression alterations that can be used as a surrogate for the activity of a pathway. In yeast, for example, individual MAP kinase pathways yield characteristic gene expression signatures as judged by either genetic or pharmacological disruption of the pathway (54). Part of our gene expression profiling program, therefore, is to build a compendium of gene expression measurements derived from normal and malignant lymphocytes that are at various stages of differentiation, activated by a variety of cytokines and other extracellular signals, or manipulated experimentally to alter key signaling pathways (16, 53, 55–57). Application of hierarchical clustering to this dataset groups together genes that are modulated in expression by a particular signaling pathway. By recognizing these patterns, it is possible to develop hypotheses about the activity of signaling pathways in cancer cells, which then require direct experimental verification.

The search for novel molecular targets in DLBCL should be directed particularly at activated B–like DLBCL, given the dismal overall survival when these patients are treated with current multiagent chemotherapy regimens (1). As we begin to apply our molecular diagnostic methods for lymphoma clinically, it will be vital to offer patients assigned to a poor prognostic category new therapeutic options. The term "activated B–like DLBCL" was adopted to describe this subset of DLBCL patients because their tumor biopsy specimens expressed many genes that are normally upregulated in blood B cells in response to mitogenic stimulation. In particular, several known downstream targets of the NF-κB transcription factors were expressed highly in many cases of activated B–like DLBCL and not germinal center B–like DLBCL (58). The NF-κB family is a group of homo- and heterodimeric transcription factors that play critical roles in development, lymphocyte activation, and the prevention of apoptosis (59). NF-κB transcription factors are latent in the cytoplasm of cells in a complex with a member of the IκB family of inhibitory proteins. IκBs become phosphorylated by an IκB kinase (IKK) complex in response to signaling through diverse pathways. This phosphorylation is the trigger for ubiquitination of IκB and its destruction by the proteasome.

Upon IκB degradation, NF-κB family members are released to travel into the nucleus and activate transcription. Two cell-line models of activated B–like DLBCL were found to have nuclear NF-κB resulting from constitutive activity of IKK (58). Most importantly, interference with the NF-κB pathway killed the activated B–like DLBCL cell lines, but not germinal center B–like DLBCL cell lines. These findings establish the NF-κB pathway as a new therapeutic target for those DLBCL cases that are refractory to current therapies.

PERSPECTIVES

The concept of a molecularly defined cancer type is being refined by gene expression profiling studies of the lymphoid malignancies. The example of DLBCL demonstrates that some of the current diagnostic categories lump together molecularly distinct diseases that presumably have distinct normal cellular counterparts and characteristic mechanisms of malignant transformation. For these cases, the medical community should rapidly adopt a new diagnostic framework that recognizes these molecular differences. From this perspective, it no longer makes sense to design a clinical trial in DLBCL without obtaining the gene expression data necessary to distinguish germinal center B–like and activated B–like DLBCL. This could be done either by DNA microarray analysis or by quantitative RT-PCR analysis of the genes that are most differentially expressed between the DLBCL subtypes (listed at http://llmpp.nih.gov/lymphoma/images/sfigure3.html). The ongoing analysis of gene expression in larger numbers of DLBCL samples will undoubtedly refine the molecular classification of DLBCL into homogenous disease entities that can be iteratively incorporated into clinical diagnosis.

Gene expression profiling revealed CLL to be a single disease, but two clinically important molecular variants were easily discerned. A clinical quantitative RT-PCR assay for the expression of 1–3 genes could be easily adopted and would provide valuable prognostic information for CLL patients.

The most important endpoint in the molecular classification of cancer is to identify effective therapies for all patients. In the case of DLBCL, gene expression profiling has been instrumental in identifying which patients will respond well to current multiagent chemotherapy regimens. The expression of NF-κB target genes revealed the importance of this signaling pathway in activated B–like DLBCL, raising the intriguing possibility that pharmacological interference with the NF-κB pathway may benefit a currently incurable group of patients. The gene expression profile of Ig-unmutated CLL suggests that the leukemic cells may be receiving growth and/or survival signals through the B cell antigen receptor. The signaling cascades downstream of the B cell antigen receptor are well understood and are attractive potential targets for therapy of the more aggressive subset of CLL cases.

The gene expression profiling studies reviewed above provide a glimpse into the molecular oncology of the near future, in which homogenous diseases are defined in precise molecular terms and are treated with specific, nontoxic therapies tailored to the causative oncogenic mechanisms. What will be required to bring these molecular diagnoses into common clinical practice? First, oncologists, pathologists, and molecular biologists must reach a consensus as to which genes are most useful in discriminating subtypes of lymphomas and leukemias. We can be optimistic about achieving this goal, since previous consensus conferences have successively improved the pathological and clinical diagnosis of lymphomas (10–12). Second, an experimental platform must be developed that will allow these molecular diagnoses to be widely tested. Possibly, DNA microarrays themselves will be used to make these diagnoses. Initially, academic laboratories with expertise in this technology will carry out these studies, but eventually, companies may perform DNA microarray analysis as a service. If the number of genes needed to make a molecular diagnosis is sufficiently small, quantitative RT-PCR may be a feasible alternative to DNA microarrays. Third, the clinical utility and reproducibility of gene expression profiling should be confirmed in multicenter phase III clinical trials. If such large-scale clinical research validates the utility of gene expression profiling, the U.S. Food and Drug Administration may then have sufficient information to approve gene expression profiling as a clinical diagnostic test. Ultimately, the molecular diagnosis of cancer by gene expression profiling will be widely adopted when treatment decisions are based on the diagnosis. With the advent of cancer therapeutics targeting specific signaling pathways, we can expect these molecular diagnostic methods to become increasingly relevant to the practicing oncologist.

ACKNOWLEDGMENTS

The work reviewed here represents the concerted efforts of many individuals in the author's laboratory and in collaborating institutions. Genomic-scale analysis of cancer requires the combined talents of many investigators, and the principal contributors to this collegial effort have coauthored the primary publications cited in this review (1, 27, 44, 58). In addition, I would like to acknowledge the Cancer Genome Anatomy Project led by Bob Strausberg and Rick Klausner for important contributions to the Lymphochip microarray. I am very grateful for the efforts and insights that my colleagues contributed to this initiative, which were instrumental in its success.

Visit the Annual Reviews home page at www.AnnualReviews.org

LITERATURE CITED

1. Alizadeh AA, Eisen MB, Davis RE, et al. 2000. Distinct types of diffuse large B-cell lymphoma identified by gene expression profiling. *Nature* 403:503–11

2. Bittner M, Meltzer P, Chen Y, et al. 2000. Molecular classification of cutaneous malignant melanoma by gene expression profiling. *Nature* 406:536–40

3. Golub TR, Slonim DK, Tamayo P, et al. 1999. Molecular classification of cancer:

class discovery and class prediction by gene expression monitoring. *Science* 286:531–37

4. Perou CM, Sorlie T, Eisen MB, et al. 2000. Molecular portraits of human breast tumours. *Nature* 406:747–52

5. Schena M, Shalon D, Davis RW, Brown PO. 1995. Quantitative monitoring of gene expression patterns with a complementary DNA microarray. *Science* 270:467–70

6. Staudt LM, Brown PO. 2000. Genomic views of the immune system. *Annu. Rev. Immunol.* 18:829–59

7. Evans WE, Relling MV. 1999. Pharmacogenomics: translating functional genomics into rational therapeutics. *Science* 286:487–91

8. Alizadeh A, Eisen M, Davis RE, et al. 1999. The Lymphochip: a specialized cDNA microarray for the genomic-scale analysis of gene expression in normal and malignant lymphocytes. *Cold Spring Harbor Symp. Quant. Biol.* 64:71–78

9. Strausberg RL, Buetow KH, Emmert-Buck MR, Klausner RD. 2000. The cancer genome anatomy project: building an annotated gene index. *Trends Genet.* 16:103–6

10. Jaffe ES, Harris NL, Diebold J, Muller-Hermelink HK. 1999. World Health Organization classification of neoplastic diseases of the hematopoietic and lymphoid tissues. A progress report. *Am. J. Clin. Pathol.* 111:S8–12

11. The Non-Hodgkin's Lymphoma Classification Project. 1997. A clinical evaluation of the international lymphoma study group classification of non-Hodgkin's lymphoma. *Blood* 89:3909–18

12. The International Non-Hodgkin's Lymphoma Prognostic Factors Project. 1993. A predictive model for aggressive non-Hodgkin's lymphoma. *N. Engl. J. Med.* 329:987–94

13. Vose JM. 1998. Current approaches to the management of non-Hodgkin's lymphoma. *Semin. Oncol.* 25:483–91

14. Fisher RI, Gaynor ER, Dahlberg S, et al. 1993. Comparison of a standard regimen (CHOP) with three intensive chemotherapy regimens for advanced non-Hodgkin's lymphoma. *N. Engl. J. Med.* 328:1002–6

15. Eisen MB, Spellman PT, Brown PO, Botstein D. 1998. Cluster analysis and display of genome-wide expression patterns. *Proc. Natl. Acad. Sci. USA* 95:14863–68

16. Ma C, Staudt LM. 2001. Molecular definition of the germinal centre stage of B-cell differentiation. *Philos. Trans. R. Soc. London B Biol. Sci.* 356:83–89

17. Lossos IS, Alizadeh AA, Eisen MB, et al. 2000. Ongoing immunoglobulin somatic mutation in germinal center B cell-like but not in activated B cell-like diffuse large cell lymphomas. *Proc. Natl. Acad. Sci. USA* 97:10209–13

18. Bahler DW, Levy R. 1992. Clonal evolution of a follicular lymphoma: evidence for antigen selection. *Proc. Natl. Acad. Sci. USA* 89:6770–74

19. Falini B, Fizzotti M, Pucciarini A, et al. 2000. A monoclonal antibody (MUM1p) detects expression of the MUM1/IRF4 protein in a subset of germinal center B cells, plasma cells, and activated T cells. *Blood* 95:2084–92

20. Angelin-Duclos C, Cattoretti G, Lin KI, Calame K. 2000. Commitment of B lymphocytes to a plasma cell fate is associated with Blimp-1 expression in vivo. *J. Immunol.* 165:5462–71

21. Weller S, Faili A, Garcia C, et al. 2001. CD40-CD40L independent Ig gene hypermutation suggests a second B cell diversification pathway in humans. *Proc. Natl. Acad. Sci. USA* 98:1166–70

22. Klein U, Rajewsky K, Kuppers R. 1998. Human immunoglobulin (Ig)M+IgD+ peripheral blood B cells expressing the CD27 cell surface antigen carry somatically mutated variable region genes: CD27 as a general marker for somatically mutated (memory) B cells. *J. Exp. Med.* 188:1679–89

23. Rai KR, Peterson BL, Appelbaum FR, et al. 2000. Fludarabine compared with

chlorambucil as primary therapy for chronic lymphocytic leukemia. *N. Engl. J. Med.* 343:1750–57

24. Hamblin TJ, Davis Z, Gardiner A, et al. 1999. Unmutated Ig V(H) genes are associated with a more aggressive form of chronic lymphocytic leukemia. *Blood* 94:1848–54

25. Damle RN, Wasil T, Fais F, et al. 1999. Ig V gene mutation status and CD38 expression as novel prognostic indicators in chronic lymphocytic leukemia. *Blood* 94:1840–47

26. Fais F, Ghiotto F, Hashimoto S, et al. 1998. Chronic lymphocytic leukemia B cells express restricted sets of mutated and unmutated antigen receptors. *J. Clin. Invest.* 102:1515–25

27. Rosenwald A, Alizadeh AA, Widhopf GF, et al. 2001. Relation of gene expression phenotype to immunoglobulin mutation genotype in B-cell chronic lymphocytic leukemia. *J. Exp. Med.* In press

28. Johnson TA, Rassenti LZ, Kipps TJ. 1997. Ig VH1 genes expressed in B cell chronic lymphocytic leukemia exhibit distinctive molecular features. *J. Immunol.* 158:235–46

29. Widhopf GF 2nd, Kipps TJ. 2001. Normal B cells express 51p1-encoded Ig heavy chains that are distinct from those expressed by chronic lymphocytic leukemia B cells. *J. Immunol.* 166:95–102

30. Broker BM, Klajman A, Youinou P, et al. 1988. Chronic lymphocytic leukemic (CLL) cells secrete multispecific autoantibodies. *J. Autoimmun.* 1:469–81

31. Sthoeger ZM, Wakai M, Tse DB, et al. 1989. Production of autoantibodies by CD5-expressing B lymphocytes from patients with chronic lymphocytic leukemia. *J. Exp. Med.* 169:255–68

32. Borche L, Lim A, Binet JL, Dighiero G. 1990. Evidence that chronic lymphocytic leukemia B lymphocytes are frequently committed to production of natural autantibodies. *Blood* 76:562–69

33. Aguilar-Santelises M, Mellstedt H, Jondal M. 1994. Leukemic cells from progressive B-CLL respond strongly to growth stimulation in vitro. *Leukemia* 8:1146–52

34. Staudt LM, Dent AL, Shaffer AL, Yu X. 1999. Regulation of lymphocyte cell fate decisions and lymphomagenesis by BCL-6. *Int. J. Immunol.* 18:381–403

35. Cattoretti G, Chang C-C, Cechova K, et al. 1995. Bcl-6 protein is expressed in germinal-center B cells. *Blood* 86:45–53

36. Onizuka T, Moriyama M, Yamochi T, et al. 1995. BCL-6 gene product, a 92- to 98-kD nuclear phosphoprotein, is highly expressed in germinal center B cells and their neoplastic counterparts. *Blood* 86:28–37

37. Allman D, Jain A, Dent A, et al. 1996. BCL-6 expression during B-cell activation. *Blood* 87:5257–68

38. Dent AL, Shaffer AL, Yu X, et al. 1997. Control of inflammation, cytokine expression, and germinal center formation by BCL-6. *Science* 276:589–92

39. Fukuda T, Yoshida T, Okada S, et al. 1997. Disruption of the Bcl6 gene results in an impaired germinal center formation. *J. Exp. Med.* 186:439–48

40. Ye BH, Cattoretti G, Shen Q, et al. 1997. The BCL-6 proto-oncogene controls germinal-centre formation and Th2-type inflammation. *Nat. Genet.* 16:161–70

41. Deweindt C, Albagli O, Bernardin F, et al. 1995. The LAZ3/BCL6 oncogene encodes a sequence-specific transcriptional inhibitor: a novel function for the BTB/POZ domain as an autonomous repressing domain. *Cell Growth Differ.* 6:1495–503

42. Chang CC, Ye BH, Chaganti RS, Dalla-Favera R. 1996. BCL-6, a POZ/zinc-finger protein, is a sequence-specific transcriptional repressor. *Proc. Natl. Acad. Sci. USA* 93:6947–52

43. Seyfert VL, Allman D, He Y, Staudt LM. 1996. Transcriptional repression by the proto-oncogene BCL-6. *Oncogene* 12:2331–42

44. Shaffer AL, Yu X, He Y, et al. 2000.

BCL-6 represses genes that function in lymphocyte differentiation, inflammation, and cell cycle control. *Immunity* 13:199–212

45. Kelsoe G. 1995. In situ studies of the germinal center reaction. *Adv. Immunol.* 60:267–88

46. MacLennan IC. 1994. Germinal centers. *Annu. Rev. Immunol.* 12:117–39

47. Turner CA Jr, Mack DH, Davis MM. 1994. Blimp-1, a novel zinc finger-containing protein that can drive the maturation of B lymphocytes into immunoglobulin-secreting cells. *Cell* 77:297–306

48. Reljic R, Wagner SD, Peakman LJ, Fearon DT. 2000. Suppression of signal transducer and activator of transcription 3-dependent B lymphocyte terminal differentiation by BCL-6. *J. Exp. Med.* 192:1841–48

49. Polyak K, Kato JY, Solomon MJ, et al. 1994. p27Kip1, a cyclin-Cdk inhibitor, links transforming growth factor-beta and contact inhibition to cell cycle arrest. *Genes Dev.* 8:9–22

50. Toyoshima H, Hunter T. 1994. p27, a novel inhibitor of G1 cyclin-Cdk protein kinase activity, is related to p21. *Cell* 78:67–74

51. Papavasiliou FN, Schatz DG. 2000. Cell-cycle-regulated DNA double-stranded breaks in somatic hypermutation of immunoglobulin genes. *Nature* 408:216–21

52. Bross L, Fukita Y, McBlane F, et al. 2000. DNA double-strand breaks in immunoglobulin genes undergoing somatic hypermutation. *Immunity* 13:589–97

53. Staudt LM. 2001. Gene expression physiology and pathophysiology of the immune system. *Trends Immunol.* 22:35–40

54. Roberts CJ, Nelson B, Marton MJ, et al. 2000. Signaling and circuitry of multiple MAPK pathways revealed by a matrix of global gene expression profiles. *Science* 287:873–80

55. Alizadeh A, Eisen M, Botstein D, et al. 1998. Probing lymphocyte biology by genomic-scale gene expression analysis. *J. Clin. Immunol.* 18:373–79

56. Feske S, Giltnane J, Dolmetsch R, et al. 2001. Gene regulation mediated by calcium signals in T lymphocytes. *Nat. Immunol.* 2:316–24

57. Alizadeh AA, Staudt LM. 2000. Genomic-scale gene expression profiling of normal and malignant immune cells. *Curr. Opin. Immunol.* 12:219–25

58. Davis RE, Brown K, Siebenlist U, Staudt LM. 2001. Constitutive NF-κB activity is required for survival of activated B-like diffuse large B-cell lymphoma cells. Submitted

59. Ghosh S, May MJ, Kopp EB. 1998. NF-kappa B and Rel proteins: evolutionarily conserved mediators of immune responses. *Annu. Rev. Immunol.* 16:225–60

Annu. Rev. Med. 2002. 53:319–36

LIPOTOXIC DISEASES

Roger H. Unger

Gifford Laboratories, Touchstone Center for Diabetes Research, Department of Internal Medicine, University of Texas Southwestern Medical Center, Dallas, Texas 75390-8854; Veterans Affairs Medical Center, Dallas, Texas 75216; e-mail: roger.unger@utsouthwestern.edu

Key Words   lipotoxicity, metabolic syndrome, lipoapoptosis, apoptosis, fatty acid homeostasis, ceramide

■ **Abstract**   I review evidence that leptin is a liporegulatory hormone that controls lipid homeostasis in nonadipose tissues during periods of overnutrition. When adipocytes store excess calories as triacylglycerol (TG), leptin secretion rises so as to prevent accumulation of lipids in nonadipose tissues, which are not adapted for TG storage. Whenever leptin action is lacking, whether through leptin deficiency or leptin resistance, overnutrition causes disease of nonadipose tissues with generalized steatosis, lipotoxicity, and lipoapoptosis. Examples of such disorders of liporegulation include generalized lipodystrophies, mutations of leptin and leptin receptor genes, and diet-induced obesity. Lipotoxicity of pancreatic β-cells, myocardium, and skeletal muscle leads, respectively, to type 2 diabetes, cardiomyopathy, and insulin resistance. In humans this constellation of abnormalities is referred to as the metabolic syndrome, a major health problem in the United States. When lipids overaccumulate in nonadipose tissues during overnutrition, fatty acids enter deleterious pathways such as ceramide production, which, through increased nitric oxide formation, causes apoptosis of lipid-laden cells, such as β-cells and cardiomyocytes. Lipoapoptosis can be prevented by caloric restriction, by thiazolidinedione treatment, and by administration of nitric oxide blockers. There is now substantial evidence that complications of human obesity may reflect lipotoxicity similar to that described in rodents.

INTRODUCTION

Obesity has reached epidemic proportions in the United States and threatens to impose unprecedented disease burdens on our population. This review focuses on one physiologic obligation of adipocytes: to protect nonadipocytes from lipid overload during periods of overnutrition and storage of triacylglycerol (TG), the putative cause of the disease consequences of obesity. To fulfill this duty, adipocytes evolved a hormone, leptin (1), which appears to play a vital antisteatotic role (2). I review the evidence that implicates failure of leptin-mediated liporegulation as a major factor in health problems associated with obesity (3–5) and the strategies for their prevention and treatment.

ROLES OF FATTY ACIDS

To understand normal intracellular liporegulation and the liporegulatory diseases that are becoming increasingly prevalent as our population becomes fatter, it is critical to appreciate the obligatory roles of long-chain fatty acids (FA) in all cells— from the most primitive single-cell organisms to the most complex of mammalian cells. The primary, essential role of FA is to form the phospholipid bilayers of the cell membranes and the phospholipid messengers that transmit vital intracellular signals. Without FA there could be no cellular life. A small reservoir of FA, stored in the form of TG (Figure 1*a*), exists in all cells, presumably to maintain the integrity of their membranes and messengers. In the paramecium, for example, the FA species in their intracellular TG reservoir are similar to those of their phospholipid membranes (6), consistent with the idea of a housekeeping role for stored FA. If so, such precious FA stores must somehow have been spared from use as a fuel, and thus conserved for the vital cellular functions (Figure 1*b*). Not until the evolution of adipocytes, which provided a "storage bin" for FA, would it have been practical to employ FA for oxidative metabolism. Prior to this, cellular life was entirely dependent on external food sources.

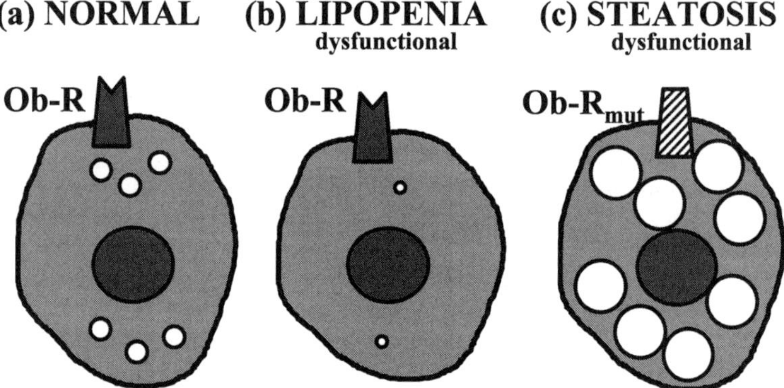

Figure 1   Intracellular fatty acid (FA) homeostasis in nonadipose cells. (*a*) Normal: A small reserve of FA in the form of triacylglycerol (TG) is present for maintenance of phospholipid membranes and messengers. (*b*) Lipopenia: During severe caloric restriction, this TG stockpile may be depleted. The function of certain cells will be compromised unless FA are provided. (*c*) Steatosis: When FA influx into cells exceeds their oxidative requirements, the unoxidized surplus enters pathways of nonoxidative metabolism and TG content rises. Although TG itself may not be harmful to the cells, TG hydrolysis may feed FA into more deleterious nonoxidative pathways, the products of which may result in dysfunction and death of the cells. Since a mutation in the leptin receptor isoform, OB-Rb, can cause steatosis, cells are depicted as having either normal or mutated OB-Rb.

THE ADIPOCYTE

The advent of adipocytes was therefore one of the most transforming of all evolutionary developments. These were the only cells specifically adapted to store large quantities of FA as TG and to release them as a fuel on demand. The adipocyte-bearing species of the world could now roam freely, independently of their food sources, and migrate across barren terrain to fertile areas. Without the evolution of the adipocyte, it is doubtful whether many of today's mammals could have survived the cycles of famine that have always plagued them (7).

THE ENDOCRINOLOGY OF THE ADIPOCYTE

Adipocytes have traditionally been regarded as a passive storage bin for excess calories deposited as TG. They do, in fact, serve as a portable fuel supply system that prolongs survival during famine and provides a ready source of fuel in situations of fight and flight. Today, however, the adipocyte is also recognized as an extremely versatile and complex endocrine gland, in which at least 17 polypeptides have thus far been identified as secretory products of adipocytes and preadipocytes (8, 9). Intuitively, one would imagine that adipocytes are endocrinologically heterogeneous. Indeed, the fact that serum leptin in man is higher in subcutaneous obesity than in visceral obesity (10) suggests that subcutaneous fat has more leptin-expressing adipocytes than visceral fat has. This fact may well explain the familiar clinical fact that lipotoxic complications are more common in visceral obesity (11).

ROLE OF LEPTIN

Initially, it was believed that the role of leptin was to prevent obesity by regulating food intake and thermogenesis via actions on the hypothalamus (11–13). More recent work suggests that, although leptin may indeed influence hypothalamic functions in normal lean animals, it does not prevent obesity in overnourished rodents (14) or humans; indeed, most normal humans and rodents become obese when offered a high-fat/high-carbohydrate diet despite plasma leptin levels that rise (15) within 24 h of the start of overnutrition (2). Evidence that leptin levels above 10 ng/ml, as occur in obese rats, exceed the blood-brain barrier transport threshold (16) suggests that the role of the hyperleptinemia of obesity may be to act directly on peripheral nonadipose tissues throughout the body (17–19), to permit obesity to exist in adipocytes without the deleterious consequences of ectopic FA overload in nonadipose tissues.

If leptin is deficient, or if its target tissues become unresponsive during overnutrition, generalized steatosis will occur (Figure 1c). This leads ultimately to so-called lipotoxicity, i.e., dysfunction of nonadipose tissues such as the pancreatic β-cells (20, 21), myocardium (22), and skeletal muscle (23, 24), and may culminate in FA-induced apoptosis (lipoapoptosis) (21, 25). Just as insulin regulates intracellular glucose homeostasis and thereby prevents glucotoxicity (26), so leptin regulates intracellular FA homeostasis and prevents lipotoxicity.

DISORDERS OF INTRACELLULAR FATTY ACID HOMEOSTASIS: LIPOTOXICITY ("METABOLIC SYNDROME")

When rodents lack leptin action, whether as a consequence of aleptinemia or of leptin resistance, they develop hyperphagia and obesity. Generalized steatosis develops in liver, heart, pancreatic islets, kidneys, skeletal muscle, and perhaps other nonadipose tissues (4). The neutral fat itself is probably relatively innocuous, but it provides an intracellular source of FA in excess of the oxidative needs of the cell. The surplus fatty acyl CoA from this and other sources may enter the nonoxidative metabolic pathways believed to be responsible for lipotoxicity and, ultimately, lipoapoptosis (21, 25) (see below). The net result is the constellation of lipotoxic disorders mentioned above and referred to in humans as the metabolic syndrome X (27, 28). In rodents without leptin or functioning leptin receptors, these manifestations are severe and develop at an early age (6). By contrast, in diet-induced obesity the rate of development of such complications is far more variable than in congenital disorders of liporegulation.

Table 1 provides classification of all known clinical syndromes believed to be the result of ectopic overaccumulation of lipids and lipotoxicity. The adipocyte mass ranges from absent to massive, but the common feature in all of these steatotic syndromes is lack of leptin action.

Genetic Causes of Lipotoxicity

LIPODYSTROPHIES   Generalized congenital lipodystrophy is probably the most severe lipotoxic disorder. The lack of adipose tissue from birth creates a congenital

TABLE 1   Disorders of liporegulation

Disorder	Adipocytes	Leptin action	Tolerance to caloric excess	Lipotoxicity
Congenital generalized lipodystrophy	None	None	None	Very severe
ob/ob	Too many	None	Minimal	Moderately severe
fa/fa	Too many	None	Minimal	Severe
db/db	Too many	None	Minimal	Severe
Diet-induced obesity	Too many	Initially normal but gradually wanes	Variable (good to poor)	Variable (none to severe)

deficiency of leptin, thereby depriving nonadipose tissues of leptin-mediated protection against steatosis (29). Moreover, the voracious appetite secondary to the lack of leptin promotes a mismatch between caloric intake and caloric requirements. Because there is no adipose tissue in which to store the surplus FA, their only destination is nonadipose tissues, where they are esterified to TG or enter lipotoxic pathways. The functional consequences of this become clinically apparent early in life in the form of severe hyperlipidemia, cardiomyopathy, insulin resistance, and diabetes (30, 31), the familiar components of the metabolic syndrome.

MUTATIONS OF THE LEPTIN AND LEPTIN RECEPTOR GENES   In rodents, mutations in the ob gene (3) or in the genes encoding the leptin receptor, OB-R, can cause, respectively, leptin deficiency and leptin unresponsiveness. The *ob/ob* mouse is an example of the former (3), and the *db/db* mouse (32) and the *fa/fa* rat (33, 34) are examples of the latter. These models all exhibit hyperphagia, driven by the lack of leptin action on appetite centers in the hypothalamus (35, 36). In addition, the lack of leptin action on the thermogenic centers in the hypothalamus (11–13) leads rapidly to obesity. In these models, the mismatch between caloric intake and energy expenditure is associated not only with an increase in the adipose tissue mass but also with a progressive increase in lipid deposition in nonadipose tissues as a consequence of the lack of antisteatotic protection. Thus, these unleptinized animals exhibit early in life the full metabolic syndrome, including hyperlipidemia, elevated free FA levels, hepatic steatosis, steatosis of heart, skeletal muscle, and pancreatic islets even on a modest 6% dietary fat intake (6). In normal animals, by contrast, the hyperleptinemia of obesity minimizes TG deposition in nonadipose tissues, even on a high-fat diet (60%) (Figure 2) (4, 37).

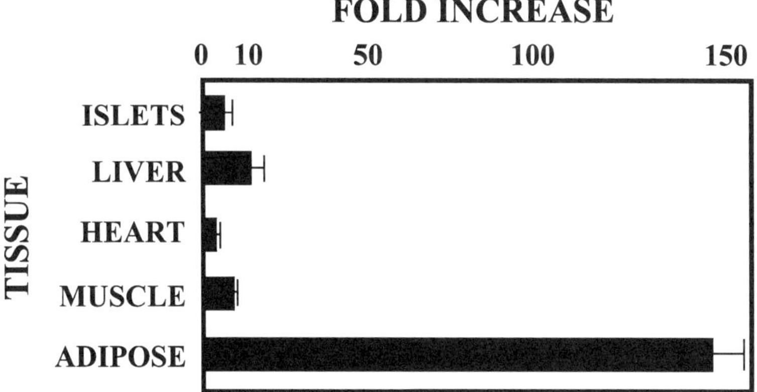

Figure 2   Antisteatotic protection in normal animals. After the feeding of a 60% fat diet for 8 weeks, a 150-fold increase in body fat, estimated by magnetic resonance spectroscopy (MRS), has occurred, but nonadipose tissues exhibit only a minimal rise in their triacylglycerol content.

Similar mutations resulting in leptin deficiency or leptin unresponsiveness have been described in humans (38, 39).

Nongenetic Causes of Lipotoxicity

HIV-1 PROTEASE INHIBITOR-INDUCED LIPODYSTROPHY   Many patients receiving HIV-1 protease inhibitors develop lipodystrophy. This syndrome involves a redistribution of body fat (40, 41) rather than the near-total loss of fat observed in congenital generalized lipodystrophy. The magnitude of the ectopic lipid deposition and its disease consequences in a given patient may depend, in large part, on the quantity of residual adipose tissue and the food intake. If the orexigenic effect of hypoleptinemia is attenuated by the severe underlying illness, mismatch between caloric intake and expenditure may be minimized, in which case lipotoxic complications in peripheral tissues will be prevented. Nevertheless, cardiomyopathy, insulin resistance, and diabetes have been reported in a substantial number of such patients.

DIET-INDUCED OBESITY   With more than half of Americans now regarded as overfed and overweight (42), diet-induced obesity may well be the most common of all American diseases. A progressive rise in body weight began in the United States soon after the end of World War II, at which time high-fat, high-carbohydrate foods were aggressively promoted and made easily available, whereas physical activity decreased as a result of the introduction of sedentary technologies. This combination of environmental changes provided the optimal recipe for a national epidemic of obesity.

Initially, in diet-induced obesity, a progressive rise in plasma leptin levels (4) permits the storage of large quantities of fat in adipose tissues without pathogenically significant ectopic fat deposition in nonadipose tissues. Ultimately, however, resistance to the antisteatotic action of leptin appears to occur. Although its cause is not understood, it could well be age-related, since severe leptin resistance occurs in normal nonobese aging rodents (43). The same may occur in humans; whereas young humans exhibit a strong correlation between body fat and plasma leptin, in middle-aged and elderly humans, the ages in which the complications of obesity are most likely to develop, the correlation is lost (44).

IS LEPTIN REALLY AN ANTISTEATOTIC HORMONE?

Teleologically, the idea that leptin functions as an antisteatotic hormone rather than an antiobesity hormone is consistent with both evolutionary considerations and actual clinical observations; however, it is as yet not generally accepted.

Recently, evidence favoring an antisteatotic role for leptin has been obtained (2). In normal rats fed a high-fat diet (60%), plasma concentration of leptin rises within 24 h and increases progressively in remarkable correlation with the increase in body fat, consistent with an antisteatotic function (Figure 3*a*). As shown in Figure 2, on a 60% fat diet, lipid deposition in heart, liver, islets, and skeletal muscle rises only minimally, despite the massive 150-fold expansion of adipocyte fat. By contrast, in rodents lacking leptin action, either because of leptin deficiency or nonfunctional leptin receptors, nonadipose tissues rapidly accumulate abnormal quantities of lipids even on a normal fat intake (6%) (Figure 3*b*). Finally, in Zucker Diabetic Fatty (ZDF) rats with nonfunctional leptin receptors, transfer by adenovirus of the normal full-length leptin receptor gene (*OB-Rb*) to the liver keeps the hepatic TG content below that of the controls (Figure 3*c*), but has no effect on the TG content of other tissues (2). These results, summarized in Figure 3, compellingly support the premise that a major function of the hyperleptinemia induced by overnutrition is to protect nonadipose tissues from lipid overaccumulation.

MECHANISMS OF INTRACELLULAR OVERACCUMULATION OF LIPIDS IN UNLEPTINIZED TISSUES

Increased Lipogenesis

The lipid excess observed in the islets of ZDF (*fa/fa*) rats is largely the result of increased lipogenesis, although decreased FA oxidation also contributes (45, 46). Whereas in normal animals FA enter nonadipose tissues as required to meet their oxidative requirements (Figure 4*a*; see color insert), in underleptinized animals this relationship is impaired and FA are present in excess of needs (Figure 4*b*). A major source of the surplus is the elevation in plasma levels of free FA and TG. At high concentrations, FA may enter cells by "flip-flopping" across the lipid bilayers (47), rather than through the FA transporters that provide facilitated uptake at lower levels (48, 49). Additionally, FA are released from the high levels of circulating lipoproteins, flooding these cells with FA far in excess of their oxidative needs (50).

A second cause of the increased lipid content of unleptinized islets is increased de novo FA synthesis from glucose. Unleptinized islet cells overexpress a battery of proteins involved in FA synthesis: sterol regulatory element binding protein (SREBP)-1c (51) and peroxisome proliferator-activated receptor (PPAR)-γ, crucial lipogenic transcription factors, and their lipogenic target enzymes, acetyl CoA carboxylase (ACC), fatty acid synthetase (FAS), liver-type fatty acyl CoA synthase (L-ACS), and glycerol phosphate acyl transferase (GPAT) (46). When leptin action is lacking, de novo lipogenesis in nonadipose tissues is inappropriately high, irrespective of FA availability.

Decreased Compensatory β-Oxidation of Fatty Acids

When normal islets are exposed to a surplus of FA, FA oxidation rises above the actual oxidative needs of the cell (Figure 5*a,b*). This compensatory oxidation is probably triggered by the FA themselves, which serve as a ligand for PPARγ

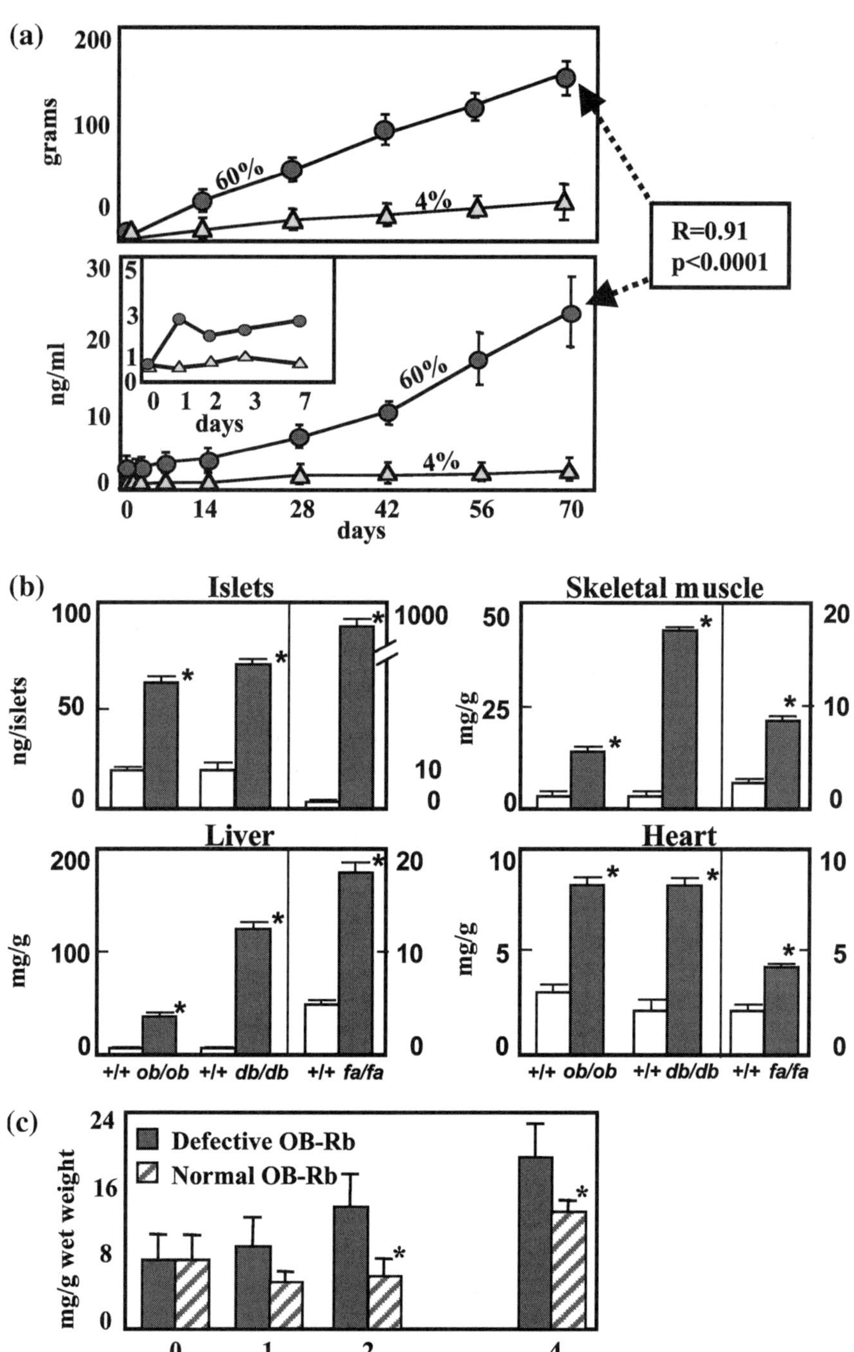

(a)
grams
200
100
0
60%
4%
R=0.91
p<0.0001
30
20
10
0
ng/ml
5
3
1
0
0 1 2 3 7
days
60%
4%
0 14 28 42 56 70
days
(b)
Islets
100
50
0
ng/islets
1000
10
0
*
*
*
Skeletal muscle
50
25
0
mg/g
20
10
0
*
*
*
Liver
200
100
0
mg/g
20
10
0
*
*
*
Heart
10
5
0
mg/g
10
5
0
*
*
*
+/+ ob/ob   +/+ db/db   +/+ fa/fa
(c)
24
16
8
0
mg/g wet weight
Defective OB-Rb
Normal OB-Rb
*
*
0 1 2 4
Time post-treatment (weeks)

(52–54) and thereby increase expression of its target enzymes of FA oxidation, carnitine palmitoyl transferase 1 (CPT-1) and ACO (55). Thus, the oxidative machinery for disposal of the excess is upregulated. Recently, however, the key role of the lipogenic enzyme, ACC-2, which catalyzes the production of malonyl-CoA in FA oxidation, has become increasingly apparent (56); McGarry et al. discovered in 1978 that its product, malonyl CoA, inhibits long-chain FA oxidation by suppressing CPT-1 activity (57). Thus, deletion (56) or inhibition of ACC-2 (58) will, by reducing malonyl CoA, increase CPT-1 activity and raise the rate of FA oxidation; this strategy can be tested as a means of reducing body fat. Leptin lowers ACC mRNA in association with increased expression of UCP-2 (59), which implies that the leptin-dependent compensatory oxidation generates heat rather than ATP. When the leptin receptor is defective from birth, as in ZDF *fa/fa* rats, 1 mM FA fails to elicit compensatory oxidation (55). Failure of FA to suppress appropriately the high levels of lipogenic enzymes, ACC and FAS, results in a progressive intracellular accumulation of FA and their nonoxidative metabolites (Figure 5*c*). This seriously compromises cellular function, leading to apoptosis via mechanisms discussed below. Exciting new work points to inhibitors of ACC and FAS as promising drugs for preventing obesity (60, 61).

MECHANISMS OF LIPOAPOPTOSIS

When compensatory oxidation of excess FA fails, the FA surplus must ultimately enter pathways of nonoxidative metabolism. Initially, TG appear to be the major lipid product, but they probably do little to the cell. Ultimately, however, hydrolysis of the TG stores will increase the already expanded FA pool, providing additional substrate for nonoxidative FA metabolism (Figure 5*c*). In pancreatic islet cells (21) and in cardiac myocytes (22), the ceramide pathway seems to be the most important

---

Figure 3   (*a*) Relationship of body fat (*upper panel*), measured by magnetic resonance spectroscopy, and plasma leptin (*lower panel*) concentration in normal rats fed a diet containing either 4% or 60% fat. The prompt rise in leptin at the start of overnutrition and the high degree of correlation between the two are consistent with an antisteatotic role for the hormone. (*b*) Comparison of triacylglycerol (TG) content of nonadipose tissues in normal rodents and rodents with leptin deficiency resulting from a mutation in the leptin gene (*ob/ob* mice) or with a loss-of-function mutation in the leptin receptor gene (*db/db* mice and *fa/fa* rats). All animals were on a diet containing only 6% fat (i.e., 10% of the fat content fed to normal rats in Figure 2). $p < 0.001$. (*c*) Effect on hepatic steatosis of adenovirus transfer of the gene encoding a functional leptin receptor (OB-Rb) to the livers of obese *fa/fa* ZDF rats with loss-of-function mutations in their OB-Rb. There was a reduction of TG in livers expressing normal OB-Rb. Steatosis in other tissues was unaffected (data not shown). $p < 0.05$. (From Reference 2 with permission.)

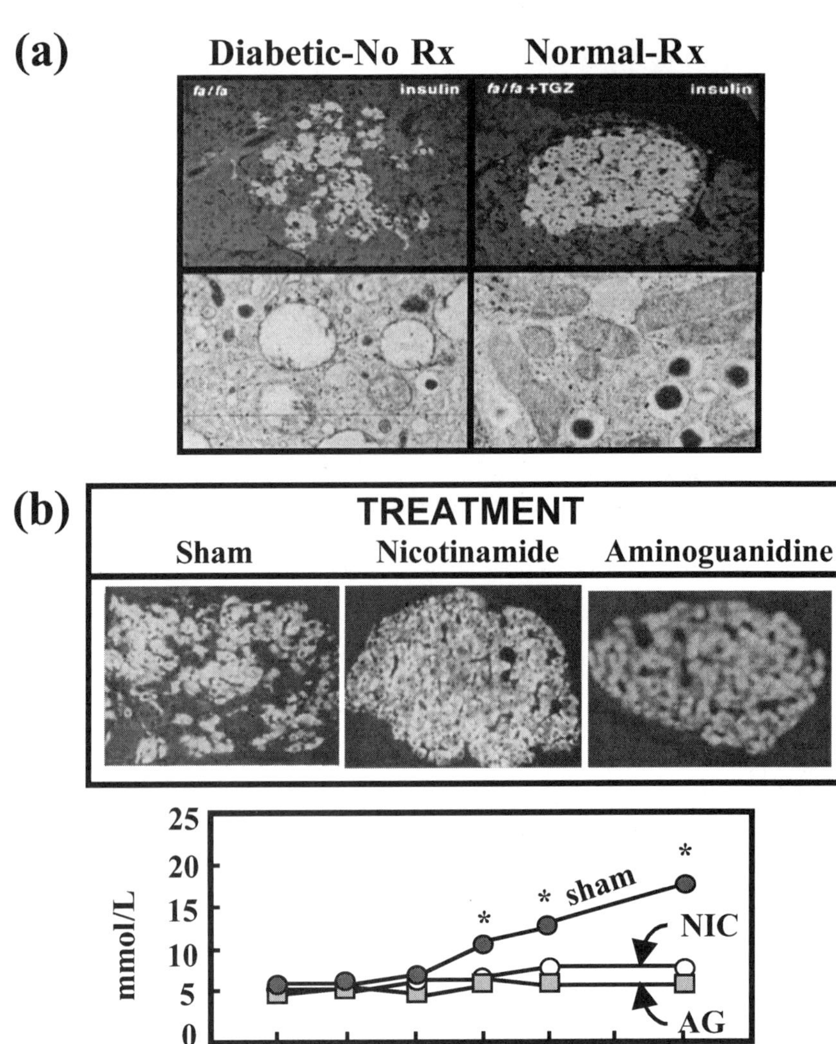

Figure 5   Effects of 7 weeks of TGZ treatment of obese ZDF (*fa/fa*) rats compared with untreated littermates. (*a*) Effects of TGZ treatment on insulin-positive β-cells (*upper panels*) and electron microscopy appearance of mitochondria (*lower panels*). (*b*) Effects of iNOS inhibitory therapy for 6 weeks. Immunofluorescent staining of pancreas of sham-, NIC- and AG-treated obese *fa/fa* ZDF rats and on blood glucose levels of obese prediabetic *fa/fa* ZDF rats compared to untreated + controls. Values represent the mean ± SEM of three to six animals. Significant differences are marked as follows: $p < 0.05$ vs. untreated lean *fa/+* ZDF group. (From References 22 and 69 with permission.)

(a) NORMAL (FA) HOMEOSTASIS

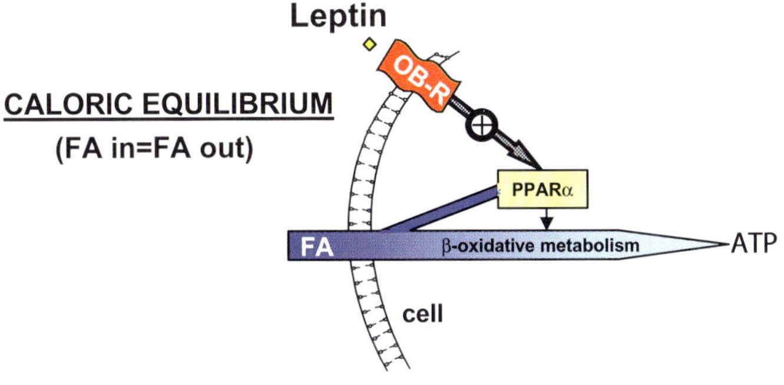

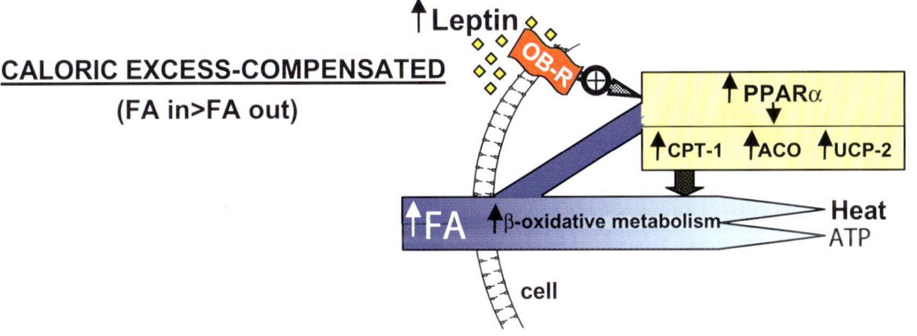

See text page C-2

(b) UNCOMPENSATED CALORIC EXCESS

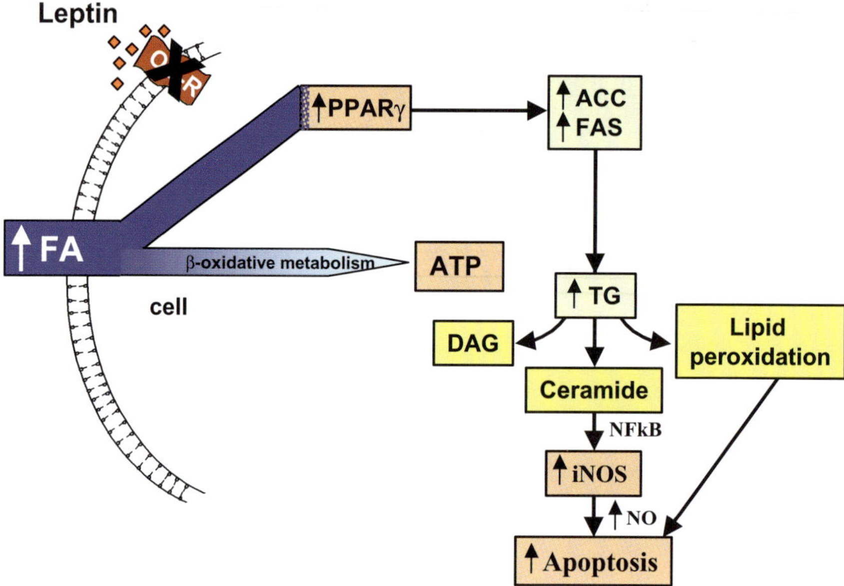

Figure 4 (*a*) Normal fatty acid (FA) homeostasis in nonadipose tissues. Caloric equilibrium: FA supplied and FA used in nonadipose tissues are equal, leaving no unoxidized FA.
Compensated caloric excess: During caloric excess, the FA supply to nonadipose tissues
may exceed their oxidative needs; however, upregulation of PPARα, the transcription factor for enzymes of FA oxidation (CPT-1 and ACO) will promote compensatory oxidation
of the surplus FA, and the unneeded energy will be dissipated as heat, thanks to upregulation of uncoupling protein (UCP)-2. This compensatory system requires the presence of
leptin and a normal leptin receptor (OB-R). (*b*) Uncompensated caloric excess: In the
absence of leptin or its receptor OB-R, hyperphagia results in a caloric intake exceeding
caloric requirements. FA storage occurs not only in adipocytes but also in nonadipocytes,
causing lipotoxicity. Since PPARα expression is reduced and PPARγ increased, the surplus FA influx presumably binds to the latter, which increases transcription of the
lipogenic enzymes ACC and FAS. This causes increased nonoxidative FA metabolism and
lipoapoptosis.

of the deleterious routes (62), although alternative pathways have not been excluded. When leptin action is lacking, the enzyme serine palmitoyl transferase (SPT) (63) is expressed at high levels (64), thereby increasing the condensation of palmitoyl CoA and serine to form dihydrosphingosine, the first step in de novo ceramide biosynthesis (Figure 5c). In the pancreatic β-cells of untreated leptinless *fa/fa* ZDF rats, profound mitochondrial alterations (Figure 6a) (65) and apoptosis appear. Apoptosis is believed to result from excessive ceramide formation coupled with underexpression of the antiapoptotic factor, Bcl$_2$ (66). This does not exclude the possibility that other pathways of lipotoxicity dominate in other tissues (67).

Preventing Lipotoxicity

Any maneuver that reduces ectopic deposition of lipid appears to prevent lipotoxicity, including caloric restriction (68) and thiazolidinedione (TZD) treatment (65). In islets, it decreases SPT expression and upregulates Bcl$_2$ (66), changes that reduce ceramide formation and prevent apoptosis. In vivo treatment of prediabetic *fa/fa* ZDF rats with the TZD troglitazone prevents the overaccumulation of lipids, mitochondrial degeneration, and apoptosis in the islets (Figure 6a) (65); it also prevents all changes in the heart (22). Treatment with inhibitors of inducible nitric oxide synthase (iNOS) both in vivo and in vitro prevents apoptosis in islets of ZDF rats. In vivo treatment protects them from diabetes (Figure 6b) (69), suggesting that iNOS upregulation by FA and high levels of NO production may be a factor in the apoptosis.

NATURAL HISTORY OF LIPOTOXIC DISEASES

Lipotoxic β-Cell Disease

In the ZDF (*fa/fa*) rat, the onset of obesity occurs at $\sim$4 weeks of age. The pattern of β-cell response to the lipid overload is biphasic. Initially, as intraislet lipid content rises from normal to $\sim$10$\times$ normal, there is increased proliferation of β-cells and a fourfold increase in β-cell mass, along with increased secretion of insulin (70, 71) (Figure 7a). The hyperinsulinemia is secondary to the increased number of β-cells due to enhanced replication. This means that, in these islets, insulin release at basal and even subbasal levels of glucose is far above normal. This combination of changes provides sufficient insulin production to maintain normoglycemia in the face of rising insulin resistance and thus to compensate for it (Figure 7a).

As this prediabetic stage of obesity progresses in the ZDF *fa/fa* rats, the intraislet lipid content rises even further (Figure 7b). The β-cells that are the most lipid-laden develop severe mitochondrial alterations, and there is an approximately tenfold increase in DNA laddering, signifying a marked increase in apoptosis (65). At this stage the rate of apoptosis must exceed the rate of β-cell replication, since there is a net loss of β-cells (Figure 7c) and a decline in insulin production to below the

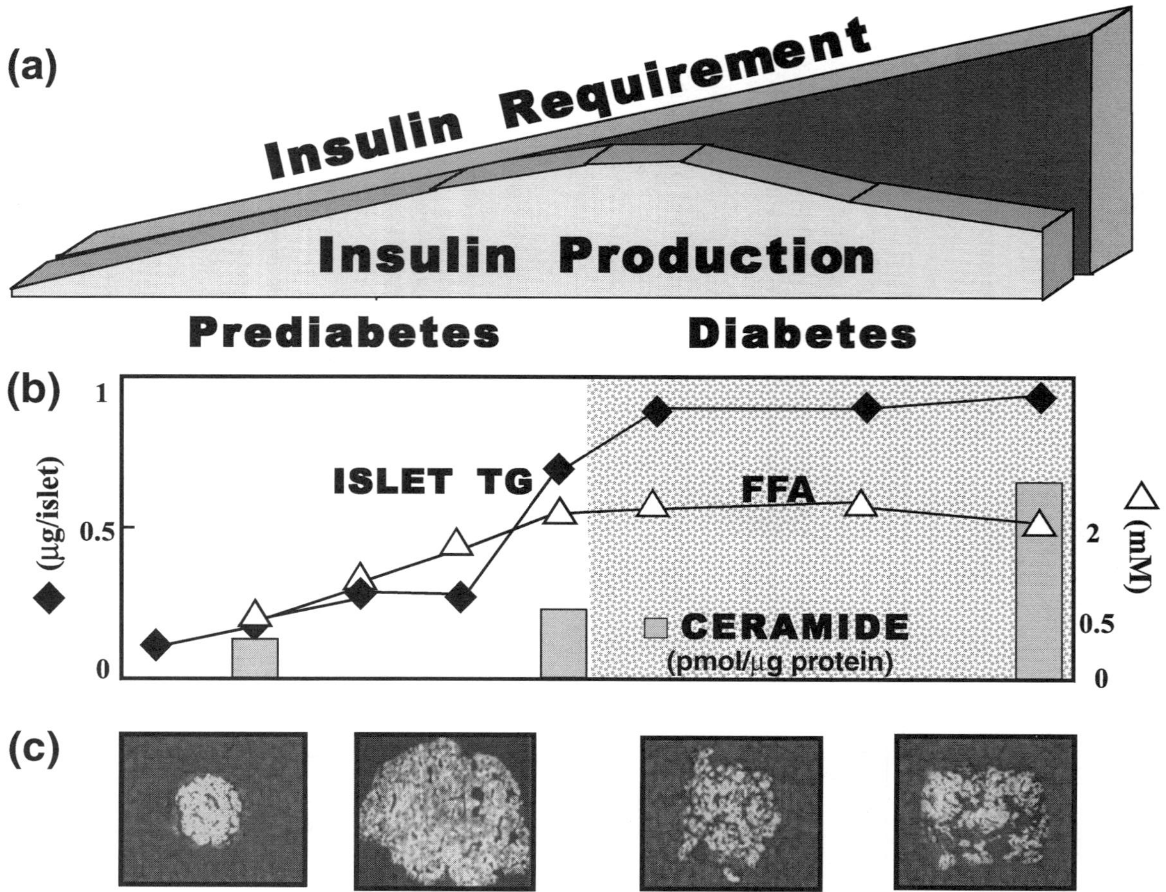
(a)
Insulin Requirement
Insulin Production
Prediabetes
Diabetes
(b)
1
(µg/islet)
ISLET TG
FFA
(mM)
0.5
2
CERAMIDE
(pmol/µg protein)
0.5
0
0
(c)

levels required to compensate for insulin resistance (Figure 7*a*) (4). With insulin resistance continuing to increase, overt diabetes appears. Ultimately, the mass of β-cells recedes to approximately the level it had maintained during the preobese stage of the disease, i.e., the fourfold increase in β-cell mass observed during the compensated stage of β-cell hyperplasia disappears (Figure 7*c*).

Lipotoxic Heart Disease

The ectopic deposition of lipids in ZDF *fa/fa* rats appears to be a generalized phenomenon not limited to any particular organ. It is not surprising, therefore, that lipotoxic changes in their islets are paralleled by lipotoxic changes in their heart. As the obese ZDF *fa/fa* animals age from 7 weeks to 20 weeks, they develop echocardiographic evidence of impaired myocardial contractility (Figure 7*a*) (22). This functional loss has been ascribed to gradual loss of cardiomyocytes through apoptosis; indeed, DNA laddering, an index of apoptosis, is more than 7 times that of wild-type controls at 7 weeks of age, even though contractility still appears normal (Figure 7*b*). However, at 20 weeks of age, when laddering is approximately 30 × that of wild-type controls, contractility has declined to less than 50% of controls (Figure 7*a*) (22), almost certainly a consequence of progressive dropout of myocardial cells. Myocardial TG content is significantly increased above control values at 7 weeks of age and it rises progressively thereafter (Figure 7*c*). A statistically significant increase in ceramide content (Figure 7*c*) suggests that this product of nonoxidative FA metabolism may be involved in the myocardial apoptosis (22). Similar conclusions were drawn from a mouse model of lipotoxic cardiomyopathy, in which myocardiocyte-specific overexpression of acyl-CoA synthase caused an increase in cardiac TG and ceramide and resulted in lipid cardiomyopathy (67).

Remarkably, treatment of obese ZDF rats with troglitazone, beginning at 7 weeks of age, prevents these changes. It reduces myocardial TG, measured both biochemically and by morphometry of lipid droplets. It also lowers ceramide content and prevents the loss of contractile function of the heart (Figure 7) (22). These findings imply that the protective effect of troglitazone on cardiac function is mediated by its antisteatotic effect, which lowers ceramide and lipoapoptosis.

Figure 6   The natural history of lipotoxic disease of islets in obese ZDF (*fa/fa*) rats. (*a*) Relationship between insulin resistance and insulin production from 4 weeks to 12 weeks of age. Parallelism between the two maintains normoglycemia despite the mounting insulin resistance secondary to the obesity. By about 12 weeks of age, insulin production no longer keeps pace with the insulin resistance and overt diabetes begins. (*b*) The relationships between plasma FFA (*white*) and the TG content of islets (*black*) and ceramide content (*gray*). (*c*) The appearance of islets stained for insulin during a 16-week observation, showing at left a perfectly normal islet in the preobese phase of the disorder, a hyperplastic islet during the obese, prediabetic (compensated) phase of the disorder, and severely damaged islet depleted of insulin-staining cells in rats with overt diabetes. (From Reference 4 with permission.)

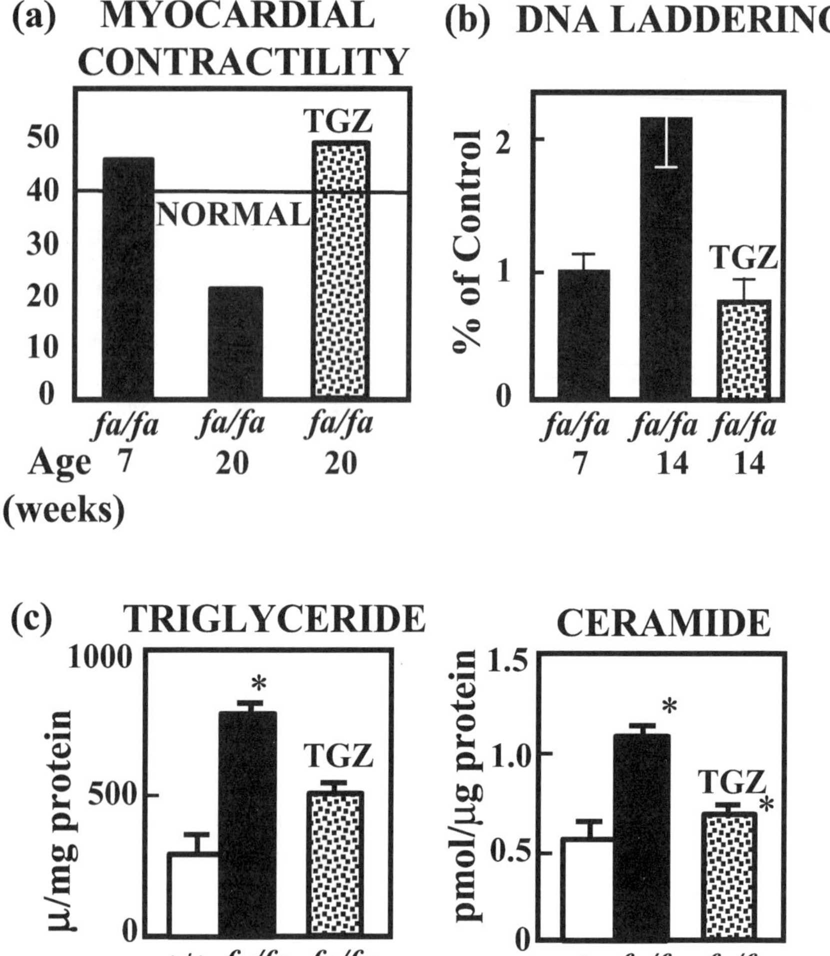

Figure 7   (*a*) Quantification of myocardial contractility, showing functional loss in 20-week-old *fa/fa* rats prevented by treatment with the antisteatotic drug troglitazone (TGZ). (*b*) DNA laddering, an index of apoptosis, is increased in heart of obese *fa/fa* ZDF rats at age 14 weeks. The increase in laddering and the loss of contractility are entirely blocked by treatment of the rats for 6 weeks with TGZ, beginning at 7 weeks of age. Data are expressed as fold change from the 7-week-old baseline in *fa/fa* rats, which is 10× that of lean +/+ rats at that age. (*c*) Cardiac triacylglycerol (TG) and ceramide content of 14-week-old ZDF (*fa/fa*) rats and wild-type controls (+/+). There is a statistically significant increase in both TG and ceramide content. TGZ treatment for 6 weeks significantly reduces TG and ceramide content toward normal. $p < 0.01$.

Thus, at least in ZDF rats, metabolic abnormalities associated with their heart disease mimic to a remarkable degree those observed in their islets, and in both organs the metabolic changes and functional evidence of disease can be completely prevented by the antisteatotic agent troglitazone.

Do Obese Humans Develop Lipotoxicity?

Again, there is no proof that complications of a monogenic disorder of intracellular lipid homeostasis in the ZDF rodent model of obesity reflect the islet and cardiac abnormalities associated with diet-induced, nongenetic human obesity and its metabolic syndrome. Nevertheless, it would be prudent to assume that they are the same until proven otherwise, because (*a*) there are clinical similarities between rodent lipotoxicity and the human metabolic syndrome; (*b*) half of the American population now classified as overweight is at high risk for developing components of the metabolic syndrome; (*c*) cardiac lipotoxicity is currently unrecognized by American clinicians as a clinical entity, despite abundant evidence that cardiac steatosis does occur (71–73); (*d*) thiazolidinediones prevent both type 2 diabetes and cardiac lipotoxicity in obese ZDF rats, suggesting that lipotoxic complications in the heart and islets of obese humans could be prevented if treated early; and (*e*) the work of L. S. Szczepaniak, R. L. Dobbins, G. Metzger, and R. G. Victor (personal communication) indicates that myocardial fat can now be estimated noninvasively using nuclear magnetic resonance.

These facts justify a rigorous survey to determine if human cardiac lipotoxicity really exists and, if so, whether currently available drugs, such as a nontoxic thiazolidinedione, would arrest its progression. A careful study of this issue now seems imperative to develop effective strategies to cope with what could well turn out to be this nation's most prevalent heart disease.

Visit the Annual Reviews home page at www.AnnualReviews.org

LITERATURE CITED

1. Zhang Y, Proenca R, Mafei M, et al. 1994. Positional cloning of the mouse obese gene and its human homologue. *Nature* 372: 425–32

2. Lee Y, Wang M-Y, Kakuma T, et al. 2001. Liporegulation in diet-induced obesity. The antisteatotic role of hyperleptinemia. *J. Biol. Chem.* 276:5629–35

3. Unger RH, Zhou Y-T, Orci L. 1999. Regulation of fatty acid homeostasis in cells: novel role of leptin. *Proc. Natl. Acad. Sci. USA* 96:2327–32

4. Unger RH, Orci L. 2001. Diseases of liporegulation: new perspective on obesity and related disorders. *FASEB J.* 15:312–21

5. Unger RH. 2000. Leptin physiology: a second look. *Regul. Pep.* 92:87–95

6. Hennessey TM, Andrews D, Nelson DL. 1983. Biochemical studies of the excitable membrane of *Paramecium tetraurelia*. VII. Sterols and other neutral lipids of cells and cilia. *J. Lipid Res.* 24:575–87

7. Neel J-V. 1999. The "thrifty genotype" in 1998. *Nutr. Rev.* 57:S2–9

8. Ahima RS, Flier JS. 2000. Adipose tissue as an endocrine organ. *Trans. Endocrinol. Metab.* 11:327–32

9. Ailhaud G. 2000. Adipose tissue as an endocrine organ. *Int. J. Obes. Relat. Metab. Disord.* (Suppl. 2):S1–3

10. Minocci A, Savia G, Lucantoni R, et al. 2000. Leptin plasma concentrations are dependent on body fat distribution in obese patients. *Int. J. Obes. Relat. Metab. Disord.* 24:1139–44

11. Halaas JL, Gajiwaia KS, Maffel M, et al. 1995. Weight-reducing effects of the plasma protein encoded by the obese gene. *Science* 269:543–46

12. Pelleymounter MA, Cullen MJ, Baker MB, et al. 1995. Effects of the obese gene product on body weight regulation in *ob/ob* mice. *Science* 269:540–43

13. Campfield LA, Smith FJ, Guisez Y, et al. 1995. Recombinant mouse OB protein: evidence for a peripheral signal linking adiposity and central neural networks. *Science* 269:546–49

14. Surwit RS, Edwards CL, Murthy S, Peters AE. 2000. Transient effects of long-term leptin supplementation in the prevention of diet-induced obesity in mice. *Diabetes* 49:1203–8

15. Caro JF, Sinha MK, Roslaczynski JW, et al. 1996. Leptin: the tale of an obesity gene. *Diabetes* 45:1455–62

16. Wang Z-W, Zhou Y-T, Kakuma T, et al. 1999. Comparing the hypothalamic and extrahypothalamic actions of endogenous hyperleptinemia. *Proc. Natl. Acad. Sci. USA* 96:100373–78

17. Shimabukuro M, Koyama K, Chen G, et al. 1997. Direct antidiabetic effect of leptin through triglyceride depletion of tissues. *Proc. Natl. Acad. Sci. USA* 94:4637–41

18. Wang M-Y, Koyama K, Shimabukuro M, et al. 1998. OB-Rb gene transfer to leptin-resistant islets reverses diabetogenic phenotype. *Proc. Natl. Acad. Sci. USA* 95:714–18

19. Wang M-Y, Koyama K, Shimabukuro M, et al. 1998. Overexpression of leptin receptors in pancreatic islets of Zucker diabetic fatty rats restores GLUT-2, glucokinase and glucose-stimulated insulin secretion. *Proc. Natl. Acad. Sci. USA* 95:11921–26

20. Lee Y, Hirose H, Ohneda M, et al. 1994. β-cell lipotoxicity in the pathogenesis of non-insulin-dependent diabetes mellitus of obese rats: impairment in adipocyte-β-cell relationships. *Proc. Natl. Acad. Sci. USA* 91:10878–82

21. Shimabukuro M, Zhou Y-T, Levi M, Unger RH. 1998. Fatty acid-induced β-cell apoptosis: a link between obesity and diabetes. *Proc. Natl. Acad. Sci. USA* 95:2498–502

22. Zhou Y-T, Grayburn P, Karim A, et al. 2000. Lipotoxic heart disease in obese rats: implications for human obesity. *Proc. Natl. Acad. Sci. USA* 97:1784–89

23. McGarry JD. 1992. What if Minkowski had been ageusic? An alternative angle on diabetes. *Science* 258:766–70

24. Koyama K, Chen G, Lee Y, Unger RH. 1997. Tissue triglycerides, insulin resistance and insulin production: implications for hyperinsulinemia of obesity. *Am. J. Physiol.* 273:E708–13

25. Shimabukuro M, Zhou Y-T, Lee Y, Unger RH. 1998. Troglitazone lowers islet fat and restores β-cell function of Zucker diabetic fatty rats. *J. Biol. Chem.* 273:3547–50

26. Unger RH, Grundy S. 1985. Hyperglycaemia as an inducer as well as a consequence of impaired islet cell function and insulin resistance: implications for the management of diabetes. *Diabetologia* 28:119–21

27. Reaven GM. 1993. Role of insulin resistance in human disease (syndrome X): an expanded definition. *Annu. Rev. Med.* 44:121–31

28. Reaven GM. 1995. Pathophysiology of insulin resistance in human disease. *Physiol. Rev.* 75:473–86

29. Shimomura I, Hammer RE, Ikemoto S, et al. 1999. Leptin reverses insulin resistance and diabetes mellitus in mice with congenital lipodystrophy. *Nature* 401:73–76

30. Seip M, Trygstad O. 1996. Generalized lipodystrophy, congenital and acquired (lipoatrophy). *Acta Paediatr. Suppl.* 413: 2–28

31. Bjornstad PG, Foerster A, Ihlen H. 1996. Cardiac findings in generalized lipodystrophy. *Acta Paediatr. Suppl.* 413:39–43

32. Lee GH, Proenca R, Montez JM, et al. 1996. Abnormal splicing of the leptin receptor in diabetic mice. *Nature* 379:632–35

33. Iida M, Murakami T, Ishida K, et al. 1996. Substitution at codon 269 (glutamine?proline) of the leptin receptor (OB-R) cDNA is the only mutation found in the Zucker fatty (*fa/fa*) rat. *Biochem. Biophys. Res. Commun.* 224:597–604

34. Phillips MS, Liu Q, Hammond HA, Dugan V, Hey PJ, et al. 1996. Leptin receptor missense mutation in the fatty Zucker rat. *Nat. Genet.* 13:18–19

35. Stephens T, Baskinski M, Bristow PK, et al. 1995. The role of neuropeptide Y in the antiobesity action of the obese gene product. *Nature* 377:530–32

36. Vaisse C, Halaas JL, Horvath CM, et al. 1996. Leptin activation of Stat 3 in the hypothalamus of wild-type and *ob/ob* mice but not *db/db* mice. *Nat. Genet.* 14:95–97

37. Unger RH, Zhou Y-T. 2001. Lipotoxicity of β-cells in obesity and in other causes of fatty acid spillover. *Diabetes* 50(Suppl. 1):S118–21

38. Montague T, Farooqi IS, Whitehead JP, et al. 1997. Congenital leptin deficiency is associated with severe early-onset obesity in humans. *Nature* 387:903–8

39. Clement K, Vaisse C, Lahlou N, et al. 1998. A mutation in the human leptin receptor gene causes obesity and pituitary dysfunction. *Nature* 392:398–401

40. Madge S, Kinloch-de-loes S, Mercey D, et al. 1999. Lipodystrophy in patients naïve to HIV protease inhibitors. *AIDS* 13:735–37

41. Kakuda TN, Brundich RC, Anderson PL, Fletcher CV. 1999. Nucleocide reverse transcriptase inhibitor-induced mitochondrial toxicity as an etiology for lipodystrophy. *AIDS* 13:2311–12

42. Spiegelman DM, Flier JS. 2001. Obesity and irregulation of energy balance. *Cell* 104:531–43

43. Wang Z-W, Pan W-T, Lee Y, et al. 2001. The role of leptin resistance in the lipid abnormalities of aging. *FASEB J.* 15:108–14

44. Moller N, O'Brien P, Nair KS. 1998. Disruption of the relationship between fat content and leptin levels with aging in humans. *J. Clin. Endocrinol. Metab.* 83:931–34

45. Lee Y, Hirose H, Zhou Y-T, et al. 1997. Increased lipogenic capacity of the islets of obese rats. A role in the pathogenesis of NIDDM. *Diabetes* 46:408–13

46. Zhou Y-T, Shimabukuro M, Lee Y, et al. 1998. Enhanced *de novo* lipogenesis in the leptin-unresponsive pancreatic islets of prediabetic Zucker diabetic fatty rats. Role in the pathogenesis of lipotoxic diabetes. *Diabetes* 47:1904–8

47. Hamilton JA. 1998. Fatty acid transport: difficult or easy? *J. Lipid Res.* 39:467–81

48. Abumrad N, Harmon C, Ibrahimi A. 1998. Membrane transport of long-chain fatty acids: evidence for a facilitated process. *J. Lipid Res.* 39:2309–18

49. Hirsch D, Stahl A, Lodish HF. 1998. A family of fatty acid transporters conserved from mycobacterium to man. *Proc. Natl. Acad. Sci. USA* 95:8625–29

50. Kim JK, Fillmore JJ, Chen Y, et al. 2001. Tissue specific overexpression of lipoprotein lipase causes tissue specific insulin resistance. *Proc. Natl. Acad. Sci. USA* 98:7522–27

51. Kakuma T, Lee Y, Higa M, et al. 2000. Leptin, troglitazone and the expression of sterol regulatory element binding proteins in liver and pancreatic islets. *Proc. Natl. Acad. Sci. USA* 97:8536–41

52. Keller H, Dreyer C, Medin J, et al. 1993. Fatty acids and retinoids control lipid metabolism through activation of peroxisome proliferator-activated receptor-retinoid X receptor heterodimers. *Proc. Natl. Acad. Sci. USA* 90:2160–64

53. Kliewer SA, Forman BM, Blumberg B, et al. 1994. Differential expression and activation of a family of murine peroxisome proliferator-activated receptors. *Proc. Natl. Acad. Sci. USA* 91:7355–59

54. Schoonjans K, Staels B, Auwerx J. 1996. The peroxisome proliferator-activated receptors (PPARs) and their effects on lipid metabolism and adipocyte differentiation. *Biochim. Biophys. Acta* 1302:93–109

55. Zhou Y-T, Shimabukuro M, Wang M-Y, et al. 1998. Role of peroxisome proliferator-activated receptor α in disease of pancreatic β-cells. *Proc. Natl. Acad. Sci. USA* 95:8898–903

56. Abu-Elheiga L, Matzuk MM, Abo-Hashema KAH, Wakil SJ. 2001. Continuous fatty acid oxidation and reduced fat storage in mice lacking acetyl-CoA carboxylase 2. *Science* 291:2613–16

57. McGarry JD, Mannaerts GP, Foster DW. 1977. A possible role for malonyl-CoA in the regulation of hepatic fatty acid oxidation and ketogenesis. *J. Clin. Invest.* 60:265–70

58. Henin N, Vincent MF, Gruber HE, Van den Berghe G. 1995. Inhibition of fatty acid and cholesterol synthesis of AMP-activated protein kinase. *FASEB J.* 9:541–46

59. Ricquier D, Bouillaud F. 2000. The uncoupling protein homologues: UCP-1, UCP-2, UCP-3, StUCP and AtUCP. *Biochem. J.* 345:161–79

60. Bergeron R, Previs SF, Cline GW, et al. 2001. Effect of 5-aminoimidazole-4-carboxamide-1-β-D-ribofuranside infusion on *in vivo* glucose and lipid metabolism in lean and obese Zucker rats. *Diabetes* 50:1076–82

61. Loftus TM, Jaworsky DE, Frehywot GL, et al. 2000. Reduced food intake and body weight in mice treated with fatty acid synthase inhibitors. *Science* 288:2379–81

62. Obeid LM, Linardic CM, Karolak LA, Hannun YA. 1993. Programmed cell death induced by ceramide. *Science* 259:1769–71

63. Weiss B, Stoffel W. 1997. Human and murine serine-palmitoyl-COA transferase: cloning, expression and characterization of the key enzyme in sphingolipid synthesis. *Eur. J. Biochem.* 249:239–47

64. Shimabukuro M, Higa M, Zhou Y-T, et al. 1998. Lipoapoptosis in β-cells of obese prediabetic *fa/fa* rats. Role of serine palmitoyltransferase overexpression. *J. Biol. Chem.* 273:32487–90

65. Higa M, Zhou Y-T, Ravazzola M, et al. 1999. Troglitazone prevents mitochondrial alterations, β-cell destruction and diabetes in obese prediabetic rats. *Proc. Natl. Acad. Sci. USA* 96:11513–18

66. Shimabukuro M, Wang M-Y, Zhou Y-T, et al. 1998. Protection against lipoapoptosis of β-cells through leptin-dependent maintenance of Bcl-2 expression. *Proc. Natl. Acad. Sci. USA* 95:9558–61

67. Chiu HC, Kovaks A, Ford BA, et al. 2001. Novel mouse model of lipotoxic cardiomyopathy. *J. Clin. Invest.* 107:813

68. Ohneda M, Inman LR, Unger RH. 1995. Caloric restriction in obese pre-diabetic rats prevents beta-cell depletion, loss of beta-cell GLUT-2 and glucose incompetence. *Diabetologia* 38:173–79

69. Shimabukuro M, Ohneda M, Lee Y, Unger RH. 1997. Role of nitric oxide in obesity-induced β-cell disease. *J. Clin. Invest.* 100:290–95

70. Milburn JL, Hirose H, Lee YH, et al. 1995. Pancreatic β-cells in obesity: evidence for induction of functional, morphologic and metabolic abnormalities by increased long-chain fatty acids. *J. Biol. Chem.* 270:1295–99

71. Alexander JK. 1985. The cardiomyopathy of obesity. *Prog. Cardiovasc. Dis.* 27:325–34

72. Alpert MA, Hashimi MW. 1993. Obesity and the heart. *Am. J. Med. Sci.* 306:117–23

73. Alpert MA. 2001. Obesity cardiomyopathy: pathophysiology and evolution of the clinical syndrome. *Am. J. Med. Sci.* 321:225–36

Annu. Rev. Med. 2002. 53:337–54

DIRECTIONS OF DRUG DISCOVERY IN OSTEOPOROSIS

Gregory R. Mundy
*Department of Medicine/Endocrinology, University of Texas Health Science Center,
7703 Floyd Curl Drive, San Antonio, Texas 78229-3900; e-mail: mundy@uthscsa.edu*

Key Words   osteoporosis, statins, leptin, bone growth factors, bisphosphonates

■ **Abstract**   Osteoporosis is a condition of increasing importance and prevalence in all parts of the world and particularly in Asia. Recent advances have led to the introduction of effective drugs that decrease bone resorption and stabilize bone mass. However, these drugs have been identified by serendipity rather than rational drug design and are not ideal because of limited bioavailability, mode of administration, or other unwanted effects. There is still a place for even more suitable and effective resorption inhibitors than those currently available. The more compelling need in this field is an acceptable drug that is anabolic for bone, that safely and acceptably increases bone mass and improves the disturbances in bone microarchitecture that characterize established and advanced osteoporosis. Possible approaches to identifying more effective resorption inhibitors and new anabolic agents are discussed.

INTRODUCTION

Osteoporosis is one of the most common conditions in the aging population and is certain to become even more common in the next 50 years. The availability of new therapies has markedly changed the management of this condition in the past 20 years. As a group, patients treated with the most effective antiresorptive agents for several years can expect a 50% reduction in fracture rate. However, current therapy is not ideal, and the individual patient with advanced disease may see little benefit. Despite the need for better therapeutic agents, there are many hurdles for pharmaceutical companies attempting to get new drugs to the market in this area.

An ideal agent for patients with established osteoporosis would inhibit osteoclastic bone resorption and stimulate new bone formation. No known therapeutic agent convincingly achieves both effects. The currently available resorption inhibitors (estrogen and related compounds, bisphosphonates, and calcitonin) have negligible to very modest effects on bone formation over prolonged periods. As a consequence, they may prevent further bone loss and stabilize bone mass but do not substantially increase bone mass. Currently, no acceptable bone formation stimulator is widely available.

0066-4219/02/0218-0337$14.00   **337**

NEW APPROACHES TO RESORPTION INHIBITION

Modifications of Existing Drugs

Three classes of bone resorption inhibitors are currently used extensively to treat or prevent osteoporosis. These are estrogen, calcitonin, and the bisphosphonates. Estrogen has been used for over 50 years, although evidence for its efficacy dates back only about 20 years. Estrogen reverses the accelerated phase of bone loss associated with the postmenopausal period, and it is helpful even if used for the first time 20 or more years after the menopause. Unfortunately, not all women will accept estrogen therapy, and in many it is contraindicated. Only 30%–40% of the patients who should be taking estrogen will in fact take it. In the next few years, the contraindications for estrogen therapy will continue to be clarified and hopefully reduced. Modes of administration such as transdermal patches that limit unwanted side effects hold promise, but their use has not been as widespread as hoped (1).

Estrogen's exact mode of action to inhibit bone resorption remains unclear. During the past 10 years, the effects of estrogen to regulate production of cytokines such as interleukin (IL)-6, IL-1, and tumor necrosis factor (2–6) have been demonstrated, and functional estrogen receptors in osteoclasts confirmed (7). Whether the major effects of estrogen on bone are direct or indirect remains unclear at this time.

Over the past 10 years, much attention has focused on an interesting series of compounds known as antiestrogens, and several companies are now actively involved in the development of compounds in this category. These compounds are now more widely known as selective estrogen response modifiers (SERMs). Theoretically, the ideal antiestrogen would have all the beneficial effects of estrogen on bone and on the cardiovascular system, including appropriate lowering of blood lipids, without the deleterious effects of estrogen on the uterus and the breast. Although some of these compounds clearly fit this category, the status of others remains unclear. The potential market is enormous, potentially even greater than the current estrogen market in postmenopausal women. The forerunner of this group of drugs is raloxifene. It has become the gold standard against which other antiestrogens are compared, since it was the first to be evaluated for this use (8) and so far seems to be the most effective.

The molecular mechanism by which SERMs can exert estrogen-like effects in some tissues and antiestrogen-like effects in others is not clear (9). Interactions between the estrogen receptor, which is a transcription factor for estrogen-target proteins, and its ligands, as well as its downstream gene targets, are still being unraveled (10, 11). There are a number of levels for potential specificity. One of these is at the receptor itself, with different domains that may be differentially activated in different tissues. In part, this may be associated with coactivator and suppressor proteins involved in estrogen receptor action (12). However, the involvement of the different estrogen receptors and these associated proteins in the antiestrogen effects is unknown.

SERMs cannot be considered as one class but probably represent novel and distinct compounds with different molecular actions. Raloxifene has been clearly shown to prevent bone loss, reduce fracture rates, and lower serum cholesterol in ovariectomized rats without any uterotrophic activity (8). The effects on bone and lipids are most likely comparable to those of estrogen. Estrogen and related compounds enhance TGFβ production in bone cells. Yang et al. (13) believe that raloxifene (and possibly other related compounds) may have a preferential effect on TGFβ III in bone.

Calcitonin is not as effective as estrogen or the bisphosphonates as an inhibitor of osteoclastic bone resorption. It has not been widely used in the United States but has very large markets in Japan, where estrogens are not popular, and in Italy. The use of intranasal preparations has improved patient acceptability, although expense remains a problem. Moreover, calcitonin's effects on inhibition of bone resorption may be transient and its effects to increase bone mass are modest.

The bisphosphonates are now established as agents of first choice for use in osteoporosis, as well as for other causes of increased bone resorption. Etidronate in short-term studies was initially thought to improve fracture risk (14), although its effects on bone mass are very modest, like those of other resorption inhibitors. Newer bisphosphonates (most notably alendronate and risedronate) are more potent and less toxic, and their usefulness, particularly in situations where estrogen cannot be used, is now well-established. Bisphosphonates have been reviewed extensively in recent years, particularly for their use in osteoporosis (14a).

The flavanoids, in particular ipriflavone, have received considerable attention recently as inhibitors of bone resorption, especially in Italy and Japan. These orally active compounds have been tested experimentally in Paget's disease of bone, primary hyperparathyroidism, and osteoporosis. They inhibit bone resorption by mechanisms that are not entirely clear, and both clinical and experimental studies indicate that their effects on bone resorption are relatively modest (either as resorption inhibitors or formation stimulators) (15). Ipriflavone has been used in patients in Europe with promising effects on markers of bone turnover, although no data on effects on fracture rate are available as yet (16). A recent study reported in preliminary form showed no effect (17).

During the next few years, continued efforts will be made to improve the efficacy of current bone resorption inhibitors. In the case of calcitonin, this will mean improvements in the mode of administration by, for example, intranasal aerosols or rectal suppositories. Transdermal estrogen patches avoid the first-pass effect of the liver and reduce estrogenic side effects, since estradiol concentration can be maintained in the systemic circulation using a very low dosage (18). Current experience suggests that transdermal estrogens may be preferable to oral estrogen, offering the same benefits for bone but avoiding some undesirable metabolic effects by circumventing the hepatic first pass effect. Although it seems unlikely that bisphosphonates will be improved, it is possible that better understanding of their mechanism of action will allow identification of even more suitable resorption inhibitors (see below).

Identification of New Resorption Inhibitors

Although current resorption inhibitors are effective, they are far from ideal. The beneficial effects of the currently available resorption inhibitors on bone resorption were discovered by serendipity rather than by rational drug discovery and development. However, as information on the cellular and molecular mechanisms involved in bone resorption accumulates, it may be possible to develop more rational therapeutic approaches to inhibiting osteoclast function (19, 20). For example, it is now realized that several tyrosine kinases are essential for both normal osteoclast formation and osteoclast action. The colony-stimulating factor-1 (CSF-1) receptor, also known as the c-fms oncogene, is a receptor tyrosine kinase (21–23). The src proto-oncogene, which is required for normal osteoclast ruffled-border formation, is a nonreceptor tyrosine kinase that may be inhibited by certain low-molecular-weight compounds such as the antibiotic herbimycin A (24, 25). Recently, several pharmaceutical and biotechnology companies have developed large programs to identify low-molecular-weight inhibitors of the src tyrosine kinase for their potential in treating osteoporosis. Recent studies have shown that a number of adhesion proteins [peptide (25a), small molecule (25b)] are important for normal osteoclastic bone resorption. Integrin antagonists have been evaluated as resorption inhibitors, and several appear promising. Selectivity of the effects and absence of toxicity will remain issues. These antagonists effectively bind the $\alpha_4\beta_3$ integrin and not only block bone resorption by osteoclasts in vitro but also prevent bone loss in ovariectomized rats. These proteins depend on the availability of arginine-glycine-aspartic acid (RGD) sequences in attachment proteins (26). Peptide antagonists for RGD sequences may be effective inhibitors of osteoclastic bone resorption. Similarly, other cytoskeletal inhibitors may be useful in treating enhanced osteoclast activity. Recent research has clarified the molecular mechanisms by which protons are generated within osteoclasts and then pumped across the ruffled border. These mechanisms involve carbonic anhydrase isoenzyme type II as well as a complex vacuolar ATPase that represents the osteoclast proton pump. Inhibitors of both the proton pump mechanism and carbonic anhydrase have been identified, and these agents inhibit osteoclastic bone resorption in vitro. Finally, proteolytic enzymes responsible for bone matrix degradation during osteoclastic bone resorption, including an array of lysosomal enzymes as well as collagenase, may be inhibited by different agents (27, 28). Cathepsin K is a critical cysteine protease involved in osteoclastic bone resorption, and it has been purified and characterized in osteoclasts (28a,b). Small molecule compounds that inhibit this enzyme could be promising approaches to new bone resorption inhibitors.

Antagonists to RANK ligand, the central cytokine involved in osteoclastic bone resorption, are extremely powerful inhibitors of bone resorption, the most powerful yet described. Two of these are being evaluated as potential pharmacologic agents, namely osteoprotegerin, the endogenous decoy receptor for RANK ligand, and a soluble antagonist to RANK, which comprises the extracellular domain of the receptor. These compounds are both peptide antagonists, and to enhance their pharmacokinetic acceptability, they have been linked to a fragment of the human immunoglobulin molecule to form a chimeric hybrid compound (called RANK.Fc in the case of the RANK antagonist). These agents are likely to be effective in osteoporosis (28c), but since they are peptides, they are not likely to be successful for chronic diseases such as osteoporosis. On the other hand, they may be very helpful in situations that call for a more short-acting and powerful effect, such as hypercalcemia or osteolysis associated with cancer (28d).

Osteopetrosis provides an ideal model for identifying drug targets for screening antiresorptive agents for osteoporosis. Osteopetrosis results when gene defects or deficiencies cause specific impairment of osteoclastic resorption. There are a number of murine models, and in each case where the molecular mechanism has been characterized, it is clear that this particular molecular mechanism is required for normal osteoclastic resorption. It therefore provides a molecular target for high-throughput screening. The various murine examples of osteopetrosis may involve either an impairment in osteoclast formation or a defect in osteoclast action. The best example of the latter is targeted disruption of the src proto-oncogene (24, 29). There are many examples of osteoclast formation impairment, occurring at different stages in the osteoclast lineage. The ideal molecular target is one that involves an impairment of osteoclast formation or function but does not involve the monocyte-macrophage lineage, and therefore is likely to lead to inhibition of important monocyte/macrophage functions. Disruption of genes such as NF-κB and PU.1 are more likely to lead to disruption of earlier cells in the lineage, whereas specific defects in osteoclast mediators such as RANK ligand expression disrupt cells later in the osteoclast-lineage (30).

However, the utility of these approaches and techniques notwithstanding, the critical issue for pharmaceutical companies is the investment involved in developing a new antiresorptive agent. The costs of drug discovery and development in this arena are so high that many companies will consider the costs are not worth the potential reward.

Bisphosphonate Modes of Action

The molecular mechanism by which bisphosphonates inhibit osteoclast function has been clarified considerably in recent years. This increased understanding of how these drugs mediate their effects raises the possibility of identifying even better drugs that use this same molecular mechanism. The bisphosphonates are clearly efficacious and relatively free from side effects, but their pharmacokinetics and poor oral absorption are major problems, since <5% of any dose administered is absorbed and patients are required to take elaborate precautions to optimize absorption.

Recently, several groups have shown that bisphosphonates affect osteoclasts by inhibiting farnesyl diphosphate synthase, an enzyme in the cholesterol biosynthesis pathway that enhances prenylation of small GTP-containing proteins and thereby is important in osteoclast cytoskeletal function and possibly other activities

(31–33). Inhibition of this enzyme leads to impairment of osteoclastic resorption. Thus, farnesyl diphosphate synthase is a potential target for further drug discovery, since drugs that inhibit this enzyme and have more suitable pharmacokinetic properties without deleterious side effects would be superior to the bisphosphonates. Farnesyl diphosphate synthase appears to be an ideal molecular target to which a high-throughput screening system could be devised, and defined chemical libraries and collections of natural products could be screened using this target to identify suitable drug candidates.

Such an approach would be taken by a pharmaceutical company only if calculations showed that the costs involved in drug discovery and development would make it a profitable exercise. One of the major disadvantages for the osteoporosis field is that the costs and time involved in identifying new agents and bringing them through the development pipeline are so great that these calculations are critical for any company to embark on such a venture.

STIMULATORS OF BONE FORMATION

In aging patients with osteoporosis, there is a decrease in osteoblast function characterized by an impairment in the capacity of osteoblasts to completely fill in the defects left by osteoclastic resorption with new bone. Bone histomorphometrists call this "decreased mean wall thickness" (34). The agents known to have a stimulatory effect on new bone formation are fluoride, low-dose intermittent parathyroid hormone, and the peptide growth factors.

Current Anabolic Agents

By anabolic agents, bone histomorphometrists mean agents that directly or indirectly stimulate osteoblasts to increase their bone-forming activity.

FLUORIDE   Fluoride has been widely used in the treatment of postmenopausal osteoporosis for many years. It has always been a controversial drug because many physicians have doubted its efficacy and have been concerned by the frequency of side effects, particularly the risk of increased bone fragility. This issue remains unresolved. New preparations such as monofluorophosphate and slow-release sodium fluoride may reduce some of these side effects. However, most investigators remain unconvinced by the available data that fluoride therapy in nontoxic doses reduces vertebral fracture rates.

Fluoride therapy undoubtedly increases bone formation. These effects are seen predominantly in spinal trabecular bone rather than cortical bone. The mechanism by which fluoride stimulates bone formation is not clear. One group has suggested that fluoride acts directly on bone cells to inhibit the activity of an osteoblast acid phosphatase that is responsible for the dephosphorylation of tyrosine kinases (35, 36). Such an effect would enhance tyrosine kinase activity and potentially enhance the effects of growth factor to cause proliferation of bone cells. An alternative theory, proposed by Burgener et al. (37), is that fluoride increases tyrosine kinase activity in osteoblasts, and this effect is potentiated by small amounts of aluminum (38). Although bone formation dramatically increases in response to fluoride therapy, the new bone may be structurally abnormal when higher doses are used. Fluoride is incorporated into the mineral phase of bone. Newly formed bone frequently shows evidence of mineralization defects. Bone tends to be spongy and irregular and mineralizes poorly. If supplemental oral calcium and vitamin D are given along with fluoride, this mineralization defect does not occur.

Fluoride therapy increases bone mass in the vertebrae in approximately 70% of osteoporotic patients. Bone mass is increased by 10% per year as measured by bone mineral density. Thus, increase is both dramatic and progressive without a plateau. Similar effects are not produced by any other current form of therapy. The responses may be even greater when assessed by quantitative computerized tomography. Many uncontrolled studies have reported the benefits of fluoride therapy. However, randomized, controlled studies show that there may be an increased risk of fractures in the appendicular skeleton, and fracture rates are unchanged in the vertebrae (39, 40). This has led to considerable skepticism regarding the benefits of fluoride. Some investigators (40a) attribute these negative results to an excessive dose of fluoride in these studies and recommend lower doses or alternative forms of therapy, including slow-release sodium fluoride and sodium monofluorophosphate.

In recent years, investigators have emphasized the formulation of fluoride used. Three different preparations of fluoride have been studied: sodium fluoride, sodium monofluorophosphate, and slow-release sodium fluoride. The latter two are associated with fewer gastrointestinal side effects and are probably safer compounds than sodium fluoride. The bioavailability of the preparation is important because the therapeutic window for fluoride is very narrow (41, 42). The use of concomitant oral calcium and vitamin D is necessary to prevent osteomalacia. Although there have been claims that slow-release fluoride has far superior beneficial effects (43), the U.S. Food and Drug Administration has remained unconvinced, and no fluoride preparation has been approved for osteoporosis.

LOW-DOSE PARATHYROID HORMONE   Parathyroid hormone (PTH), when administered intermittently and in low doses, has long been known to have an anabolic or bone-forming effect in rodents, dogs, and humans (44). This anabolic effect is probably mediated by the production of peptide bone growth factors such as insulin-like growth factor I and transforming growth factor β by bone cells in response to PTH (45). In contrast, when PTH is administered continuously in high doses, the major effect is an increase in bone turnover, with a prominent increase in osteoclastic bone resorption. The effect seems to occur predominantly on cancellous bone in the axial skeleton. Studies have been in progress for some years to determine if the anabolic effect of PTH can be therapeutically useful in patients with osteoporosis (46–48). Several pharmaceutical companies have developmental programs with PTH, parathyroid hormone-related peptide (PTHrP), or synthetic analogs as potential anabolic agents. The anabolic effect of PTH may be enhanced by a concomitant administration of 1,25-dihydroxyvitamin D. Current data suggest that beneficial effects in patients may plateau after several years and then decline, particularly in cortical bone.

Unresolved issues concerning PTH therapy include the long-term effects on cortical bone, the optimal timing and dosage schedule, the need for concomitant administration of 1,25-dihydroxyvitamin D, whether the effects are mediated through the same receptor responsible for osteoclastic bone resorption, and whether the anabolic effects can be mimicked by oral agents. The status of PTH as a potential therapeutic agent has been reviewed (49), and the potential for PTH-rP or analogs (50) has been summarized (51).

STRONTIUM RANELATE   Strontium ranelate, potentially both a resorption inhibitor and formation stimulator, has recently been receiving attention (51a). Its effects in preclinical studies appear promising (51b), but its precise molecular mechanism of action is entirely unknown. It is now undergoing phase III studies.

PEPTIDE GROWTH FACTORS   In recent years, increased understanding of the peptide growth regulatory factors in bone that control the cellular events of bone formation has led to the real possibility that these factors may be potential drugs for stimulating bone growth in patients with bone loss. Although this area of study is still very young, sufficient progress has been made in recent years to suggest that the introduction of such agents in the relatively near future is not so far-fetched.

Nevertheless, many potential problems are associated with the use of peptide growth factors in the therapy of osteoporosis. The obvious major problem is that of delivery. Because all the peptide growth factors are potent peptides with short half-lives, they must be administered parenterally, a serious limitation to their use in patients with chronic diseases such as osteoporosis. Moreover, most of the peptide growth factors identified so far affect the functions of many cells outside bone. Consequently, systemic administration could well lead to deleterious side effects such as hypoglycemia (for IGF-I) or fibrosis due to mesenchymal cell proliferation (TGFβ). This suggests that their usefulness may be limited to local administration unless they can be targeted to bone (for example, by linking them to bone-seeking bisphosphonates) or unless low-molecular-weight compounds are developed that could be administered orally but could modulate their local production in the bone cell microenvironment. Statins (see below) exert their effects on bone formation via this latter mechanism.

Identification of New Anabolic Agents for Bone

In the identification of an anabolic agent that will stimulate bone formation and be useful for treating patients with established osteoporosis, the first step is to select a molecular target that is critical to bone formation and that can be readily regulated such that the consequence is osteoblast proliferation, differentiation, and the formation by maturing osteoblasts of a differentiated and normal mineralized bone matrix. Without a suitable target, further work is likely to be fruitless. If an appropriate target is identified, then all further steps should be rather routine should the resources for high-throughput screening and medicinal chemistry be available.

SELECTION OF A MOLECULAR TARGET   Less is known about the specific genes involved in controlling bone formation by osteoblasts than is known about the parallel process of osteoclastic bone resorption. Nevertheless, in recent years, substantial advances in our understanding of the process of bone formation have occurred. For example, a critical transcription factor expressed uniquely by osteoblasts and centrally involved in osteoblast differentiation has been identified. This transcription factor, CBFA1, is a member of the runt family. Absence of expression leads to complete impairment of bone formation, although there is normal development of a cartilage skeleton as well as normal patterning (52–54). CBFA1, therefore, is an ideal potential target for controlling the process of osteoblast differentiation and bone formation.

Other recently identified transcription factors could also be important. For example, overexpression of Fra-1 or ^{a}FosB, two members of the BP-1 subfamily of leucine zipper-containing transcription factors, cause generalized increases in bone formation in vivo (55, 56). However, this review focuses on growth regulatory factors that are important in bone formation.

The normal process of bone formation on endosteal bone surfaces follows bone resorption and occurs specifically at resorption sites. Bone formation begins with chemotaxis of osteoblast precursors to sites of resorption defects, followed by proliferation of these precursors to form a team of maturing osteoblasts. With further maturation, the osteoblasts form cells capable of laying down a mineralized bone matrix, expressing the structural proteins of the bone matrix, and then mineralizing this bone matrix. This is a prolonged process that is highly coordinated with other events occurring in the bone microenvironment, and it is obviously under the control of powerful growth regulatory factors. Most of these factors are incorporated into the bone matrix, are released in active form when bone is resorbed (57), and are available locally to control all the events involved in bone formation. Current evidence suggests that these growth factors are released as a cascade to initially control osteoblast precursor proliferation and chemotaxis, possibly apoptosis of osteoclasts, and ultimately osteoblast differentiation. Specific growth factors have unique and defined roles in this cascade.

Unique among these growth factors are the bone morphogenetic proteins (BMPs). Although they are members of the transforming growth factor β (TGFβ) superfamily, their effects on osteoblasts are very different from those of TGFβ. The BMPs enhance osteoblast differentiation, whereas TGFβ stimulates osteoblast proliferation but decreases differentiation. Current evidence suggests that TGFβ is more important in the early events of osteoblast function than during the process of bone formation, whereas the BMPs are involved later.

Over the past 10 years, we have characterized in particular the BMP-2 and BMP-4 promoters, identified response elements and response regions in these promoters, and characterized their effects in normal osteoblast differentiation (57a). We found that BMP-2 acts as an autocrine factor in osteoblast proliferation. For example, BMP-2 is expressed by differentiating normal osteoblasts (58); it enhances its own expression (59). BMP-2 stimulates osteoblast differentiation (59) and is required for osteoblast differentiation (58). This is shown by experiments in which osteoblast differentiation can be impaired by rendering osteoblasts unresponsive to BMP-2 through the use of mutant BMP receptors or antagonists such as noggin. Thus, BMP-2 is an autocrine factor that controls osteoblast differentiation as well as enhancing the expression of the structural proteins of the bone matrix, such as type-1 collagen, osteopontin, osteocalcin, and bone sialoprotein. It also enhances the expression of the transcription factor CBFA1 and stimulates osteoblast proliferation.

This expanding body of information on BMP-2 has been utilized to explore the stimulation of its expression as a potential target for enhancing osteoblast differentiation, based on the premise that small molecules that enhance BMP-2 expression by osteoblasts would promote bone formation. The extraordinarily complex BMP-2 promoter has been characterized. It contains several transcription start sites. Using the $-2736/+114$ region of the left prime flanking region of the BMP-2 gene, we developed a cell-based screening assay in which this region of the murine BMP-2 gene is stably transfected into osteoblasts linked to the firefly luciferase reporter gene, and screened an extensive library of defined chemical compounds, as well as a natural products collection (60).

STATINS AS POTENTIAL ANABOLIC AGENTS   Among the natural products, the statins, compounds that inhibit the enzyme 3-hydroxy-3-methylglutaryl coenzyme A reductase (HMG Co-A reductase), the first step in cholesterol biosynthesis, were identified as specific stimulators of the BMP-2 promoter. A series of counterscreens using other promoters such as serum response element and the cytomegalovirus promoter were also examined. The BMP-4 promoter showed that the effects of statins on the BMP-2 promoter were specific.

Next, the capacity of statins to stimulate bone formation was tested. The most potent of the newer statins, both as inhibitors of HMG Co-A reductase and stimulators of bone formation, were atorvastatin and cerivastatin, which were several orders of magnitude more potent in their effects on bone than mevastatin, lovastatin, simvastatin, or fluvastatin. The only statin in which there was no effect was pravastatin, a synthetic compound that does not exist in the prodrug (closed ring or lactone) form. Pravastatin is less lipophilic than the other statins, and this property may be responsible for its lack of efficacy on bone cells.

Our initial tests found that statins increased bone formation when cultured with explants of neonatal murine calvaria. Each of the statins caused a marked increase in osteoblast accumulation and new bone formation in doses of 1–5 μM over 4–7 days of bone organ culture. The effect was even more obvious when the bones were exposed to statins for only 6 h and the cultures were examined 12 days later.

The effects of statins were also tested on bone in vivo. In the first series of experiments, they were injected into the subcutaneous tissue over the murine calvaria and examined the effects on the underlying bone. There was a 30%–60% increase in cortical bone width after only 5 days' exposure to lovastatin and simvastatin, similar to the effects of recombinant human BMP-2 and recombinant human fibroblast growth factor (FGF)-1 applied in this manner (61). There were no stimulatory effects on osteoclasts, which are readily detectable in this assay.

Finally, statins' effects in normal intact rats and in rat models of osteoporosis were tested. These models included rats that were ovariectomized at the time of statin administration (modeling the perimenopausal woman) as well as rats that had been ovariectomized several months before statins were administered (modeling the older woman with established osteoporosis). In each case, the statins were administered orally for one month.

Following 35 days of administration of lovastatin or simvastatin by oral gavage in doses of 5–10 mg/kg body weight/day, there was a marked increase in trabecular bone area in both intact and ovariectomized rats associated with increases in bone formation and mineral apposition rate. Similar effects were found whether rats were ovariectomized at the time of statin administration or had been ovariectomized for several months. The treated animals also showed a decrease in osteoclast numbers, suggesting that the statins may have reduced bone resorption.

More recently, we attempted to determine how statins stimulate the BMP-2 promoter. It is apparent that there is a perfect correlation between the potency of statins as inhibitors of HMG Co-A reductase and their capacity to stimulate BMP-2 expression and bone formation. Moreover, the addition of mevalonate and other downstream metabolites of the mevalonate pathway to bone organ cultures to which statins have been added inhibits the effects of statins on bone formation and BMP-2 transcription. These two lines of evidence suggest that the mechanisms by which statins stimulate bone formation is mediated through HMG Co-A reductase. However, they do not show how HMG Co-A reductase inhibition enhances BMP-2 expression. Statins are known to affect other biological processes through effects not mediated by changes in serum cholesterol. In ischemic stroke, statins mediate their effects through enhanced production of eNOS mRNA and ultimately impairment of prenylation of GTP-containing proteins. Similar mechanisms are probably present in bone cells, because specific inhibitors of eNOS block the effects of statins on bone formation, whereas statins enhance nitric oxide generation and eNOS expression at the protein and mRNA levels (61a). Further studies will be necessary to show the mechanism by which they stimulate BMP-2 expression in bone.

However, it is clear that statins mediate their effects on bone formation by enhanced BMP-2 expression. Transgenic mice that are unresponsive to BMP-2 by means of a truncated mutant BMP type 1B receptor targeted to the osteoblast lineage do not respond to BMP-2 or lovastatin but respond normally to acidic FGF (62), which was determined by utilizing the local calvarial injection technique

(60). This indicates the critical role of the BMP-2 signal transduction pathway for statin effects on bone.

Carefully marketed statins are poorly delivered to the periphery because they have been selected by their capacity to be extracted by the liver to inhibit cholesterol biosynthesis. Many of them are also subject to first-pass metabolism in the liver whereby they become inactive metabolites. To bypass the liver, the effects of topical application of statins to rats have been examined. When statins are administered topically, blood levels of statin are higher and are maintained longer with less variability. These results are typical of mechanisms that bypass first-pass metabolism. These higher statin levels in the blood are paralleled by increased biological effects on bone. Effects of lovastatin on bone formation are pronounced with only five days of therapy. This shows a very marked increase not only in bone volume but also in bone formation rates.

The observation that statins stimulate bone formation in rodents has led to retrospective examinations of large databases to determine if there is any evidence for correlation between statin usage and bone mineral density or subsequent development of fractures. Of the six published reports of observational studies that examine these associations, five are positive and one is negative. However, several abstracts presented in the past year or so also reported no effects of statins on bone mass or subsequent development of fractures. The most recent report (63) was accompanied by an editorial (64) stating that, in view of all available studies, it is certainly possible that statins have a beneficial effect on fracture risk and bone mineral density, but it is also possible that the results are due to a confounding variable that has not yet been identified. This issue can be resolved only by a randomized, controlled trial using the appropriate statin in the correct dose and mode of administration.

Administration of statins in this context is not a straightforward issue in itself. Some statins, such as pravastatin, are water-soluble; they do not enter bone cells and so cause no biological effect on bone. Moreover, laboratory data suggest that like PTH, statins are more effective when administered intermittently in low doses, and therefore it is important that careful preclinical studies be performed to determine the appropriate dose and mode of administration.

Proteasome Inhibitors

In examining other mechanisms by which important growth regulatory factors and transcription factors that control bone formation can be modulated, the effects of specific inhibitors of the ubiquitin-proteasome pathway on BMP-2 expression and bone formation were examined. The rationale for this approach was that expression of decapentaplegic (dpp), the homolog of the BMP-2 and BMP-4 genes in *Drosophila*, is controlled by the ubiquitin-proteasome pathway. Expression of dpp is regulated by the transcription factor cubitus interruptus, so that the larger form of this transcription factor is degraded by a proteasomal process that can be inhibited by proteasome inhibitors. The cleaved form of cubitus interruptus suppresses dpp transcription. Based on this reasoning, it was determined if proteasome inhibitors would enhance BMP-2 and BMP-4 expression in osteoblasts. It was found that specific inhibitors of the LMP7/X component of the chymotrypsin-like activity of the 20S proteasome stimulated BMP-2 expression and impaired degradation of Gli3, the homolog of cubitus interruptus in mammalian osteoblasts. Specific inhibitors of this subunit of the 20S proteasome stimulated bone formation and BMP-2 expression in concentrations as low as 1 nM. These compounds were tested for their effects on bone formation in bone organ cultures, by utilizing local injection over the murine calvaria and by systemic administration to normal intact mice. The compounds stimulated bone formation dramatically, with increases in bone formation rates of >70% after only 5 days of treatment persisting for at least 2 weeks following final exposure to the drug. These are much greater responses than are seen with any other known stimulator of bone formation, including PTH.

Leptin and Its Relationship to Bone Mass

Recently, a link has been suggested between the polypeptide hormone leptin and bone mass (65). This is of particular interest because leptin is secreted by adipocytes for control of body weight, and it has long been known that there is a negative correlation between obesity and bone mass. Osteoporosis is one of those unusual situations where obesity is protective (66, 67). It occurs most frequently in thin and slightly built Caucasian women (68).

The relationship between adipose tissue and bone mass, however, does not stop there. There is also a clear inverse relationship between adipogenesis and osteogenesis in the bone marrow. Adipocytes and osteoblasts share a common stem cell precursor, and there appears to be preferential differentiation along the adipocyte lineage in conditions such as aging and estrogen withdrawal, which favor adipocyte generation in the bone marrow cavity (69, 70). This may in part be related to BMP-2 receptor expression and responsivity. We have found that BMP-2 induces osteoblast differentiation through the BMP type 1B receptor pathway and adipocyte differentiation through the BMP receptor type 1A pathway (58).

The findings of Ducy et al. (65) suggest that leptin may be the key to understanding the molecular mechanism linking bone mass and body weight. They examined two murine models of obesity, the leptin-deficient ob/ob mice and the leptin-receptor–deficient db/db mice. In both cases, the mice have a phenotype associated with increased bone formation rates and high bone mass. The authors demonstrated reversal of the high-bone-mass phenotype in ob/ob mice that were leptin-deficient following intracerebroventricular infusions of leptin, although they could not demonstrate leptin receptors on osteoblasts. They concluded that leptin modulates bone mass by a central effect, and suggest leptin deficiency or insensitivity is responsible for the decreased bone mass in these mice.

What does this mean for potential drug therapy? Based on these data, it is possible that inhibition of leptin action enhances bone mass. Ducy et al. (65) propose that the increased bone mass associated with obesity may be related to leptin insensitivity, in the same way that non–insulin-dependent diabetes mellitus is caused by insulin insensitivity. Thus, antagonists to leptin action may have potential utility as stimulators of increased bone mass.

CONCLUSION

Osteoporosis represents a vast therapeutic market that has been recognized by the medical profession and pharmaceutical industry only recently. Finding appropriate therapies is not straightforward, since osteoporosis is a chronic disease of complex pathophysiology that is associated sometimes with increases in bone resorption and sometimes with decreases in bone formation. Drugs that target only bone-resorbing or bone-forming cells will not necessarily be appropriate for all patients. Currently, the best available drugs inhibit osteoclastic bone resorption and are best utilized for maintaining bone mass and preventing further bone loss. It is hoped that future therapies will rebuild bone that has been resorbed and restore trabecular bone microarchitecture. Although are no known available agents achieve this goal, it appears likely that, as a consequence of the intense interest in this area, one or more will soon be available.

Visit the Annual Reviews home page at www.AnnualReviews.org

LITERATURE CITED

1. Stevenson JC. 1993. E.R.T. New generation transdermal patches. *4th Int. Symp. Osteoporosis and Consens. Dev. Conf., Hong Kong*, p. 763 (Abstr.)
2. Pacifici R, Rifas L, Teitelbaum S, et al. 1987. Spontaneous release of interleukin-1 from human blood monocytes reflects bone formation in idiopathic osteoporosis. *Proc. Natl. Acad. Sci. USA* 84:4616–20
3. Pacifici R, Rifas L, McCracken R, et al. 1991. Ovarian steroid treatment blocks a postmenopausal increase in blood monocyte interleukin-1 release. *Proc. Natl. Acad. Sci. USA* 86:2398–402
4. Girasole G, Jilka RL, Passeri G, et al. 1992. 17-β estradiol inhibits interleukin-6 production by bone marrow–derived stromal cells in osteoblasts in vitro: a potential mechanism for the anti-osteotropic effect of estrogens. *J. Clin. Invest.* 89:883–91
5. Jilka RL, Hangoc G, Girasole G, et al. 1992. Increased osteoclast development after estrogen loss—mediation by interleukin-6. *Science* 257:88–91
6. Ammann P, Rizzoli R, Bonjour JP, et al. 1997. Transgenic mice expressing soluble tumor necrosis factor–receptor are protected against bone loss caused by estrogen deficiency. *J. Clin. Invest.* 99:1699–703
7. Oursler MJ, Osdoby P, Pyfferoen J, et al. 1991. Avian osteoclasts as estrogen target cells. *Proc. Natl. Acad. Sci. USA* 88:6613–17
8. Black LJ, Sato M, Rowley ER. 1994. Raloxifene (LY139481 HCI) prevents bone loss and reduces serum cholesterol without causing uterine hypertrophy in ovariectomized rats. *J. Clin. Invest.* 93:63–69
9. Pennisi E. 1996. Drugs' link to genes reveals estrogen's many sides. *Science* 273:1171

10. McDonnell DP, Vegeto E, O'Malley BW. 1992. Identification of a negative regulatory function for steroid receptors. *Proc. Natl. Acad. Sci. USA* 89:10563–67

11. Tzukerman MT, Esty A, Santiso-Mere D, et al. 1994. Human estrogen receptor transcriptional capacity is determined by both cellular and promoter context and mediated by two functionally distinct intramolecular regions. *Mol. Endocrinol.* 8: 21–30

12. O'Malley BW, Onate SA, Tsai SY, et al. 1995. Sequence and characterization of a coactivator for the steroid hormone receptor superfamily. *Science* 270:1354–57

13. Yang NN, Venugopalan M, Hardikar S, et al. 1996. Identification of an estrogen response element activated by metabolites of 17β-estradiol raloxifene. *Science* 273:1222–25

14. Storm T, Thamsborg G, Steiniche T, et al. 1990. Effect of intermittent cyclical etidronate therapy on bone mass and fracture rate in women with postmenopausal osteoporosis. *N. Engl. J. Med.* 322:1265–71

14a. Fleisch H. 2000. *Bisphosphonates in Bone Disease—From the Laboratory to the Patient.* San Diego: Academic. 4th ed.

15. Miyauchi A, Notoya K, Taketomi S. 1996. Novel ipriflavone receptors coupled to calcium influx regulate osteoclast differentiation and function. *Endocrinology* 137:3544–50

16. Brandi ML. 1993. New treatment strategies: ipriflavone, strontium, vitamin D metabolites. *4th Int. Symp. Osteoporosis and Consens. Dev. Conf., Hong Kong,* pp. 443–45

17. Alexandersen P, Toussaint A, Reginster J, et al. 2000. Ipriflavone has no effect on bone metabolism and causes lymphopenia in osteopenic women. *J. Bone Miner. Res.* 15(1), Abstr. 1240

18. Balfour JA, McTavish D. 1992. Transdermal estradiol—a review of its pharmacological profile, and therapeutic potential in the prevention of postmenopausal osteoporosis. *Drugs and Aging* 2:487–507

19. Mundy GR. 1993. Cytokines of bone. In *Physiology and Pharmacology of Bone: Handbook of Experimental Pharmacology,* ed. GR Mundy, TJ Martin, pp. 185–214. Berlin: Springer-Verlag

20. Baron R. 1993. Biology of the osteoclast. In *Physiology and Pharmacology of Bone. Handbook of Experimental Pharmacology,* ed. GR Mundy, TJ Martin, pp. 111–47. Berlin: Springer-Verlag

21. Yoshida H, Hayashi SI, Kunisada T, et al. 1990. The murine mutation osteopetrosis is in the coding region of the macrophage colony stimulating factor gene. *Nature* 345:442–44

22. Felix R, Cecchini MG, Hofstetter W, et al. 1990. Impairment of macrophage colony-stimulating factor production and lack of resident bone marrow macrophages in the osteopetrotic op/op mouse. *J. Bone Miner. Res.* 5:781–89

23. Kodama H, Yamasaki A, Nose M, et al. 1991. Congenital osteoclast deficiency in osteopetrotic op/op mice is cured by injections of macrophage colony stimulating factor. *J. Exp. Med.* 173:269–72

24. Soriano P, Montgomery C, Geske R, et al. 1991. Targeted disruption of the c-src proto-oncogene leads to osteopetrosis in mice. *Cell* 64:693–702

25. Yoneda T, Lowe C, Lee CH, et al. 1993. Herbimycin A, a pp60[c-src] tyrosine kinase inhibitor, inhibits osteoclastic bone resorption in vitro and hypercalcemia in vivo. *J. Clin. Invest.* 91:2791–95

25a. Fisher JE, Caulfield MP, Sato M, et al. 1993. Inhibition of osteoclastic bone resorption in vivo by echistatin an "arginyl-glycyl-aspartyl" (RDG) containing peptide. *Endocrinology* 132:1411–13

25b. Engleman VW, Nickols GA, Ross FP, et al. 1997. A peptidomimetic antagonist of the $\alpha_v\beta_3$ integrin inhibits bone resorption in vitro and prevents osteoporosis in vivo. *J. Clin. Invest.* 99:2284–92

26. Horton MA, Davies J. 1989. Perspectives—adhesion receptors in bone. *J. Bone Miner. Res.* 4:803–8

27. Vaes E. 1968. The action of parathyroid hormone on the excretion and synthesis of lysosomal enzymes and on the extracellular release of acid by bone cells. *J. Cell. Biol.* 39:676–97

28. Eilon G, Raisz LG. 1978. Comparison of the effects of stimulators and inhibitors of resorption on the release of lysosomal enzymes and radioactive calcium from fetal bone in organ culture. *Endocrinology* 103:1969–75

28a. Bossard MJ, Tomaszek TA, Thompson SK, et al. 1996. Proteolytic activity of human osteoclast cathepsin K—expression, purification, activation, and substrate identification. *J. Biol. Chem.* 271:12517–24

28b. Drake FH, Dodds RA, James IE, et al. 1996. Cathepsin K, but not cathepsin B, L, or S, is abundantly expressed in human osteoclasts. *J. Biol. Chem.* 271:12511–16

28c. Min H, Morony S, Sarosi I, et al. 2000. Osteoprotegerin reverses osteoporosis by inhibiting endosteal osteoclasts and prevents vascular calcification by blocking a process resembling osteoclastogenesis. *J. Exp. Med.* 192:463–74

28d. Oyajobi BO, Anderson DM, Traianedes K, et al. 2001. Therapeutic efficacy of soluble RANK-IgG Fc (RANK.Fc) fusion protein in suppressing bone resorption and hypercalcemia in a model of humoral hypercalcemia of malignancy. *Cancer Res.* 61:2572–78

29. Boyce BF, Yoneda T, Lowe C, et al. 1992. Requirement of pp60c-src expression for osteoclasts to form ruffled borders and resorb bone in mice. *J. Clin. Invest.* 90(4):1622–27

30. Abu-Amer Y, Tondravi MM. 1997. NK-kappaB and bone: the breaking point. *Nat. Med.* 3:1189–90

31. Van Beek E, Pieterman E, Cohen L, et al. 1999. Nitrogen-containing bisphosphonates inhibit isopentenyl pyrophosphate isomerase/farnesyl pyrophosphate synthase activity with relative potencies corresponding to their antiresorptive potencies in vitro and in vivo. *Biochem. Biophys. Res. Commun.* 255:491–94

32. Reszka AA, Halasy-Nagy JM, Masarachia PJ, Rodan GA. 1999. Bisphosphonates act directly on the osteoclast to induce caspase cleavage of Mst1 kinase during apoptosis. *J. Biol. Chem.* 274:34967–73

33. Benford HL, Frith JC, Auriola S, et al. 1999. Farnesol and geranylgeraniol prevent activation of caspases by aminobisphosphonates: biochemical evidence for two distinct pharmacological classes of bisphosphonate drugs. *Mol. Pharmacol.* 56(1):131–40

34. Darby AJ, Meunier PJ. 1981. Mean wall thickness and formation periods of trabecular bone packets in idiopathic osteoporosis. *Calcif. Tissue Int.* 33:199–204

35. Lau KH, Farley JR, Freeman TK, et al. 1989. A proposed mechanism of the mitogenic action of fluoride on bone cells: inhibition of the activity of an osteoblastic acid phosphatase. *Metabolism* 38:858–68

36. Farley JR, Wergedal JE, Baylink DJ. 1983. Fluoride directly stimulates proliferation and alkaline phosphatase activity of bone-forming cells. *Science* 222:330–32

37. Burgener D, Bonjour JP, Caverzasio J. 1995. Fluoride increases tyrosine kinase activity in osteoblast-like cells: regulatory role for the stimulation of cell proliferation and Pi transport across the plasma membrane. *J. Bone Miner. Res.* 10:164–71

38. Caverzasio J, Imai T, Ammann P, et al. 1996. Aluminum potentiates the effect of fluoride on tyrosine phosphorylation and osteoblast replication in vitro and bone mass in vivo. *J. Bone Miner. Res.* 11:46–55

39. Riggs BL, Hodgson SF, O'Fallon WM, et al. 1990. Effect of fluoride treatment on the fracture rate in postmenopausal

women with osteoporosis. *N. Engl. J. Med.* 322:802–9

40. Kleerekoper M, Peterson EL, Nelson DA, et al. 1991. A randomized trial of sodium fluoride as a treatment for postmenopausal osteoporosis. *Osteoporosis Int.* 1:155–61

40a. Riggs BL, Hodgson SF, O'Fallon WM, et al. 1990. Effect of fluoride treatment on the fracture rate in postmenopausal women with osteoporosis. *N. Engl. J. Med.* 322:802–9

41. Pak C, Sakhaee K, Zerwekh JE, et al. 1989. Safe and effective treatment of osteoporosis with intermittent slow release sodium fluoride: augmentation of vertebral bone mass and inhibition of fractures. *J. Clin. Endocrinol. Metab.* 68:150–59

42. Nagant C, Devogelaer JP, Stein F. 1990. Fluoride treatment for osteoporosis. *Lancet* 336:48–49

43. Pak CY, Sakhaee K, Adams-Huet B, et al. 1995. Treatment of postmenopausal osteoporosis with slow-release sodium fluoride. Final report of a randomized controlled trial. *Ann. Intern. Med.* 123(6):466–67

44. Parsons JA, Potts JT Jr. 1972. Physiology and chemistry of parathyroid hormone. *Clin. Endocrinol. Metab.* 1:33–78

45. Canalis E, Centrella M, Burch W, et al. 1989. Insulin-like growth factor I mediates selective anabolic effects of parathyroid hormone in bone cultures. *J. Clin. Invest.* 8:60–65

46. Reeve J, Meunier PJ, Parsons JA, et al. 1980. Anabolic effect of human parathyroid hormone fragment on trabecular bone in involutional osteoporosis: a multicentre trial. *BMJ* 280:1340–44

47. Reeve J, Davie U, Arlot M, et al. 1989. Parathyroid peptide (hPTH-1-34) in the treatment of osteoporosis. In *Clinical Disorders of Bone and Mineral Metabolism*, ed. M Kleerekoper, SM Krane, pp. 621–27. New York: Mary Ann Liebert

48. Slovik DM, Rosenthal DI, Doppelt SH, et al. 1986. Restoration of spinal bone in osteoporotic men by treatment with human parathyroid hormone (1-34) and 1,25-dihydroxyvitamin D. *J. Bone Miner. Res.* 1:377–81

49. Reeve J. 1996. PTH: A future role in the management of osteoporosis? *J. Bone Miner. Res.* 11:440–45

50. Vickery BH, Avnur Z, Cheng Y, et al. 1996. RS-66271, a C-terminally substituted analog of human parathyroid hormone-related protein (1-34), increases trabecular and cortical bone in ovariectomized, osteopenic rats. *J. Bone Miner. Res.* 11:1943–53

51. Stewart AF. 1996. PTHrP(1-36) as a skeletal anabolic agent for the treatment of osteoporosis. *Bone* 19:303–6

51a. Marie PJ, Hott M, Modrowski D, et al. 1993. An upcoupling agent containing strontium prevents bone loss by depressing bone resorption and maintaining bone formation in estrogen-deficient rats. *J. Bone Miner. Res.* 8:607–15

51b. Grynpas MD, Hamilton E, Cheung R, et al. 1996. Strontium increases vertebral bone volume in rats at a low dose that does not induce mineralization defect. *Bone* 18:253–59

52. Komori T, Yagi H, Nomura S, et al. 1997. Targeted disruption of Cbfa1 results in a complete lack of bone formation owing to maturational arrest of osteoblasts. *Cell* 89(5):755–64

53. Ducy P, Zhang R, Geoffroy V, et al. 1997. Osf2/Cbfa1: a transcriptional activator of osteoblast differentiation. *Cell* 89(5):747–54

54. Otto F, Thornell AP, Crompton T, et al. 1997. Cbfa1, a candidate gene for cleidocranial dysplasia syndrome, is essential for osteoblast differentiation and bone development. *Cell* 89(5):767–71

55. Jochum W, David JP, Elliott C, et al. 2000. Increased bone formation and osteosclerosis in mice overexpressing the transcription factor Fra-1. *Nat. Med.* 6:980–84

56. Sabatakos G, Sims NA, Chen J, et al. 2000. Overexpression of β FosB transcription factor(s) increases bone formation

and inhibits adipogenesis. *Nat. Med.* 6:985–90

57. Pfeilschifter J, Mundy GR. 1987. Modulation of transforming growth factor β activity in bone cultures by osteotropic hormones. *Proc. Natl. Acad. Sci. USA* 84: 2024–28

57a. Ghosh-Choudhury N, Harris MA, Feng JQ, et al. 1994. Expression of the BMP 2 gene during bone cell differentiation. *Crit. Rev. Eukaryot. Gene Expr.* 4:345–55

58. Chen D, Ji X, Harris MA, et al. 1998. Differential roles for bone morphogenetic protein (BMP) receptor type IB and IA in differentiation and specification of mesenchymal precursor cells to osteoblast and adipocyte lineages. *J. Cell. Biol.* 142 (1):295–305

59. Harris SE, Sabatini M, Harris MA, et al. 1994. Expression of bone morphogenetic protein messenger RNA in prolonged cultures of fetal rat calvarial cells. *J. Bone Miner. Res.* 9(3):389–94

60. Mundy GR, Garrett IR, Harris SE, et al. 1999. Stimulation of bone formation in vitro and in rodents by statins. *Science* 286:1946–49

61. Dunstan CR, Boyce R, Boyce BF, et al. 1999. Systemic administration of acidic fibroblast growth factor (FGF-1) prevents bone loss and increases new bone formation in ovariectomized rats. *J. Bone Miner. Res.* 14(6):953–59

61a. Garrett IR, Gutierrez G, Escobedo A, et al. 2001. Statins stimulate bone formation through their effects on eNOS. *J. Bone Miner. Res.* In press

62. Garrett IR, Esparza J, Chen D, et al. 2000. Statins mediate their effects on osteoblasts by inhibition of HMG-CoA reductase and ultimately BMP-2. *J. Bone Miner. Res.* 15(1):F378 (Abstr.)

63. Van Staa TP, Wegman S, de Vries F, et al. 2001. Use of statins and risk of fractures. *JAMA* 285(14):1850–55

64. Hennessy S, Strom BL. 2001. Statins and fracture risk. *JAMA* 285(14):1888–89

65. Ducy P, Amling M, Takeda S, et al. 2000. Leptin inhibits bone formation through a hypothalamic relay: a central control of bone mass. *Cell* 100:197–207

66. Felson DT, Zhang Y, Hannan MT, Anderson JJ. 1993. Effects of weight and body mass index on bone mineral density in men and women: the Framingham Study. *J. Bone Miner. Res.* 8:567–73

67. Tremollieres FA, Pouilles JM, Ribot C. 1993. Vertebral postmenopausal bone loss is reduced in overweight women: a longitudinal study in 155 early postmenopausal women. *J. Clin. Endocrinol. Metab.* 77:683–86

68. Ravn P, Cizza G, Bjarnason NH, et al. 1999. Low body mass index is an important risk factor for low bone mass and increased bone loss in early postmenopausal women. *J. Bone Miner. Res.* 14:1622–27

69. Martin RB, Chow BD, Lucas PA. 1990. Bone marrow fat content in relation to bone remodeling and serum chemistry in intact and ovariectomized dogs. *Calcif. Tissue Int.* 46:189–94

70. Meunier PJ, Aaron J, Edouard C, Vignon G. 1971. Osteoporosis and the replacement of cell populations of the marrow by adipose tissue: a quantitative study of 84 iliac bone biopsies. *Clin. Orthop. Rel. Res.* 80:147–54

Annu. Rev. Med. 2002. 53:355–68

EARLY MANAGEMENT OF PROSTATE CANCER:
How to Respond to an Elevated PSA?

Eduardo I. Canto and Kevin M. Slawin
Scott Department of Urology, Baylor College of Medicine, Houston, Texas 77030;
e-mail: ecanto@bcm.tmc.edu, kslawin@bcm.tmc.edu

Key Words screening, digital rectal exam, biopsy, free PSA, benign prostatic hyperplasia

■ **Abstract** Support for prostate cancer screening efforts is provided by observational studies reporting decreases in prostate cancer–specific mortality in areas where screening is performed with digital rectal exam (DRE) and measurement of serum prostate-specific antigen (PSA) levels. The combination of PSA and DRE is an excellent cancer-screening tool with sensitivity and positive predictive value superior to that of mammography and breast exam. Use of percent free PSA further improves the specificity of PSA testing, particularly in the range of 4–10 ng/ml, at which most false positive PSA tests occur. Men older than 50 with a >10-year life expectancy should be considered for prostate cancer screening. Those with an abnormal DRE or a PSA above 4 ng/ml should be referred to a urologist for further discussion of the risks and benefits of a prostate biopsy. Furthermore, those with a significant change in either DRE or PSA results, or those at higher risk for prostate cancer with a PSA level above 2.5 ng/ml, should also be referred for evaluation.

WHY SCREEN FOR PROSTATE CANCER?

Prostate cancer is the most common cancer and the second most common cause of cancer death in men. In 2001, it is estimated that 198,100 men will be diagnosed with it and 31,500 will succumb to it. In 1998, half of all men dying of prostate cancer were between 60 and 79 years of age (1). The burden of suffering from prostate cancer is significant. Nevertheless, prostate cancer screening in the United States remains controversial. Several organizations have issued guidelines regarding prostate cancer screening, and these recommendations vary. The Guide to Clinical Preventive Services issued by the U.S. Preventive Services Task Force (USPSTF) argues against any prostate cancer screening at all, either by digital rectal exam (DRE) or by measurement of serum prostate-specific antigen (PSA) (2). The American College of Preventive Medicine recommends that men aged 50 or older with a >10-year life expectancy be informed about the risks and potential benefits of prostate cancer screening and be allowed to make their own decision (3). The American Urological Association (AUA), the American College of Radiology, the American Foundation for Urologic Disease, and the American Cancer Society (ACS) have taken a more proactive stance (4–6). The AUA recommends that all men older than 50 with a >10-year life expectancy be offered prostate cancer screening with PSA and DRE. African-American men, or men with a first-degree relative with prostate cancer and a >10-year life expectancy, should be offered prostate cancer screening at an earlier age because they are at increased risk of developing prostate cancer (6). The ACS sets 40 as the age at which to begin screening these men with higher risk (5). The American Association of Family Physicians has not developed specific guidelines for prostate cancer screening (7).

The lack of consensus in favor of routine prostate cancer screening is not due to a lack of morbidity and mortality associated with prostate cancer, a lack of curative treatments, or even a lack of a good screening test. The number of deaths per year from prostate cancer is comparable to that of breast cancer. The mean age at death from prostate cancer is only 10–15 years older than that of breast cancer (1). For patients with organ-confined prostate cancer, radical prostatectomy has a greater than 90% cure rate (8). As screening tools, combined PSA and DRE compare favorably with mammography and breast exam. Combined PSA and DRE have an estimated sensitivity in the 70%–80% range and a positive predictive value (PPV) of 30%–40% (9–12). A suspicious PSA or DRE is followed by a needle biopsy of the prostate. This relatively safe procedure is carried out in the office without the need for anesthetic, and its specificity is near 100%. Combined mammography and breast exam are also 70%–80% sensitive, but their PPV is 9%–22%, depending on age and family history (13). Mammograms are significantly more expensive than serum PSA measurement.

The lack of consensus about prostate cancer screening is due to the wide variability in the biologic potential of the disease. Prostate cancer diagnosed at an early stage may not become symptomatic for an average of 10 years (11). Nevertheless, more than 50% of men diagnosed with early-stage, moderately differentiated prostate cancer who live 15 years after diagnosis will die of metastatic disease (14). This means that in order to assess the survival benefit that results from a therapeutic intervention, patients need to be followed for at least 15 years.

Differences in screening recommendations exist mainly because of differences in the level of evidence required by various organizations to make a positive recommendation, rather than because of differences in interpretation of the available data. The USPSTF favors only interventions proven, by randomized controlled trials, to reduce morbidity and mortality (2). Because of this rigorous standard, the USPSTF will argue against prostate cancer screening until data from randomized controlled studies demonstrate that screening decreases mortality. Other organizations, exemplified by the AUA and ACS, base their recommendations on a periodic review of all available data, including nonrandomized studies. In May 2000, an ACS workshop reviewed data generated since it last revised its prostate cancer screening guidelines in 1997 (5). Similarly, the AUA restated its prostate cancer screening guidelines in a two-part "Best Practice Policy" statement published in the February 2001 issue of *Urology* (6). Both organizations base their recommendations favoring DRE and PSA screening on recent nonrandomized prostate cancer mortality data (15, 16).

In the United States, the overall prostate cancer mortality rate increased significantly in the mid-1980s and began to decrease in 1991, with the current age-adjusted mortality rate now similar to that recorded in the late 1970s (1). Whereas the previous increase in prostate cancer–specific mortality is most likely a result of attribution bias, the subsequent decrease in mortality is not explained by this and could be consistent with either an improvement in therapeutic outcomes or more widespread treatment. The prostate cancer mortality rate followed a similar trend in Olmsted County, Minnesota, where the decrease in prostate cancer mortality was preceded by a decrease in the incidence of advanced disease (17). An analysis of the Surveillance, Epidemiology, and End Results (SEER) Program of the National Cancer Institute (NCI) database indicates that the 1997 prostate cancer mortality rate in males 60–79 years of age was lower than in any year since 1950. In addition, the incidence of metastatic disease has decreased and the incidence of nonmetastatic, high-grade disease has increased (18, 19). This is consistent with a screening program that identifies clinically significant disease at an early stage.

The best observational data supporting prostate cancer screening come from Tyrol, Austria. Prostate cancer screening with DRE and PSA in Tyrol began in 1993 (15, 16). Mortality from prostate cancer in men 40–79 years old remained constant from 1970 to 1993 but has decreased 42% since 1993 in Tyrol. In other parts of Austria, where screening is not performed, prostate cancer mortality remained constant.

The decrease in prostate cancer–specific mortality in the United States is probably due to a combination of screening and better therapies, including identification and treatment of advanced disease, improvements in prostatectomy technique, the introduction of conformational external beam radiotherapy, and the introduction in the late 1980s of gonadotropin-releasing hormone analogues and androgenic receptor blockers. However, the Tyrol data support the hypothesis that instituting generalized prostate cancer screening can reduce mortality independently of the improvements in therapy that have occurred over the past decade.

A final assessment of the benefits of prostate cancer screening and current therapies is expected to come from ongoing large, randomized, controlled trials. In the United States, the Prostate Cancer Intervention vs. Observation Trial and the Prostate, Lung, Colorectal, and Ovarian Cancer screening trial are designed to address the benefits of therapy and screening, respectively (20, 21). In Europe, the European Randomized Study for Screening for Prostate Cancer is expected to enroll 239,000 men in 10 countries and be completed in 2008 (22). Although physicians and patients alike eagerly await the results of the various ongoing randomized prostate cancer screening trials, these are not without flaws. There will probably be a significant degree of contamination of the control arm by study participants who find it easy to undergo PSA testing outside of the study. Furthermore, for patients diagnosed with prostate cancer, treatment protocols and treatment efficacy vary widely across locations depending on local resources and expertise (4, 22).

Who should be screened for prostate cancer? On the basis of currently available data, patients over 50 years of age who have a >10-year life expectancy should be offered yearly prostate cancer screening with PSA and DRE. Men with at least one first-degree relative diagnosed with prostate cancer at an early age, and men of African-American descent, should be offered screening starting at age 45. Men with multiple first-degree relatives diagnosed with prostate cancer at an early age may benefit from screening at age 40 (5, 6).

BASICS OF PSA

PSA is a 33-kDa serine protease of the kallikrein family. It was initially identified in prostatic tissue extracts in 1970 and was cloned in 1987 (23, 24). It is made primarily by the prostatic epithelium and periurethral glands in males, but it has also been detected in endometrium, breast tissue, breast cancer, breast milk, and female serum (25). In the normal prostate, the prostatic epithelium secretes PSA into the seminal fluid, where it reaches mg/ml concentrations and is involved in the degradation of seminal plasma motility inhibitor precursor/semenogelin I, the predominant protein in human ejaculate (26).

In the normal male, PSA enters the circulation through an unknown mechanism and reaches ng/ml concentrations. PSA is organ-specific but not cancer-specific, since normal, hyperplastic, and neoplastic prostate epithelial cells all manufacture it. PSA production per gram of tissue is influenced by testosterone levels and the variable epithelium-to-stroma ratio of the prostate (27, 28).

Prostatic epithelium produces more than one molecular form of PSA. For example, recent studies have found that the PSA produced by the transitional zone epithelium of prostates with nodular benign prostatic hypertrophy (BPH) has a higher percentage of PSA molecules that have been clipped at amino-acid residues Lys145–146 and Lys182–183 than PSA produced by either prostate cancer or normal transition-zone and peripheral-zone epithelial cells (29–31). This enzymatically inactive form of PSA has been named BPSA.

Prostate cancer has also been found to produce more than one molecular form of PSA. Mikolajczyk et al. found that prostate cancer produces PSA with either two or four unclipped amino acids from its leader sequence (32). This pPSA is not present in transitional-zone epithelium, where BPH occurs.

Approximately three quarters of the PSA found in serum is irreversibly bound to the protease inhibitor alpha-1-antichymotrypsin. Serum PSA is also found bound to alpha-2-macroglobulin. Measured PSA in serum is 5%–50% unbound (33). Although alpha-2-macroglobulin-bound PSA may retain part of its enzymatic activity, both unbound and alpha-1-antichymotrypsin-bound PSA are enzymatically inactive (34).

PSA has five immune reactive sites. Two of these epitopes are hidden on alpha-1-antichymotrypsin-bound PSA, allowing commercial immunoassays to differentiate bound from free PSA. All five epitopes are hidden in alpha-2-macroglobulin-bound PSA. Therefore, the total PSA measured by commercial assays corresponds to unbound PSA (free PSA) plus alpha-1-antichymotrypsin-bound PSA (33, 35).

ROLE OF PSA IN EARLY PROSTATE CANCER DETECTION

Combined use of DRE and PSA is the best available prostate cancer screening tool. The combination of DRE and PSA is better than either alone; each identifies cancers not detected by the other (9, 36). Most information available about the accuracy of PSA is based on screening studies of nonrandomized, self-selected populations of men. Because not all men had their prostates pathologically analyzed or biopsied, it is difficult to calculate a true sensitivity or negative predictive value for combined DRE and PSA. We can calculate the PPV for the population of men screened, defined as the rate of cancer detection in men with elevated PSA or abnormal DRE. Furthermore, because prostate cancer is diagnosed by core needle biopsies, sampling error is unavoidable. Only by serial biopsy over time can we measure the true PPV (the rate at which cancer is present in men with elevated PSA) and specificity. Using a quadrant core biopsy technique (one core per quadrant of prostate), Catalona et al. (9) found that 26% of 6630 men who volunteered for prostate cancer screening had either an abnormal DRE or a PSA above 4 ng/ml. Of these, 23% were found on biopsy to have cancer. By rebiopsying men with elevated PSA levels (between 4 and 10 ng/ml) but negative initial biopsies, Catalona showed that 19% of these men had prostate cancer that was missed on the initial biopsy (37). This percent-positive biopsy rate achieved with serial biopsy has been approached on initial biopsy in recent studies by increasing the sampling at biopsy from 4 cores to 10 or 12 cores (10, 38) (Table 1).

About 40% of cystoprostatectomy specimens from unscreened men are found to have prostate cancer on microscopic examination (39, 40). As noted above, in prostate cancer screening programs, about 20%–30% of those tested have either an abnormal DRE or a PSA above 4.0 ng/ml. Of these, only 30%–40% are found to have cancer (9, 10, 36, 38, 41, 42). It may seem that prostate cancer screening with

TABLE 1 Cancer detection rates in men not previously biopsied ($n = 264$)

| | PSA (ng/ml) | | | | | | | |
| | <4.0 | | 4.0–10.0 | | >10.0 | | Overall | |
DRE results	Total patients	Patients with cancer	Total patients	Patients with cancer	Total patients	Patients with cancer	Total patients	Patients with cancer
Normal	18	5 (27.8%)	123	51 (41.5%)	19	12 (63.2%)	160	68 (42.5%)
Abnormal	43	8 (18.6%)	53	30 (56.6%)	8	6 (75.0%)	104	44 (42.3%)

From Reference 10, p. 1556, with permission.

DRE and PSA is no better than randomly biopsying the general population, since the rate of cancer detection in males with abnormal screening tests is comparable to the prevalence of prostate cancer in the population being screened. However, only 10%–20% of prostate cancers found on cystoprostatectomy series are clinically significant (39, 40). In contrast, 90% of prostate cancers diagnosed as a result of PSA and DRE screening are clinically significant (40). Therefore, PSA- and DRE-based prostate cancer screening can detect 70%–80% of all clinically significant prostate cancers at the expense of biopsying only 20%–30% of the population screened (9, 40). This is much better than randomly biopsying the entire population. On the other hand, at a cost of about $1500 per person for transrectal prostate needle biopsy, there is a clear need for increasing the specificity and PPV of combined PSA and DRE screening.

Because most false negative results of PSA screening are in men with serum PSA lower than 10 ng/ml, most efforts at improving PSA specificity target this PSA range. Current attempts to improve the specificity of PSA screening are based on five observations related to the biological properties of PSA: (*a*) The total amount of prostatic glandular epithelium increases with BPH and results in a higher serum PSA, even in the absence of cancer; (*b*) the prevalence of BPH increases with age; (*c*) the presence of prostate cancer correlates with a lower fraction of unbound to alpha-1-antichymotrypsin-bound PSA; (*d*) as prostate cancer progresses, the serum PSA concentration increases; (*e*) prostate cancer releases 10 times more PSA into the serum per gram of tissue than normal or BPH epithelium (43, 44).

On the basis of observations that the total amount of prostatic glandular epithelium increases with BPH and that prostate cancer releases 10 times more PSA into the serum per gram of tissue than normal or BPH epithelium, Benson et al. introduced the use of PSA density in 1992 to correct for the effect of prostate volume (43). This test is intended for men with a PSA level of 4–10 ng/ml and a normal DRE. PSA density is calculated by dividing the total serum PSA level (ng/ml) by the prostate volume as measured by transrectal ultrasonography. PSA density has not found wide application because it is limited by the variability in prostate volume measurement by ultrasound, the stroma-to-epithelium ratio in BPH, and the need to perform transrectal ultrasonography to obtain a value (44, 45). Furthermore, studies using PSA density have obtained conflicting results (41, 46). These studies may have been confounded by the fact that using only quadrant or sextant biopsies may favor finding prostate cancer in smaller prostates in which there is less sampling error (10).

Using data from the Baltimore Longitudinal Aging study, Carter et al. showed that an average rate of change in the serum PSA greater than 0.75 ng/ml per year could differentiate between men with and without prostate cancer as early as nine years before diagnosis (11). The formula for PSA velocity is $\frac{1}{2}[(\text{PSA2} - \text{PSA1}/\text{time in years}) + (\text{PSA3} - \text{PSA2}/\text{time in years})]$. In this formula, PSA1, PSA2, and PSA3 equal the first, second, and third serum PSA measurements, respectively. In clinical practice, the applicability of PSA velocity is limited by the use of different laboratories by the same patient from one year to the next and the need for three PSA measurements spanning at least a two-year period. PSA velocity is more specific (90% vs. 60% in patients with BPH) but less sensitive (78% vs. 72%) than the standard cutoff PSA value of 4 ng/ml (11). PSA velocity is useful when deciding whether or not to perform a second biopsy in a patient with an elevated PSA or to perform a biopsy in a concerned, young patient with a rising PSA that is not yet above 4.

In an effort both to correct for the natural development of BPH as men age and to increase the sensitivity of PSA in younger men, Oesterling and colleagues proposed the use of age-based serum PSA reference ranges (47). Large studies have shown that the use of age-specific PSA reference ranges increases the number of cancers detected in men younger than 60 and decreases the biopsy rate of older men at the expense of missing only an additional 3%–4% of cancers. More than 75% of the additional cancers detected in men younger than 60 had favorable pathological features. More than 90% of the cancers missed in older men had favorable pathological features (48, 49). However, the use of age-specific PSA ranges remains controversial. Two studies have shown the standard 4.0 ng/ml PSA cutoff to be optimal for all age groups screened (9, 50).

The observation that the concentration of unbound serum PSA as a fraction of the total serum PSA is lower in men with cancer has prompted the use of the percent free PSA to increase the specificity of serum PSA measurement (33). In a large multicenter study using the Tandem-E PSA assay (Hybritech, Inc., San Diego, California), Catalona and associates found that if men with a percent free PSA of >25 did not undergo biopsy, the number of unnecessary biopsies would be reduced by 20%, and 95% of the cancers that would have been detected by biopsying everyone with a PSA of 4–10 ng/ml would still be detected (42). These results have been reproduced, and the U.S. Food and Drug Administration consequently has approved the use of percent free PSA for the early detection of prostate cancer (51, 52).

Of men with a normal DRE and total PSA of 2.6–4 ng/nl, 13%–20% will develop clinically detectable prostate cancer within five years (53). Percent free PSA has also been tested in this population in an effort to improve surgical cure rates by diagnosing prostate cancer at an earlier stage. Vashi et al., using the AxSYM PSA assay (Abbott Laboratories, Abbott Park, Illinois), found that by obtaining a biopsy in patients with a percent free PSA below 19% and total PSA of 3–4 ng/ml, they detected 90% of cancers that would have been found if all men with a total PSA within this range had undergone a biopsy (54). Using this free PSA cutoff, they detected 1 cancer per 1.7 biopsies. Catalona et al., using the Tandem-E PSA assay, reported similar rates of prostate cancer detection using a free PSA cutoff of 27% in patients with total PSA of 2.6–4 ng/ml (55). In this study, 83% of the cancers diagnosed were considered clinically significant, yet 81% of patients who underwent surgery had organ-confined disease.

In addition to its use in the diagnosis of prostate cancer, percent free PSA may also be useful in tumor staging. In a prospective study comparing preoperative percent free PSA to postprostatectomy pathology in patients with disease clinically staged as T1c (tumor confined to the prostate, not palpable, and identified only by needle biopsy), a multivariate logistic regression analysis found that percent free PSA was the strongest predictor of postoperative pathological stage (56). Of patients with free PSA levels of >15%, 75% had small tumors (occupying 10% or less of the prostate volume), tumors with Gleason sum less than 7, and organ-confined disease, compared with only 34% of patients with free PSA of <15%. By analyzing blood samples collected as part of the Baltimore Longitudinal Aging study, Carter and associates demonstrated a statistically significant difference in percent free PSA levels between aggressive cancers (that have either extracapsular extension, metastasis, Gleason 7 score or greater, or positive margins at prostatectomy) and nonaggressive cancers 12 years prior to diagnosis (when total PSA levels were the same) (57).

In the primary health care setting, the most effective way to improve the specificity of PSA and DRE screening in men with PSA of 4–10 ng/ml is by using the free-PSA fraction, which allows for further stratification of prostate cancer risk. Patients with a free-PSA fraction of >25% (based on the Tandem-E PSA assay) have a <10% chance of being diagnosed with prostate cancer on biopsy, whereas patients with a low free-PSA fraction (<10%) have a >50% chance (42, 57). Similarly, the specificity of PSA between 2.6 and 4.0 ng/ml can be improved by measurement of the free-PSA fraction. A cutoff of 27%, using the Tandem-E assay, has been suggested to reduce the number of unnecessary biopsies (55).

FROM ELEVATED PSA TO PROSTATE BIOPSY

Although the most common noncancerous condition responsible for elevation in serum PSA levels is BPH, other factors influence the results of a serum PSA test. Vigorous prostatic massage or ejaculation may result in clinically relevant elevations in serum PSA (twofold increases have been reported). However, DRE is less likely to affect serum PSA measurements (12, 58, 59).

Some medications have been shown to affect serum PSA levels. The best-studied is finasteride. Finasteride at 5 mg/day has been shown to decrease total PSA, on average, by 50% after a 6-month course (60, 61). Nevertheless, on an individual basis, finasteride can cause the PSA to change anywhere from −80% to +20% (60). Percent free PSA appears to be unaffected by use of finasteride (61). In young, healthy males, use of Propecia (finasteride 1mg/day) has been noted to decrease serum PSA by 0.2ng/ml (62). Alpha 1-adrenergic antagonists, on the other hand, have not been associated with changes in serum PSA (63). Nutritional supplements or even home-prepared teas, such as those from aloe, may contain estrogens that may also artificially reduce the serum PSA concentration and mask the presence of prostate cancer (64).

Infectious or noninfectious prostatitis and urinary retention can significantly increase serum total PSA. In general, the serum PSA returns to normal within one month after the symptoms of prostatitis have resolved. The serum PSA may return to normal sooner after the relief of urinary retention (65).

Handling of specimens may affect measured free PSA concentrations. When blood is stored at 4°C or room temperature, 60%–90% of free PSA is degraded per month. This ex vivo preferential degradation of free PSA can be prevented by storage at −20°C. If the specimen will not be processed within 24 h, it is best stored at −70°C (66).

Urologic procedures such as cystoscopy and needle biopsy of the prostate may cause significant elevations in serum PSA (67). Needle biopsy has been shown to increase serum PSA values by a median of 7.9 ng/ml within 24 h after biopsy. After needle biopsy of the prostate, some patients may have a persistent elevation lasting up to a month, but in most patients, serum PSA returns to normal 14–17 days after biopsy. Although one study revealed a fourfold increase in serum PSA after cystoscopy, routine urethral catheterization has not been associated with elevations in serum PSA (12).

What is the proper response to an elevated PSA? To answer this question, one must first define "elevated" PSA. A serum total PSA greater than 4.0 ng/ml generally is regarded as abnormal. However, current data support the use of a PSA cutoff of 2.6 ng/ml in men who (a) have a life expectancy of more than 15 years, are between 45 and 50 years old, and have one first-degree relative who developed prostate cancer at an early age or (b) are of African-American descent (5, 6). Men with multiple first-degree relatives who developed prostate cancer at an early age should be screened at age 40. If their PSA is <1.0 ng/ml, no additional testing is needed until age 45. If the PSA is 1.0–2.5 ng/ml, yearly testing is advisable. If the PSA is 2.6 ng/ml or greater, biopsy is recommended (5). It is reasonable, given current data, to obtain a free-PSA fraction to improve the test's specificity and PPV. When the Hybritech assay is used, percent free PSA cutoffs of 27% and 25% in patients with PSA of 2.6–4 ng/ml and 4–10 ng/ml, respectively, have been suggested (42, 55).

Once a PSA level is found to be elevated according to the established criteria, the possibility of non-neoplastic causes should be excluded. By far the most common non-neoplastic cause of an elevated PSA is BPH. Because one cannot reliably measure prostate volume on DRE, a percent free PSA may be obtained in patients with a PSA of 4–10 ng/ml who are of advanced age or are suspected to have BPH. If the patient is potent, the time relation of testing to ejaculation should be ascertained. If the blood was drawn within 48 h after ejaculation, repetition of the study can be considered. Any history of urinary instrumentation in the days prior to the PSA test should be elicited. The patient should also be questioned about symptoms of acute or chronic prostatitis. If this diagnosis is suspected, prostatic secretions should be inspected for the presence of inflammatory cells. If prostatitis is diagnosed, the patient should be treated appropriately and the study repeated a month after symptoms have subsided. This more comprehensive evaluation is often best performed by a urologist, who may consider performing a transrectal ultrasound-guided biopsy after consultation with the patient.

THE FUTURE OF PROSTATE CANCER SCREENING

Since the introduction of PSA testing into clinical practice, the entire spectrum of prostate cancer, from diagnosis to staging and monitoring of response to therapy, has been altered profoundly. Whereas an elevated PSA increases the probability of prostate cancer diagnosis, other benign conditions of the prostate may also elevate the PSA level. An elevated or rising PSA level is often an indication of prostatic disease and should prompt evaluation by a urologist. The identification of disease-associated molecular forms of PSA, and of assays to measure them specifically, holds the promise of maintaining the high sensitivity of PSA-based screening for prostate cancer while improving the specificity.

Nevertheless, it is likely that in the near future, we will have the ability to better identify patients at high risk of developing prostate cancer at an early age by genetic testing. Although the identity of the genetic susceptibility gene remains controversial (68), segregation analysis suggests the presence of a dominant prostate cancer susceptibility gene that may be responsible for 9% of all prostate cancers and for 43% of prostate cancer cases in males <55 years old. Carriers of this allele have an estimated 88% probability of developing prostate cancer by age 85 (69). The situation may be similar to that of BRCA1 in breast cancer. BRCA1 accounts for 84% of the early onset hereditary breast cancer. Approximately 10% of breast cancers are believed to be hereditary (70). Gene-based testing may therefore allow for targeted PSA-based screening of males who are at higher risk of developing prostate cancer at an early age and would, therefore, benefit from therapeutic intervention.

ACKNOWLEDGMENT

Special thanks to Carolyn Schum for her excellent editorial assistance.

Visit the Annual Reviews home page at www.AnnualReviews.org

LITERATURE CITED

1. Greenlee RT, Hill-Harmon MB, Murray T, et al. 2001. Cancer statistics, 2001. *CA Cancer J. Clin.* 51:15–36

2. DiGuiseppi C, ed. 1996. *U.S. Preventive Services Task Force. Guide to Clinical Prevetive Services.* Baltimore: Williams & Wilkins

3. Ferrini R, Woolf SH. 1998. American College of Preventive Medicine practice policy. Screening for prostate cancer in American men. *Am. J. Prev. Med.* 15:81–84

4. Cookson MM. 2001. Prostate cancer: screening and early detection. *Cancer Control* 8:133–40

5. Smith DS, von Eschenbach AC, Wender R, et al. 2001. American Cancer Society guidelines for the early detection of cancer: update on early detection guidelines for prostate, colorectal, and endometrial cancers. *CA Cancer J. Clin.* 51:38–75

6. Carroll P, Coley C, McLeod D, et al. 2001. Prostate-specific antigen best practice policy. I. Early detection and diagnosis of prostate cancer. *Urology* 57:217–24

7. Zoorob R, Anderson R, Cefalu C, et al.

2001. Cancer screening guidelines. *Am. Fam. Physician* 63:1101–12

8. Hull GW, Rabbani F, Abbas F, et al. 2001. Cancer control with radical prostatectomy alone in 1000 consecutive patients. *J. Urol.* In press

9. Catalona WJ, Richie JP, Ahmann FR, et al. 1994. Comparison of digital rectal examination and serum prostate specific antigen in the early detection of prostate cancer: results of a multicenter clinical trial of 6,630 men. *J. Urol.* 151:1283–90

10. Gore JL, Shariat SF, Miles BJ, et al. 2001. Optimal combinations of systematic sextant and laterally directed biopsies for the detection of prostate cancer. *J. Urol.* 165:1554–59

11. Carter HB, Pearson JD, Metter EJ, et al. 1992. Longitudinal evaluation of prostate-specific antigen levels in men with and without prostate disease. *JAMA* 267:2215–20

12. Stamey TA, Yang N, Hay AR, et al. 1987. Prostate-specific antigen as a serum marker for adenocarcinoma of the prostate. *N. Engl. J. Med.* 317:909–16

13. Kerlikowske K, Grady D, Barclay J, et al. 1993. Positive predictive value of screening mammography by age and family history of breast cancer. *JAMA* 270:2444–50

14. Aus G. 1994. Prostate cancer. Mortality and morbidity after non-curative treatment with aspects on diagnosis and treatment. *Scand. J. Urol. Nephrol. Suppl.* 167:1–41

15. Bartsch G, Horninger W, Klocker H, et. al. 2000. Decrease in prostate cancer mortality following introduction of prostate specific antigen (PSA) screening in the federal state of Tyrol, Austria. *Annu. Meet. Am. Urol. Assoc., Atlanta* (Abstr.), ed. JY Gillenwater. Hagerstown, MD: Lippincott Williams Wilkins

16. Reissigl A, Horninger W, Fink K, et al. 1997. Prostate carcinoma screening in the county of Tyrol, Austria: experience and results. *Cancer* 80:1818–29

17. Roberts RO, Bergstralh EJ, Katusic SK, et al. 1999. Decline in prostate cancer mortality from 1980 to 1997, and an update on incidence trends in Olmsted County, Minnesota. *J. Urol.* 161:529–33

18. Ries LAG, Eisner MP, Kosary CL, et al., eds. 2000. *SEER Cancer Statistics Review, 1973–1998.* Bethesda, MD: Natl. Cancer Inst.

19. Tarone RE, Chu KC, Brawley OW. 2000. Implications of stage-specific survival rates in assessing recent declines in prostate cancer mortality rates. *Epidemiology* 11:167–70

20. Wilt TJ, Brawer MK. 1997. The Prostate Cancer Intervention Versus Observation Trial (PIVOT). *Oncology* 11:1133–39; discussion 9–40, 43

21. Prorok PC, Andriole GL, Bresalier RS, et al. 2000. Design of the Prostate, Lung, Colorectal and Ovarian (PLCO) Cancer Screening Trial. *Control Clin. Trials* 21:273S–309S

22. Beemsterboer PM, de Koning HJ, Kranse R, et al. 2000. Prostate specific antigen testing and digital rectal examination before and during a randomized trial of screening for prostate cancer: European randomized study of screening for prostate cancer, Rotterdam. *J. Urol.* 164:1216–20

23. Ablin RJ, Soanes WA, Bronson P, Witebsky E. 1970. Precipitating antigens of the normal human prostate. *J. Reprod. Fertil.* 22:573–74

24. Lundwall A, Lilja H. 1987. Molecular cloning of human prostate specific antigen cDNA. *FEBS Lett.* 214:317–22

25. Diamandis EP. 1996. Prostate specific antigen—new applications in breast and other cancers. *Anticancer Res.* 16:3983–84

26. Robert M, Gibbs BF, Jacobson E, Gagnon C. 1997. Characterization of prostate-specific antigen proteolytic activity on its major physiological substrate, the sperm motility inhibitor precursor/semenogelin I. *Biochemistry* 36:3811–19

27. Goldfarb DA, Stein BS, Shamszadeh M, Petersen RO. 1986. Age-related changes in tissue levels of prostatic acid phosphatase

and prostate specific antigen. *J. Urol.* 136: 266–69

28. Henttu P, Liao SS, Vihko P. 1992. Androgens up-regulate the human prostate-specific antigen messenger ribonucleic acid (mRNA), but down-regulate the prostatic acid phosphatase mRNA in the LNCaP cell line. *Endocrinology* 130:766–72

29. Mikolajczyk SD, Millar LS, Wang TJ, et al. 2000. "BPSA," a specific molecular form of free prostate-specific antigen, is found predominantly in the transition zone of patients with nodular benign prostatic hyperplasia. *Urology* 55:41–45

30. Wang TJ, Slawin KM, Rittenhouse HG, et al. 2000. Benign prostatic hyperplasia-associated prostate-specific antigen (BPSA) shows unique immunoreactivity with anti-PSA monoclonal antibodies. *Eur. J. Biochem.* 267:4040–45

31. Mikolajczyk SD, Millar LS, Marker KM, et al. 2000. Seminal plasma contains "BPSA," a molecular form of prostate-specific antigen that is associated with benign prostatic hyperplasia. *Prostate* 45: 271–76

32. Mikolajczyk SD, Millar LS, Wang TJ, et al. 2000. A precursor form of prostate-specific antigen is more highly elevated in prostate cancer compared with benign transition zone prostate tissue. *Cancer Res.* 60:756–59

33. Stenman UH, Leinonen J, Alfthan H, et al. 1991. A complex between prostate-specific antigen and alpha 1-antichymotrypsin is the major form of prostate-specific antigen in serum of patients with prostatic cancer: assay of the complex improves clinical sensitivity for cancer. *Cancer Res.* 51:222–26

34. Huber PR, Mattarelli G, Strittmatter B, et al. 1995. In vivo and in vitro complex formation of prostate specific antigen with alpha 1-anti-chymotrypsin. *Prostate* 27:166–75

35. Vessella RL, Lange PH. 1997. Issues in the assessment of prostate-specific antigen immunoassays. An update. *Urol. Clin. North Am.* 24:261–68

36. Bretton PR. 1994. Prostate-specific antigen and digital rectal examination in screening for prostate cancer: a community-based study. *South. Med. J.* 87:720–23

37. Keetch DW, Catalona WJ, Smith DS. 1994. Serial prostatic biopsies in men with persistently elevated serum prostate specific antigen values. *J. Urol.* 151:1571–74

38. Bahnson RR, Niemann TH. 2001. Extended sector biopsy for detection of carcinoma of the prostate. *Urol. Oncol.* 6:91–93

39. Stamey TA, Freiha FS, McNeal JE, et al. 1993. Localized prostate cancer. Relationship of tumor volume to clinical significance for treatment of prostate cancer. *Cancer* 71:933–38

40. Ohori M, Wheeler TM, Dunn JK, et al. 1994. The pathological features and prognosis of prostate cancer detectable with current diagnostic tests. *J. Urol.* 152:1714–20

41. Catalona WJ, Richie JP, deKernion JB, et al. 1994. Comparison of prostate specific antigen concentration versus prostate specific antigen density in the early detection of prostate cancer: receiver operating characteristic curves. *J. Urol.* 152:2031–36

42. Catalona WJ, Partin AW, Slawin KM, et al. 1998. Use of the percentage of free prostate-specific antigen to enhance differentiation of prostate cancer from benign prostatic disease: a prospective multicenter clinical trial. *JAMA* 279:1542–47

43. Benson MC, Whang IS, Pantuck A, et al. 1992. Prostate specific antigen density: a means of distinguishing benign prostatic hypertrophy and prostate cancer. *J. Urol.* 147:815–16

44. Stamey TA, Kabalin JN, McNeal JE, et al. 1989. Prostate specific antigen in the diagnosis and treatment of adenocarcinoma of the prostate. II. Radical prostatectomy treated patients. *J. Urol.* 141:1076–83

45. Partin AW, Carter HB, Chan DW, et al. 1990. Prostate specific antigen in the staging of localized prostate cancer: influence of tumor differentiation, tumor volume and benign hyperplasia. *J. Urol.* 143:747–52

46. Brawer MK, Aramburu EA, Chen GL, et al. 1993. The inability of prostate specific antigen index to enhance the predictive value of prostate specific antigen in the diagnosis of prostatic carcinoma. *J. Urol.* 150:369–73

47. Oesterling JE, Jacobsen SJ, Chute CG, et al. 1993. Serum prostate-specific antigen in a community-based population of healthy men. Establishment of age-specific reference ranges. *JAMA* 270:860–64

48. Reissigl A, Pointner J, Horninger W, et al. 1995. Comparison of different prostate-specific antigen cutpoints for early detection of prostate cancer: results of a large screening study. *Urology* 46:662–65

49. Partin AW, Criley SR, Subong EN, et al. 1996. Standard versus age-specific prostate specific antigen reference ranges among men with clinically localized prostate cancer: a pathological analysis. *J. Urol.* 155:1336–39

50. Littrup PJ, Kane RA, Mettlin CJ, et al. 1994. Cost-effective prostate cancer detection. Reduction of low-yield biopsies. nvestigators of the American Cancer Society National Prostate Cancer Detection Project. *Cancer* 74:3146–58

51. Luderer AA, Chen YT, Soriano TF, et al. 1995. Measurement of the proportion of free to total prostate-specific antigen improves diagnostic performance of prostate-specific antigen in the diagnostic gray zone of total prostate-specific antigen. *Urology* 46:187–94

52. Partin AW, Catalona WJ, Southwick PC, et al. 1996. Analysis of percent free prostate-specific antigen (PSA) for prostate cancer detection: influence of total PSA, prostate volume, and age. *Urology* 48:55–61

53. Gann PH, Hennekens CH, Stampfer MJ. 1995. A prospective evaluation of plasma prostate-specific antigen for detection of prostatic cancer. *JAMA* 273:289–94

54. Vashi AR, Wojno KJ, Henricks W, et al. 1997. Determination of the "reflex range" and appropriate cutpoints for percent free prostate-specific antigen in 413 men referred for prostatic evaluation using the AxSYM system. *Urology* 49:19–27

55. Catalona WJ, Smith DS, Ornstein DK. 1997. Prostate cancer detection in men with serum PSA concentrations of 2.6 to 4.0 ng/mL and benign prostate examination. Enhancement of specificity with free PSA measurements. *JAMA* 277:1452–55

56. Southwick PC, Catalona WJ, Partin AW, et al. 1999. Prediction of post–radical prostatectomy pathological outcome for stage T1c prostate cancer with percent free prostate specific antigen: a prospective multicenter clinical trial. *J. Urol.* 162:1346–51

57. Carter HB, Partin AW, Luderer AA, et al. 1997. Percentage of free prostate-specific antigen in sera predicts aggressiveness of prostate cancer a decade before diagnosis. *Urology* 49:379–84

58. Tchetgen MB, Song JT, Strawderman M, et al. 1996. Ejaculation increases the serum prostate-specific antigen concentration. *Urology* 47:511–16

59. Chybowski FM, Bergstralh EJ, Oesterling JE. 1992. The effect of digital rectal examination on the serum prostate specific antigen concentration: results of a randomized study. *J. Urol.* 148:83–86

60. Guess HA, Heyse JF, Gormley GJ, et al. 1993. Effect of finasteride on serum PSA concentration in men with benign prostatic hyperplasia. Results from the North American phase III clinical trial. *Urol. Clin. North Am.* 20:627–36

61. Pannek J, Marks LS, Pearson JD, et al. 1998. Influence of finasteride on free and total serum prostate specific antigen levels in men with benign prostatic hyperplasia. *J. Urol.* 159:449–53

62. Overstreet JW, Fuh VL, Gould J, et al. 1999. Chronic treatment with finasteride daily does not affect spermatogenesis or semen production in young men. *J. Urol.* 162:1295–300

63. Roehrborn CG, Oesterling JE, Olson PJ, Padley RJ. 1997. Serial prostate-specific

antigen measurements in men with clinically benign prostatic hyperplasia during a 12-month placebo-controlled study with terazosin. HYCAT Investigator Group. Hytrin Community Assessment Trial. *Urology* 50:556–61

64. Telefo PB, Moundipa PF, Tchana AN, et al. 1998. Effects of an aqueous extract of *Aloe buettneri, Justicia insularis, Hibiscus macranthus, Dicliptera verticillata* on some physiological and biochemical parameters of reproduction in immature female rats. *J. Ethnopharmacol.* 63:193–200

65. Dalton DL. 1989. Elevated serum prostate-specific antigen due to acute bacterial prostatitis. *Urology* 33:465

66. Woodrum D, French C, Shamel LB. 1996. Stability of free prostate-specific antigen in serum samples under a variety of sample collection and sample storage conditions. *Urology* 48:33–39

67. Deliveliotis C, Alivizatos G, Stavropoulos NJ, et al. 1994. Influence of digital examination, cystoscopy, transrectal ultrasonography and needle biopsy on the concentration of prostate-specific antigen. *Urol. Int.* 53:186–90

68. Xu J, Zheng SL, Chang B, et al. 2001. Linkage of prostate cancer susceptibility loci to chromosome 1. *Hum. Genet.* 108:335–45

69. Carter BS, Beaty TH, Steinberg GD, et al. 1992. Mendelian inheritance of familial prostate cancer. *Proc. Natl. Acad. Sci. USA* 89:3367–71

70. Nathanson KN, Wooster R, Weber BL. 2001. Breast cancer genetics: what we know and what we need. *Nat. Med.* 7:552–56

Annu. Rev. Med. 2002. 53:369–81

RECENT ADVANCEMENTS IN THE TREATMENT OF CHRONIC MYELOGENOUS LEUKEMIA

Michael E. O'Dwyer, Michael J. Mauro, and Brian J. Druker
*Leukemia Center, Oregon Cancer Institute, Oregon Health & Science University,
3181 SW Sam Jackson Park Road, Portland, Oregon 97201;
e-mail: odwyerm@ohsu.edu, maurom@ohsu.edu, drukerb@ohsu.edu*

Key Words   CML, tyrosine kinase, Bcr-Abl, STI571, tyrosine kinase inhibitor

■ **Abstract**   Chronic myelogenous leukemia (CML) is a clonal hematopoetic stem cell disorder characterized by the Philadelphia chromosome and resultant production of the constitutively activated Bcr-Abl tyrosine kinase. Characterized clinically by marked myeloid proliferation, it invariably terminates in an acute leukemia. Conventional therapeutic options include interferon-based regimens and stem cell transplantation, with stem cell transplantation being the only curative therapy. Through rational drug development, STI571, a Bcr-Abl tyrosine kinase inhibitor, has emerged as a paradigm for gene product targeted therapy, offering new hope for expanded treatment options for patients with CML.

INTRODUCTION

Chronic myelogenous leukemia (CML) is a myeloproliferative disorder resulting from the clonal expansion of a transformed hematopoetic stem cell. Following an initial chronic phase lasting a median of 4–5 years, CML progresses through a poorly defined accelerated phase to a terminal acute leukemia (blast crisis). An understanding of the molecular pathogenesis of CML has fostered the development of specific, molecularly targeted treatments that may fundamentally alter the way physicians approach this disease. This article provides an overview of CML, including basic biology and standard treatment approaches, before focusing on the recent development of STI571, a rationally designed, targeted therapy, and the implications of this new drug for future treatment algorithms.

CLINICAL FEATURES

CML is a malignant, clonal hematopoietic stem cell disorder (1). CML accounts for 20% of all cases of leukemia, with an annual incidence of 1–1.5 cases per 100,000. Although CML affects all age groups, data from the Surveillance, Epidemiology, and End Results Program (SEER) for the United States lists the median age at death for all patients with CML as 70.0 years (2). Thus, the median age at diagnosis for patients not selected by referral is probably close to 60 years of age. Clinically, the course of CML is divided into three phases: a chronic phase, lasting an average of 4–5 years, an accelerated phase lasting 6–18 months, and a blast phase lasting 3–6 months. The chronic phase of CML is characterized by myeloid hyperplasia with marked leukocytosis and circulating immature cells of the granulocytic series. Thrombocytosis is common and there is invariably some degree of basophilia. During the chronic phase, leukemic cells retain the capacity to differentiate normally. At diagnosis up to 50% of patients are asymptomatic and are identified through routine blood tests. Common presenting symptoms include fatigue, night sweats, and splenomegaly with abdominal discomfort and early satiety. With disease progression there is increasing myeloid immaturity as cells lose the capacity to terminally differentiate. Eventually the disease terminates in an acute leukemia or blast phase that can be either myeloid or lymphoid phenotype. The accelerated phase is an intermediate stage during which patients show signs of disease progression, including a rising percentage of blasts (15%–30%) and basophils (>20%) in the peripheral blood or bone marrow, without meeting the criteria of an acute leukemia (3).

MOLECULAR BASIS

The majority of cases of CML are associated with the presence of a specific chromosomal translocation (9; 22) (q34;q11) (4). This reciprocal translocation between the long arms of chromosomes 9 and 22 results in a shortened chromosome 22, commonly known as the Philadelphia chromosome (Ph) (5; for a personal perspective on the discovery of the Ph chromosome, please refer to Peter Nowell's prefatory chapter in this volume) . The molecular consequence of this translocation event is the fusion of the c-*abl* oncogene from chromosome 9 to sequences from chromosome 22, the breakpoint cluster region (*bcr*), giving rise to a chimeric *bcr-abl* gene (6). This gene encodes a fusion protein, of varying size, depending on the site of the breakpoint in Bcr (Figure 1). The two most common fusion proteins produced are termed p185 (185 kDa) and p210 (210 kDa). The p210 protein is seen in ~95% of patients with CML and up to 20% of adult patients with de novo acute lymphocytic leukemia (ALL), whereas the p185 form is seen in ~10% of adult patients with ALL and in the majority of pediatric patients with Ph-positive ALL (5% of pediatric ALL cases). These fusion proteins have constitutive tyrosine kinase activity, which is essential for their transforming ability (7). Conclusive evidence for their role in leukemogenesis is the demonstration that introduction of *bcr-abl* into murine hematopoietic stem cells followed by transplantation of these stem cells into syngeneic mice produces a CML-like syndrome (8, 9). Similarly, transgenic mice expressing Bcr-Abl develop leukemia (10). Although Bcr-Abl is thought to be the initial disease-transforming event in CML, the acquisition of other molecular and cytogenetic abnormalities is likely to be responsible for disease progression.

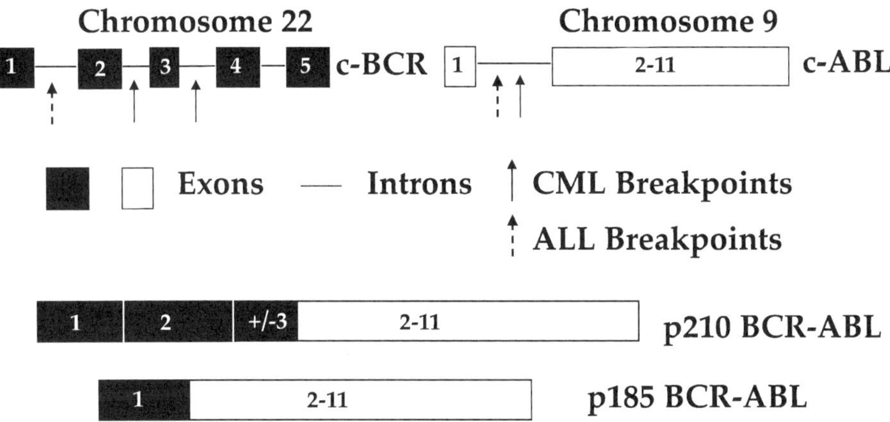

Figure 1 Common breakpoints in chronic myelogenous leukemia (CML) and Ph-positive acute lymphocytic leukemia (ALL) and the molecular consequences of these rearrangements. In CML and Ph-positive ALL, a break occurs between the first and second exon of c-abl. Thus, virtually all of the c-abl locus is translocated to chromosome 22, into the *bcr* gene. In CML, the breakpoints in *bcr* occur after what was historically called the second or third exon, resulting in a chimeric mRNA and protein of 210 kDa. In Ph-positive ALL, the breakpoints in the *bcr* gene occur after the first exon, creating a smaller fusion mRNA and protein, termed p185Bcr-Abl.

The constitutive tyrosine kinase activity of Bcr-Abl causes activation of a variety of intracellular signaling pathways leading to alterations in the proliferative, adhesive, and survival properties of CML cells (11). However, all these events depend on the tyrosine kinase activity of the Bcr-Abl protein. It is clear, therefore, that inhibition of the tyrosine kinase activity of Bcr-Abl should be an effective treatment of CML, since Bcr-Abl is present in the majority of patients with CML, it is the causative abnormality of the disease, and its kinase activity is essential for transformation.

STANDARD TREATMENT OPTIONS

Standard treatment options for patients in the chronic phase of CML are allogeneic stem cell transplantation, hydroxyurea, busulfan, or interferon-α-based regimens (12). Initial cytoreductive therapy often uses hydroxyurea. This agent, a ribonucleotide reductase inhibitor, is effective at controlling blood counts in a majority of patients. Hydroxyurea is generally well tolerated, but unfortunately cytogenetic responses (a reduction in the percentage of Ph-positive bone marrow metaphases) are rare and the onset to blast crisis is not delayed, with transformation occurring within a median of 4–6 years.

Allogeneic stem cell transplantation, using myeloablative doses of chemotherapy and/or radiation followed by infusion of allogeneic stem cells, remains the only proven curative therapy for CML. For young (age <40 years) chronic-phase patients undergoing HLA-matched transplants within 1 year of diagnosis, long-term survival rates of up to 70%–80% have been reported. With advances in molecular HLA typing and improvements in infectious and graft-versus-host disease prophylaxis, outcomes for related and unrelated donor transplants are similar (13). Outcome from transplant is superior during earlier-stage disease and within the first year after diagnosis. Other factors that predict poorer outcomes from an allogeneic stem cell transplant include increasing age and poorer-quality matches (14). Transplantation exploits the immunologically mediated graft-versus-leukemia effect, which is best demonstrated by the success of donor lymphocyte infusions in inducing lasting remissions in patients with recurrent CML after allogeneic stem cell transplantation (15). Irrespective of the type of transplant, donor availability is a major problem: Approximately 65% of younger patients do not have an HLA-matched sibling donor, and although matched unrelated donors are found in ~85% of cases, molecular typing (HLA A, B, C; DRB1; DQB1) identifies perfect matches in less than half of these (16). Therefore, for the majority of patients with CML, allogeneic stem cell transplantation is not an option. Whether this will change with the use of less toxic nonmyeloablative approaches remains to be seen. Such regimens use less intensive conditioning therapy than the standard allogeneic stem cell transplantation. The primary aim of nonmyeloablative approaches is the induction of sufficient immunosuppression in the recipient to allow durable engraftment of both donor stem cells and donor lymphocytes, which can then exert a potent graft-versus-leukemia effect (17). However, graft-versus-host disease remains a major limiting factor of this approach.

Interferon-α is a member of a family of glycoproteins that have antiviral and antiproliferative properties. It was first shown to be an active agent in CML in the early 1980s and since then has become the nontransplant treatment of choice for chronic-phase patients (18). In several large, prospective, randomized trials, interferon-α increased survival when administered in chronic phase, and a meta-analysis of several major trials showed a significant survival advantage for interferon-α over hydroxyurea and busulfan (19). In this meta-analysis, five-year survival rates were 57% and 42% for interferon-α and chemotherapy, respectively. Although hematologic responses are seen in the majority (80%) of patients treated with interferon-α, cytogenetic responses are seen in 30%–50% of patients, with complete cytogenetic responses in only 10%–20% of interferon-treated patients. This group of patients with complete cytogenetic responses gains the greatest survival advantage and has a median survival of over eight years. The optimal dose of interferon-α is not defined, but evidence from clinical trials supports a dose-response effect. Unfortunately, many patients (up to 20%) tolerate interferon-α poorly, necessitating discontinuation of treatment.

Investigators have sought to improve on the success of treatment with interferon-α alone by adding cytosine arabinoside (ara-C), which has significant antileukemic activity. A randomized trial of the combination showed significantly improved response rates over interferon-α alone, which translated into an overall survival advantage (20). A subsequent study found improved response rates but no survival advantage for the combination (21). In addition, the combination of interferon-α and cytarabine is associated with increased gastrointestinal and marrow toxicity, and not surprisingly, many patients tolerate it poorly. Another potential problem with the use of interferon-α is that it may compromise the outcome of subsequent transplantation owing to an increase in graft rejection or graft-versus-host disease unless it has been discontinued at least three months prior to the procedure (22).

DEVELOPMENT OF STI571

As noted, the deregulated tyrosine kinase activity of Bcr-Abl is known to be the essential transforming event in CML. Tyrosine kinases regulate numerous cellular processes, including growth and survival through the phosphorylation of substrate proteins. An agent that specifically blocked Abl tyrosine kinase activity would be predicted to be an ideal targeted drug for CML (Figure 2). The first synthetic tyrosine kinase inhibitors, the tyrphostins, were described in 1988 (23). Working in parallel, scientists at Ciba-Geigy (now Novartis) identified a

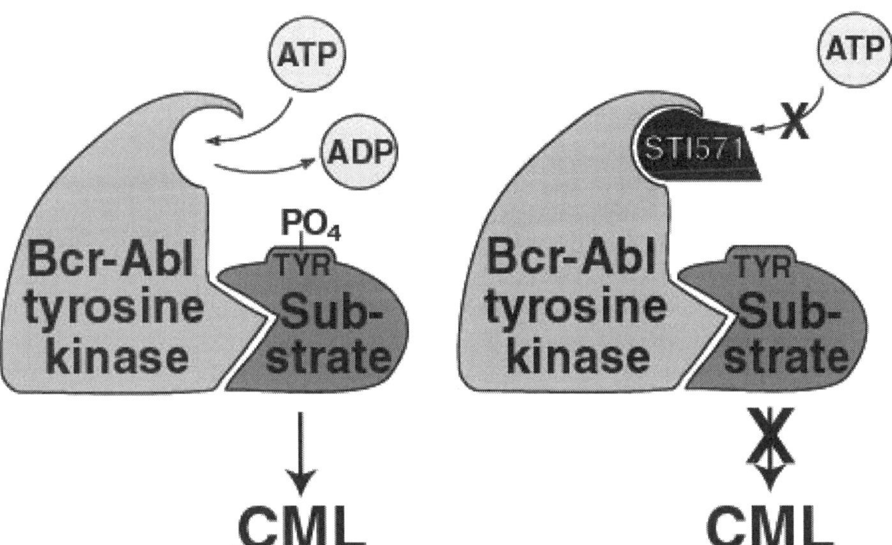

Figure 2 The Bcr-Abl tyrosine kinase is a constitutively active kinase that functions by binding ATP and transferring phosphate from ATP to tyrosine residues on various substrates. This activity causes the excess proliferation of myeloid cells characteristic of CML. STI571 functions by blocking the binding of ATP to the Bcr-Abl tyrosine kinase, thus inhibiting the activity of the kinase. In the absence of tyrosine kinase activity, substrates required for Bcr-Abl function cannot be phosphorylated.

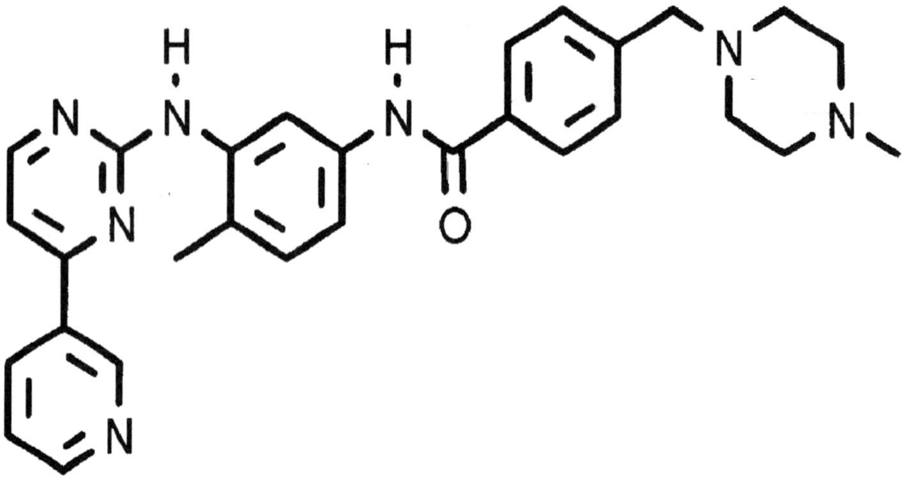

Figure 3   Structure of STI571

2-phenylaminopyrimidine as a lead tyrosine kinase inhibitor by screening a large library of compounds. Using structure-activity relationships, compounds of increasing potency and specificity were synthesized (24). STI571 (formerly CGP57148B, now imatinib mesylate or Gleevec) was initially developed as a specific platelet-derived growth factor receptor (PDGF-R) inhibitor but was also found to be a potent Abl tyrosine kinase inhibitor (Figure 3). Further testing revealed that it was relatively selective for Abl tyrosine kinases, including Bcr-Abl. Besides the PDGF-R, the only other tyrosine kinase inhibited by STI571 is c-Kit. Preclinical studies in our laboratory showed that STI571 specifically inhibits the proliferation of cell lines containing p210 Bcr-Abl and clonal growth of myeloid cells from CML patients (25). Similar findings have been seen in many other CML cell lines and patient samples that express either p210 or p185 Bcr-Abl (26–29). Long-term culture of marrow cells has shown that prolonged exposure over many weeks has a sustained inhibitory effect on CML progenitors with little toxicity to normal cells (30). Studies in mice also showed that STI571 had in-vivo activity against Bcr-Abl-expressing cells and that continuous exposure to STI571 was necessary to eradicate the tumors, suggesting this would be important for optimal antileukemic effects (25, 31). Prior to clinical testing, STI571 was shown to have an acceptable animal toxicology profile.

CLINICAL TRIALS OF STI571

A phase I clinical trial with STI571 started in June 1998. This trial was a dose escalation study, designed to establish the maximum tolerated dose with a secondary endpoint of clinical efficacy. Patients were eligible if they were in the chronic phase of CML and had failed therapy with interferon-α. STI571 was administered as once-daily oral therapy and no other cytoreductive agents were allowed. Once doses of 300 mg or greater were reached, 53 of 54 patients achieved a complete hematologic response (32). Responses were typically seen within the first 3 weeks of therapy and have been maintained in 51 of 53 patients, with a median duration of follow-up of 310 days. At this dose level ($>$300 mg) cytogenetic responses were seen in 53% of patients, with 13% achieving a complete cytogenetic response. Side effects have been minimal, with no dose-limiting toxicities encountered. The most common side effects have been nausea, vomiting, fluid retention, muscle cramps, and arthralgias. Grade 2 and 3 myelosuppression was observed at a dose $>$300 mg in 21% and 8% of patients, respectively. The myelosuppression might be consistent with a therapeutic effect, since the majority of hematopoiesis in these patients is contributed by the Ph-positive clone. Pharmacokinetic studies showed that the half-life of STI571 is 13–16 h, which is sufficiently long to permit once-daily dosing. Although the follow-up on this group of patients is relatively short, these data indicate that an Abl-specific tyrosine kinase inhibitor has significant activity in CML, even in interferon-refractory patients. This trial also demonstrates the essential role of Bcr-Abl tyrosine kinase activity in CML.

Given the effectiveness of STI571 in chronic-phase patients who had failed interferon, the phase I studies were expanded to include CML patients in myeloid and lymphoid blast crisis and patients with relapsed or refractory Ph-positive ALL (33). Patients have been treated with daily doses of 300–1000 mg of STI571. Out of 38 patients with myeloid blast crisis, 21 (55%) responded to therapy, defined by a decrease in percentage of marrow blasts to less than 15%, and 8 of 38 (21%) had clearance of blasts from their marrows to less than or equal to 5%. Out of 20 patients with lymphoid phenotype disease, CML in lymphoid blast crisis, or Ph-positive ALL, 14 (70%) responded, with 11 of them (55%) clearing their marrow blasts to $<$5%. Unfortunately, all but one of the lymphoid phenotype patients relapsed between days 42 and 123. However, 7 (18%) of the 38 myeloid blast crisis patients continue on STI571, in remission, with follow-up ranging from 101 to 349 days. Thus, STI571 has remarkable single-agent activity in CML blast crisis and Ph-positive ALL, but responses tend not to be durable. However, these studies demonstrate that in the majority of cases, the leukemic clone in Bcr-Abl-positive acute leukemias, including CML blast crisis, remains at least partially dependent on Bcr-Abl kinase activity for survival.

The success of the phase I studies prompted phase II studies; single-agent STI571 was tested further in interferon-refractory and interferon-intolerant patients as well as in accelerated-phase patients and patients with CML in myeloid blast crisis and Ph-positive ALL. These studies accrued over 1000 patients at 27 centers in 6 countries over a period of 6–9 months, and interim results were presented at the American Society of Hematology meeting in December 2000 (34–36). The results confirmed those seen in the phase I trials and served as the basis for accelerated U.S. Food and Drug Administration approval of STI571. A phase III randomized study comparing STI571 with interferon plus cytarabine in newly diagnosed patients accrued over 1000 patients in a six-month period, and data collection is ongoing.

OTHER THERAPEUTIC TARGETS FOR STI571

In addition to inhibiting the Abl kinase, STI571 inhibits the PDGF-R and c-kit tyrosine kinases (24). Given the utility of STI571 in CML, it is logical to try STI571 in other diseases in which these kinases are activated. The PDGF-R is activated as a consequence of its fusion to the Tel transcription factor in a subset of patients with chronic myelomonocytic leukemia (37), and preclinical data support the use of STI571 in this setting (28). Glioblastomas have been reported to have autocrine activation of PDGF-R, and recent studies using glioblastoma cell lines suggest that STI571 could have utility in this malignancy (38). Numerous other malignancies have also been reported to have autocrine activation of PDGF-R, including non–small cell lung, breast, and prostate cancer, but the data supporting a role for PDGF-R activation in these diseases are less compelling (39). However, clinical trials with STI571 in these diseases could be envisioned to test this hypothesis.

c-kit has been implicated in the pathophysiology of a variety of human tumors, including mastocytosis/mast cell leukemia, germ cell tumors, small cell lung cancer, gastrointestinal stromal tumors (GIST), AML, neuroblastoma, melanoma, ovarian cancer, and breast cancer. In GIST, c-kit is activated by point mutation in the majority of cases, and this event is believed to be a critical pathogenetic event (40–43). Early results demonstrate that STI571 also has dramatic activity in this tumor, which has previously been highly refractory to chemotherapy (44–46).

The majority of cases of systemic mastocytosis have a mutation of aspartic acid 816 to valine (D816V) in the kinase domain of c-kit, resulting in activation of c-kit (47). Unfortunately, the kinase activity of the D816V mutant isoform was recently shown to be resistant to STI571 (48). Thus, STI571 is unlikely to be useful in this disorder. Autocrine activation of c-kit has been reported in small cell lung cancer, but the precise role of c-kit activation in the pathogenesis of small cell lung cancer is less clear. Two groups have recently reported activity of STI571 against small cell lung cancer cell lines (49, 50), and clinical trials are planned.

FUTURE DIRECTIONS IN THE THERAPY
OF CHRONIC MYELOGENOUS LEUKEMIA

STI571 is still at a relatively early stage of clinical development and much has yet to be learned. From the experience with chronic-phase and blast-crisis patients, it is clear that STI571 works best when used early in the disease course. Whether it will work even better in early chronic-phase patients or should replace interferon-α-based regimens in patients not eligible for stem cell transplant remains to be determined from the phase III study. Because *bcr-abl* may be the sole molecular abnormality in early chronic-phase patients, it is conceivable that in these patients, STI571 alone may prove to be sufficient therapy. In late chronic-phase disease, however, STI571 alone may fail to achieve an optimal therapeutic response. For example, $\sim$50% of patients who fail interferon do not achieve a cytogenetic response after six months of therapy with STI571.

Resistance to STI571 is clearly a documented problem, particularly in advanced disease. This may be multifactorial and could include mechanisms such as clonal evolution, *bcr-abl* gene amplification or mutation and development of a multidrug resistance phenotype. There are now several reports of *bcr-abl* gene amplification as a mechanism of resistance in CML cell lines (51–53), and analysis of a small number of blast crisis patients who relapsed while on STI571 have shown either Bcr-Abl amplification or Bcr-Abl kinase domain mutations (54). Additional studies are ongoing to determine whether these or other mechanisms are present in the majority of patients who relapse while on therapy with STI571.

Preclinical data demonstrate that the addition of STI571 to other antileukemic agents such as cytarabine, interferon-α, and daunorubicin enhances the antiproliferative effect (55, 56). A combination of STI571 with these conventional antileukemic agents may be useful to improve the durability of responses in patients with advanced disease by avoiding in vivo selection of CML clones harboring additional genetic abnormalities. However, the ultimate goal of combination therapy would be to further improve the rate and durability of complete cytogenetic responses in patients with chronic-phase CML. Clinical trials using STI571 in combination with interferon and with low-dose cytarabine are ongoing in chronic-phase patients. For blast crisis and Ph-positive ALL, STI571 is being tested in combination with standard induction chemotherapy regimens.

It must be reemphasized that allogeneic stem cell transplantation is still the only treatment known to cure CML. However, the availability of improved nontransplant treatment options and the concerns regarding toxicity from transplant make the decision regarding initial therapy difficult. Although transplantation results are best when patients are transplanted within one year of diagnosis, it is unknown whether initial treatment with STI571 would compromise the outcome of a delayed transplant. Pending the availability of additional data, individual decisions regarding the choice and timing of transplantation will continue to depend on factors such as patient age, availability of a well-matched donor, individual prognostic factors, and of course, patient preference. Our current algorithm is to recommend stem cell transplantation to younger patients with suitably matched donors and nontransplant therapies to older patients or patients who lack donors. The age cutoff for these recommendations depends in part on whether patients present with low- or high-risk features for disease progression to blast phase (57) and on an assessment of the risk of transplant mortality (14). This issue is discussed in greater detail elsewhere (58).

CONCLUSIONS

STI571 is an example of a rationally designed, molecularly targeted therapy based on the specific abnormality present in a human malignancy. It promises to be an important advance in the treatment of CML, and its successful development represents a new paradigm in cancer drug development, which we hope will be followed by other specific targeted therapies in oncology.

Visit the Annual Reviews home page at www.AnnualReviews.org

LITERATURE CITED

1. Sawyers CL. 1999. Chronic myeloid leukemia. *N. Engl. J. Med.* 340:1330–40

2. Ries LAG, Eisner MP, Kosary CL, et al., eds. 2001. *SEER Cancer Statistics Review, 1973–1998*. Bethesda, MD: Natl. Cancer Inst.

3. Faderl S, Talpaz M, Estrov Z, et al. 1999. Chronic myelogenous leukemia: biology and therapy. *Ann. Intern. Med.* 131:207–19

4. Rowley JD. 1973. A new consistent abnormality in chronic myelogenous leukaemia identified by quinacrine fluorescence and giemsa staining. *Nature* 243:290–93

5. Nowell PC, Hungerford DA. 1960. A minute chromosome in human chronic granulocytic leukemia. *Science* 132:1497–501

6. Shtivelman E, Lifshitz B, Gale RP, Canaani E. 1985. Fused transcript of abl and bcr genes in chronic myelogenous leukaemia. *Nature* 315:550–54

7. Lugo TG, Pendergast AM, Muller AJ, Witte ON. 1990. Tyrosine kinase activity and transformation potency of bcr-abl oncogene products. *Science* 247:1079–82

8. Daley GQ, Van Etten RA, Baltimore D. 1990. Induction of chronic myelogenous leukemia in mice by the P210bcr/abl gene of the Philadelphia chromosome. *Science* 247:824–30

9. Kelliher MA, McLaughlin J, Witte ON, Rosenberg N. 1990. Induction of a chronic myelogenous leukemia-like syndrome in mice with v-abl and BCR/ABL. *Proc. Natl. Acad. Sci. USA* 87:6649–53

10. Heisterkamp N, Jenster G, ten Hoeve J, et al. 1990. Acute leukaemia in bcr/abl transgenic mice. *Nature* 344:251–53

11. Deininger MW, Goldman JM, Melo JV. 2000. The molecular biology of chronic myeloid leukemia. *Blood* 96:3343–56

12. Silver RT, Woolf SH, Hehlmann R, et al. 1999. An evidence-based analysis of the effect of busulfan, hydroxyurea, interferon, and allogeneic bone marrow transplantation in treating the chronic phase of chronic myeloid leukemia: developed for the American Society of Hematology. *Blood* 94:1517–36

13. Hansen JA, Gooley TA, Martin PJ, et al. 1998. Bone marrow transplants from unrelated donors for patients with chronic myeloid leukemia. *N. Engl. J. Med.* 338:962–68

14. Gratwohl A, Hermans J, Goldman JM, et al. 1998. Risk assessment for patients with chronic myeloid leukaemia before allogeneic blood or marrow transplantation. Chronic Leukemia Working Party of the European Group for Blood and Marrow Transplantation. *Lancet* 352:1087–92

15. Kolb HJ, Schattenberg A, Goldman JM, et al. 1995. Graft-versus-leukemia effect of donor lymphocyte transfusions in marrow grafted patients. European Group for Blood and Marrow Transplantation Working Party Chronic Leukemia. *Blood* 86:2041–50

16. Petersdorf EW, Gooley TA, Anasetti C, et al. 1998. Optimizing outcome after unrelated marrow transplantation by comprehensive matching of HLA class I and II alleles in the donor and recipient. *Blood* 92:3515–20

17. Carella AM, Champlin R, Slavin S, et al. 2000. Mini-allografts: ongoing trials in humans. *Bone Marrow Transpl.* 25:345–50

18. Talpaz M, McCredie KB, Mavligit GM, Gutterman JU. 1983. Leukocyte interferon-induced myeloid cytoreduction in chronic myelogenous leukemia. *Blood* 62:689–92

19. Chronic Myeloid Leukemia Trialists' Collaborative Group. 1997. Interferon alfa versus chemotherapy for chronic myeloid leukemia: a meta-analysis of seven randomized trials. *J. Natl. Cancer Inst.* 89:1616–20

20. Guilhot F, Chastang C, Michallet M, et al. 1997. Interferon alfa-2B combined with

cytarabine versus interferon alone in chronic myelogenous leukemia. *N. Engl. J. Med.* 337:223–29

21. Rosti G, Bonifazi F, De Vivo A, et al. 1999. Cytabarine increases karyotypic response and survival in αIFN treated chronic myelogenous leukemia patients: results of a national prospective randomized trial of the Italian cooperative study group on CML. *Blood* 94:600a (Abstr.)

22. Hehlmann R, Hochhaus A, Kolb HJ, et al. 1999. Interferon-alpha before allogeneic bone marrow transplantation in chronic myelogenous leukemia does not affect outcome adversely, provided it is discontinued at least 90 days before the procedure. *Blood* 668–77

23. Yaish P, Gazit A, Gilon C, Levitzki A. 1988. Blocking of EGF-dependent cell proliferation by EGF receptor kinase inhibitors. *Science* 242:933–35

24. Druker BJ, Lydon NB. 2000. Lessons learned from the development of an abl tyrosine kinase inhibitor for chronic myelogenous leukemia. *J. Clin. Invest.* 105:3–7

25. Druker BJ, Tamura S, Buchdunger E, et al. 1996. Effects of a selective inhibitor of the ABL tyrosine kinase on the growth of BCR-ABL positive cells. *Nat. Med.* 2:561–66

26. Deininger MW, Goldman JM, Lydon N, Melo JV. 1997. The tyrosine kinase inhibitor CGP57148B selectively inhibits the growth of BCR-ABL-positive cells. *Blood* 90:3691–98

27. Gambacorti-Passerini C, le Coutre P, Mologni L, et al. 1997. Inhibition of the ABL kinase activity blocks the proliferation of BCR/ABL+ leukemic cells and induces apoptosis. *Blood Cells Mol. Dis.* 23:380–94

28. Carroll M, Ohno-Jones S, Tamura S, et al. 1997. CGP 57148, a tyrosine kinase inhibitor, inhibits the growth of cells expressing BCL-ABL, TEL-ABL and TEL-PDGFR fusion proteins. *Blood* 90:4947–52

29. Beran M, Cao X, Estrov Z, et al. 1998. Selective inhibition of cell proliferation and BCR-ABL phosphorylation in acute lymphoblastic leukemia cells expressing Mr 190,000 BCR-ABL protein by a tyrosine kinase inhibitor (CGP-57148). *Clin. Cancer Res.* 4:1661–72

30. Kasper B, Fruehauf S, Schiedlmeier B, et al. 1999. Favorable therapeutic index of a p210(BCR-ABL)-specific tyrosine kinase inhibitor; activity on lineage-committed and primitive chronic myelogenous leukemia progenitors. *Cancer Chemother. Pharmacol.* 44:433–38

31. le Coutre P, Mologni L, Cleris L, et al. 1999. In vivo eradication of human BCR/ABL-positive leukemia cells with an ABL kinase inhibitor. *J. Natl. Cancer Inst.* 91:163–68

32. Druker BJ, Talpaz M, Resta D, et al. 2001. Efficacy and safety of a specific inhibitor of the BCR-ABL tyrosine kinase in chronic myeloid leukemia. *N. Engl. J. Med.* 344:1031–37

33. Druker BJ, Sawyers CL, Kantarjian H, et al. 2001. Activity of a specific inhibitor of the Bcr-Abl tyrosine kinase in the blast crisis of chronic myeloid leukemia and acute lymphoblastic leukemia with the Philadelphia chromosome. *N. Engl. J. Med.* 344:1038–42

34. Kantarjian H, Sawyers C, Hochhaus A, et al. 2000. Phase II study of STI571, a tyrosine kinase inhibitor, in patients with resistant or refractory Philadelphia chromosome positive chronic myeloid leukemia. *Blood* 96:470a (Abstr.)

35. Sawyers CL, Hochhaus A, Feldman E, et al. 2000. A Phase II study to determine the safety and anti-leukemic effects of STI571 in patients with Philadelphia chromosome positive chronic myeloid leukemia in myeloid blast crisis. *Blood* 96:503a (Abstr.)

36. Talpaz M, Silver RT, Druker BJ, et al. 2000. A Phase II study of STI571 in adult patients with Philadelphia chromosome positive chronic myeloid leukemia in accelerated phase. *Blood* 96:469a (Abstr.)

37. Golub TR, Barker GF, Lovett M, Gilliland DG. 1994. Fusion of PDGF receptor beta

to a novel ets-like gene, tel, in chronic myelomonocytic leukemia with t(5;12) chromosomal translocation. *Cell* 77:307–16

38. Kilic T, Alberta JA, Zdunek PR, et al. 2000. Intracranial inhibition of platelet-derived growth factor-mediated glioblastoma cell growth by an orally active kinase inhibitor of the 2-phenylaminopyrimidine class. *Cancer Res.* 60:5143–50

39. Kolibaba KS, Druker BJ. 1997. Protein tyrosine kinases and cancer. *Biochim. Biophys. Acta* 1333:F217–48

40. Lux ML, Rubin BP, Biase TL, et al. 2000. KIT extracellular and kinase domain mutations in gastrointestinal stromal tumors. *Am. J. Pathol.* 156:791–95

41. Hirota S, Isozaki K, Moriyama Y, et al. 1998. Gain-of-function mutations of c-kit in human gastrointestinal stromal tumors. *Science* 279:577–80

42. Nishida T, Hirota S. 2000. Biological and clinical review of stromal tumors in the gastrointestinal tract. *Histol. Histopathol.* 15:1293–301

43. Nishida T, Hirota S, Taniguchi M, et al. 1998. Familial gastrointestinal stromal tumours with germline mutation of the KIT gene. *Nat. Genet.* 19:323–24

44. Joensuu H, Roberts PJ, Sarlomo-Rikala M, et al. 2001. Effect of the tyrosine kinase inhibitor STI571 in a patient with a metastatic gastrointestinal stromal tumor. *N. Engl. J. Med.* 344:1052–56

45. Blanke CD, von Mehren M, Joensuu H, et al. 2001. Evaluation of the safety and efficacy of an oral molecularly-targeted therapy, STI571, in patients with unresectable or metastatic gastrointestinal stromal tumors (GISTS) expressing c-KIT (CD117). *Proc. Am. Soc. Clin. Oncol.* 20:1a (Abstr.)

46. Van Oosterom AT, Judson I, Verweij J, et al. 2001. STI571, an active drug in metastatic gastrointestinal stromal tumors (GIST), an EORTC Phase I study. *Proc. Am. Soc. Clin. Oncol.* 20:1a (Abstr.)

47. Longley BJ, Metcalfe DD. 2000. A proposed classification of mastocytosis incorpo-rating molecular genetics. *Hematol. Oncol. Clin. North Am.* 14:697–701

48. Heinrich MC, Wait CL, Yee KWH, Griffith DJ. 2000. STI571 inhibits the kinase activity of wild type and juxtamembrane c-kit mutants but not the exon 17 D816V mutation associated with mastocytosis. *Blood* 96:173b (Abstr.)

49. Krystal GW, Honsawek S, Litz J, Buchdunger E. 2000. The selective tyrosine kinase inhibitor STI571 inhibits small cell lung cancer growth. *Clin. Cancer Res.* 6:3319–26

50. Wang WL, Healy ME, Sattler M, et al. 2000. Growth inhibition and modulation of kinase pathways of small cell lung cancer cell lines by the novel tyrosine kinase inhibitor STI 571. *Oncogene* 19:3521–28

51. le Coutre P, Tassi E, Varella-Garcia M, et al. 2000. Induction of resistance to the Abelson inhibitor STI571 in human leukemic cells through gene amplification. *Blood* 95:1758–66

52. Weisberg E, Griffin JD. 2000. Mechanism of resistance to the ABL tyrosine kinase inhibitor STI571 in BCR/ABL-transformed hematopoietic celllines. *Blood* 95:3498–505

53. Mahon FX, Deininger MW, Schultheis B, et al. 2000. Selection and characterization of BCR-ABL positive cell lines with differential sensitivity to the tyrosine kinase inhibitor STI571: diverse mechanisms of resistance. *Blood* 96:1070–79

54. Gorre ME, Mohammed M, Ellwood K, et al. 2001. Clinical resistance to STI-571 cancer therapy caused by BCR-ABL gene mutation or amplification. *Science* 93:876–80

55. Thiesing JT, Ohno-Jones S, Kolibaba KS, Druker BJ. 2000. Efficacy of an Abl tyrosine kinase inhibitor in conjunction with other anti-leukemic agents against Bcr-Abl positive cells. *Blood* 96:3195–99

56. Fang G, Kim CN, Perkins CL, et al. 2000. CGP57148B (STI-571) induces differentiation and apoptosis and sensitizes Bcr-Abl-positive human leukemia cells to apoptosis

due to antileukemic drugs. *Blood* 96:2246–53

57. Hasford J, Pfirrmann M, Hehlmann R, et al. 1998. A new prognostic score for survival of patients with chronic myeloid leukemia treated with interferon alfa. Writing Committee for the Collaborative CML Prognostic Factors Project Group. *J. Natl. Cancer Inst.* 90:850–58

58. Goldman JM, Druker BJ. 2001. Chronic myeloid leukemia: current treatment options. *Blood* 98: In press

Annu. Rev. Med. 2002. 53:383–91

SURGICAL MANAGEMENT OF HEART FAILURE: An Overview

David Zeltsman[1] and Michael A. Acker[2]

[1]Section of Cardiac Surgery, Division of Cardiothoracic Surgery, Department of Surgery, University of Medicine and Dentistry of New Jersey, Robert Wood Johnson Medical School, New Brunswick, New Jersey 08901; [2]Section of Cardiac Surgery, Division of Cardiothoracic Surgery, Department of Surgery, University of Pennsylvania School of Medicine, Philadelphia, Pennsylvania 19104; e-mail: michael.acker@uphs.upenn.edu

Key Words   mechanical circulatory support, transplantation, Dor procedure, mitral valve repair

■ **Abstract**   Cardiac transplantation remains the gold standard of surgical therapies for advanced and end-stage heart failure. However, this very limited option trades one disease for another and can benefit only a small minority of patients. Heart failure is currently considered secondary to a structural increase in ventricular chamber volume or remodeling. Surgical therapies formerly contraindicated for the failing heart, as well as new therapies, can successfully affect ventricular remodeling and improve cardiac function. Surgical revascularization for patients with ejection fractions <20% is becoming common. Mitral valve repair is being explored, with surprisingly low operative mortality and encouraging intermediate results. Direct surgical approaches to restoring normal geometry and size to failing hearts, such as left ventricular reduction (Batista procedure), endoventricular patch plasty (Dor procedure), cardiomyoplasty, and prosthetic external constraints are under clinical investigation. Developments in mechanical assist therapy and a new generation of implantable intracorporeal assist devices are also discussed.

INTRODUCTION

Cardiac failure remains the leading cause of death in the United States, affecting more than five million people and causing >700,000 deaths annually. Approximately a third of heart failure patients are in New York Heart Association (NYHA) class III/IV. The growing cost of caring for these patients approaches $50 billion per year.

Traditionally, heart failure has been thought secondary to impaired left ventricular pump performance. According to this view, systolic dysfunction is secondary to contractile failure. Currently systolic dysfunction is thought secondary to a structural increase in ventricular chamber volume. Instead of contractile failure leading to chamber dilatation, chamber dilatation occurs as an early response to decreased wall motion, which is mandated to generate a normal stroke volume from a larger end diastolic volume. Remodeling is the term used to refer to the pathologic change in chamber length and shape not related to a preload-mandated increase in sacromere length. As the heart remodels and dilates, the radius of curvature increases. The resulting greater wall tension increases myocardial oxygen consumption, decreases subendocardial blood flow, impairs energetics, and increases arrhythmias. Overall, poor prognosis directly correlates with the degree of remodeling (1).

According to this view, remodeling, not contractile failure, is the key to the severity of depression of ejection fraction and poor prognosis. The remodeling process has been shown to be reversible. Current therapies that improve mortality, such as angiotensin-converting enzyme inhibitors and new-generation beta-blockers, can inhibit progressive chamber remodeling and improve survival. Trials such as the Survival and Ventricular Enlargement trial (SAVE) (2), Acute Infarction Ramipril Efficacy study (AIRE) (3), and Trandolapril Cardiac Evaluation (TRACE) (4) all demonstrated improved mortality, which was attributed to the administration of angiotensin-converting enzyme (ACE) inhibitors in the early post-infarction period. Recently, beta-blockers have also been prospectively evaluated in multiple large-scale studies, such as the first and second Cardiac Insufficiency Bisoprolol Study (CIBIS and CIBIS II) (5, 6), Metoprolol CR/XL Randomized Intervention Trial in Heart Failure (MERIT-HF) (7), and Carvedilol Heart Failure Study (8, 9). In these studies, beta-blockers consistently improved left ventricular function and long-term outcomes, significantly decreased all-cause hospitalization rate, and reduced mortality. Further data suggest that survival benefits attributed to ACE inhibitors (10, 11) and beta-blockers (12) can be attributed to the reversed remodeling properties of these drug groups.

Nevertheless, despite significant advances in the pharmacological support of the failing heart, the results are far from perfect. Mortality remains high and hospitalization costly. There is a growing understanding that in addition to new and evolving surgical approaches, old surgical therapies formerly contraindicated for the failing heart can combat ventricular remodeling and improve cardiac function.

HEART TRANSPLANTATION

Cardiac transplantation remains the gold standard of surgical therapies for advanced and end-stage heart failure. The one-year survival after heart transplantation is 85% and at five years survival is 68.5% (13, 14). It is offered at 142 cardiac transplant centers nationwide and >2000 heart transplants are performed annually. However, the Achilles heel of heart transplantation is the persistent and worsening shortage of organ donors. Although 4296 patients were on the United Network for Organ Sharing (UNOS) national patient waiting list as of April 2001, only 49% will proceed to heart transplantation (15). The number of donors has persistently decreased over the past several years from 2426 in 1997 to 2197 in 2000, representing almost a 10% decrease. Because of the unavailability of a donor heart, 709 patients died while on the cardiac transplant waiting list (15). Despite its success, transplantation is epidemiologically trivial. It will remain a very limited option that trades one disease for another and can only be applied to a small number of patients who potentially could benefit. Therefore, an aggressive search for alternative surgical management of end-stage heart disease must be undertaken.

SURGICAL REVASCULARIZATION

The most frequently reported indication for heart transplantation in the United States is coronary artery disease, accounting for 44.6% of the patients (13). Surgical revascularization for patients with ejection fractions of <20% to recruit hibernating myocardium is becoming commonplace (16). These patients are generally sicker with more perioperative risk factors and, despite increased hospital mortality of ~4%–6%, they enjoy 90% one-year survival and 64% five-year survival (17). Patients with ischemic cardiomyopathy, evidence of viable myocardium, and bypassable vessels can be revascularized with permissible risk, achieving 88% perioperative survival with 72% of the patients alive at one year. These results are reproducible and have been reported by different authors (18–21).

CORRECTION OF MITRAL INSUFFICIENCY

Mitral valve repair for both primary and secondary severe mitral regurgitation in dilated cardiomyopathic ventricles with ejection fraction of <30% is being actively pursued. Mitral insufficiency, an important complication of dilative cardiomyopathy, results from enlargement of the mitral annular-ventricular apparatus with ensuing loss of valve leaflet coaptation (22–24). As the annular dilation progresses, a centrally located functional regurgitant jet develops despite structural preservation of the chordal and papillary muscle complex (24). Ischemic mitral regurgitation appears to be more complex, resulting from deformational changes in the ventricular geometry, annular dilatation, and papillary muscle dysfunction. Often the posterior leaflet becomes functionally restricted owing to ventricular enlargement. Among patients with significant (>2+) secondary mitral regurgitation, mitral valve repair should be considered in NYHA class III/IV patients with dilated cardiomyopathies. Bolling has demonstrated operative mortality <5% with significant improvement in NYHA class symptoms, as well as good survival rates at one and two years (23, 24). The annuloplasty is generally performed with a complete (encircling) ring that undersizes the mitral annulus and offers effective correction of mitral regurgitation in heart failure patients. The procedure is well tolerated, and the elimination of mitral regurgitation helps to reverse remodeling with restoration of elliptical left ventricular contour and decreased sphericity (24). If mitral valve repair is not possible, it is essential that mitral valve replacement be performed with retention of the subchordal attachments. Preservation of both the anterior and posterior chorded attachments to the papillary muscles helps to maintain normal ventricular geometry and function following mitral valve replacement (25–28).

REVERSAL OF THE REMODELING PROCESS

The concept of surgically reversing the remodeling process—partial left ventriculectomy—for patients with NYHA class IV idiopathic dilated cardiomyopathies was introduced by Batista et al. in 1996. They described an operation in which normal muscle between the anterior and posterior papillary muscles is resected, along with mitral valve repair/replacement, so as to restore the ventricle to a more normal volume/mass/diameter relationship. The reduction in ventricular diameter, according to LaPlace's law, results in decreased ventricular wall tension and thus improved systolic performance (29, 30). Although many patients improved markedly, perioperative mortality was high (>20%) in many reports. In the largest and best-controlled series from the Cleveland Clinic, perioperative mortality was only 3.2% but 16% of patients required left ventricular assist devices following the procedure. Many patients improved enough to allow removal from the transplant list, but freedom from death, need for left ventricular assist device, need for transplant or return to class IV heart failure symptoms was only 50% and 37% at one and two years, respectively. After initial success, many patients redilated (31, 32). Overall enthusiasm for the procedure has waned. Selection criteria need to improve before the role of partial left ventriculectomy for end-stage heart failure patients can be determined.

Direct surgical restoration of left ventricular geometry with reduction in left ventricular size and shape has evolved over the past few years from partial left ventriculectomy to a modification of the Dor procedure for left ventricular aneurysm (33) called endoventricular circular patch plasty or surgical ventricular restoration (SVR). This procedure is considered for patients who have ischemic cardiomyopathies with status post large anterior wall myocardial infarctions, resulting in dilated spherical left ventricles associated with an area of anterior akinesia or dyskinesia. An endoventricular dacron patch is used to exclude akinetic or dyskinetic portions of the anterior wall and septum, so as to restore a more normal size and shape to the left ventricle. This results in more normal ventricular geometry (elliptical instead of spherical) and improved systolic performance. A recent study on the results of this procedure, usually combined with coronary artery bypass grafting in 586 patients, reported overall mortality of 7.7%; left ventricular and systolic volume index decreased from 98 ± 95 to 64 ± 40 ml/m^2 and left ventricular ejection function improved from 29.5% to 40% postoperatively (34–36).

Carefully controlled studies are needed to determine if decreased ventricular size results in diastolic compromise, if the increase in ejection fraction in smaller ventricles translates to an increase in stroke volume, and if further remodeling occurring after the operation limits its overall long-term success (36). A National Institutes of Health–sponsored, multicentered, randomized trial is planned for patients with heart failure and coronary artery disease amenable to surgical revascularization (STICH). In patients with reported left ventricular dysfunction, SVR and surgical revascularization will be randomized to either surgical revascularization alone or surgical revascularization and SVR to determine its impact on cardiac function and overall survival.

Recently, new girdling devices have been evaluated to limit or to reverse ventricular remodeling. Lessons learned from the clinical experience with dynamic cardiomyoplasty revealed that much of its benefit was derived from the girdling effect of the muscle wrap and not from an increase in stroke volume as originally conceived. Use of the prosthetic external constraint CardioCor (Acorn Cardiovascular, Inc.), currently under active clinical investigation, is based on the belief that heart failure is primarily the result of ongoing ventricular remodeling. Preclinical evaluation in canine models of chronic dilated cardiomyopathy and heart failure has demonstrated a halting or reversal of ventricular remodeling and preservation or improvement of cardiac function. In addition, improved myocyte contraction and relaxation, enhanced inotropic response, and altered gene expression have been demonstrated (37–42). In more than 60 European patients who have had the Acorn jacket placed, no evidence of coronary or ventricular constriction has been seen for up to two years (43). Currently a randomized, prospective, multicentered phase II U.S. Food and Drug Administration (FDA) study is under way in patients with NYHA class III heart failure, comparing the efficacy of the Acorn jacket in dilated left ventricles with and without mitral insufficiency. In the future, this device or something similar may be used prophylactically in patients with large myocardial infarctions to prevent subsequent remodeling and heart failure.

MECHANICAL ASSISTANCE

Mechanical ventricular assistance as a bridge to transplantation is an established therapy. Seventy percent of individuals are successfully transplanted after implantation of a left ventricular assist device. The TCI HeartMate is the most successful device, having the lowest incidence of stroke despite patients being managed on only one aspirin daily. Patients can be sent home to wait for a suitable heart to become available. These devices allow patients in cardiogenic shock not only to live but to be mobile and rehabilitated prior to their transplant. The expert use of a variety of ventricular assist devices for left, right, and biventricular support is mandatory for any cardiac transplant center today (44–47).

Several investigators have reported prolonged (weeks to months) use of left ventricular assist devices as a bridge to recovery. Muller reports improvement in patients with dilated cardiomyopathy after weeks to months of left ventricular unloading (48). Others feel that this approach in patients with chronic heart failure is very unpredictable and rarely successful (49). In patients presenting with fulminant acute myocarditis, however, such support has been particularly successful, resulting in full cardiac recovery in many cases (50, 51).

The success of the TCI HeartMate as a bridge to transplantation has led to its consideration as a permanent or destination device. This application is currently being studied in class IV patients who are not transplant candidates in a multicentered, prospective, randomized study (REMATCH) (52). Although this study is still ongoing, the disadvantage of this and other present-day devices may turn out to be a high incidence of infection—driveline exit site, pump pocket, or true endocarditis. Until this complication is drastically reduced, these devices cannot be considered for permanent placement (53).

A new generation of assist devices will soon be entering initial phase I and II studies. Axial flow pumps have been developed that are tiny compared with present general pulsatile pumps, yet still capable of up to 10 liters of flow. The LionHeart (Arrow International), currently undergoing phase I FDA evaluation, is a destination device that is totally intracorporeal, LVAD, powered by transcutaneous energy transmission with no driveline crossing the skin. Total artificial hearts (Abiocor—Abiomed) will very soon enter clinical trials (54).

SUMMARY

An aggressive approach to surgical revascularization, correction of mitral insufficiency, or reversal of left ventricular remodeling by new girdling devices (or the Dor procedure in end-stage heart failure) should be considered in any patient who has exhausted pharmacologic therapy. Such therapies are best performed in large heart failure/transplant centers having specialized expertise with these procedures in patients with end-stage heart failure. The development and clinical use of a new generation of totally intracorporeal assist devices, permanently implanted in patients with end-stage heart failure who are not transplant candidates, which overcome the current problems of thromboembolism, infection, and large size, will be a clinical reality within the near future.

Visit the Annual Reviews home page at www.AnnualReviews.org

LITERATURE CITED

1. Cohn JN. 1995. Structural basis for heart failure. *Circulation* 91:2504–7
2. Pfeffer MA, Braunwald E, Moye LA, et al. 1992. Effect of captopril on mortality and morbidity in patients with left ventricular dysfunction after myocardial infarction. Results of the survival and ventricular enlargement trial. The SAVE Investigators. *N. Engl. J. Med.* 327:669–77
3. The Acute Infarction Ramipril Efficacy (AIRE) Study Investigators. 1993. Effects of ramipril on mortality and morbidity of survivors of acute myocardial infarction with clinical evidence of heart failure. *Lancet* 342:821–28
4. Kober L, Torp-Pedersen C, Carlsen JE, et al. 1995. A clinical trial of the angiotensin-converting-enzyme inhibitor trandolapril in patients with left ventricular dysfunction after myocardial infarction. Trandolapril Cardiac Evaluation (TRACE) Study Group. *N. Engl. J. Med.* 21; 333(25): 1670–81
5. CIBIS Investigators and Committee. 1994. A randomized trial of beta-blockade in heart failure: the Cardiac Insufficiency Bisoprolol Study (CIBIS). *Circulation* 94: 1765–73
6. CIBIS II Investigators and Committees. 1999. The Cardiac Insufficiency Bisoprolol

Study (CIBIS II): a randomized trial. *Lancet* 353:9–13

7. MERIT-HF Study Group. 1999. Effects of metoprolol CR/XL in chronic heart failure: metoprolol CR/XL randomized trial in congestive heart failure. *Lancet* 353:2001–7

8. Packer M, Bristow MR, Cohn JN, et al. 1996. The effect of carvedilol on morbidity and mortality in patients with chronic heart failure. U.S. Carvedilol Heart Failure Study Group. *N. Engl. J. Med.* 334:1349–55

9. Yancy CW, Fowler MB, Colucci WS, et al. for U.S. Carvedilol Heart Failure Study Group. 2001. Race and the response to adrenergic blockade with carvedilol in patients with chronic heart failure. *N. Engl. J. Med.* 344:1358–65

10. Aikawa Y, Rohde L, Plehn J, et al. 2001. Regional wall stress predicts ventricular remodeling after anteroseptal myocardial infarction in the Healing and Early Afterload Reducing Trial (HEART): an echocardiography-based structural analysis. *Am. Heart J.* 141:234–42

11. Konstam MA, Kronenberg MW, Rousseau MF, et al. 1993. Effects of the angiotensin converting enzyme inhibitor enalapril on the long-term progression of left ventricular dilatation in patients with asymptomatic systolic dysfunction. SOLVD (Studies of Left Ventricular Dysfunction) Investigators. *Circulation* 88:2277–83

12. Australia/New Zealand Heart Failure Research Collaborative Group. 1997. Randomized, placebo-controlled trial of carvedilol in patients with congestive heart failure due to ischemic heart disease. *Lancet* 349:375–80

13. Keck BM, Bennet LE, Rosendale J, et al. 2000. Worldwide thoracic organ transplantation: a report from the UNOS/ISHLT International Registry for Thoracic Organ Transplantation. In *Clinical Transplants 1999*, ed. JM Cecka, PI Terasaki, pp. 35–49. Richmond, VA: United Network of Organ Sharing

14. 2000. Annual Report of the U.S. Scientific Registry of Transplant Recipients and the Organ Procurement and Transplantation Network: transplant data 1989–2000. Rockville, MD and Richmond, VA: HHS/HRSA/OSP/DOT and UNOS. http://www.unos.org/Data/anrpt_main.htm

15. 2001. Transplant patient data source. Richmond, VA: United Network for Organ Sharing. http://www.patients.unos.org/data.htm

16. Pagano D, Bonser RS, Camici PG. 1999. Myocardial revascularization for the treatment of post-ischemic heart failure. *Curr. Opin. Cardiol.* 14:506–9

17. Trachiotis GD, Weintraub WS, Johnston TS, et al. 1998. Coronary artery bypass grafting in patients with advanced left ventricular dysfunction. *Ann. Thorac. Surg.* 66(5):1632–39

18. Dreyfus GD, Duboc D, Blasco A, et al. 1994. Myocardial viability assessment in ischemic cardiomyopathy: benefits of coronary revascularization. *Ann. Thorac. Surg.* 57(6):1402–7

19. Tjan TD, Kondruweit M, Scheld HH, et al. 2000. The bad ventricle—revascularization versus transplantation. *Thorac. Cardiovasc. Surg.* 48(1):9–14

20. Lansman SL, Cohen M, Galla JD, et al. 1993. Coronary bypass with ejection fraction of 0.20 or less using centigrade cardioplegia: long-term follow-up. *Ann. Thorac. Surg.* 56(3):480–85

21. Kaul TK, Agnihotri AK, Fields BL, et al. 1996. Coronary artery bypass grafting in patients with an ejection fraction of twenty percent or less. *J. Thorac. Cardiovasc. Surg.* 111(5):1001–12

22. Hendren WG, Nemec JJ, Lytle BW, et al. 1991. Mitral valve repair for ischemic mitral insufficiency. *Ann. Thorac. Surg.* 52(6):1246–51

23. Bolling SF, Pagani FD, Deeb GM, Bach DS. 1998. Intermediate-term outcome of mitral reconstruction in cardiomyopathy. *J. Thorac. Cardiovasc. Surg.* 115(2):381–86

24. Smolens IA, Pagani FD, Bolling SF. 2000. Mitral valve repair in heart failure. *Eur. J. Heart Fail.* 2(4):365–71

25. Sintek CF, Pfeffer TA, Kochamba G, et al. 1995. Preservation of normal left ventricular geometry during mitral valve replacement. *J. Heart Valve Dis.* 4(5):471–75

26. Sarris GE, Cahill PD, Hansen DE, et al. 1988. Restoration of left ventricular systolic performance after reattachment of the mitral chordae tendineae. The importance of valvular-ventricular interaction. *J. Thorac. Cardiovasc. Surg.* 95(6):969–79

27. Natsuaki M, Itoh T, Tomita S, et al. 1996. Importance of preserving the mitral subvalvular apparatus in mitral valve replacement. *Ann. Thorac. Surg.* 61(2):585–90

28. Komeda M, David TE, Rao V, et al. 1994. Late hemodynamic effects of the preserved papillary muscles during mitral valve replacement. *Circulation* 90(5 Pt 2):II190–94

29. Batista RJ, Santos JL, Takeshita N, et al. 1996. Partial left ventriculectomy to improve left ventricular function in end-stage heart disease. *J. Cardiovasc. Surg.* 11(2): 96–97

30. Batista RJ, Verde J, Nery P, et al. 1997. Partial left ventriculectomy to treat end-stage heart disease. *Ann. Thorac. Surg.* 64 (3):634–38

31. McCarthy JF, McCarthy PM, Starling RC, et al. 1998. Partial left ventriculectomy and mitral valve repair for end-stage congestive heart failure. *Eur. J. Cardiothorac. Surg.* 13 (4):337–43

32. Etoch SW, Koenig SC, Laureano MA, et al. 1999. Results after partial left ventriculectomy versus heart transplantation for idiopathic cardiomyopathy. *J. Thorac. Cardiovasc. Surg.* 117(5):952–59

33. Dor V, Saab M, Coste P, et al. 1989. Left ventricular aneurysm: a new surgical approach. *Thorac. Cardiovasc. Surg.* 37(1): 11–19

34. Athanasuleas CL, Stanley AW Jr, Buckberg GD, et al. 2001. Surgical anterior ventricular endocardial restoration (SAVER) in the dilated remodeled ventricle after anterior myocardial infarction. RESTORE group. Reconstructive endoven-tricular surgery, returning torsion original radius elliptical shape to the LV. *J. Am. Coll. Cardiol.* 37(5):1199–209

35. Dor V, Sabatier M, Di Donato M, et al. 1998. Efficacy of endoventricular patch plasty in large postinfarction akinetic scar and severe left ventricular dysfunction: comparison with a series of large dyskinetic scars. *J. Thorac. Cardiovasc. Surg.* 116:50–59

36. Di Donato M, Sabatier M, Dor V, et al. 2001. Effects of the Dor procedure on left ventricular dimension and shape and geometric correlates of mitral regurgitation one year after surgery. *J. Thorac. Cardiovasc. Surg.* 121(1):91–96

37. Sabbah HN, Sharov VG, Chaudhry PA, et al. 2001. Chronic therapy with the Acorn Cardiac Support Device in dogs with chronic heart failure: three and six months hemodynamic, histologic and ultrastructural findings. *J. Heart Lung Transplant.* 20:189 (Abstr.)

38. Sabbah HN, Gupta RC, Sharov VG, et al. 2001. Prevention of progressive left ventricular dilation with the Acorn Cardiac Support Device down regulates stretch-response proteins and improves sarcoplasmic reticulum recycling in dogs with chronic heart failure. *J. Am. Coll. Cardiol.* 1:37 (Suppl. A):474A (Abstr.)

39. Saavedra F, Tunin R, Mishima T, et al. 2000. Reverse remodeling and enhanced adrenergic reserve from a passive external ventricular support in experimental dilated heart failure. *Circulation* 102(Suppl.): 11:501 (Abstr.)

40. Sabbah HN, Gupta RC, Sharov VG, et al. 2000. Prevention of progressive left ventricular dilation with the Acorn Cardiac Support Device (CSD) down regulates stretch-mediated p21ras, attentuates myocyte hypertrophy and improves sarcoplasmic reticulum calcium cycling in dogs with heart failure. *Circulation* 102 (Suppl.): 11–683 (Abstr.)

41. Chaudry PA, Mishima T, Sharov VG, et al. 2000. Passive epicardial containment

prevents ventricular remodeling in heart failure. *Ann. Thorac. Surg.* 70:1275–80

42. Gupta RC, Sharov VG, Mishra S, et al. 2001. Chronic therapy with the Acorn Cardiac Support Device (CSD) attentuates cardiomyocyte apoptosis in dogs with heart failure. *J. Am. Coll. Cardiol.* 37 (Suppl. A): 478A (Abstr.)

43. Kleber FX, Sonntag S, Krebs H, et al. 2001. Follow-up on passive cardiomyoplasty in congestive heart failure: influence on the Acorn Cardiac Support Device on left ventricular function. *J. Am. Coll. Cardiol.* 37 (Suppl. A) 143A (Abstr.)

44. Goldstein DJ, Oz MC. 2000. Mechanical support for postcardiotomy cardiogenic shock. *Semin. Thorac. Cardiovasc. Surg.* 12(3):220–28

45. McCarthy PM, Portner PM, Tobler HG, et al. 1991. Clinical experience with the Novacor ventricular assist system. Bridge to transplantation and the transition to permanent application. *J. Thorac. Cardiovasc. Surg.* 102(4):578–86

46. Levin HR, Chen JM, Oz MC, et al. 1994. Potential of left ventricular assist devices as outpatient therapy while awaiting transplantation. *Ann. Thorac. Surg.* 58(5):1515–20

47. Sun BC, Catanese KA, Spanier TB, et al. 1999. 100 long-term implantable left ventricular assist devices: the Columbia Presbyterian interim experience. *Ann. Thorac. Surg.* 68(2):688–94

48. Muller J, Wallukat G, Weng YG, et al. 1997. Weaning from mechanical cardiac support in patients with idiopathic dilated cardiomyopathy. *Circulation* 15;96(2):542–49

49. Mancini DM, Beniaminovitz A, Levin H, et al. 1998. Low incidence of myocardial recovery after left ventricular assist device implantation in patients with chronic heart failure. *Circulation* 98:2383–89

50. McCarthy RE, Boehmer JP, Hruban RH, et al. 2000. Long-term outcome of fulminant myocarditis as compared with acute (nonfulminant) myocarditis. *N. Engl. J. Med.* 342(10):690–95

51. Acker MA. 2001. Mechanical circulatory support for patients with acute/fulminant myocarditis. *Ann. Thorac. Surg.* 71(3 Suppl.):S73–76; discussion S82–85

52. Rose EA, Moskowitz AJ, Packer M, et al. 1999. The REMATCH trial: rationale, design, and end points. Randomized Evaluation of Mechanical Assistance for the Treatment of Congestive Heart Failure. *Ann. Thorac. Surg.* 67(3):723–30

53. Mann DL, Willerson JT. 1998. Left ventricular assist devices and the failing heart: a bridge to recovery, a permanent assist device, or a bridge too far? *Circulation* 98(22):2367–69

54. Frazier OH. Future directions of cardiac assistance. *Semin. Thorac. Cardiovasc. Surg.* 12(3):220–28

Annu. Rev. Med. 2002. 53:393–407

NEPHRON-SPARING SURGERY FOR RENAL CELL CARCINOMA

Andrew C. Novick

Urological Institute, The Cleveland Clinic Foundation, 9500 Euclid Avenue, Cleveland, Ohio 44195; e-mail: novicka@ccf.org

Key Words kidney, organ-sparing, cancer, nephrectomy, conservative

■ **Abstract** Nephron-sparing surgery (NSS) provides effective curative therapy for patients with localized renal cell carcinoma. In patients with imperative indications, it represents an alternative to renal replacement therapy. For selected patients with systemic comorbidities that threaten global renal function, NSS preserves unaffected nephrons with excellent cancer-specific survival. Elective partial nephrectomy for patients with a small ($\leq$4 cm), unifocal tumor and a normal contralateral kidney is associated with a low risk (0%–3%) of local recurrence and cancer-specific survival rates of 90%–100%. Comparisons between radical and partial nephrectomy demonstrate equivalent cancer control over five years. Minimally invasive techniques of NSS are feasible but await improved technologies and long-term outcome data before they become fully acceptable treatment options.

INTRODUCTION

Epithelial tumors of the kidney account for approximately 3% of all solid neoplasms, with an incidence roughly equal to that of all forms of leukemia combined. Adenocarcinoma or renal cell carcinoma (RCC) represents nearly 85% of newly diagnosed malignancies of the kidney, occurring at an estimated rate of 4.4–11.1 per 100,000 person years. Recent data from the U.S. Surveillance Epidemiology and End Results (SEER) program demonstrate a steady rise in RCC rates of 2.3%–4.3% annually between 1975 and 1995 (1). This can be attributed in part to early detection through the widespread use of noninvasive imaging techniques, although incidental detection alone cannot fully explain the upward trend. Despite the lack of effective medical therapy, a small but significant improvement in overall five-year survival has been noted. This has been primarily due to early detection and advances in surgical management of the disease rather than improvements in systemic therapy.

Surgical resection remains the cornerstone of treatment for RCC. The classic concept of wide excision of the affected kidney outside of its investing (Gerota's) fascia, to include the perirenal fat and ipsilateral adrenal gland, has governed surgical thinking and management of this tumor for over a half a century. The rationale for choosing this approach over simple nephrectomy is based on the philosophy of maintaining anatomic planes of resection to obtain the widest surgical margin possible, recognizing that extrarenal involvement of the adjacent perirenal fat and adrenal may contribute to surgical failure. Today, a better understanding of the biology of RCC, standardized staging, and changing patterns of presentation for patients with this tumor permit a refined surgical approach, limiting potential long-term morbidity by maximizing preservation of functional renal parenchyma.

Partial nephrectomy for excision of tumorous renal lesions dates back as far as 1884, when Wells described the technique for removal of a perirenal fibrolipoma. Czerny was the first to use partial nephrectomy for therapy of a renal malignancy in 1897; however, excessive postoperative morbidity limited its application until the 1950s, when Vermooten suggested that peripheral encapsulated renal neoplasms could be locally excised, leaving a margin of normal parenchyma around the tumor. The role of partial nephrectomy was subsequently challenged by Robson et al., who demonstrated in 1969 that early ligation of the renal vessels decreased the risk of hematologic spread when accompanied by removal of the perinephric fat and excision of all regional lymph nodes (2). Since that time, radical nephrectomy has remained the standard against which all other forms of surgical treatment for RCC must be measured.

Enthusiasm for nephron-sparing surgery (NSS) has been stimulated by several trends, including advances in renal imaging, improved surgical techniques and methods to prevent ischemic renal injury, better postoperative management including renal replacement therapy, and long-term prospective cancer-free survival data. Extended experience has now established that NSS can be performed safely, with low morbidity, preservation of renal function, low local recurrence rates, and high patient satisfaction.

CURRENT INDICATIONS

NSS is indicated if radical nephrectomy would render the patient anephric, with subsequent immediate need for dialysis. This encompasses patients with bilateral RCC or RCC involving a solitary functioning kidney. The latter circumstance may result from unilateral renal agenesis, prior removal of the contralateral kidney, or irreversible impairment of contralateral renal function. NSS is also indicated in patients with unilateral RCC and a functioning opposite kidney, when the opposite kidney is affected by a condition that might threaten its future function, such as calculus disease, chronic pyelonephritis, renal artery stenosis, ureteral reflux, or systemic diseases such as diabetes and nephrosclerosis (3).

Recent studies have clarified the role of NSS in patients with localized unilateral RCC and a normal contralateral kidney. The data indicate that radical nephrectomy and NSS provide equally effective curative treatment for such patients who present with a single, small (≤4 cm), and clearly localized RCC. More recent data further suggest that NSS provides a long-term renal functional advantage over radical nephrectomy in patients with a normal opposite kidney. The results of NSS are less satisfactory in patients with larger (≥4 cm) or multiple localized RCCs, and radical nephrectomy remains the treatment of choice in such cases when the opposite kidney is normal.

PREOPERATIVE EVALUATION

Evaluation of patients with RCC prior to NSS must include a detailed history and physical examination, a laboratory evaluation including serum creatinine, liver function tests, and urinalysis or urine dipstick check to screen for preoperative proteinuria. Radiographic testing is used to rule out locally extensive or metastatic disease, including chest X-ray and abdominal computed tomography (CT) as well as possible bone scan and chest or head CT depending on the clinical circumstances.

NSS is technically more challenging than en bloc removal of the kidney by radical nephrectomy and therefore requires a more detailed understanding of renal anatomy. Knowledge of the relationship of the tumor and its vascular supply to the collecting system and adjacent normal renal parenchyma is essential for preoperative assessment, which must include a plan for complete tumor removal and reconstruction of the renal remnant. Therefore, more extensive and invasive preoperative imaging studies are often obtained before NSS than before radical nephrectomy. In some instances, these include arteriography and occasionally venography.

Arteriography has been used to delineate the intrarenal vasculature and may aid in excision of the tumor while minimizing blood loss and injury to normal adjacent parenchyma. It is most useful for nonperipheral tumors encompassing two or more renal arterial segments. Selective renal venography is performed in patients with large or centrally located tumors to evaluate for the presence of intrarenal venous thrombosis and assess adequacy of venous drainage of the planned renal remnant. However, these radiographic studies provide only two-dimensional views, and the risks and costs of conventional arteriography and venography are significant. Furthermore, these studies yield limited information on anatomic spatial relationships between the tumor, normal parenchyma, collecting system, and vascular supply.

Advances in helical CT and computer technology now allow production of high-quality three-dimensional images of the renal vasculature and soft tissue anatomy in any plane. New volume-rendering software allows real-time interactive stereoscopic viewing of these images and provides a topographical map of the renal surface and multiplanar views of the intrarenal anatomy. This permits evaluation of the complex renal anatomy using a single, unified study in a format that is familiar to the surgeon and consistent with intraoperative findings, thereby obviating the need for mental reconstruction of several two-dimensional imaging studies. A detailed prospective study at the Cleveland Clinic demonstrated the utility of three-dimensional volume-rendering CT in accurately depicting the renal parenchyma and vascular anatomy necessary for the performance of NSS (4). The data from three-dimensional CT integrate essential information from angiography, venography, excretory urography, and conventional two-dimensional CT into a single preoperative staging test that diminishes the need for more invasive imaging. The use of a 3–5-minute videotape in the operating room provides concise, accurate, and immediate three-dimensional information to the surgeon during the dissection, allowing him or her to anticipate the subtleties of the anatomy. Three-dimensional volume-rendered CT has become the imaging modality of choice prior to NSS, allowing hilar dissection, tumor removal, and reconstruction to proceed quickly and confidently.

OPERATIVE TECHNIQUE

It is usually possible to perform NSS for malignancy in situ by using an operative approach that optimizes exposure of the kidney and by combining meticulous surgical technique with an understanding of the renal vascular anatomy in relation to the tumor. At the Cleveland Clinic, we use an extraperitoneal flank incision through the bed of the eleventh or twelfth rib for almost all of these operations; we occasionally use a thoracoabdominal incision for very large tumors involving the upper portion of the kidney. These incisions allow the surgeon to operate on the mobilized kidney almost at skin level and provide excellent exposure of the peripheral renal vessels. With an anterior subcostal transperitoneal incision, the kidney is invariably located in the depth of the wound, and the surgical exposure is simply not as good. Extracorporeal surgery is rarely necessary in these patients today.

A variety of surgical techniques are available for performing partial nephrectomy in patients with malignancy. These include polar (apical and basilar) segmental nephrectomy, wedge resection, and transverse resection. All of these techniques require adherence to basic principles of early vascular control, avoidance of ischemic renal damage, complete tumor excision with free margins, precise closure of the collecting system, careful hemostasis, and closure or coverage of the renal defect with adjacent fat, fascia, peritoneum, or Oxycel. Whichever technique is used, the tumor is removed with a small surrounding margin of grossly normal renal parenchyma. Intraoperative ultrasonography is very helpful in achieving accurate tumor localization, particularly for intrarenal lesions that are not visible or palpable from the external surface of the kidney. A recent prospective study demonstrated that intraoperative ultrasonography is of limited value for detecting occult multicentric tumors in the kidneys (5).

In patients with RCC, NSS is contraindicated in the presence of lymph node metastasis because the prognosis for these patients is poor. Enlarged or suspicious-looking lymph nodes should be biopsied before initiating the renal resection. When NSS is performed, after excision of all gross tumor, absence of malignancy in the remaining portion of the kidney should be verified intraoperatively by frozen-section examinations of biopsy specimens obtained at random from the renal margin of excision. It is unusual for such biopsies to demonstrate residual tumor but, if they do, additional renal tissue must be excised.

Some RCCs are surrounded by a distinct pseudocapsule of fibrous tissue, and simple enucleation has been used in such cases to achieve tumor removal. Initial reports indicated satisfactory short-term clinical results after enucleation, with good patient survival and a low rate of local tumor recurrence. However, most recent studies have linked enucleation with a higher risk of leaving residual malignancy in the kidney. Several carefully done histopathologic studies have demonstrated frequent microscopic tumor penetration of the pseudocapsule that surrounds the neoplasm. These data indicate that it is not always possible to be assured of complete tumor encapsulation prior to surgery. Local recurrence of tumor in the treated kidney is a grave complication of partial nephrectomy for RCC, and every attempt should be made to prevent it. Therefore, it is the author's view that a surrounding margin of normal parenchyma should be removed with the tumor whenever possible. This provides an added margin of safety against the development of local tumor recurrence and, in most cases, does not appreciably increase the technical difficulty of the operation. The technique of enucleation is currently used only in occasional patients with von Hippel–Lindau disease who have multiple low-stage encapsulated tumors involving both kidneys.

CLINICAL RESULTS

The technical success rate with NSS is excellent, and long-term patient survival free of cancer is comparable to that obtained after radical nephrectomy, particularly for low-stage RCC (Table 1) (7–10). The major disadvantage of NSS for RCC is the risk of postoperative local tumor recurrence in the operated kidney, which has occurred in 3%–6% of patients. These local recurrences are most likely a manifestation of undetected microscopic multifocal RCC in the remnant kidney. The risk of local tumor recurrence after radical nephrectomy has not been studied but is presumably very low.

We recently reviewed the results of NSS for treatment of localized sporadic RCC in 485 patients treated at the Cleveland Clinic prior to December 1996 (10). A technically successful operation with preservation of function in the treated kidney was

TABLE 1   Results of nephron-sparing surgery for renal cell carcinoma

Patients	Number of recurrence	Local tumor survival	5-Year cancer-specific reference
121	4.1%	90%	7
185	5.9%	89%	8
146	2.7%	93%	9
485	3.2%	92%	10

achieved in 476 patients (98%). The overall and cancer-specific five-year patient survival rates were 81% and 93%, respectively. Recurrent RCC developed postoperatively in 44 of 485 patients (10%). Sixteen patients (3.2%) developed local recurrence in the remnant kidney, and 28 patients (5.8%) developed metastatic disease.

More recently, we received the long-term (10-year) results of NSS in 107 patients with localized sporadic RCC treated prior to 1988 (11). All patients were followed for at least 10 years or until death. Cancer-specific survival was 88.2% at 5 years and 73% at 10 years. Long-term preservation of renal function was achieved in 100 patients (93%). These results attest that NSS is an effective therapy for localized RCC, providing both long-term tumor control and preservation of renal function.

NEPHRON-SPARING SURGERY WITH A NORMAL CONTRALATERAL KIDNEY

Although radical nephrectomy remains the standard treatment for localized RCC in patients with an anatomically and functionally normal opposite kidney, a growing number of authors are reporting excellent results with NSS in this setting. A recent review article detailed the outcome of NSS in 315 patients with unilateral localized RCC and a normal opposite kidney (12). The mean cancer-specific survival rate was 95% at approximately three years of follow-up, and there were only two cases of postoperative tumor recurrence. Significantly, the mean tumor size in most of these reports was <3.5 cm. Clearly, patient selection on the basis of small tumor size was a significant factor accounting for favorable outcome after NSS in these studies.

A Cleveland Clinic study reviewed the outcome of NSS in 216 patients with sporadic RCC (13). Our findings confirmed that cancer-free survival was significantly extended in patients with small (<4 cm) tumors relative to those with larger ones. Other factors associated with significantly improved survival were unilateral renal involvement, low pathologic tumor stage, and the presence of a single tumor. There were no postoperative tumor recurrences and the cancer-specific five-year survival rate was 100% in patients with small (<4 cm), unilateral stage $T_{1-2}N_0M_0$ RCC.

The above data suggested that NSS may be an acceptable therapeutic approach in patients who have a single, small (<4 cm) RCC and a normal contralateral kidney. To test this hypothesis, we conducted a subsequent study wherein the outcome following radical nephrectomy versus NSS was evaluated in 88 patients with a single, small (<4 cm), localized, unilateral, sporadic RCC (14). The radical ($n = 42$) and nephron-sparing ($n = 46$) surgical groups were well-matched for patient age, sex, renal function, diabetes, hypertension, tumor size, tumor location, and tumor stage. All patients in both groups had low–pathologic-tumor-stage RCC. A single patient in each group developed recurrent RCC postoperatively. The cancer-specific five-year survival rates for patients in the radical and nephron-sparing surgical groups were 97% and 100%, respectively. More recently, Lerner and associates from the Mayo Clinic reported the results of a similar study comprising patients with solitary, small (<4 cm), low-stage RCC; the five-year cancer-specific survival rates following radical nephrectomy versus NSS were 96% and 92%, respectively (8). A subsequent Cleveland Clinic study showed that there are no significant biologic differences between centrally versus peripherally located small, solitary, unilateral RCCs and that treatment with NSS or radical nephrectomy is equally effective regardless of tumor location in these patients (15).

The data from these studies affirm that radical nephrectomy and NSS provide equally effective curative treatment for patients with a single, small, unilateral, localized RCC. Other studies have further shown that the cost of NSS is equivalent to that of radical nephrectomy (16) and that quality of life is improved following NSS in these patients (17). Finally, recent data comparing the long-term (>10 years) development of renal dysfunction following elective NSS versus radical nephrectomy now suggest that progressive renal insufficiency is significantly less after NSS in patients with a normal contralateral kidney (18). Therefore, patients with a single, small, unilateral, localized RCC may now be considered suitable candidates for NSS even when the opposite kidney is completely normal.

FOLLOW-UP

Patients who undergo NSS for RCC are advised to return for initial follow-up 4–6 weeks postoperatively. At that time, a serum creatinine measurement and intravenous pyelogram are obtained to document renal function and anatomy; in patients with impaired overall renal function, a renal ultrasound or magnetic resonance imaging (MRI) study is obtained instead of an intravenous pyelogram.

The Cleveland Clinic recently completed a detailed analysis of tumor recurrence patterns after NSS for sporadic localized RCC in 327 patients (19). The purpose of this study was to develop appropriate guidelines for long-term surveillance after NSS for RCC. RCC recurred postoperatively in 38 patients (11.7%), including 13 patients (4.0%) who developed local tumor recurrence and 25 patients (7.6%) who developed metastatic disease. The incidence of postoperative local tumor recurrence and metastatic disease according to initial pathologic tumor stage was as follows: 0% and 4.4% for T_1RCC, 2.0% and 5.3% for T_2RCC, 8.2% and 11.5% for T_{3a}RCC, and 10.6% and 14.9% for T_{3b}RCC. The peak postoperative intervals for developing local tumor recurrence were 6–24 months (in T_3RCC patients) and >48 months (in T_2RCC patients).

The above data indicate that surveillance for recurrent malignancy after NSS for RCC can be tailored according to the initial pathologic tumor stage. The recommended surveillance scheme is depicted in Table 2. All patients should be evaluated annually with a medical history, physical examination, and selected blood studies including serum calcium, alkaline phosphatase, liver function tests, blood urea nitrogen, serum creatinine, and electrolytes. A 24-h urinary protein measurement should be obtained in patients with a solitary remnant kidney to screen for hyperfiltration nephropathy (20). Patients with proteinuria may be treated with a low-protein diet and a converting enzyme inhibitor agent, which appear to help prevent glomerulopathy caused by reduced renal mass (21).

TABLE 2   Recommended postoperative surveillance after nephron-sparing surgery for sporadic localized renal cell carcinoma

Pathologic tumor stage	History, exam, chest blood tests[*]	X-Ray	Abdominal CT scan
T_1	Yearly	—	—
T_2	Yearly	Yearly	Every 2 years
T_3	Yearly	Yearly	Every 6 months for 2 years, then every 2 years

[*]Medical history, physical examination, and measurement of serum calcium, alkaline phosphatase, liver function, and renal function.

The need for postoperative radiographic surveillance studies varies according to the initial pathologic tumor (pT) stage (Table 2). Patients who undergo NSS for pT_1RCC do not require radiographic imaging postoperatively in view of the very low risk of recurrent malignancy. A yearly chest radiograph is recommended after NSS for pT_2 or pT_3RCC because the lung is the most common site of postoperative metastasis in both groups. Abdominal or retroperitoneal tumor recurrence is uncommon in pT_2 patients, particularly early after NSS, and these patients require only occasional follow-up abdominal CT scanning. Patients with pT_3RCC have a higher risk of developing local tumor recurrence, particularly during the first two years after NSS, and they may benefit from more frequent follow-up abdominal CT scanning initially.

VON HIPPEL LINDAU DISEASE

Treatment of RCC in patients with von Hippel–Lindau disease (VHL) differs significantly from that of patients with sporadic renal neoplasms primarily due to the tendency of lesions in VHL to be bilateral, multifocal, and often microscopic. This reflects the changes in the germline of the VHL gene located on the short arm of chromosome 3 (3p25–26). For this reason, RCC occurs at a much younger age in patients with VHL and the entire renal parenchyma has a higher lifetime risk for developing subsequent tumors. Additionally, the malignant potential of cysts is often underappreciated on ultrasound or CT in patients with VHL, and histologically these cysts frequently contain either frank carcinoma or a hyperplastic clear cell lining that may represent incipient tumor (22). Adequate surgical treatment of localized RCC in VHL therefore requires complete excision of all solid and cystic renal lesions. Available options include NSS, with close surveillance and subsequent resection of recurrent disease, or bilateral radical nephrectomy, which renders the patient anephric with the potential for subsequent transplantation (23).

The utility of NSS to preserve renal function and avoid or postpone dialysis in patients with VHL has recently been examined (24). In a multicenter study of 49 VHL patients undergoing NSS for RCC, the 5- and 10-year cancer-specific survival rates were 100% and 81%, respectively. During a mean follow-up of 68 months, half the patients (51%) treated with NSS experienced local recurrence; most were salvaged with either repeat NSS or removal of the renal remnant. Whether these recurrences represent de novo tumors or microscopic, clinically undetected foci present at the time of the original surgery is not known. Survival free of local recurrence was 71% at 5 years but only 15% at 10 years. These data underscore the need for diligent surveillance in these patients. NSS is therefore feasible in well-selected patients with VHL and can preserve renal function without compromising cancer-free survival in most patients.

NEPRHON-SPARING SURGERY WITH COEXISTENT RENAL ARTERY DISEASE

Occasionally, preoperative history and radiographic imaging reveal both RCC and renal artery stenosis (RAS) in the same patient. This can complicate the clinical picture. When RCC and RAS are found in the same kidney and a normal contralateral kidney is present, the treatment of choice is radical nephrectomy. Involvement of all functional renal parenchyma by either or both of these processes poses a more difficult therapeutic dilemma. Management of such cases must be individualized to achieve maximal cancer control while balancing the need to preserve overall renal function.

Campbell et al. reviewed their experience in the management of 34 patients with concurrent RCC and RAS affecting all of the functioning renal parenchyma (25). The mean patient age was 67 and the majority of cases of RAS were due to atherosclerotic disease (88%). Patients were divided into four groups: (a) a solitary kidney with RCC and RAS, (b) bilateral RCC and bilateral RAS, (c) unilateral RCC and contralateral RAS, and (d) unilateral RCC and bilateral RAS. All patients underwent complete surgical excision of their tumor and a NSS approach was employed in 88%. Eight patients underwent simultaneous partial or radical nephrectomy and surgical renal revascularization with excellent cancer-free survival and maintenance of renal function in all but one patient, who ultimately required dialysis. In recent years, improved endovascular management of RAS has increased the number of therapeutic options available for the management of patients with RCC and coexisting renal artery disease (26).

ADVANCED RENAL CELL CARCINOMA

NSS in patients with locally advanced or metastatic disease is primarily indicated in two instances: (a) to avoid rendering the patient anephric and in need of renal replacement therapy, and (b) to obtain tissue for adoptive immunotherapy. Under these circumstances, it is possible to provide symptomatic relief for locally advanced disease and in some cases to aggressively resect all clinically evident tumor while maintaining acceptable renal function. Few studies have examined the role of partial nephrectomy in these selected circumstances. Angermeier et al. reviewed nine patients who underwent partial nephrectomy for tumor with venous involvement in a solitary kidney (27). Although all cases were technically successful and renal function was preserved, many patients developed local or distant metastasis. Krishnamurthi et al. reviewed the clinical outcome of 15 patients with metastatic RCC who underwent NSS and surgical or systemic treatment of metastases (28). All cases were technically successful and the need for renal replacement therapy was obviated in all but one patient. In patients with metachronous metastases in a solitary kidney, death from disease occurred later than in patients with synchronous lesions resected from the kidney and other soft tissues. Although these preliminary data are from highly selected patient populations, they suggest that partial nephrectomy can occasionally provide effective treatment for patients with locally advanced or completely resected metastatic RCC.

MINIMALLY INVASIVE NEPHRON-SPARING SURGERY

New minimally invasive technologies are currently being applied to the field of NSS in an effort to decrease operative time, pain, morbidity, and hospital stay. Foremost among these is the burgeoning role of laparoscopy with tumor destruction or complete in vivo resection by various techniques. The primary modalities in clinical use today are laparoscopic cryoablation and laparoscopic partial nephrectomy. Most initial reports include only highly selected patients with unifocal, small, exophytic, peripheral lesions away from the collection system (29–34). As experience with these techniques increases, larger and more difficult lesions are being approached laparoscopically with promising anecdotal results (35–36).

Laparoscopic access to the kidney may be intra- or retroperitoneal. Whether the approach is open or laparoscopic, complete tumor destruction with maximal preservation of unaffected nephrons remains the goal. Laparoscopic tumor destruction differs primarily in the energy source being used.

Laparoscopic cryoablation may represent a reasonable alternative for nephron-sparing management of these tumors. In some respects, the kidney is an anatomically favored site for cryoablative therapy, since it can readily be dissected away from adjacent organs and usually gives rise to unifocal malignancy. This is in contrast to the prostate, which is intimately opposed to the rectum and sphincter and tends to harbor multifocal carcinoma.

During cryoablation, the tumor is supercooled to a core temperature no higher than $-40°C$ using a liquid nitrogen–based cryoprobe. Normal and neoplastic renal tissues are ablated and rendered necrotic at $-20°C$ (37). To assure complete tumor destruction, the advancing iceball is monitored laparoscopically and ultrasonographically. A dual freeze-thaw cycle is used. Initial experimental studies at the

Cleveland Clinic evaluated the efficacy of intraparenchymal cryoablative therapy with or without renal artery occlusion in mongrel dogs (38). Effective renal tissue ablation was confirmed at the treatment site in all instances. Renal artery occlusion did not significantly alter the freezing process and provided no practical advantage.

Relatively few laparoscopic renal cryoablation procedures have been performed worldwide to date. Our group at the Cleveland Clinic reported the initial series of 10 patients in 1988, and our experience now comprises over 50 carefully selected patients with localized RCC. These have all been patients with a single, small (<4 cm), solid, peripheral renal tumor not involving the intrarenal collecting system.

We recently reviewed our experience with laparoscopic renal cryoablation in the initial 50 patients with localized RCC who met the above criteria. All 50 operations were technically successful and there were no significant postoperative complications. The mean operative time was 2.6 h and the mean blood loss was 51 cc. Hospital stay was <23 h for most patients and the median time for complete recovery was two weeks. Renal function was preserved in all treated kidneys. Sequential postoperative MRI scans demonstrated a gradual contraction in the size of the cryolesion; in some patients, the cryolesion was no longer visible radiographically at one year. Thirty-one patients have undergone CT-directed percutaneous biopsy of the cryoablated renal tumor site six months postoperatively; all but one of these biopsies have all been negative for cancer. There have been no cases of renal fossa or metastatic tumor recurrence with follow-up of up to three years.

Laparoscopic renal cryoablation is potentially an attractive addition to the nephron-sparing armamentarium for treating RCC. Our preliminary experience suggests that this approach is technically feasible with minimal patient morbidity. A major criticism of the technique is that histologic documentation of complete tumor destruction is not currently available. Meticulous long-term clinical and radiographic follow-up of these patients is ultimately needed to validate the efficacy of this minimally invasive approach for treating renal malignancy.

Newer energy sources for tumor ablation include high-intensity focused ultrasound (HIFU) (39, 40), interstitial radiofrequency ablation (RFA), and laser and microwave coagulators (41). These modalities may eventually permit tumor destruction by minimally invasive or completely extracorporeal methods. However, each is limited by the ability to image the destructive process precisely as it is being administered, thereby minimizing injury to normal adjacent parenchyma while assuring complete destruction of the lesion. Theoretic and experimental evidence indicate that the primary mechanism of tissue destruction by both HIFU and RFA is thermonecrosis. These modalities have been shown to induce cavitary defects of animal and human renal lesions in a safe and reproducible manner while limiting collateral injury to the unaffected parenchyma.

In HIFU, beams of the required frequency (a few megahertz) are generated by resonant electrical excitation of the thin plates of a piezoceramic. The beam is then focused on the lesion at F2 using a bowel or lens system similar to that used by lithotriptors (extracorporeal shockwave lithotripsy; ESWL) (40). The acute effects of HIFU on the kidney include localized hemorrhage, fiber rupture, and coagulation necrosis with resultant infiltration of acute and chronic inflammatory cells (39, 42, 43).

Currently, there is considerably more experience with tissue destruction using RFA, which has been successfully used to treat benign prostatic enlargement in an outpatient setting (44). Radiofrequency energy causes high-frequency current flow from the needle electrode into the surrounding tissue. This causes ionic agitation, molecular friction, and cellular warming with rapid desiccation and cell death (45). The size and configuration of the lesion are related to the amount of energy delivered, ablation time, tissue impedance, electrolyte content of the tissue, and surface area of the electrode (46). Although it is technically difficult to control for each of these variables independently, limited success has been reported using RFA to ablate small renal tumors in a rabbit model (45, 47).

In order to gain a place among the armamentarium of nephron-sparing approaches, HIFU and RFA must demonstrate clinical and pathologic success approaching that of open partial nephrectomy. Moreover, the initial use of these technologies must be in well-selected and highly motivated patients, and the data must be reported and interpreted in that context.

The technique of laparoscopic partial nephrectomy for the treatment of RCC is in its very early stages. The cumulative experience reported in the literature comprises fewer than 100 cases, and these have been confounded by a lack of standardized technique and variable experience (29–31, 33–35, 48–50). Although both intra- and retroperitoneal laparoscopic partial nephrectomies have been successfully performed, it has been difficult to reproduce the essential elements of open partial nephrectomy using contemporary laparoscopic instrumentation. Despite advanced techniques, including the use of a harmonic scalpel and biologic tissue adhesives such as fibrin glue (49, 50), laparoscopic partial nephrectomy has resulted in longer operative times and higher complication rates than open partial nephrectomy.

At the Cleveland Clinic, we have recently developed a technique for laparoscopic partial nephrectomy that duplicates established open surgical principles. The key technical steps include (*a*) preparation of the renal hilum, (*b*) renal mobilization preserving the perinephric fat covering the tumor, (*c*) laparoscopic flexible ultrasonography, (*d*) scoring of the renal parenchyma along the proposed line of resection, (*e*) intravenous mannitol, (*f*) clamping of the renal artery and vein, (*g*) ice-slush hypothermia (if needed), (*h*) excision of the tumor using cold- and/or hot-cutting, (*i*) suturing of the collecting system, if necessary, and (*j*) repair of the parenchymal defect using surgicel bolsters and mattress sutures. A purely laparoscopic technique, involving intracorporeal free-hand suturing, is employed.

Since August 1999, laparoscopic partial nephrectomy has been performed in 36 patients with small, exophytic renal tumors. Mean tumor size was 2.9 cm (range 1.4–7.0 cm). The operation was successful in all cases without any open conversions. Mean operative time was 2.9 h, warm ischemia was 20 min, and blood loss was 237 ml. Formal calyceal suture repair was performed in seven patients. Mean hospital stay was 1.7 days. The final pathology revealed RCC in 20 patients and other tumors in the remainder. All margins of resection were negative for tumor.

Our initial experience suggests that laparoscopic partial nephrectomy can be performed for small exophytic renal tumors with adherence to established principles and techniques of the open surgical approach. Although both the instrumentation and technique are being refined, it is too early to consider laparoscopic partial nephrectomy a reproducible cancer operation that is appropriate outside of a specialized tertiary care institution.

Visit the Annual Reviews home page at www.AnnualReviews.org

LITERATURE CITED

1. Chow WH, Devesa SS, Warren JL, Fraumeni JF Jr. 1999. Rising incidence of renal cell cancer in the United States. *JAMA* 281:1628–31

2. Robson CJ, Churchill BM, Anderson W. 1969. The results of radical nephrectomy for renal cell carcinoma. *J. Urol.* 101:297–301

3. Licht MR, Novick AC. 1993. Nephron-sparing surgery for renal cell carcinoma. *Urology* 149:1–7

4. Coll DM, Uzzo RG, Herts BR, et al. 1999. 3-dimensional volume rendered computerized tomography for preoperative evaluation and intraoperative treatment of patients undergoing nephron-sparing surgery. *J. Urol.* 161:1097–102

5. Campbell SC, Fichtner J, Novick AC, et al. 1996. Intraoperative evaluation of renal cell carcinoma: a prospective study of the role of ultrasonography and histopathological frozen sections. *J. Urol.* 155:1191–95

6. Campbell SC, Novick AC, Streem SB, et al. 1994. Complications of nephron-sparing surgery for renal tumors. *J. Urol.* 151:1177–80

7. Steinbach F, Stockle M, Muller SC, et al. 1992. Conservative surgery of renal cell tumors in 140 patients: 21 years of experience. *J. Urol.* 148:24–29, discussion 29–30

8. Lerner SE, Hawkins CA, Blute ML, et al. 1996. Disease outcome in patients with low stage renal cell carcinoma treated with nephron sparing or radical surgery. *J. Urol.* 155:1868–73

9. Belldegrun A, Tsui KH, deKernion JB, Smith RB. 1999. Efficacy of nephron-sparing surgery for renal cell carcinoma: analysis based on the new 1997 Tumor-Node-Metastasis Staging System. *J. Clin. Oncol.* 17:2868–75

10. Hafez KS, Fergany AF, Novick AC. 1999. Nephron-sparing surgery for localized renal cell carcinoma: impact of tumor size on patient survival, tumor recurrence, and TNM staging. *J. Urol.* 162:1930–33

11. Fergany AF, Hafez KS, Novick AC. 2000. Long-term results of nephron-sparing surgery for localized renal cell carcinoma: 10-year follow-up. *J. Urol.* 163:442–45

12. Novick AC. 1995. Partial nephrectomy for renal cell carcinoma. *Urology* 36:149–52

13. Licht MR, Novick AC, Goormastic M. 1994. Nephron-sparing surgery in incidental versus suspected renal cell carcinoma. *J. Urol.* 152:39–42

14. Butler BP, Novick AC, Miller DP, et al. 1995. Management of small unilateral renal cell carcinomas: radical versus nephron-sparing surgery. *Urology* 45:34–40, discussion 40–41

15. Hafez KS, Novick AC, Butler BP. 1998. Management of small solitary unilateral renal cell carcinomas: impact of central versus peripheral tumor location. *J. Urol.* 159:1156–60

16. Uzzo RG, Wei JT, Hafez K, et al. 1999.

Comparison of direct hospital costs and length of stay for radical nephrectomy versus nephron-sparing surgery in the management of localized renal cell carcinoma. *Urology* 54:994–98

17. Clark PE, Schover LR, Uzzo RG, et al. 2000. Quality of life and psychological adaptation following surgery for localized renal cell carcinoma: impact of the amount of remaining renal tissue. *J. Urol.* 163:157

18. Lau W, Blute ML, Zincke H. 2000. Matched comparison of radical nephrectomy versus elective nephron-sparing surgery for renal cell carcinoma: evidence for increased renal failure rate on long-term follow-up (>10 years). *J. Urol.* 163:153

19. Hafez KS, Novick AC, Campbell SC. 1997. Patterns of tumor recurrence and guidelines for follow-up after nephron-sparing surgery for sporadic renal cell carcinoma. *J. Urol.* 157:2067–70

20. Novick AC, Gephardt G, Guz B, et al. 1991. Long-term follow-up after partial removal of a solitary kidney. *N. Engl. J. Med.* 325:1058–62

21. Novick AC, Schreiber JM Jr. 1995. Effect of angiotensin-converting enzyme inhibition on nephropathy in patients with a remnant kidney. *Urology* 46:785–89

22. Christenson PJ, Craig JP, Bibro MC, O'Connell KJ. 1982. Cysts containing renal cell carcinoma in von Hippel–Lindau disease. *J. Urol.* 128:798–800

23. Goldfarb DA, Neumann HP, Penn I, Novick AC. 1997. Results of renal transplantation in patients with renal cell carcinoma and von Hippel–Lindau disease. *Transplant* 64:1726–29

24. Steinbach F, Novick AC, Zincke H, et al. 1995. Treatment of renal cell carcinoma in von Hippel–Lindau disease. A multicenter study. *J. Urol.* 153:1812–16

25. Campbell SC, Novick AC, Streem SB, Klein EA. 1993. Management of renal cell carcinoma with coexistent renal artery disease. *J. Urol.* 150:808–13

26. Hafez KS, Krishnamurthi V, Campbell SC, Novick AC. 2000. Contemporary management of renal cell carcinoma with coexistent renal artery disease: update of the Cleveland Clinic experience. *Urology* 56:382–86

27. Angermeier KW, Novick AC, Streem SB, Montie JE. 1990. Nephron-sparing surgery for renal cell carcinoma with venous involvement. *J. Urol.* 144:1352–55

28. Krishnamurthi V, Novick AC, Bukowski R. 1996. Nephron-sparing surgery in patients with metastatic renal cell carcinoma. *J. Urol.* 156:36–39

29. de Cannière L, Michel LA, Lorge F, et al. 1997. Direct carbon dioxide insufflation of the retroperitoneum under laparoscopic control for renal and adrenal surgery. *Eur. J. Surg.* 163:339–44

30. Janetschek G, Daffner P, Peschel R, Bartsch G. 1998. Laparoscopic nephron sparing surgery for small renal cell carcinoma. *J. Urol.* 159:1152–55

31. McDougall EM, Elbahnasy AM, Clayman RV. 1998. Laparoscopic wedge resection and partial nephrectomy—the Washington University experience and review of the literature. *J. Soc. Laparoendoscopic Surg.* 2:15–23

32. Gill IS, Novick AC, Soble JJ, et al. 1998. Laparoscopic renal cryoablation: initial clinical series. *Urology* 52:543–51

33. Gasman D, Saint F, Barthelemy Y, et al. 1996. Retroperioneoscopy: a laparoscopic approach for adrenal and renal surgery. *Urology* 47:801–6

34. Winfield HN, Donovan JF, Lund GO, et al. 1995. Laparoscopic partial nephrectomy: initial experience and comparison to the open surgical approach. *J. Urol.* 153:1409–14

35. Hoznek A, Solomon L, Antiphon P, et al. 1999. Partial nephrectomy with retroperitoneal laparoscopy. *J. Urol.* 162:1922–26

36. About CC, Hoznek A, Salomon L, et al. 1999. Is open surgery for partial nephrectomy an obsolete surgical procedure? *Curr. Opin. Urol.* 9:383–89

37. Chosy SG, Nakada SY, Lee FTJ, Warner TF. 1998. Monitoring renal cryosurgery:

predictors of tissue necrosis in swine. *J. Urol.* 159:1370–74

38. Campbell SC, Krishnamurthi V, Chow G, et al. 1998. Renal cryosurgery: experimental evaluation of treatment parameters. *Urology* 52:29–33, discussion 33–34

39. Adams JB, Moore RG, Anderson JH, et al. 1996. High intensity focused ultrasound ablation of rabbit kidney tumors. *J. Endourol.* 10:71–75

40. Hill CR, ter Haar GR. 1995. High intensity focused ultrasound—potential for cancer treatment. *Br. J. Radiol.* 68:1296–303

41. Wolf JS Jr. 1998. Evaluation and management of solid and cystic renal masses. *J. Urol.* 159:1120–33

42. Kóehrman KU, Michel M, Fruhauf J, et al. 2000. High intensity focused ultrasound for non-invasive tissue ablation in the kidney, prostate and uterus. *J. Urol.* 163:698A (Abstr.)

43. Watkins NA, Morris SB, Rivens I, ter Haar GR. 1997. High intensity focused ultrasound ablation of the kidney in a large animal model. *J. Endourol.* 11:191–96

44. Dixon CM. 1995. Transurethral needle ablation for the treatment of benign prostatic hyperplasis. *Urol. Clin. N. Am.* 22:441–44

45. Polascik TJ, Hamper U, Lee BR, et al. 1999. Ablation of renal tumors in a rabbit model with interstitial saline-augmented radiofrequency energy: preliminary report of a new technology. *Urology* 53:465–72, discussion 470–72

46. Ziotta AR, Schulman CC. 1999. Ablation of renal tumors in a rabbit model with interstitial saline-augmented radiofrequency energy. *Urology* 54:382–83

47. Patel VR, Leveille RJ, Hoey MF, et al. 2000. Radiofrequency ablation of rabbit kidney using liquid electrode: acute and chronic observations. *J. Endourol.* 14:155–59

48. Abbou CC, Janetschek G, Jeschke K, Rassweiler J. 2000. Laparoscopic partial nephrectomy for renal cell carcinoma: the European experience. *J. Urol.* 163:77A (Abstr.)

49. Kletscher BA, Lauvetz RW, Segura JW. 1995. Nephron-sparing laparoscopic surgery: techniques to control the renal pedicle and manage parenchymal bleeding. *J. Endourol.* 9:23–30

50. Elashry OM, Wolf JSJ, Rayala HJ, et al. 1997. Recent advances in laparoscopic partial nephrectomy: comparative study of electrosurgical snare electrode and ultrasound dissection. *J. Endourol.* 11:15–22

Annu. Rev. Med. 2002. 53:409–35

THE MECHANISMS OF ACTION OF PPARS

Joel Berger and David E. Moller
*Department of Molecular Endocrinology, Merck Research Laboratories, P.O. Box 2000,
Rahway, New Jersey 07065; e-mail: joel_berger@merck.com; david_moller@merck.com*

Key Words   PPAR, nuclear receptors, diabetes, dyslipidemia

■ **Abstract**   The peroxisome proliferator-activated receptors (PPARs) are a group
of three nuclear receptor isoforms, PPARγ, PPARα, and PPARδ, encoded by different
genes. PPARs are ligand-regulated transcription factors that control gene expression
by binding to specific response elements (PPREs) within promoters. PPARs bind as
heterodimers with a retinoid X receptor and, upon binding agonist, interact with co-
factors such that the rate of transcription initiation is increased. The PPARs play a
critical physiological role as lipid sensors and regulators of lipid metabolism. Fatty
acids and eicosanoids have been identified as natural ligands for the PPARs. More
potent synthetic PPAR ligands, including the fibrates and thiazolidinediones, have
proven effective in the treatment of dyslipidemia and diabetes. Use of such ligands
has allowed researchers to unveil many potential roles for the PPARs in pathological
states including atherosclerosis, inflammation, cancer, infertility, and demyelination.
Here, we present the current state of knowledge regarding the molecular mechanisms
of PPAR action and the involvement of the PPARs in the etiology and treatment of
several chronic diseases.

INTRODUCTION

The peroxisome proliferator-activated receptors (PPARs) form a subfamily of the
nuclear receptor superfamily. Three isoforms, encoded by separate genes, have
been identified thus far: PPARγ, PPARα, and PPARδ. The PPARs are ligand-
dependent transcription factors that regulate target gene expression by binding to
specific peroxisome proliferator response elements (PPREs) in enhancer sites of
regulated genes. Each receptor binds to its PPRE as a heterodimer with a retinoid
X receptor (RXR). Upon binding an agonist, the conformation of a PPAR is altered
and stabilized such that a binding cleft is created and recruitment of transcriptional
coactivators occurs. The result is an increase in gene transcription.

The first cloning of a PPAR (PPARα) occurred in the course of the search for
the molecular target of hepatic peroxisome proliferating agents in rodents. Since
then, numerous fatty acids and their derivatives, including a variety of eicosanoids
and prostaglandins, have been shown to serve as ligands of the PPARs. It has
therefore been suggested that these receptors play a central role in sensing nutrient
levels and in modulating their metabolism. Recently, it has been demonstrated that

the PPARs are the primary targets of numerous classes of synthetic compounds used in the successful treatment of diabetes and dyslipidemia. As such, a significant understanding of the molecular and physiological characteristics of these receptors has become extremely important to those engaged in the development or utilization of drugs used to treat metabolic disorders. In addition, owing to the great interest within the research community, additional putative roles for the PPARs have been proposed. Various researchers have put forth data supporting regulatory roles for PPARγ and PPARα in a wide range of events involving the vasculature, including atherosclerotic plaque formation and stability, vascular tone, and angiogenesis. PPARγ has also demonstrated significant anti-inflammatory action in models of colon inflammation. PPARδ, γ, and α have each been implicated in regulating both normal cellular differentiation and the pathophysiology of carcinogenesis. Another potentially exciting area of research is the central nervous system (CNS), where PPARδ has been linked to myelinogenesis and glial cell maturation. Finally, PPARδ has been shown to affect embryo implantation and therefore fertility. Such observations, discussed in greater detail below, may eventually lead to important new therapeutic uses for PPAR ligands.

RECEPTOR STRUCTURE

PPARs, like other nuclear receptors, possess a modular structure composed of functional domains (1). The DNA binding domain (DBD) and the ligand binding domain (LBD) are the most highly conserved regions across the receptor isoforms. The DBD consists of two zinc fingers that specifically bind PPREs in the regulatory region of PPAR-responsive genes. The LBD, located in the C-terminal half of the receptor, has been shown by crystallographic studies to be composed of 13 α-helices and a small 4-stranded β-sheet (Figure 1, see color insert). The ligand binding "pocket" of PPARs appears to be quite large in comparison with that of other nuclear receptors (2, 3). This difference may allow the PPARs to interact with a broad range of structurally distinct natural and synthetic ligands. Located in the C terminus of the LBD is the ligand-dependent activation domain, AF-2. This region is intimately involved in the generation of the receptors' coactivator binding pocket (2). A ligand-independent activation function, AF-1, is found in close proximity to the N terminus of the receptor in the A/B domain (4).

RXR AND HETERODIMERIZATION

Unlike the steroid hormone receptors, which function as homodimers, PPARs form heterodimers with the retinoid X receptor (RXR) (5). Like PPARs, RXR exists as three distinct isoforms: RXRα, β, and γ, all of which are activated by the endogenous agonist 9-*cis* retinoic acid (6). No specific roles have yet been elaborated for these different isoforms within the PPAR:RXR complex. However, synthetic RXR agonists ("rexinoids") can activate the complex and thereby obtain antidiabetic outcomes similar to those seen with PPAR agonists in mouse models of type 2 diabetes (7).

PEROXISOME PROLIFERATOR RESPONSE ELEMENT

Peroxisome proliferator response elements (PPREs) are direct repeat (DR)-1 elements consisting of two hexanucleotides with the consensus sequence AGGTCA separated by a single nucleotide spacer. Such a sequence, or a similar one, has been found in numerous PPAR-inducible genes including acyl-CoA oxidase and adipocyte fatty acid-binding protein (8). *Cis* elements adjacent to the PPRE core site (especially 5′) appear to play a role in defining the binding selectivity of these response elements (8). Interestingly, PPAR:RXR binds the PPRE with a reverse polarity in comparison with vitamin D receptor (VDR):RXR and thyroid receptor (TR):RXR heterodimers on DR-3 and DR-4 elements, respectively (9).

COACTIVATORS

Several cofactor proteins, coactivators, and corepressors that mediate the ability of nuclear receptors to initiate (or suppress) the transcription process were recently identified (10). Coactivators interact with nuclear receptors in an agonist-dependent manner through a conserved LXXLL motif (where X is any amino acid) (11, 12). This coactivator domain is oriented by a "charge clamp" formed by residues within helix 3 and the AF-2 of helix 12 of the LBD. It can then bind to a hydrophobic cleft in the surface of the receptor formed by helices 3, 4, and 5 and the AF-2 helix (2). Agonist-induced alterations in the conformation of PPAR have been demonstrated by comparing the protease digest patterns of the apo- and agonist-bound receptor (13). Several coactivators, including CBP/p300 and steroid receptor coactivator (SRC)-1 (14), possess histone acetylase activity that can re-model chromatin structure. A second group, represented by the members of the DRIP/TRAP complex such as PPAR binding protein (PBP)/TRAP220 (15), form a bridge between the nuclear receptor and the transcription initiation machinery. The precise role of a third group, including PGC-1 (16), RIP140 (17), and ARA70 (18), is not well understood at the molecular level. At its most simple, a sequence of events can be envisioned in which coactivators with histone acetylase activity complex with liganded, PPRE-bound PPAR/RXR receptors, disrupt nucleosomes, and "open-up" chromatin structure in the vicinity of the regulatory region of a gene (Figure 2, see color insert). Complexes such as DRIP/TRAP are then recruited and provide a direct link to the basal transcription machinery. As a result, initiation of transcription is induced.

The binding of a partial agonist to PPARγ was recently shown to cause the receptor to interact with CBP or SRC-1 in a less efficacious manner than a full agonist (19). Such distinctive PPAR:cofactor interactions may be a critical element in transmitting signals that result in unique gene regulatory activity and could therefore prove useful in identifying and characterizing selective PPAR modulators with novel physiological actions.

LIGAND SCREENING ASSAYS

Several assays have been developed to identify and characterize PPAR ligands (Figure 2). Transactivation assays involve cotransfection of cells with a PPAR expression vector and a reporter construct containing a PPRE-driven gene reporter (20). An agonist will increase the reporter gene signal in such assays. Alternatively, chimeric receptors consisting of the PPAR LBD and the yeast transcription factor Gal4 DBD have been utilized with a Gal4-responsive reporter plasmid (21). Radio-labeled thiazolidinediones (TZDs) and subsequently developed non-TZDs have been used in competitive PPAR ligand binding assays (13, 20). PPAR scintillation proximity assays (SPAs), using receptor LBDs attached to scintillant-containing beads, allowed for high-throughput screening for ligands (22). Most recently, a novel fluorescent energy transfer assay was implemented to evaluate the ability of ligands to induce PPAR-cofactor interaction in a rapid, cell-free format (23).

NATURAL LIGANDS

Owing to the critical role PPARs play in lipid metabolism, the search for natural ligands began with fatty acids and eicosanoids. In fact, such metabolites have been identified as bona fide natural ligands of the PPARs. Cell-based transactivation assays and, more recently, direct binding studies have been used to characterize these endogenous receptor effectors.

Fatty acids and eicosanoid derivatives bind and activate PPARγ at micromolar concentrations. PPARγ clearly prefers polyunsaturated fatty acids, including the essential fatty acids linoleic acid, linolenic acid, arachidonic acid, and eicosapentaenoic acid (3). The micromolar affinity of these metabolites is in line with their serum levels. However, their intracellular concentration ranges are unknown. Conversion of linoleic acid to 9-HODE and 13-HODE by 15-lipoxygenase can provide additional micromolar PPARγ agonists (24). A PGD2-derivative, 15-deoxy-$\Delta^{12,14}$-prostaglandin J$_2$ (15d-PGJ2), was demonstrated to be a relatively weak (2–5 μM) PPARγ ligand and agonist (25, 26), although the physiological relevance of this ligand is unclear because cellular concentrations cannot be accurately determined. More recently, an oxidized alkyl phospholipid, hexadecyl azelaoyl phosphatidylcholine, was shown to bind PPARγ with a K_d of $\sim$40 nM; it activated the receptor with a similar EC$_{50}$ (27). These affinities, which are the highest thus far reported for a natural PPAR ligand, are similar to those of the potent synthetic ligand rosiglitazone. This work provides a new and perhaps important link between oxidized low-density lipoproteins, PPARγ activation, and the physiology of atherosclerotic plaques.

PPARα can be activated by a wide variety of saturated and unsaturated fatty acids, including palmitic acid, oleic acid, linoleic acid, and arachidonic acid (28). A number of fatty acids have been found to bind the receptor directly with micromolar affinities (29, 30). As discussed above, it is unclear whether the concentrations at which binding has been noted are physiologically relevant. The lipoxygenase metabolite 8(S)-HETE was identified as a submicromolar ligand for PPARα (31) but is apparently not present at high enough levels in the cell to be classified as a true natural ligand. In lieu of high-affinity endogenous ligands, it is plausible that PPARα functions primarily as a sensor of free fatty acid levels in the tissues where it is expressed.

Like other PPARs, PPARδ interacts with saturated and unsaturated fatty acids; its ligand selectivity is intermediate between that of PPARγ and PPARα (3). Notably, the polyunsaturated fatty acids dihomo-γ-linolenic acid, EPA, and arachidonic acid had low micromolar affinities for PPARδ (30). Palmitic acid and its metabolically stable analogue, 2-bromopalmitic acid, were also identified as PPARδ agonists (32). A number of eicosanoids, including PGA1 and PGD2, have been shown to activate PPARδ (31). Carbaprostacyclin, a semisynthetic prostaglandin, is also a micromolar PPARδ agonist (30). The physiological levels of its naturally occurring precursor, prostacyclin, however, are unknown because of its metabolic instability.

SYNTHETIC LIGANDS

Several key observations made in the mid-1990s regarding thiazolidinedione (TZD) antidiabetic agents have allowed researchers to determine their primary molecular site of action. Such compounds had been developed over the preceding 15 years on the basis of their insulin-sensitizing effects in pharmacological studies in animals. TZDs were found to induce adipocyte differentiation and increase expression of adipocyte genes, including the adipocyte fatty acid-binding protein aP2 (33, 34). Independently, Spiegelman and colleagues reported that PPARγ interacted with a regulatory element within the 5' flanking region of the *aP2* gene that controlled its adipocyte-specific expression (35). These seminal observations were the precursor to additional experiments, which determined that TZDs such as rosiglitazone, pioglitazone, englitazone, and ciglitazone were, in fact, PPARγ ligands and agonists (13, 20, 36). Rosiglitazone was shown to bind the receptor with a high affinity (K_d of $\sim$40 nM), whereas pioglitazone, englitazone, and ciglitazone were less potent ligands. Such characterization of these antidiabetic agents also demonstrated a definite correlation between the in vivo PPARγ binding and agonist activities of these compounds and their in vivo insulin-sensitizing actions (13, 36).

TZDs were developed primarily to improve the antidiabetic actions of the fibrate hypolipidemic agents. Several TZDs, including troglitazone, rosiglitazone, and pioglitazone, have insulin-sensitizing and antidiabetic activity in humans with type 2 diabetes or impaired glucose tolerance (37, 38). AL-294, the first significant lead compound, evolved into both the TZDs and the parallel α-alkoxyphenylproprionates (39). Select compounds of this latter class have shown potent PPARγ activity as well as significant PPARα activity. TZDs have also been identified that are dual PPARγ/α agonists; KRP-297 is representative of this compound class (40). Previously, we presented a novel class of phenylacetic acid derivatives, such as L-796449, which are potent agonists of all three PPARs, and L-805645, which is a PPARγ selective compound (21,41). GW2570 is a very potent non-TZD PPARγ-selective agonist that was recently shown to have antidiabetic efficacy in humans (38). In addition to these potent PPARγ ligands, a subset of the non-steroidal anti-inflammatory drugs (NSAIDs), including indomethacin, fenoprofen, and ibuprofen, have displayed weak PPARγ and PPARα activities (42). The PPARγ antagonist GW0072 was recently reported to interact with different amino acid residues within the LBD of the receptor versus full agonists; in cell culture experiments, the antagonist blocked adipocyte differentiation (19).

The fibrates, amphipathic carboxylic acids that have been proven useful in the treatment of hypertriglyceridemia, are PPARα ligands. Clofibrate is a prototype for this class, which was developed before PPARs were identified, using in vivo assays in rodents to assess lipid-lowering efficacy (43). This compound was later found to induce peroxisome proliferation in rodents (44). Since the identification of clofibrate, research efforts have expanded considerably, and this class of lipid-lowering agents has been further characterized. Clofibrate and fenofibrate have been shown to activate PPARα with a tenfold selectivity over PPARγ (38). Bezafibrate acted as a pan-agonist that showed similar potency on all three PPAR isoforms. WY-14643, the 2-arylthioacetic acid analogue of clofibrate, was a potent murine PPARα agonist as well as a weak PPARγ agonist. In humans, fibrates must all be used at high doses (300–1200 mg/day) to achieve efficacious lipid-lowering activity. Recently, the ureidofibrate, GW2331, was found to be a nanomolar PPARα and PPARγ ligand (45), whereas the closely related GW9578, a ureidobutyric acid, was reported to be a potent PPARα-selective agonist with robust hypolipidemic activity in vivo (46).

In order to define the physiological role of PPARδ, efforts have been made to develop novel compounds that activate this receptor in a selective manner. Among the α-substituted carboxylic acids described previously (21), the potent PPARδ ligand L-165041 demonstrated $\sim$30-fold agonist selectivity for this receptor over PPARγ; additionally, it was inactive on murine PPARα. This compound was found to increase high-density lipoprotein levels in rodents (47). Recently, Oliver et al. reported that GW501516 was a potent, highly selective PPARδ ligand and agonist (48). In obese, insulin-resistant rhesus monkeys, this compound afforded beneficial changes in serum lipid parameters.

PPARγ

Cloning and Characterization

Three homologous PPARs, classified as PPARα, β (δ), and γ, were cloned from a *Xenopus* cDNA library in 1992 (49). PPARγ was subsequently cloned from several mammalian species including human (50). Two PPARγ isoforms are expressed at the protein level in mouse (51) and human (52), $\gamma 1$ and $\gamma 2$. These differ only in that $\gamma 2$ has 30 additional amino acids at its N terminus due to differential promoter usage within the same gene and subsequent alternative RNA processing. PPAR$\gamma 2$ is expressed primarily in adipose tissue (53). PPAR$\gamma 1$ is expressed in a broad range of tissues including heart, skeletal muscle, colon, small and large intestines, kidney, pancreas, and spleen.

Physiologic Effects and Mechanisms of Insulin Sensitization

PPARγ is necessary and sufficient to differentiate adipocytes. It was first shown to interact directly with the *cis* element that regulates adipocyte-specific expression of the fatty acid-binding protein aP2 (54). Introduction of PPARγ into fibroblasts in the presence of weak PPAR ligands induced differentiation of the cells into adipocytes (55). Recently, several groups of researchers reported that PPARγ heterozygous null mice had reduced amounts of adipose tissue (56–58). Barak et al. (56) described a homozygous null mouse that exhibited extreme lipodystrophy. PPARγ dominant-negative mutants have been generated (59–61). When expressed in 3T3-L1 cells, such mutants inhibited their differentiation into adipocytes (59, 60). In adipocytes, PPARγ regulates the expression of numerous genes (Table 1) involved in lipid metabolism, including aP2 (35), PEPCK (62), acyl-CoA synthase (63), and LPL (64). PPARγ has also been shown to control expression of FATP-1 (65) and CD36 (66), both involved in lipid uptake into adipocytes. These genes have all been shown to possess PPREs within their regulatory regions.

PPARγ also regulates genes that control cellular energy homeostasis (Table 1). It has been shown to increase expression of the mitochondrial uncoupling proteins, UCP-1, UCP-2, and UCP-3 in vitro and in vivo (67). The physiological outcomes of these alterations are not yet understood. In contrast to its positive action on the UCPs, PPARγ downregulates leptin, a secreted, adipocyte-selective protein that inhibits feeding and augments catabolic lipid metabolism (68, 69). This receptor activity might explain the increased caloric uptake and storage noted in vivo upon treatment with PPARγ agonists.

PPARγ has been associated with several genes that affect insulin action. TNFα, a pro-inflammatory cytokine that is expressed by adipocytes, has been associated with insulin resistance (70) and diminished insulin signal transduction (71). PPARγ agonists inhibited expression of TNFα in adipose tissue of obese rodents (72) and TNFα-induced insulin resistance (73). They also ablated the actions of TNFα in adipocytes in vitro (74). Activation of PPARγ has been shown to increase expression of c-CBL-associated protein in cultured adipocytes (75). This protein, which appears to play a positive role in the insulin signaling pathway, contains a functional PPRE within the 5′ regulatory region of its gene (76). Expression of IRS-2, a protein with a proven role in insulin signal transduction in insulin-sensitive tissue, was also increased in cultured adipocytes and human adipose tissue incubated with PPARγ agonists (77). Recently, we have demonstrated that PPARγ

TABLE 1   Genes regulated in vivo by PPARγ agonists[*]

Gene	Regulation	Potential function(s)
aP2—adipocyte fatty acid binding protein	↑ WAT	Intracellular fatty acid binding
Acyl-CoA synthetase	↑ WAT	Lipogenesis and/or catabolism
PEPCK—phosphoenolpyruvate carboxykinase	↑ WAT	Glycerol synthesis (for triglycerides)
LPL-lipoprotein lipase	↑ WAT	Hydrolysis of triglyceride-containing particles
CD36	↑ WAT	Cell surface fatty acid transporter
FATP-1	↑ WAT ↓ muscle	Cell surface fatty acid transporter
Uncoupling protein 1—UCP1	↑ BAT ↑ WAT	Uncouple mitochondrial respiration
UCP3 (+/−UCP2)	↑ WAT	Uncouple mitochondrial respiration
Carnitine palmitoyl transferase1 CPT1	↑ WAT	Translocation of fatty acids into mitochondria
c-CBL-associated protein	↑ WAT	Insulin signaling toward glucose transport
Insulin receptor substrate-2—IRS-2	↑ WAT	Insulin receptor-mediated signaling
Pyruvate dehydrogenase kinase 4—PDK4	↑ WAT ↓ muscle	Inhibition of pyruvate dehydrogenase (inhibition of glucose oxidation)
Adipocyte complement-related factor 30—Acrp30	↑ WAT	Fat-specific secreted protein; beneficial metabolic effects on liver/muscle (?)
TNFα	↓ WAT	Pro-inflammatory cytokine; potential mediator of insulin resistance
Leptin	↓ WAT	Fat-derived hormone that inhibits food intake
11-β hydroxysteroid dehydrogenase 1—11β-HSD-1	↓ WAT (↓ liver)	Controls intracellular conversion to active cortisol

[*]Increases or decreases in mRNA expression are noted in white (WAT) or brown (BAT) adipose tissue and skeletal muscle. See text for details and references.

agonists inhibit expression of 11β-hydroxysteroid dehydrogenase 1 (11β-HSD-1) in adipocytes and adipose tissue of type 2 diabetes mouse models (41). This enzyme, which is highly expressed in adipocytes and hepatocytes, converts cortisone to the glucocorticoid agonist cortisol. Because hypercorticosteroidism exacerbates insulin resistance (78) and 11β-HSD-1 null mice are resistant to diet-induced diabetes (79), our results suggest that some of the insulin-sensitizing actions observed after activation of PPARγ may result from a decrease in adipose 11β-HSD-1 levels.

Adipocyte-related complement protein (Acrp)30 is a secreted adipocyte-specific protein that was recently shown to have in vivo effects including decreased glucose, triglycerides, and free fatty acids (80, 81). Treatment of diabetic mice with PPARγ agonists normalized low mRNA levels and increased plasma levels of Acrp30 (82). Compared with normal human subjects, patients with type 2 diabetes have reduced plasma levels of Acrp30 (83). Increases in Acrp30 plasma levels were seen in human subjects treated with rosiglitazone but not the PPARα agonist fenofibrate (82). Induction of Acrp30 by PPARγ agonists might therefore also play a key role in the mechanism of PPARγ agonist-mediated amelioration of the metabolic syndrome.

Given that PPARγ is expressed predominantly in adipose tissue, the prevailing hypothesis regarding the net in vivo efficacy of PPARγ agonists involves direct actions on adipose cells, with secondary effects in key insulin-responsive tissues such as skeletal muscle and liver. The lack of glucose-lowering efficacy of rosiglitazone in a mouse model of severe insulin resistance where white adipose tissue was essentially absent supports this notion (84). Although low levels of PPARγ are expressed in muscle, in vivo treatment of insulin-resistant rats produced acute (<24 h) normalization of adipose tissue insulin action, whereas insulin-mediated glucose uptake in muscle was not improved until several days after the initiation of therapy (85). This is consistent with the fact that PPARγ agonists can produce an increase in adipose tissue insulin action after direct in vitro incubation (86), whereas no such effect could be demonstrated using isolated in vitro incubated skeletal muscle (85). In addition, recent analysis of tissue mRNA expression reveals that selected PPRE-containing genes that are induced in adipose tissue are actually suppressed in skeletal muscle. An example is pyruvate dehydrogenase kinase 4 (87). In vivo, PPARγ-mediated suppression of this gene in muscle would be expected to produce a net increase in glucose oxidation. Therefore, as depicted in Figure 3 (see color insert), mediators of the beneficial metabolic effects of PPARγ agonists on distant tissues (muscle and liver) are likely to involve a combined effect to (*a*) enhance insulin-mediated adipose tissue uptake, storage (and potentially catabolism) of free fatty acids (88); (*b*) induce the production of adipose-derived factors with potential insulin-sensitizing activity (e.g., Acrp30); and (*c*) suppress the circulating levels and/or actions of insulin resistance-causing adipose-derived factors such as TNFα or "resistin" (89).

Inflammation

The inhibitory effects of PPARγ activation on TNFα action discussed above led several research groups to examine the anti-inflammatory properties of PPARγ agonists. Monocytes and macrophages play an important part in the inflammatory process through the release of inflammatory cytokines such as TNFα and IL-6 and the production of nitric oxide (NO) by inducible nitric oxide synthase (iNOS). Expression of PPARγ was robustly upregulated upon the differentiation of monocytes into macrophages (90). In vitro treatment of rodent macrophages with PPARγ

agonists downregulated NO production (91). Such ligands were also found to block PMA-induced synthesis of IL-6 and TNFα in primary human monocytes in spite of the low level of expression PPARγ in these cells (92). Note that the agonist concentrations used in the two aforementioned experiments did not correlate with the reported affinities of the compounds for the receptor. Furthermore, in contrast to the results described above, TZD and non-TZD PPARγ agonists, with the exception of the natural ligand 15d-PGJ2, do not inhibit LPS-induced cytokine production in cultured macrophages and db/db mice treated in vivo (93). We concluded that activation of PPARγ was not a major mechanism by which to inhibit activation of monocytic cells. In general accordance with this conclusion, the Evans group recently utilized murine PPARγ null macrophages to demonstrate that previously reported inhibitory actions of PPARγ agonists on macrophage cytokine production occur via a receptor-independent mechanism (94).

In contrast to the results above, Chinetti et al. demonstrated that rosiglitazone induced apoptosis of cultured macrophages by altering NFκB signaling at concentrations that paralleled its known affinity for PPARγ (90). This ligand has also been shown to block inflammatory cytokine synthesis in colonic cell lines by inhibiting activation of the NFκB pathway (95). This latter observation offers a possible mechanistic explanation for the observed anti-inflammatory actions of TZDs in rodent models of colitis (95).

Cancer

The interest in studying the effects of PPARγ activation on various forms of cancer is derived from previous results suggesting that PPARγ ligands inhibited cell proliferation when inducing adipocyte differentiation. For example, activation of PPARγ caused logarithmically growing fibroblasts and virally transformed HIB1B adipocytes to withdraw from the cell cycle (96). Activation of PPARγ by pioglitazone blocked the cell cycle and caused differentiation of primary liposarcoma cells in culture (97). In human subjects, the PPARγ agonist troglitazone caused differentiation of advanced liposarcomas (98). Such results support a therapeutic role for PPARγ ligands in the treatment of this often recalcitrant form of cancer. PPARγ has been shown to be expressed at significant levels in human mammary adenocarcinomas, and PPARγ agonists have been reported to reduce growth and induce differentiation of malignant breast epithelial cells (99). Such ligands have also inhibited tumor growth in mouse models of mammary carcinoma (100).

PPARγ is expressed at high levels in primary colon tumors and colon cancer cell lines (101). Incubating such transformed cells with PPARγ agonists caused them to withdraw from the cell cycle, decrease their growth rate, and demonstrate changes in morphology indicative of increased differentiation (102). Inhibitors of cyclooxygenases (COXs) have been shown to be effective in reducing the risk of colon cancer. Since the COXs metabolize fatty acids to prostaglandins and eicosanoids, it was suggested that they might promote carcinogenesis by generating PPARγ ligands. In support of this hypothesis, APC$^{min/+}$ mice (a model of inherited polyposis) treated with high doses of two TZDs displayed a small but statistically significant increase in the number of colon polyps (103, 104). However, others have found that treating mice with troglitazone inhibited growth of transplanted human colon tumors (102). In light of the above contradictory results, it is not presently possible to conclude what role PPARγ plays in the pathophysiology of colon cancer.

Hypertension

Hypertension is a complex disorder of the cardiovascular system that is associated with insulin resistance. Type 2 diabetes patients demonstrate a 1.5- to 2-fold increase in hypertension in comparison with the general population (105). Troglitazone therapy has been shown to decrease blood pressure in diabetic patients (106) as well as in obese, insulin-resistant persons (107). Since such reductions in blood pressure correlate with decreases in insulin levels (106), they may be mediated, at least in part, by an improvement in insulin sensitivity.

Genetic Variation

Several groups have reported nucleotide sequence polymorphisms within the coding exons of the PPARγ gene (108–111); however, there are no known spontaneous mutations affecting PPARγ in nonhuman species. A silent polymorphism (C $\rightarrow$ T) in the sixth exon common to PPARγ1 and PPARγ2 (109, 111) was suggested to distinguish the relationship between body mass index (BMI) and plasma leptin levels in subjects with the CC genotype versus those with the T allele (CT or TT). Thus, genetic variation in or near the PPARγ locus could modulate leptin levels in response to variable degrees of body adiposity.

More important was the discovery of a polymorphism encoding the substitution of Ala for Pro at amino acid 12, as initially reported by Yen et al. (109). The Ala^{12} allele frequency varies from 0.03 to 0.12 in several populations and was initially shown to be associated with increasing degrees of obesity (112). In several additional studies, the Ala^{12} allele was associated with lower BMI, improved insulin sensitivity, and reduced incidence of type 2 diabetes (108, 113). In one large study, the more common Pro^{12} allele was associated with a 1.25-fold increase in risk of type 2 diabetes (113). In contrast, other groups failed to detect an association of Ala^{12} with altered metabolic parameters (114, 115). Importantly, the recombinant receptor bearing this single amino acid change was apparently defective with respect to DNA binding and its ability to mediate ligand-stimulated transactivation in transfected cells (108). Because this variant is relatively prevalent, it may contribute to altered physiology of fat metabolism in humans.

A second PPARγ polymorphism, encoding a Pro^{115} $\rightarrow$ Gln substitution, was present in 4 of 121 obese German subjects (mean BMI 33.9) but was absent in each of 237 normal-weight controls (mean BMI 25) (110). Interestingly, this polymorphism is adjacent to Ser^{114}, which may be an important site of negative regulation via growth factor-mediated phosphorylation (116). Thus, like an artificial

Ser[114] → Ala mutant (116), the naturally occurring Gln[115] mutant resulted in a greater degree of adipogenesis than wild-type PPARγ when studied in overexpressing cells (110).

In contrast to the more subtle potential effects of the Ala[12] or Gln[115] polymorphisms, Barroso et al. recently reported on two families with a phenotype of severely insulin-resistant type 2 diabetes in association with heterozygous PPARγ mutations—either Pro[467] → Leu or Val[290] → Met (117). Interestingly, hypertension was reported as an additional associated phenotype. Importantly, in both families, these mutant receptors were shown to have severely impaired function with potential dominant-negative effects when studied in transfected cells.

PPARα

Cloning and Characterization

Murine PPARα was the first member of this nuclear receptor subclass to be cloned (118). It has subsequently been cloned from frog (49), rat (119), rabbit (120), and human (121). Human PPARα has been mapped to chromosome 22 adjacent to the region 22q12-q13.1 (121). In rodents and humans, PPARα is expressed in numerous metabolically active tissues including liver, kidney, heart, skeletal muscle, and brown fat (122, 123). It is also present in monocytic (90), vascular endothelial (124), and vascular smooth muscle cells (125).

PPARα serves as the receptor for a structurally diverse class of compounds, including hypolipidemic fibrates, that induce hepatic peroxisome proliferation, hepatomegaly, and hepatocarcinogenesis in rodents (118). Remarkably, these toxic effects are lost in humans, although the same compounds activate PPARα across species (126). Several explanations have been proffered for the differential effects of PPARα agonists. Hepatic expression of wild PPARα is expressed at levels tenfold higher in rodent liver than in human liver (127). The PPREs of genes involved in peroxisome proliferation, including acetyl CoA oxidase (ACO), have been shown to differ between rodents and humans. The human enhancer sequence of ACO could not be activated by PPARα in transactivation experiments (128).

PPARα has been shown to play a critical role in the regulation of cellular uptake, activation, and β-oxidation of fatty acids. PPARα induces expression of the fatty acid transport protein (FATP) (65) and FAT (129), two proteins that transport fatty acids across the cell membrane. Activation of PPARα also directly upregulates transcription of long chain fatty acid acetyl-CoA synthase (63) as well as ACO (49, 130), enoyl-CoA hydratase/dehydrogenase multifunctional enzyme (131), and keto-acyl-CoA thiolase (132) enzymes in the peroxisomal β-oxidation pathway. Carnitine palmitoyltransferase I (CPT I) catalyzes the rate-limiting step in the translocation of activated fatty acids into the inner membrane of the mitochondria where the most productive step in their catabolism occurs. This enzyme is strongly induced by PPARα ligands (133), and a functional PPRE has been identified in the 5′ flanking region of its gene (134–136). Other PPARα-responsive genes in this mitochondrial metabolic pathway have also been reported, including various acyl-CoA dehydrogenases (137, 138) and hydroxymethylglutaryl-CoA synthase (139). The CYP4A subclass of cytochrome P450 enzymes catalyzes the ω-hydroxylation of fatty acids, a pathway that is particularly active in the fasted and diabetic states. Fibrates and other peroxisome proliferators activate expression of the CYP4As, and functional PPREs have been found in the regulatory regions of CYP4A genes (140, 141). In sum, PPARα is an important lipid sensor and regulator of cellular energy-harvesting metabolism. Potent genetic proof for this conclusion is offered by Lee et al., who reported that PPARα null mice had depressed levels of numerous fatty acid metabolizing enzymes and were unresponsive to the actions of peroxisome proliferating agents (142).

Dyslipidemia and Atherosclerosis

Atherosclerosis is a very prevalent disease in westernized societies. In addition to a strong association with elevated LDL cholesterol, dyslipidemia characterized by elevated triglyceride-rich particles and low levels of HDL cholesterol is commonly associated with other aspects of a metabolic syndrome that includes obesity, insulin resistance, type 2 diabetes, and an increased risk of coronary artery disease (143). Thus, in 8500 men with known coronary artery disease, 38% were found to have low HDL (<35 mg/dL) and 33% had elevated triglycerides (>200 mg/dL) (144). Treatment of these patients with fibrates such as gemfibrozil and fenofibrate, which are weak PPARα agonists, resulted in substantial triglyceride lowering and modest HDL-raising efficacy (145). More importantly, a recent large prospective trial proved that treatment with gemfibrozil produced a 22% reduction in cardiovascular events or death (145, 146). Thus PPARα agonists can effectively improve cardiovascular risk factors and have a net benefit to improve cardiovascular outcomes.

Mechanisms by which PPARα activation causes triglyceride lowering are likely to include the effects of agonists to suppress hepatic apo-CIII gene expression while also stimulating LPL gene expression (64, 147). Moreover, the triglyceride-lowering activity of fibrates and related compounds is ablated in PPARα null mice (148). The effect of fibrates to increase HDL levels has been suggestively associated with an increase in apo-AI gene expression, although this finding is not universally observed (149); thus, additional mechanisms may be involved (discussed below).

The presence of PPARα and/or PPARγ expression in vascular cell types including macrophages, endothelial cells, and vascular smooth muscle cells suggests that direct vascular effects might contribute to potential antiatherosclerosis efficacy (143). As discussed above, PPARγ agonists have been reported to produce variable antiinflammatory effects in monocyte-macrophages. In addition, several lines of evidence have shown that PPARα agonists have potentially relevant local or systemic antiinflammatory effects, particularly in vascular smooth muscle cells (see below). A particular effect of either PPARα (150) or PPARγ (151–153) activation to inhibit cytokine-induced vascular cell adhesion and to suppress monocyte-macrophage migration has also been recently reported as a possible mechanism of antiatherosclerosis efficacy.

Two recent studies have suggested that either PPARα (154) or PPARγ (154, 155) activation in macrophages can induce the expression of a cholesterol efflux "pump" known as ABC-A1. Since ABC-A1 is a target gene for the liver-X-receptor (LXR), these investigators also showed a modest induction of LXR expression, which may represent the indirect mechanism by which PPAR activation can upregulate ABC-A1.

Although the net effect of fibrates to reduce cardiovascular risk in humans is now well accepted, the potential for an antiatherosclerosis effect of PPARγ agonists (e.g., TZDs) remains unexplored in humans. Several recent studies have shown that PPARγ-selective compounds have the capacity to reduce arterial lesion size in animal models of atherosclerosis. In LDL-receptor null mice, rosiglitazone, troglitazone, and a potent non-TZD PPARγ agonist were shown to inhibit lesion formation (156, 157). In addition, troglitazone was shown to suppress lesion formation in atherosclerosis-prone apo-E null mice (158) and in Wantanabe hyperlipidemic rabbits (159). Furthermore, troglitazone treatment of apo-E–deficient mice for 7 days was sufficient to attenuate monocyte-macrophage homing to arterial lesions in vivo (153). Thus, via multifactorial mechanisms including improvements in circulating lipids, systemic and local anti-inflammatory effects, and, potentially, inhibition of vascular cell proliferation, both PPARα and PPARγ agonists show strong promise for use in the treatment or prevention of atherosclerosis.

Inflammation

PPARα was first proposed to be a modulator of inflammation when leukotriene B4 (LTB4), a potent chemotactic agent, was found to be a ligand and agonist for the receptor (160). It was suggested that activation of PPARα inhibited the inflammatory action of such eicosanoids by augmenting expression of hepatic enzymes involved in their metabolism. This argument was fortified when it was observed that PPARα null mice have more extended inflammatory responses than their wild-type littermates in response to LTB4 or its precursor arachidonic acid.

Other, nonhepatic, anti-inflammatory mechanisms have been described for PPARα ligands that may be important in maintaining vascular health. Treatment of cytokine-activated human macrophages with PPARα agonists induced apoptosis of the cells by interfering with the antiapoptotic NFκB signaling pathway (90). Staels et al. reported that PPARα but not PPARγ agonists inhibited activation of aortic smooth muscle cells in response to inflammatory stimuli by repressing NFκB signaling (125). In hyperlipidemic patients, fenofibrate treatment decreased the plasma concentrations of the inflammatory cytokine interleukin-6 (125). Additional work showed that IκBα levels were induced in vascular smooth muscle cells by fibrates, thereby offering another anti-inflammatory mechanism for PPARα agonists (161). In contrast with these results, increased plasma TNFα levels were observed in fibrate-treated endotoxemic mice (162). This undesirable effect may be associated with PPARα-induced hepatic peroxisome proliferation. Clearly, additional research is needed to further investigate these provocative results and to deepen our knowledge of PPARα's role in the physiopathology of the inflammatory process, especially as it affects the vascular system.

Genetic Variation

The existence of a few sequence variants in the human PPARα gene was first reported by Tugwood; these included Thr^{71} → Met, Lys^{123} → Met, Ala^{268} → Val, Gly^{296} → Ala, and Val^{444} → Ala (163). One particular allele with Met at positions 71 and 123 as well as the Ala^{444} substitution was shown to undergo normal RXR dimerization and DNA binding but was inactive in a cell-based transactivation assay (163). Subsequently, another potentially important hPPARα polymorphism was described that lacks 203 basepairs encoding residues 508–712 at the C-terminal end of the DNA binding domain (further described above). More recently, a Leu^{162} → Val variant was shown to be associated with higher total and HDL cholesterol in a relative small cohort of human subjects (164). This polymorphism apparently has greater transcriptional activity when studied in transfected cells. In an additional study, the Leu^{162} → Val allele was associated with higher LDL and apoB levels, suggesting that it conferred increased atherosclerosis risk. Therefore, the existence of PPARα genetic variants with clear-cut functional effects and a bona fide causal relationship to metabolic alterations has yet to be discovered.

PPARδ

Cloning and Characterization

Human (165) and *Xenopus* (49) PPARδ cDNAs were cloned in the early 1990s. The receptor was subsequently cloned from mouse (166) and rat (167). Human PPARδ has been localized to chromosome 6p21.1–p21.2 (168) whereas the murine gene has been mapped to chromosome 17 (169). PPARδ is expressed in a wide range of tissues and cells, with relatively higher levels of expression noted in brain, adipose, and skin (122, 170). Thus far, no PPARδ-specific gene targets have been identified.

Dyslipidemia and Insulin Resistance

Using relatively selective PPARδ agonists such as L-165041, we determined that such compounds produced minimal, if any, significant glucose- or triglyceride-lowering activity in murine models of type 2 diabetes compared with efficacious PPARγ or PPARα agonists (21). Subsequently, a modest increase in HDL-cholesterol levels was detected with L-165041 in db/db mice (47). More recently, Oliver et al. reported that the potent and selective PPARδ agonist GW-501516 could induce a substantial increase in HDL-cholesterol levels as well as a reduction in triglyceride levels in obese Rhesus monkeys (48). In addition, elevated levels of plasma insulin (a consequence of insulin resistance) were suppressed by

GW-501516 treatment. Although these beneficial metabolic effects in a primate model have yet to be reproduced by others or with other compounds, the results point to an important therapeutic potential for PPARδ -selective compounds.

Fertility

One area in which the role of PPARδ has been examined is fertility. COX-2 null female mice are reported to display decreased fecundity, in part due to decreased blastocyte implantation and decidualization (171). COX-2 catalyzes the rate-limiting step in generating prostaglandins, including prostacyclin, the eicosanoid that appears to serve as the natural agonist for PPARδ. PPARδ was found to be expressed in implantation sites within the uterus, and was strongly upregulated during the decidualization process in a manner similar to COX-2 (172). When COX-2 null mice were treated with carboprostacyclin or our PPARδ-selective agonist L-165041, implantation was restored (172). Such results support the conclusion that PPARδ may play a role in maintaining reproductive capacity in females.

Cancer

Throughout the past decade, researchers have sought to establish the roles of the three PPAR isoforms in the pathophysiology of cancer. In 1999, He et al. identified PPARδ as a target of the tumor suppressor APC in colorectal cancer cells (173). In these cells, which possess inactivation mutations of APC, PPARδ was highly expressed, and transcription factors in the APC signaling pathway, β-catenin/Tcf-4, were found to interact directly with and activate the promoter of PPARδ. Recently, a PPAR$\delta^{-/-}$ colorectal cancer cell line was found to exhibit a greatly decreased ability to form tumors in nude mice in comparison with PPAR$^{+/-}$ cancer cells (174). Although far from conclusive, these results do suggest that PPARδ antagonists might prove beneficial in the treatment of colon cancer.

Central Nervous System

Localization studies have demonstrated that PPARδ is abundantly expressed throughout the rat CNS, with particularly high levels found in the dentate gyrus, hippocampus, telencephalic cortex, cerebellum, and thalamic nuclei (122, 175, 176). Further investigation has shown that PPARδ expression is at its highest level in the embryonic brain (stage E18.5), suggesting that it may play a critical role in regulating the differentiation of cells within the CNS (177).

We have examined the expression of PPARδ in murine brain by in situ hybridization and immunohistochemistry and found it to be expressed widely throughout murine brain but at particularly high levels in the entorhinal cortex, hypothalamus, and hippocampus as well as the corpus callosum and the neostriatum (J.W. Woods, M. Tanen, D.J. Figueroa, C. Biswas, E. Zycband, D.E. Moller, C.P. Austin & J. Berger, unpublished data). Expression of PPARδ in the caudate putamen and corpus callosum suggests its possible involvement in volitional movement

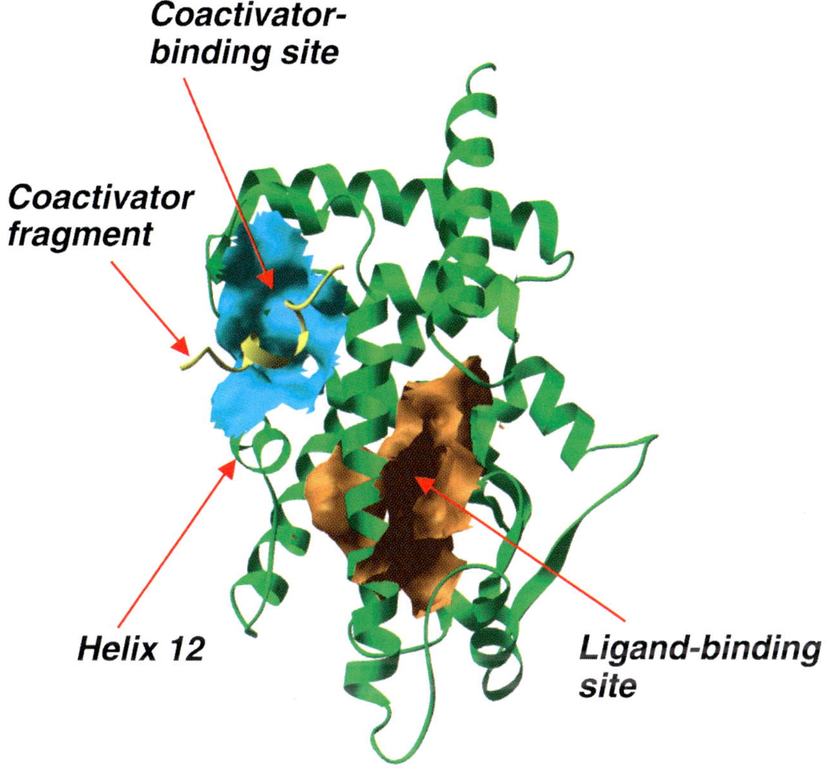

Figure 1 X-ray crystal structure of PPARγ ligand binding domain. Several key α-helices are shown along with the relative location of key functional regions.

- Molecular Mechanism

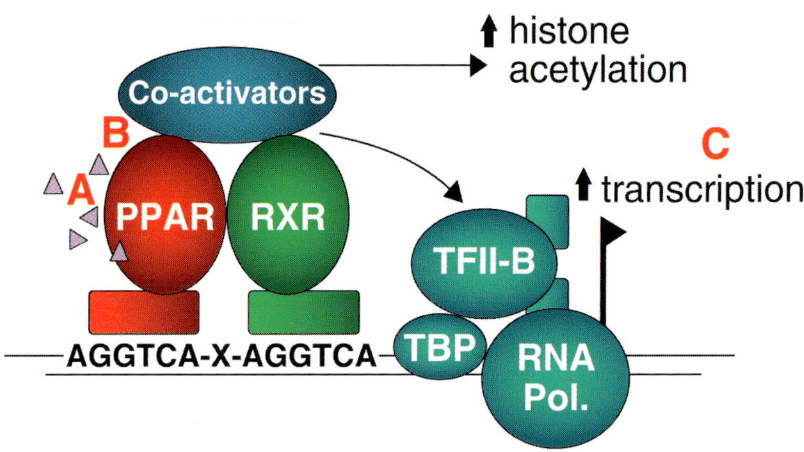

- Assay Formats
    - ♦ Ligand binding (S.P.A.)...............**A**
    - ♦ Co-activator association (H.T.R.F.).............**B**
    - ♦ Gene transcription
        - ♦ Gal4-chimeric receptors
        - ♦ COS-1 cells.......**C**

Figure 2 Mechanism of transcriptional activation by PPAR isoforms. Selected molecular components are shown relative to assay formats that can be used to characterize compound activities.

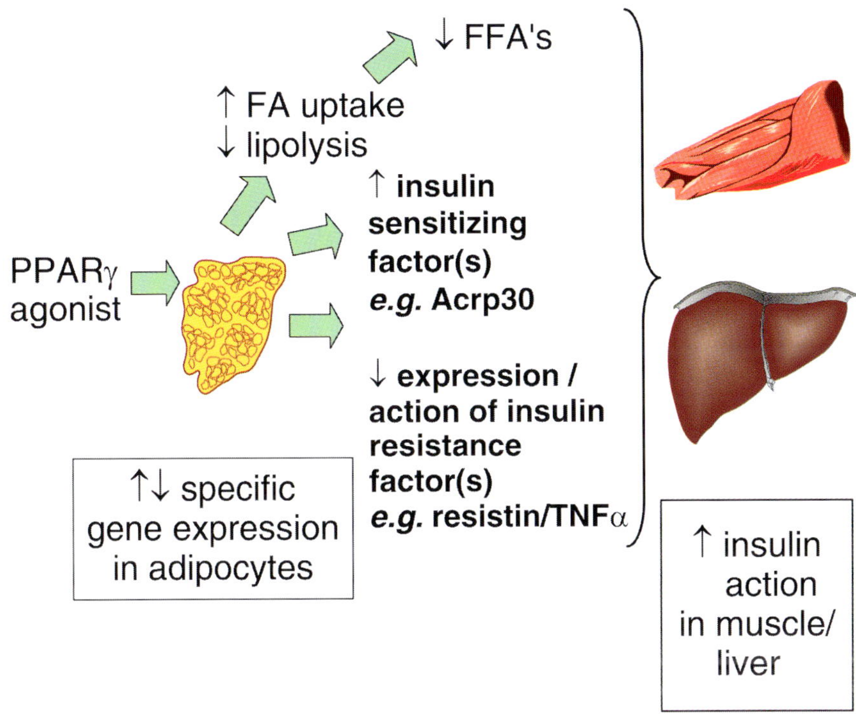

Figure 3 Working hypothesis for PPARγ-mediated increases in insulin sensitivity.

as well as cortical processing of signals from the thalamus (178). PPARδ expression in limbic regions (hypothalamus, hippocampus, and entorhinal cortex) suggests that PPARδ might also play a role in more complex emotional, circadian, and autonomic functions (179). PPARδ was highly expressed within oligodendrocytes of the corpus callosum and neurons but not in astrocytes of the caudate putamen.

High levels of PPARδ expression have recently been reported in cultured murine oligodendrocytes, and PPARδ agonists, bromopalmitate and our L-165041, were found to augment differentiation of and myelinogenesis by these cells (180, 181). It is therefore noteworthy that PPARδ null mice were found to have diminished myelination levels of the corpus callosum (182), an area normally rich in PPARδ-expressing oligodendrocytes (see above). PPARδ has also been found to be the major isotype expressed in cultured rat neurons and to be coexpressed with acyl-CoA synthase 2, an enzyme thought to play an important role in fatty acid utilization within the brain (183). Using L-165041, it was discovered that the *ACS2* gene is transcriptionally regulated by PPARδ. Together, these data suggest a role for PPARδ in myelination, neuronal signaling, and lipid metabolism in the CNS.

CONCLUSIONS AND FUTURE DIRECTIONS

Isoforms of the PPAR family of nuclear receptors are clearly involved in the systemic regulation of lipid metabolism and serve as "sensors" for fatty acids, prostanoid metabolites, eicosanoids, and related molecules. These receptors function to regulate a broad array of genes in a coordinate fashion. Important biochemical pathways that regulate peroxisomal function, lipid oxidation, metabolism of xenobiotics, lipid synthesis, adipocyte differentiation, insulin action, cell proliferation, and inflammation can be modulated by activation (or inhibition) of individual PPAR isoforms. Strong therapeutic effects of PPARα and PPARγ agonists to favorably influence systemic lipid levels, glucose homeostasis, and atherosclerosis risk (in the case of PPARα activation in humans) have recently been discovered. Although specific molecular mechanisms by which PPARα activation can effectively ameliorate dyslipidemia are now well characterized, the multifactorial mechanism by which PPARγ agonists reduce insulin resistance remains to be further elucidated. Recent observations made using PPARδ ligands suggest that this less well characterized isoform may also be an important therapeutic target for selected disorders, including cancer, infertility, and dyslipidemia.

Further assessment of the physiologic effects of individual PPARs, such as can be achieved with the use of tissue-selective knockout mice, should provide better insights into the precise roles of these receptors in individual cell types. In addition, the use of gene microarray and proteomic techniques to carefully monitor the full spectrum of gene expression and protein effects of more selective compounds has yet to be fully exploited. A more complete understanding of the potential utility (and pitfalls) of modulating individual PPAR actions should follow.

Visit the Annual Reviews home page at www.AnnualReviews.org

LITERATURE CITED

1. Laudet V, Hanni C, Coll J, et al. 1992. Evolution of the nuclear receptor gene superfamily. *EMBO J.* 11:1003–13
2. Nolte RT, Wisely GB, Westin S, et al. 1998. Ligand binding and co-activator assembly of the peroxisome proliferator-activated receptor-gamma. *Nature* 395:137–43
3. Xu HE, Lambert MH, Montana VG, et al. 1999. Molecular recognition of fatty acids by peroxisome proliferator-activated receptors. *Mol. Cell* 3:397–403
4. Werman A, Hollenberg A, Solanes G, et al. 1997. Ligand-independent activation domain in the N terminus of peroxisome proliferator-activated receptor gamma (PPARγ). Differential activity of PPARγ1 and -2 isoforms and influence of insulin. *J. Biol. Chem.* 272:20230–35
5. Miyata KS, McCaw SE, Marcus SL, et al. 1994. The peroxisome proliferator-activated receptor interacts with the retinoid X receptor in vivo. *Gene* 148:327–30
6. Mangelsdorf DJ, Borgmeyer U, Heyman RA, et al. 1992. Characterization of three RXR genes that mediate the action of 9-*cis* retinoic acid. *Genes Dev.* 6:329–44
7. Mukherjee R, Davies PJA, Crombie DL, et al. 1997. Sensitization of diabetic and obese mice to insulin by retinoid X receptor agonists. *Nature* 386:407–10
8. Wahli W, Braissant O, Desvergne B. 1995. Peroxisome proliferator activated receptors: transcriptional regulators of adipogenesis, lipid metabolism and more. *Chem. Biol.* 2:261–66
9. IJpenberg A, Jeannin E, Wahli W, Desvergne B. 1997. Polarity and specific sequence requirements of peroxisome proliferator-activated receptor (PPAR)/retinoid X receptor heterodimer binding to DNA. A functional analysis of the malic enzyme gene PPAR response element. *J. Biol. Chem.* 272:20108–17
10. Xu L, Glass CK, Rosenfeld MG. 1999. Coactivator and corepressor complexes in nuclear receptor function. *Curr. Opin. Genet. Dev.* 9:140–47
11. Heery DM, Kalkhoven E, Hoare S, Parker MG. 1997. A signature motif in transcriptional co-activators mediates binding to nuclear receptors. *Nature* 387:733–36
12. Torchia J, Rose DW, Inostroza J, et al. 1997. The transcriptional co-activator p/CIP binds CBP and mediates nuclear-receptor function. *Nature* 387:677–84
13. Berger J, Bailey P, Biswas C, et al. 1996. Thiazolidinediones produce a conformational change in peroxisomal proliferator-activated receptor-γ: binding and activation correlate with antidiabetic actions in db/db mice. *Endocrinology* 137:4189–95
14. Zhu Y, Qi C, Calandra C, et al. 1996. Cloning and identification of mouse steroid receptor coactivator-1 (mSRC-1), as a coactivator of peroxisome proliferator-activated receptor gamma. *Gene Expr.* 6:185–95
15. Zhu Y, Qi C, Jain S, et al. 1997. Isolation and characterization of PBP, a protein that interacts with peroxisome proliferator-activated receptor. *J. Biol. Chem.* 272:25500–6
16. Puigserver P, Wu Z, Park CW, et al. 1998. A cold-inducible coactivator of nuclear receptors linked to adaptive thermogenesis. *Cell* 92:829–39
17. Miyata KS, McCaw SE, Meertens LM, et al. 1998. Receptor-interacting protein 140 interacts with and inhibits transactivation by peroxisome proliferator-activated receptor alpha and liver-X-receptor alpha. *Mol. Cell. Endocrinol.* 146:69–76
18. Heinlein CA, Ting HJ, Yeh S, Chang C. 1999. Identification of ARA70 as a ligand-enhanced coactivator for the peroxisome proliferator-activated receptor gamma. *J. Biol. Chem.* 274:16147–52

19. Oberfield JL, Collins JL, Holmes CP, et al. 1999. A peroxisome proliferator-activated receptor gamma ligand inhibits adipocyte differentiation. *Proc. Natl. Acad. Sci. USA* 96:6102–6

20. Lehmann JM, Moore LB, Smith-Oliver TA, et al. 1995. An antidiabetic thiazolidinedione is a high affinity ligand for peroxisome proliferator-activated receptor γ *J. Biol. Chem.* 270:12953–56

21. Berger J, Leibowitz MD, Doebber TW, et al. 1999. Novel PPARγ and PPARδ ligands produce distinct biological effects. *J. Biol. Chem.* 274:6718–25

22. Elbrecht A, Chen Y, Adams A, et al. 1999. L-764406 is a partial agonist of human peroxisome proliferator-activated receptor gamma. The role of Cys313 in ligand binding. *J. Biol. Chem.* 274:7913–22

23. Zhou G, Cummings R, Li Y, et al. 1998. Nuclear receptors have distinct affinities for coactivators: characterization by fluorescence resonance energy transfer. *Mol. Endocrinol.* 12:1594–604

24. Nagy L, Tontonoz P, Alvarez JGA, et al. 1998. Oxidized LDL regulates macrophage gene expression through ligand activation of PPARγ. *Cell* 93:229–40

25. Forman BM, Tontonoz P, Chen J, et al. 1995. 15-deoxy-prostaglandin J2 is a ligand for the adipocyte determination factor PPARγ. *Cell* 83:803–12

26. Kliewer SA, Lenhard JM, Willson RM, et al. 1995. A prostaglandin J2 metabolite binds peroxisome proliferator-activated receptor γ and promotes adipocyte differentiation. *Cell* 83:813–19

27. Davies SS, Pontsler AV, Marathe GK, et al. 2001. Oxidized alkyl phospholipids are specific, high affinity peroxisome proliferator-activated receptor gamma ligands and agonists. *J. Biol. Chem.* 276:16015–23

28. Gottlicher M, Widmark E, Li Q, Gustafsson JA. 1992. Fatty acids activate a chimera of the clofibric acid-activated receptor and the glucocorticoid receptor. *Proc. Natl. Acad. Sci. USA* 89:4653–57

29. Kliewer SA, Sundseth SS, Jones SA, et al. 1997. Fatty acids and eicosanoids regulate gene expression through direct interactions with peroxisome proliferator-activated receptors α and γ. *Proc. Natl. Acad. Sci. USA* 94:4318–23

30. Forman BM, Chen J, Evans RM. 1997. Hypolipidemic drugs, polyunsaturated fatty acids, and eicosanoids are ligands for peroxisome proliferator-activated receptors α and δ. *Proc. Natl. Acad. Sci. USA* 94:4312–17

31. Yu K, Bayona W, Kallen CB, et al. 1995. Differential activation of peroxisome proliferator-activated receptors by eicosanoids. *J. Biol. Chem.* 270:23975–83

32. Amri E-Z, Bonino F, Ailhaud G, et al. 1995. Cloning of a protein that mediates transcriptional effects of fatty acids in preadipocytes. *J. Biol. Chem.* 270:2367–71

33. Kletzien RF, Clarke SD, Ulrich RG. 1992. Enhancement of adipocyte differentiation by an insulin-sensitizing agent. *Mol. Pharmacol.* 41:393–98

34. Harris PK, Kletzien RF. 1994. Localization of a pioglitazone response element in the adipocyte fatty acid-binding protein gene. *Mol. Pharmacol.* 45:439–45

35. Tontonoz P, Hu E, Graves R, et al. 1994. mPPARgamma 2: tissue-specific regulator of an adipocyte enhancer. *Genes Dev.* 8:1224–34

36. Willson TM, Cobb JE, Cowan DJ, et al. 1996. The structure-activity relationship between peroxisome proliferator-activated receptor gamma agonism and the antihyperglycemic activity of thiazolidinediones. *J. Med. Chem.* 39:665–68

37. Moller DE, Greene DA. 2001. Peroxisome proliferator-activated receptor (PPAR) γ agonists for diabetes. In *Drug Discovery—Advances in Protein Chemistry*, ed. E Scolnick, pp. 181–212. London: Harcourt

38. Willson TM, Brown PJ, Sternbach DD,

Henke BR. 2000. The PPARs: from orphan receptors to drug discovery. *J. Med. Chem.* 43:527–50

39. Hulin B, Newton LS, Lewis DM, et al. 1996. Hypoglycemic activity of a series of alpha-alkylthio and alpha-alkoxy carboxylic acids related to ciglitazone. *J. Med. Chem.* 39:3897–907

40. Murakami K, Tobe K, Ide T, et al. 1998. A novel insulin sensitizer acts as a coligand for peroxisome proliferator-activated receptor-alpha (PPAR-alpha) and PPAR-gamma: effect of PPAR-alpha activation on abnormal lipid metabolism in liver of Zucker fatty rats. *Diabetes* 47:1841–47

41. Berger J, Tanen M, Elbrecht A, et al. 2001. Peroxisome proliferator-activated receptor-gamma ligands inhibit adipocyte 11β-hydroxysteroid dehydrogenase type 1 expression and activity. *J. Biol. Chem.* 276:12629–35

42. Lehmann JM, Lenhard JM, Oliver BB, et al. 1997. Peroxisome proliferator-activated receptors alpha and gamma are activated by indomethacin and other non-steroidal anti-inflammatory drugs. *J. Biol. Chem.* 272:3406–10

43. Thorp JM, Waring WS. 1962. Modification and distribution of lipids by ethyl-chlorophenoxyisobutyrate. *Nature* 194:948–49

44. Hess R, Staubli W, Riess W. 1965. Nature of hepatomegalic effect produced by ethyl-chlorophenoxy-isobutyrate in the rat. *Nature* 208:856–58

45. Brown PJ, Smith-Oliver TA, Charifson PS, et al. 1997. Identification of peroxisome proliferator-activated receptor ligands from a biased chemical library. *Curr. Biol.* 4:909–18

46. Brown PJ, Winegar DA, Plunket KD, et al. 1999. A ureido-thioisobutyric acid (GW9578) is a subtype-selective PPARα agonist with potent lipid-lowering activity. *J. Med. Chem.* 42:3785–88

47. Leibowitz MD, Fievet C, Hennuyer N, et al. 2000. Activation of PPARδ alters lipid metaboism in db/db mice. *FEBS Lett.* 473:333–336

48. Oliver WR, Shenk JL, Snaith MR, et al. 2001. A selective peroxisome proliferator-activated receptor delta agonist promotes reverse cholesterol transport. *Proc. Natl. Acad. Sci. USA* 98:5306–11

49. Dreyer C, Krey G, Keller H, et al. 1992. Control of the peroxisomal beta-oxidation pathway by a novel family of nuclear hormone receptors. *Cell* 68:879–87

50. Greene ME, Blumberg B, McBride OW, et al. 1995. Isolation of the human peroxisome proliferator activated receptor gamma cDNA: expression in hematopoietic cells and chromosomal mapping. *Gene Expr.* 4:281–99

51. Zhu Y, Qi C, Korenberg JR, et al. 1995. Structural organization of mouse peroxisome proliferator-activated receptor γ (mPPARγ) gene: alternative promoter use and different splicing yield two mPPARγ isoforms. *Proc. Natl. Acad. Sci. USA* 92:7921–25

52. Elbrecht A, Chen Y, Cullinan CA, et al. 1996. Molecular cloning, expression and characterization of human peroxisome proliferator activated receptors gamma1 and gamma2. *Biochem. Biophys. Res. Commun.* 224:431–37

53. Fajas L, Auboeuf D, Raspe E, et al. 1997. The organization, promoter analysis, and expression of the human PPARgamma gene. *J. Biol. Chem.* 272:18779–89

54. Tontonoz P, Graves R, Budavari A, et al. 1994. Adipocyte-specific transcription factor ARF 6 is a heterodimeric complex of two nuclear hormone receptors, PPARg and RXRa. *Nucleic Acids Res.* 22:5628–34

55. Tontonoz P, Hu E, Spiegelman BM. 1994. Stimulation of adipogenesis in fibroblasts by PPARγ2, a lipid activated transcription factor. *Cell* 79:1147–56

56. Barak Y, Nelson MC, Ong ES, et al. 1999. PPARγ is required for placental, cardiac, and adipose tissue development. *Mol. Cell* 4:585–95

57. Kubota N, Terauchi Y, Miki H, et al. 1999. PPARγ mediates high-fat diet-induced adipocyte hypertrophy and insulin resistance. *Mol. Cell* 4:597–609

58. Rosen ED, Sarraf P, Troy AE, et al. 1999. PPARγ is required for the differentiation of adipose tissue in vivo and in vitro. *Mol. Cell* 4:611–17

59. Masugi J, Tamori Y, Kasuga M. 1999. Inhibition of adipogenesis by a COOH-terminally truncated mutant of PPARγ2 in 3T3-L1 cells. *Biochem. Biophys. Res. Commun.* 264:93–99

60. Gurnell M, Wentworth JM, Agostini M, et al. 2000. A dominant-negative peroxisome proliferator-activated receptor gamma (PPARγ) mutant is a constitutive repressor and inhibits PPARγ-mediated adipogenesis *J. Biol. Chem.* 275:5754–59

61. Berger J, Patel HV, Woods J, et al. 2000. A PPARγ mutant serves as a dominant negative inhibitor of PPAR signaling and is localized in the nucleus. *Mol. Cell Endocrinol.* 162:57–67

62. Tontonoz P, Hu E, Devine J, et al. 1995. PPARγ2 regulates adipose expression of the phosphoenolpyruvate carboxykinase gene. *Mol. Cell Biol* 15:351–57

63. Schoonjans K, Watanabe M, Suzuki H, et al. 1995. Induction of the acyl-coenzyme A synthetase gene by fibrates and fatty acids is mediated by a peroxisome proliferator response element in the C promoter. *J. Biol. Chem.* 270:19269–76

64. Schoonjans K, Peinado-Onsurbe J, Lefebvre AM, et al. 1996. PPARα and PPARγ activators direct a distinct tissue-specific transcriptional response via a PPRE in the lipoprotein lipase gene. *EMBO J.* 15:5336–48

65. Martin G, Schoonjans K, Lefebvre AM, et al. 1997. Coordinate regulation of the expression of the fatty acid transport protein and acyl-CoA synthetase genes by PPARα and PPARγ activators. *J. Biol. Chem.* 272:28210–17

66. Sfeir Z, Ibrahimi A, Amri E, et al. 1997. Regulation of FAT/CD36 gene expression: further evidence in support of a role of the protein in fatty acid binding/transport. *Prostaglandins Leukot. Essent. Fatty Acids* 57:17–21

67. Kelly LJ, Vicario P, Thompson GM, et al. 1998. Peroxisome proliferator-activated receptors γ and α mediate in vivo regulation of uncoupling protein (UCP1, UCP2, UCP3) gene expression. *Endocrinology* 139:4920–27

68. Kallen CB, Lazar MA. 1996. Antidiabetic thiazolidinediones inhibit leptin (ob) gene expression in 3T3-L1 adipocytes. *Proc. Natl. Acad. Sci. USA* 93:5793–96

69. De Vos P, Lefebvre AM, Miller SG, et al. 1996. Thiazolidinediones repress ob gene expression in rodents via activation of peroxisome proliferator-activated receptor gamma. *J. Clin. Invest.* 98:1004–9

70. Hotamisligil GS, Shargill NS, Spiegelman BM. 1993. Adipose expression of tumor necrosis factor-alpha: direct role in obesity-linked insulin resistance. *Science* 259:87–91

71. Hotamisligil GS, Murray DL, Choy LN, Spiegelman BM. 1994. Tumor necrosis factor alpha inhibits signaling from the insulin receptor. *Proc. Natl. Acad. Sci. USA* 91:4854–58

72. Hofmann C, Lorenz K, Braithwaite SS, et al. 1994. Altered gene expression for tumor necrosis factor-alpha and its receptors during drug and dietary modulation of insulin resistance. *Endocrinology* 134:264–70

73. Miles PDG, Romeo OM, Higo K, et al. 1997. TNF-alpha induced insulin resistance in vivo and its prevention by troglitazone. *Diabetes* 46:1678–83

74. Peraldi P, Xu M, Spiegelman BM. 1997. Thiazolidinediones block tumor necrosis factor-alpha-induced inhibition of insulin signaling. *J. Clin. Invest.* 100:1863–69

75. Ribon V, Johnson JH, Camp HS, Saltiel AR. 1998. Thiazolidinediones and insulin resistance: peroxisome proliferator-activated receptor gamma activation stimulates expression of the CAP gene.

Proc. Natl. Acad. Sci. USA 95:14751–56

76. Baumann CA, Chokshi N, Saltiel AR, Ribon V. 2000. Cloning and characterization of a functional peroxisome proliferator activator receptor-gamma-responsive element in the promoter of the CAP gene. *J. Biol. Chem.* 275:9131–35

77. Smith U, Gogg S, Johansson A, et al. 2001. Thiazolidinediones (PPARγ agonists) but not PPARα agonists increase IRS-2 gene expression in 3T3-L1 and human adipocytes. *FASEB J.* 15:215–20

78. Rebuffe-Scrive M, Krotkiewski M, Elfverson J, Bjorntorp P. 1988. Muscle and adipose tissue morphology and metabolism in Cushing's syndrome. *J. Clin. Endocrinol. Metab.* 67:1122–28

79. Kotelevtsev Y, Holmes MC, Burchell A, et al. 1997. 11β-hydroxysteroid dehydrogenase type 1 knockout mice show attenuated glucocorticoid-inducible responses and resist hyperglycemia on obesity or stress. *Proc. Natl. Acad. Sci. USA* 94:14924–29

80. Fruebis J, Tsao TS, Javorschi S, et al. 2001. Proteolytic cleavage product of 30-kDa adipocyte complement-related protein increases fatty acid oxidation in muscle and causes weight loss in mice. *Proc. Natl. Acad. Sci. USA* 98:2005–10

81. Berg AH, Combatsiaris TC, Du X, et al. 2001. The adipocyte-secreted protein Acrp30 enhances hepatic insulin action. *Nat. Med.* 7:947–53

82. Combatsiaris T, Berger J, Tanen M, et al. 2001. Induction of Acrp30 levels by PPARγ agonists: a potential mechanism of insulin sensitization. *Diabetes* 50:A271

83. Hotta K, Funahashi T, Arita Y, et al. 2000. Plasma concentrations of a novel, adipose-specific protein, adiponectin, in type 2 diabetic patients. *Arterioscler. Thromb. Vasc. Biol.* 20:1595–99

84. Chao L, Marcus-Samuels B, Mason MM, et al. 2000. Adipose tissue is required for the antidiabetic, but not the hypolipidemic, effect of thiazolidinediones. *J. Clin. Invest.* 106:1221–28

85. Zierath JR, Ryder JW, Doebber T, et al. 1998. Role of skeletal muscle in thiazolidinedione insulin sensitizer action. *Endocrinology* 139:5034–41

86. Berger J, Biswas C, Hayes N, et al. 1996. An antidiabetic thiazolidinedione potentiates insulin stimulation of glycogen synthase in rat adipose tissue. *Endocrinology* 137:1984–90

87. Way JM, Harrington WW, Brown KK, et al. 2001. Comprehensive messenger ribonucleic acid profiling reveals that peroxisome proliferator-activated receptor γ activation has coordinate effects on gene expression in multiple insulin-sensitive tissues. *Endocrinology* 142:1269–77

88. Oakes ND, Thalen PG, Jacinto SM, Ljung B. 2001. Thiazolidinediones increase plasma-adipose tissue FFA exchange capacity and enhance insulin-mediated control of systemic FFA availability. *Diabetes* 50:1158–65

89. Steppan CM, Bailey ST, Bhat S, et al. 2001. The hormone resistin links obesity to diabetes. *Nature* 409:307–12

90. Chinetti G, Griglio S, Antonucci M, et al. 1998. Activation of proliferator-activated receptors alpha and gamma induces apoptosis of human monocyte-derived macrophages. *J. Biol. Chem.* 273:25573–80

91. Ricote M, Li AC, Willson TM, et al. 1998. The peroxisome proliferator-activated receptor-gamma is a negative regulator of macrophage activation. *Nature* 391:79–82

92. Jiang C, Ting AT, Seed B. 1998. PPAR-gamma agonists inhibit production of monocyte inflammatory cytokines. *Nature* 391:82–86

93. Thieringer R, Fenyk-Melody JE, Le Grand CB, et al. 2000. Activation of peroxisome proliferator-activated receptor γ does not inhibit IL-6 or TNF-α responses of macrophages to LPS in vitro or in vivo. *J. Immunol.* 164:1046–54

94. Chawla A, Barak Y, Nagy L, et al. 2001. PPAR-γ dependent and independent effects on macrophage-gene expression in lipid metabolism and inflammation. *Nat. Med.* 7:48–52

95. Su CG, Wen X, Bailey ST, et al. 1999. A novel therapy for colitis utilizing PPARγ ligands to inhibit the epithelial inflammatory response. *J. Clin. Invest.* 104:383–89

96. Altiok S, Xu M, Spiegelman BM. 1997. PPARγ induces cell cycle withdrawal: inhibition of E2F/DP DNA-binding activity via down-regulation of PP2A. *Genes Dev.* 11:1987–98

97. Tontonoz P, Singer S, Forman BM, et al. 1997. Terminal differentiation of human liposarcoma cells induced by ligands for peroxisome proliferator-activated receptor gamma and the retinoid X receptor. *Proc. Natl. Acad. Sci. USA* 94:237–41

98. Demetri GD, Fletcher CD, Mueller E, et al. 1999. Induction of solid tumor differentiation by the peroxisome proliferator-activated receptor-gamma ligand troglitazone in patients with liposarcoma. *Proc. Natl. Acad. Sci. USA* 96:3951–56

99. Mueller E, Sarraf P, Tontonoz P, et al. 1998. Terminal differentiation of human breast cancer through PPARγ. *Mol. Cell* 1:465–70

100. Elstner E, Muller C, Koshizuka K, et al. 1998. Ligands for peroxisome proliferator-activated receptor gamma and retinoic acid receptor inhibit growth and induce apoptosis of human breast cancer cells in vitro and in BNX mice. *Proc. Natl. Acad. Sci. USA* 95:8806–11

101. DuBois RN, Gupta R, Brockman J, et al. 1998. The nuclear eicosanoid receptor, PPARγ, is aberrantly expressed in colonic cancers. *Carcinogenesis* 19:49–53

102. Sarraf P, Mueller E, Jones D, et al. 1998. Differentiation and reversal of malignant changes in colon cancer through PPARγ. *Nat. Med.* 4:1046–52

103. Saez E, Tontonoz P, Nelson MC, et al. 1998. Activators of the nuclear receptor PPARγ enhance colon polyp formation. *Nat. Med.* 4:1058–61

104. Lefebvre AM, Chen I, Desreumaux P, et al. 1998. Activation of the peroxisome proliferator-activated receptor gamma promotes the development of colon tumors in C57BL/6J-APCMin/$^+$ mice. *Nat. Med.* 4:1053–57

105. Simonson DC. 1988. Etiology and prevalence of hypertension in diabetic patients. *Diabetes Care* 11:821–27

106. Ogihara T, Rakugi H, Ikegami H, et al. 1995. Enhancement of insulin sensitivity by troglitazone lowers blood pressure in diabetic hypertensives. *Am. J. Hypertens.* 8:316–20

107. Nolan JJ, Ludvik B, Beerdsen P, et al. 1994. Improvement in glucose tolerance and insulin resistance in obese subjects treated with troglitazone. *N. Engl. J. Med.* 331:1188–93

108. Deeb SS, Fajas L, Nemoto M, et al. 1998. A Pro12Ala substitution in PPARγ2 associated with decreased receptor activity, lower body mass index and improved insulin sensitivity. *Nat. Genet.* 20:284–7

109. Yen C-J, Beamer BA, Negri C, et al. 1997. Molecular scanning of the human peroxisome proliferator activated receptor γ gene in diabetic Caucasians: identification of a Pro12Ala PPARγ2 missense mutation. *Biochem. Biophys. Res. Commun.* 241:270–4

110. Ristow M, Muller-Wieland D, Pfeiffer A, et al. 1998. Obesity associated with a mutation in a genetic regulator of adipocyte differentiation. *N. Engl. J. Med.* 339:953–9

111. Meirhaeghe A, Fajas L, Helbecque N, et al. 1998. A genetic polymorphism of the peroxisome proliferator-activated receptor γ gene influences plasma leptin levels in obese humans. *Hum. Mol. Genet.* 7:435–40

112. Beamer BA, Yen C-J, Anderson RE, et al. 1998. Association of the Pro12Ala variant in the peroxisome proliferator-activated

receptor $\gamma 2$ gene with obesity in two Caucasian populations. *Diabetes* 47: 1806–8

113. Altshuler D, Hirschhorn JN, Klannemark M, et al. 2000. The common PPARγ Pro12Ala polymorphism is associated with decreased risk of Type 2 diabetes. *Nat. Genet.* 26:76–80

114. Mori Y, Kim-Motoyama H, Katakura T, et al. 1998. Effect of the Pro12Ala variant of the human peroxisome proliferator-activated receptor $\gamma 2$ gene on adiposity, fat distribution, and insulin sensitivity in Japanese men. *Biochem. Biophys. Res. Commun.* 251:195–98

115. Ringel J, Engeli S, Distler A, Sharma AM. 1999. Pro12Ala missense mutation of the peroxisome proliferator activated receptor gamma and diabetes mellitus. *Biochem. Biophys. Res. Commun.* 254:450–53

116. Hu E, Kim JB, Sarraf P, Spiegelman BM. 1996. Inhibition of adipogenesis through MAP kinase-mediated phosphorylation of PPARγ. *Science* 274:2100–3

117. Barroso I, Gurnell M, Crowley VEF, et al. 1999. Dominant negative mutations in human PPARγ associated with severe insulin resistance, diabetes mellitus, and hypertension. *Nature* 402:880–83

118. Issemann I, Green S. 1990. Activation of a member of the steroid hormone receptor superfamily by peroxisome proliferators. *Nature* 347:645–49

119. Gottlicher M, Widmark E, Li Q, Gustafsson JA. 1992. Fatty acids activate the clofibric acid activated receptor and the glucocorticoid receptor. *Proc. Natl. Acad. Sci. USA* 89:4653–57

120. Guan Y, Zhang Y, Davis L, Breyer MD. 1997. Expression of peroxisome proliferator-activated receptors in urinary tract of rabbits and humans. *Am. J. Physiol. Renal Physiol.* 273:F1013–F22

121. Sher T, Yi H-F, McBride OW, Gonzalez FJ. 1993. cDNA cloning, chromosomal mapping, and functional characterization of the human peroxisome proliferator ac-

tivated receptor. *Biochemistry* 32:5598–604

122. Braissant O, Foufelle F, Scotto C, et al. 1996. Differential expression of peroxisome proliferator-activated receptor (PPARs): tissue distribution of PPAR-alpha, -beta, and -gamma in the adult rat. *Endocrinology* 137:354–66

123. Auboeuf D, Rieusset J, Fajas L, et al. 1997. Tissue distribution and quantification of the expression of mRNAs of peroxisome proliferator-activated receptors and liver X receptorα in humans. *Diabetes* 46:1319–27

124. Inoue I, Shino K, Noji S, et al. 1998. Expression of peroxisome proliferator-activated receptor alpha (PPARα) in primary cultures of human vascular endothelial cells. *Biochem. Biophys. Res. Commun.* 246:370–74

125. Staels B, Koenig W, Habib A, et al. 1998. Activation of human aortic smooth-muscle cells is inhibited by PPARα but not by PPARγ activators. *Nature* 393:790–93

126. Cattley RC, DeLuca J, Elcombe C, et al. 1998. Do peroxisome proliferating compounds pose a hepatocarcinogenic hazard to humans? *Regul. Toxicol. Pharmacol.* 27:47–60

127. Palmer CN, Hsu MH, Griffin KJ, et al. 1998. Peroxisome proliferator activated receptor-alpha expression in human liver. *Mol. Pharmacol.* 53:14–22

128. Lambe KG, Woodyatt NJ, Macdonald N, et al. 1999. Species differences in sequence and activity of the peroxisome proliferator response element (PPRE) within the acyl CoA oxidase gene promoter. *Toxicol. Lett.* 110:119–27

129. Motojima K, Passilly P, Peters JM, et al. 1998. Expression of putative fatty acid transporter genes are regulated by peroxisome proliferator-activated receptor alpha and gamma activators in a tissue- and inducer-specific manner. *J. Biol. Chem.* 273:16710–14

130. Tugwood JD, Isseman I, Anderson RG,

et al. 1992. The mouse peroxisome-proliferator-activated receptor recognizes a response element in the 5′ flanking sequence of the rat acyl CoA oxidase gene. *EMBO J.* 11:433–39

131. Marcus SL, Miyata KS, Zhang B, et al. 1993. Diverse peroxisome proliferator-activated receptors bind to the peroxisome proliferator-responsive elements of the rat hydratase/dehydrogenase and fatty acyl-CoA oxidase genes but differentially induce expression. *Proc. Natl. Acad. Sci. USA* 90:5723–27

132. Zhang B, Marcus SL, Miyata KS, et al. 1993. Characterization of protein-DNA interactions within the peroxisome proliferator-responsive element of the rat hydratase-dehydrogenase gene. *J. Biol. Chem.* 268:12939–45

133. Brady PS, Marine KA, Brady LJ, Ramsay RR. 1989. Co-ordinate induction of hepatic mitochondrial and peroxisomal carnitine acyltransferase synthesis by diet and drugs. *Biochem. J.* 260:93–100

134. Yu GS, Lu YC, Gulick T. 1998. Coregulation of tissue-specific alternative human carnitine palmitoyltransferase Ibeta gene promoters by fatty acid enzyme substrate. *J. Biol. Chem.* 273:32901–9

135. Mascaro C, Acosta E, Ortiz JA, et al. 1998. Control of human muscle-type carnitine palmitoyltransferase I gene transcription by peroxisome proliferator-activated receptor. *J. Biol. Chem.* 273:8560–63

136. Brandt JM, Djouadi F, Kelly DP. 1998. Fatty acids activate transcription of the muscle carnitine palmitoyltransferase I gene in cardiac myocytes via the peroxisome proliferator-activated receptor alpha. *J. Biol. Chem.* 273:23786–92

137. Aoyama T, Peters JM, Iritani N, et al. 1998. Altered constitutive expression of fatty acid-metabolizing enzymes in mice lacking the peroxisome proliferator-activated receptor alpha (PPARα). *J. Biol. Chem.* 273:5678–84

138. Gulick T, Cresci S, Caira T, et al. 1994. The peroxisome proliferator-activated receptor regulates mitochondrial fatty acid oxidative enzyme gene expression. *Proc. Natl. Acad. Sci. USA* 91:11012–16

139. Rodriguez JC, Gil-Gomez G, Hegardt FG, Haro D. 1994. Peroxisome proliferator-activated receptor mediates induction of the mitochondrial 3-hydroxy-3-methylglutaryl-CoA synthase gene by fatty acids. *J. Biol. Chem.* 269:18767–72

140. Aldridge TC, Tugwood JD, Green S. 1995. Identification and characterization of DNA elements implicated in the regulation of CYP4A1 transcription. *Biochem. J.* 306:473–79

141. Kroetz DL, Yook P, Costet P, et al. 1998. Peroxisome proliferator-activated receptor alpha controls the hepatic CYP4A induction adaptive response to starvation and diabetes. *J. Biol. Chem.* 273:31581–89

142. Lee SS-T, Pineau T, Drago J, et al. 1995. Targeted disruption of the α isoform of the peroxisome proliferator-activated receptor gene in mice results in abolishment of the pleiotropic effects of peroxisome proliferators. *Mol. Cell. Biol.* 15:3012–22

143. Plutzky J. 2000. Emerging concepts in metabolic abnormalities associated with coronary artery disease. *Curr. Opin. Cardiol.* 15:416–21

144. Rubins HB, Robins SJ, Collins D, et al. 1995. Distribution of lipids in 8,500 men with coronary artery disease. *Am. J. Cardiol.* 75:1196–201

145. Linton MF, Fazio S. 2000. Re-emergence of fibrates in the management of dyslipidemia and cardiovascular risk. *Curr. Atheroscler. Rep.* 2:29–35

146. Rubins HB, Robins SJ. 2000. Conclusions from the VA-HIT study. *Am. J. Cardiol.* 86:543–44

147. Staels B, Vu-Dac N, Kosykh V, et al. 1995. Fibrates down-regulate apolipoprotein C-III expression independent of induction of peroxisomal Acyl Co-enzyme A oxidase. *J. Clin. Invest.* 95:705–12

148. Peters JM, Hennuyer N, Staels B,

et al. 1997. Alterations in lipoprotein metabolism in peroxisome proliferator-activated receptor α-deficient mice. *J. Biol. Chem.* 272:27307–12

149. Schoonjans K, Staels B, Auwerx J. 1996. Role of the peroxisome proliferator-activated receptor (PPAR) in mediating the effects of fibrates and fatty acids on gene expression. *J. Lipid Res.* 37:907–25

150. Marx N, Sukhova GK, Collins T. 1999. PPARα activators inhibit cytokine-induced vascular cell adhesion molecule-1 expression in human endothelial cells. *Circulation* 99:3125–31

151. Marx N, Schonbeck U, Lazar MA, et al. 1998. Peroxisome proliferator-activated receptor gamma activators inhibit gene expression and migration in human vascular smooth muscle cells. *Circ. Res.* 83: 1097–103

152. Kintscher U, Goetze S, Wakino S, et al. 2000. Peroxisome proliferator-activated receptor and retinoid X receptor ligands inhibit monocyte chemotactic protein-1-directed migration of monocytes. *Eur. J. Pharmacol.* 410:259–70

153. Pasceri V, Wu HD, Willerson JT, Yeh ETH. 2000. Modulation of vascular inflammation in vitro and in vivo by peroxisome proliferator-activated receptor-γ activators. *Circulation* 101:235–38

154. Chinetti G, Lestavel S, Bocher V, et al. 2001. PPARγ and PPARγ activators induce cholesterol removal from human macrophage foam cells through stimulation of the ABCA1 pathway. *Nat. Med.* 7:53–58

155. Chawla A, Boisvert WA, Lee CH, et al. 2001. A PPARγ-LXR-ABCA1 pathway in macrophages is involved in cholesterol efflux and atherogenesis. *Mol. Cell* 7:161–71

156. Collins AR, Meeham WP, Kintscher U, et al. 2001. Troglitazone inhibits formation of early atherosclerotic lesions in diabetic and non-diabetic low density lipoprotein receptor-deficient mice. *Arterioscler. Thromb. Biol.* 21:365–71

157. Li AC, Brown KK, Silvestre MJ, et al. 2000. Peroxisome proliferator- activated receptor γ ligands inhibit development of atherosclerosis in LDL receptor-deficient mice. *J. Clin. Invest.* 106:523–31

158. Chen Z, Ishibashi S, Perrey S, et al. 2001. Troglitazone inhibits atherosclerosis in apoliporotein E-knockout mice. *Arterioscler. Thromb. Vasc. Biol.* 21:372–77

159. Shiomi M, Ito T, Tsukada T, et al. 1999. Combination treatment with troglitazone, an insulin action enhancer, and pravastatin, an inhibitor of HMG-CoA reductase, shows a synergistic effect on atherosclerosis of WHHL rabbits. *Atherosclerosis* 142:345–53

160. Devchand PR, Keller H, Peters JM, et al. 1996. The PPARα-leukotriene B4 pathway to inflammation control. *Nature* 384:39–43

161. Delerive P, Gervois P, Fruchart JC, Staels B. 2000. Induction of IκBα expression as a mechanism contributing to the anti-inflammatory activities of peroxisome proliferator-activated receptor-alpha activators. *J. Biol. Chem.* 275:36703–7

162. Hill MR, Clarke S, Rodgers K, et al. 1999. Effect of peroxisome proliferator-activated receptor alpha activators on tumor necrosis factor expression in mice during endotoxemia. *Infect. Immun.* 67: 3488–93

163. Tugwood JD, Aldridge TC, Lambe KG, et al. 1997. Peroxisome proliferator activated receptors: structures and function. *Ann. NY Acad. Sci.* 804:252–64

164. Flavell DM, Torra IP, Jamshidi Y, et al. 2000. Variation in the PPARa gene is associated with altered function in vitro and plasma lipid concentrations in Type II diabetic subjects. *Diabetologia* 43:673–80

165. Schmidt A, Endo N, Rutledge SJ, et al. 1992. Identification of a new member of the steroid hormone receptor superfamily that is activated by a peroxisome proliferator and fatty acid. *Mol. Endocrinol.* 6:1634–41

166. Kliewer SA, Forman BM, Blumberg

B, et al. 1994. Differential expression and activation of a family of murine peroxisome proliferator-activated receptors. *Proc. Natl. Acad. Sci. USA* 91:7355–59

167. Mukherjee R, Jow L, Noonan D, McDonnell DP. 1994. Human and rat peroxisome proliferator activated receptors (PPARs) demonstrate similar tissue distribution but different responsiveness to PPAR activators. *J. Steroid Biochem. Mol. Biol.* 51:157–66

168. Yoshikawa T, Brkanac Z, Dupont BR, et al. 1996. Assignment of the human nuclear hormone receptor, NUC1 (PPARδ), to chromosome 6p21.1-p21.2. *Genomics* 35:637–38

169. Jones PS, Savory R, Barratt P, et al. 1995. Chromosomal localisation, inducibility, tissue-specific expression and strain differences in three murine peroxisome-proliferator-activated-receptor genes. *Eur. J. Biochem.* 233:219–26

170. Amri EZ, Bonino F, Ailhaud G, et al. 1995. Cloning of a protein that mediates transcriptional effects of fatty acids in preadipocytes. Homology to peroxisome proliferator-activated receptors. *J. Biol. Chem.* 270:2367–71

171. Lim H, Paria BC, Das SK, et al. 1997. Multiple female reproductive failure in cyclooxygenase 2-deficient mice. *Cell* 91:197–208

172. Lim H, Gupta RA, Ma WG, et al. 1999. Cyclo-oxygenase-2-derived prostacyclin mediates embryo implantation in the mouse via PPARδ. *Genes Dev.* 13:1561–74

173. He TC, Chan TA, Vogelstein B, Kinzler KW. 1999. PPARδ is an APC-regulated target of nonsteroidal anti-inflammatory drugs. *Cell* 99:335–45

174. Park BH, Vogelstein B, Kinzler KW. 2001. Genetic disruption of PPARδ decreases the tumorigenicity of human colon cancer cells. *Proc. Natl. Acad. Sci. USA* 98:2598–603

175. Kremarik-Bouillaud P, Schohn H, Dauca M. 2000. Regional distribution of PPARβ in the cerebellum of the rat. *J. Chem. Neuroanat.* 19:225–32

176. Xing G, Zhang L, Heynen T, et al. 1995. Rat PPARδ contains a CGG triplet repeat and is prominently expressed in the thalamic nuclei. *Biochem. Biophys. Res. Commun.* 217:1015–25

177. Braissant O, Wahli W 1998. Differential expression of peroxisome proliferator-activated receptor-alpha, -beta, and -gamma during rat embryonic development. *Endocrinology* 139:2748–54

178. Matsumoto N, Minamimoto T, Graybiel AM, Kimura M. 2001. Neurons in the thalamic cm-pf complex supply striatal neurons with information about behaviorally significant sensory events. *J Neurophysiol.* 85:960–76

179. Quigg M, Clayburn H, Straume M, et al. 1999. Hypothalamic neuronal loss and altered circadian rhythm of temperature in a rat model of mesial temporal lobe epilepsy. *Epilepsia* 40:1688–96

180. Granneman J, Skoff R, Yang X. 1998. Member of the peroxisome proliferator-activated receptor family of transcription factors is differentially expressed by oligodendrocytes. *J. Neurosci. Res.* 51:563–73

181. Saluja I, Granneman JG, Skoff RS. 2001. PPARδ agonists stimulate oligodendrocyte differentiation in tissue culture. *Glia* 33:194–204

182. Peters JM, Lee SS, Li W, et al. 2000. Growth, adipose, brain, and skin alterations resulting from targeted disruption of the mouse peroxisome proliferator-activated receptor $\beta(\delta)$. *Mol. Cell Biol.* 20:5119–28

183. Basu-Modak S, Braissant O, Escher P, et al. 1999. Peroxisome proliferator-activated receptor beta regulates acyl-CoA synthetase 2 in reaggregated rat brain cell cultures. *J. Biol. Chem.* 274:35881–88

Annu. Rev. Med. 2002. 53:437–52

CANCER GENE THERAPY: Scientific Basis

Punit D. Wadhwa, Steven P. Zielske, Justin C. Roth, Christopher B. Ballas, Janice E. Bowman, and Stanton L. Gerson

Division of Hematology/Oncology and Comprehensive Cancer Center, University Hospitals of Cleveland and Case-Western Reserve University, Cleveland, Ohio 44106-4937; e-mail: punitwadhwa@yahoo.com; spz@po.cwru.edu; jcr9@po.cwru.edu; cbb3@po.cwru.edu; bowman_janice@yahoo.com; slg5@po.cwru.edu

Key Words   tumor suppressor genes, suicide genes, dendritic cells, angiogenesis, chemotherapy-resistance genes

■ **Abstract**   Gene therapy of cancer has been one of the most exciting and elusive areas of therapeutic research in the past decade. Critical developments have occurred in gene therapy targeting cancer cells, cancer vasculature, the immune system, and the bone marrow, itself often the target for severe toxicity from therapeutic agents. We review some recent developments in the field. In each instance, clear preclinical models validated the therapeutic approach and efforts have been made to evaluate the target impact in both preclinical and early clinical trials. Although no cures can consistently be expected from today's cancer gene therapy, the rapid progress may imply that such cures are a few short years away.

TUMOR SUPPRESSOR GENE THERAPY

Tumor suppressor genes are involved in cellular checkpoint control, preventing the passage of cells with damaged DNA or other cellular damage through the cell cycle. The p53 tumor suppressor gene plays a critical regulatory role in determining the fate of a cell after apoptotic signaling and DNA damage, through its transcriptional activation of p21, a potent inhibitor of cyclin D1–mediated G1/S transition (1). Among the tumor suppressor genes, p53 is unique in its ability to induce cellular apoptosis if DNA damage is extensive, mediated through transcriptional activation of such proapoptotic genes as bax (2) and fas (3), and transcriptional repression of bcl-2. Viral-mediated wild-type p53 gene therapy is currently being tested in clinical trials for patients with non–small cell lung cancer and head and neck cancers, as outlined in Table 1. The rationale for these trials stems from extensive preclinical data demonstrating the efficacy of p53 gene transfer in tumor suppression or inhibition of proliferation in a variety of tumors mutant in p53, both in cell-line models in vitro and in xenograft models in vivo. No current gene therapy approach is able to transduce an entire tumor mass. This limitation

TABLE 1   p53 gene therapy trials

Tumor	p53 Status	Number of patients	Study phase	Grade III–IV toxicity related to vector	Transgene transfer	Clinical response	Vector	Reference
NSC lung	Mutant	9	1	None	8/9 patients	3 PR, 3 SD	Retrovirus	72
NSC lung	Mutant	28	1	Grade III nausea (1/28)	18/21	2/25 PR 16/25 SD	Adenovirus	73
SCCHN	Mixed	17	1	None	Not evaluated	2/17 PR 6/17 SD	Adenovirus	74

PR, partial response; NSC, non–small cell lung cancer; SCCHN, squamous cell cancer of head and neck; SD, stable disease.

may be surmounted by the ability of p53 to inhibit tumor angiogenesis, thereby mediating the killing of adjacent untransduced cells in a "bystander" fashion.

Although most preclinical models have focused on tumors with a null or mutant p53 genotype, p53 gene therapy has also proven efficacious in tumors with a wild-type p53 status, especially when used in conjunction with chemotherapy or radiotherapy. Spitz et al. (4) studied the synergistic interaction between adenoviral-mediated p53 (Ad p53) gene transfer and radiation in a murine subcutaneous xenograft model of SW260 colorectal cancer. A significant suppression of tumor growth was seen in mice treated with both modalities. The delay in regrowth to a tumor size of 1000 mm^3 was 2 days for mice treated with 5 Gy alone, 15 days for mice treated with Ad p53 alone, and 37 days for mice treated with the combination, suggesting the enhancement of radiation sensitivity mediated by p53 gene transfer. A similar synergistic interaction was observed by Roth et al. (5) in an H1299 (p53 null) non–small cell lung cancer xenograft model, validating the rationale for combining the two modalities in a clinical setting. Nielsen et al. (6) demonstrated a synergy between Ad p53 and the chemotherapeutic agent paclitaxel in murine xenograft tumor models of human head and neck, ovarian, prostate, and breast cancers (characterized by a p53 null or mutant status); they reported a 60%–90% reduction in tumor burden in animals treated with both modalities as opposed to those treated with Ad p53 or paclitaxel alone.

Nishizaki et al. (7) investigated the antiangiogenic effect of Ad p53–mediated gene transfer on the mutant p53-expressing H226Br non–small cell lung cancer cell line. They observed a 75% reduction in expression of the angiogenic peptide VEGF at both the protein and the mRNA level in the cell lines transduced with Ad p53 as opposed to a control vector. Ad p53 also was found to significantly up-regulate the expression of the antiangiogenic peptide brain-specific angiogenesis inhibitor BA-I1. In an in vivo model, Ad p53–transduced H226Br cells were packed into membrane chambers, which were subsequently implanted into a dorsal air sac produced in *nu/nu* mice; significant inhibition of angiogenesis and neovascularization was observed relative to mock-transduced controls. Additionally, in vivo mixing studies with combinations of parental and Ad p53–transduced H226Br cells demonstrated a significant reduction in tumor volumes in mice injected with the mixture as opposed to mice treated with parental cells alone, confirming the presence of an in vivo bystander effect, probably mediated by the inhibition of angiogenesis as described above.

An alternative approach to targeting p53 mutant tumor cells is to introduce a virus that selectively replicates in cells with mutant p53. The adenoviral protein E1B-55K is known to bind to the tumor suppressor protein p53 and suppress p53-mediated cell cycle arrest or apoptosis. Bischoff et al. (7a) used an adenovirus with an E1B55K deletion (dl1520) to target malignancies characterized by a mutant p53 status. They surmised that this virus (ONYX-015) would replicate only in tumor cells with a mutant or null p53 status. The ONYX-015 virus has demonstrated efficacy in inducing regressions of human cervical carcinoma ($p53^{-/-}$) xenografts in nude mice, while exerting no effect on glioblastoma multiforme xenografts characterized by a wild-type p53 status. This virus is currently being tested in phase II clinical trials for patients with recurrent head and neck cancer, and it appears promising when used in conjunction with the chemotherapeutic agents cisplatin and 5-fluorouracil (7b). However, the selectivity of this approach for cancer cells mutant in p53 has been questioned by other investigators. Rothmann et al. (7c) have demonstrated replication of ONXY-015 in various tumor cell lines with wild-type p53, suggesting that replication is independent of p53 status. In addition, replication in primary human cells occurred in a multiplicity of infection (MOI)-dependent manner. The molecular basis for this discrepancy remains to be fully elucidated.

A potential consequence of repeated administration of adenoviral vectors for gene transfer is the development of neutralizing antibodies. This can be important in the anticancer response, generating an immune-mediated bystander effect, but it can reduce the efficacy of the primary viral-based therapeutic effect. In the above studies utilizing adenoviral delivery, immune responses are seen in the tumors with infiltration of both B and T cells, suggesting that the immune response may be an important component of the host response and anticancer effect of these therapies. Nonetheless, strategies to abrogate the immune response through prior oral tolerization (7d), shielding of key antigenic epitopes by coating of the virus with cationic lipid and polyethylene glycol (7e), and blockade of the costimulatory molecule CD40 ligand (7f) are being investigated.

Although most of the current clinical trials have focused on safety and toxicity issues and the efficacy of transgene transfer, some are noteworthy for clinical responses and disease stabilization in a subset of treated patients, as outlined in Table 1.

SUICIDE GENE THERAPY

Suicide genes, so called because they induce cell death, encode an enzyme product capable of converting a prodrug into a cytotoxic compound. Suicide gene therapy involves delivering the suicide gene (not normally present) to the target cells and then administering the prodrug. Delivery of the suicide gene is generally accomplished by injecting a viral vector containing the suicide gene directly into the tumor mass, thereby infecting tumor cells, though variations exist.

An inherent limitation of all viral-based cancer gene therapy protocols is the inability to transduce the entire tumor cell population. This may be overcome by the ability of suicide gene–transduced cells to mediate cytotoxicity of adjacent untransduced cells, the so-called bystander effect. Possible mechanisms for the bystander effect include direct cell-cell drug transfer via gap junctions, immune-mediated responses such as the production of TNF-α (which can induce hemorrhagic tumor necrosis) by vector-infected and/or dead tumor cells, and tumor cell phagocytosis of apoptotic vesicles containing the cytotoxic metabolite. Mesnil et al. (8) reviewed the critical role of gap junctions in the bystander effect, especially in the context of using herpes simplex virus thymidine kinase (HSV-TK) as the suicide gene and ganciclovir as the prodrug. The HSV-TK gene is possibly the best-characterized suicide gene (9), primarily because it mediates phosphorylation of the prodrug ganciclovir 1000 times more efficiently than its mammalian counterpart. The phosphorylated forms of ganciclovir bring about DNA chain termination and cause single-strand breaks, leading to cell death. Mesnil et al. noted a direct correlation between connexin expression and the potency of the bystander effect, as measured by the number of cells required to produce an equivalent amount of bystander cell killing, both in vitro and in vivo. Increasing expression of connexins either by transduction of a connexin gene or by treatment with compounds known to increase gap junctions and/or their function (such as retinoids or cAMP) may also increase the bystander effect. Still other bystander effect mechanisms may play a significant role in the antitumor effect of HSV-TK/ganciclovir and other suicide gene therapies.

Another extensively studied suicide gene is the *E. coli* cytosine deaminase gene. When expressed in mammalian cells, cytosine deaminase can convert the nontoxic compound 5 fluoro-cytosine (5FC) to the cytotoxic 5 fluoro-uracil (5FU). Both the HSV-TK and cytosine deaminase genes have been delivered to tumor cell lines in vitro and to tumor cells in vivo, either singly (10) or in combination (11), and have been shown to confer prodrug (ganciclovir and 5FC respectively) sensitivity in a dose-dependent manner. In many cases, the immune response following suicide gene–mediated tumor cell killing is a significant part of the antitumor effect, and immunologic protection against subsequent challenge by repeated tumor cell injections may ensue.

Unfortunately, the in vivo use of suicide genes for cancer therapy is not entirely advantageous in its current form. Delivery of suicide genes is imprecise at best, and normal cells may be infected or may succumb to the bystander effect, resulting in their death and possibly leading to negative consequences for normal tissue (10). However, it is likely that such detrimental effects are highly dependent on the model system being studied. Block et al. (12) found that the cytosine deaminase gene, delivered via adenovirus, primarily in tumor cells as opposed to normal tissues after systemic injection of the vector, resulted in specific killing of tumor cells and minimal effect on surrounding normal tissue. Improved targeting of tumor

TABLE 2   Suicide gene therapy trials

Tumor	Number of patients	Phase of study	Grade III–IV toxicity	Transgene transfer	Clinical response	Vector	Reference
Prostate	18	1	Grade III hepatotoxicity (1 patient)	Not evaluated	3 PR	Adenovirus	75
Mesothelioma	21	1	Grade III hepatotoxicity (2 patients)	11/20 evaluable	3 SD	Adenovirus	76
Glioblastoma	48	1–2 (adjuvant)	Seizure (1 patient) Hydrocephalus (1 patient)	Not evaluated	7/48 tumor-free at 6 months	Retrovirus	77

PR, partial response; SD, stable disease.

cells will go a long way toward making suicide gene therapy effective, especially when coupled with other approaches such as improving the activity of prodrug-converting enzymes and induction of apoptosis.

For example, Black et al. (13) used random sequence mutagenesis to create HSV-TK mutants that significantly increased the sensitivity of transduced cells to acyclovir and ganciclovir. One of these mutants, the HSV-TK 30 (14), has been tested in various human cancer cell lines; it renders these cells 9–500 times more sensitive to ganciclovir than the wild-type HSV-TK. Many such promising approaches to improving suicide gene therapy of cancer await investigation. The most promising will combine better targeting of cancer cells with maximization of cell killing, while minimizing damage to surrounding normal tissue.

Although suicide gene therapy is still in its infancy, clinical trials are already under way, most using the HSV-TK and ganciclovir system, as outlined in Table 2.

ANTIANGIOGENIC GENE THERAPY

Tumor growth and survival depend on angiogenesis to provide a path for delivery of oxygen and nutrients to tumor cells. Without this process of blood vessel recruitment, tumor growth is limited to 1–2 mm^2, the diffusion limit of oxygen. In 1971, Folkman proposed that tumor growth could be arrested by blocking angiogenesis (15). Furthermore, metastasis may also be prevented, since the formation of tumor vasculature seems to be a requisite for it. This promoted a widespread search for proangiogenic factors associated with neovascularization and tumor vessel maturation. It is widely known that the "angiogenic switch" during tumorigenesis appears to be caused by the disruption of a complex balance of two types of angiogenesis mediators, angiogenic growth factors and angiogenesis inhibitors, which fluctuate over the course of tumor development (16, 17). Blood vessel growth can be triggered by either tumor cells or accessory cells within the tumor stroma, which secrete angiogenic factors such as basic fibroblast growth factor (bFGF) and vascular endothelial growth factor (VEGF). These factors, along with platelet-derived growth factor (PDGF), transforming growth factor (TGF-β), and angiopoietins, are also involved in maturation and stabilization of newly formed vessels (18, 19).

In order to inhibit the development of tumor blood vessels, numerous endogenous inhibitors of angiogenesis have been discovered. Because of difficulties in producing large quantities of stable recombinant endogenous antiangiogenic proteins, in vivo gene therapy has become an attractive alternative. Cancer gene therapy strategies include (*a*) direct targeting of a tumor by increasing local concentrations of antiangiogenic agents within the tumor and (*b*) systemic delivery, in which the patient's normal tissues essentially function as a factory producing a particular agent (20, 21). The lack of toxicity of antiangiogenic agents increases the feasibility of the systemic delivery approach, and the effectiveness of the tumor-directed approach may depend on a tumor blood supply to deliver the gene. Most antiangiogenesis gene therapy studies to date have been pursued in murine tumor models.

VEGF, an endothelial cell–specific growth factor, is a key mediator of tumor-induced angiogenesis. VEGF can potentially be inhibited by blocking its translation or transcription. One approach to this end is to introduce a gene encoding an antisense VEGF cDNA, which will bind to the VEGF mRNA, thus inhibiting translation of the VEGF protein. Treatment of human glioma tumors subcutaneously preestablished in athymic nude mice with an adenovirus containing an antisense VEGF_{165} cDNA was shown to significantly suppress tumor growth (22). Moreover, expression of the VEGF receptor flk-1 had an antiangiogenic effect on neuroblastomas in SCID mice (23). After subcutaneous injection of neuroblastoma cells retrovirally transduced with the flk-1 transgene, tumor size was less than 33% of the average size of tumors in control mice.

Two of the most popular endothelial cell growth inhibitors are angiostatin and endostatin, which have been the subject of many of the current preclinical studies for endothelial cell–specific antiangiogenic agents. Sauter et al. (24) demonstrated that systemic administration of an adenovirus containing the murine endostatin gene into athymic nude mice with Lewis lung carcinoma xenograft tumors significantly reduced tumor burden and decreased tumor volume by 78%. In addition, treatment with the endostatin vector prevented formation of pulmonary micrometastases.

Some antiangiogenic agents have been used in combination with other agents and/or treatments. In a glioma tumor model, no significant effect on xenograft tumor growth was observed after intratumoral injection of an adenovirus encoding an angiostatin-like molecule (25). Conversely, when virus delivery was combined with irradiation treatments, tumor growth was very significantly inhibited. Furthermore, the combination improved survival rate more than virus or irradiation treatment alone. Scappaticci et al. (26) demonstrated the effectiveness of simultaneous use of two different antiangiogenic agents in inhibiting tumor growth.

In a murine leukemia model, animals received a combination of leukemia cells retrovirally transduced with the murine endostatin and angiostatin genes. Interestingly, a complete loss of tumorigenicity was observed in 40% of these mice, leading to a survival advantage over those treated with angiostatin or endostatin alone and suggesting a synergistic antitumor effect.

Gene therapy has emerged as a capable strategy for delivery of antiangiogenic agents to tumor cells. The studies described here are just a few of many demonstrating the ability of these agents to inhibit or decrease tumor growth in vivo. As a result of successful preclinical data, many antiangiogenic agents are currently being studied in clinical trials (see 27 for review), several of which use the gene therapy approach. Various tumor types clearly have different molecular mechanisms controlling angiogenesis, so the efficacy of specific antiangiogenic agents will probably vary with each tumor type. Furthermore, the effectiveness of some agents may be optimal at certain stages of tumor development and metastasis. The best protocol for gene therapy has not yet been determined, but since tumor-directed delivery may require chronic drug treatment, the systemic approach may prove more realistic. Improvements in gene vector technology and a clearer understanding of the mechanisms of angiogenesis will facilitate development of current preclinical models into clinical trials using antiangiogenic agents.

GENETIC ENHANCEMENT OF ANTITUMOR IMMUNE RESPONSES

Strategies Using Dendritic and T Cells

The major cell-based immunomodulatory strategy being investigated for effectiveness against tumors utilizes dendritic cells, modified either to present specific tumor antigens to immune effector cells or to be more efficient in activating an antitumor immune response. A second strategy involves genetic modification of T cells to alter their antigen specificity and increase their responsiveness to tumor antigens.

Dendritic cells are antigen-presenting cells that can initiate a potent immune response. After acquisition of tumor proteins, dendritic cells process and can present peptides to $CD4^+$ T cells, leading to their activation. Activated $CD4^+$ T cells express CD40 ligand, which in turn activates $CD8^+$ cytotoxic T cells, generating an antitumor response.

Dendritic cells have been pulsed with specific tumor antigen peptides or tumor extracts in an attempt to load tumor peptides into the major histocompatibility complex for presentation to T cells (28). However, the disadvantages of this method, including transient presentation of specific peptides and the requirement that the appropriate peptides be known, have prompted transduction of the tumor protein into the dendritic cell as a means to express tumor antigens for an extended period and to allow normal antigen processing and presentation of a full range of peptides from that particular tumor protein. These events should result in a more robust and sustained antigen presentation, enabling a more potent antitumor immune response than is possible by transient presentation of a single peptide.

Preclinical data have sustained these concepts, allowing them to be tested in clinical trials. Model melanoma tumor-associated antigens, such as MART-1, TRP-1, TRP-2, and gp100, have been transduced into dendritic cells to induce and enhance antitumor immunity. Transduction of dendritic cells resulted in an enhanced immune response to tumor antigens and a reduction in lung metastases in a murine melanoma model (29). In another study, mice were protected from tumor challenge after injection of dendritic cells expressing tumor-associated antigens (30). Growth of established tumors was also greatly slowed after this treatment. Additional studies showing protection from tumor challenge, slowing of tumor growth, or induction of an antitumor response have been described (31–34).

Another dendritic cell approach to enhancing the antitumor immune response involves transduction of the gene encoding CD40 ligand. CD40 ligand expression causes autoactivation by interacting with CD40 already expressed by the dendritic cell, which enables direct stimulation of antigen-specific $CD8^+$ T cells without the need for a $CD4^+$ T cell interaction. This may magnify the immune response against a tumor. Indeed, in a murine melanoma model, this technique resulted in sustained tumor regression coupled with a survival advantage (35). Intratumoral injection of modified dendritic cells can also enhance a tumor-specific cytotoxic T cell response. Coinjection into a tumor of a CD40-expressing adenoviral vector, resulting in tumor expression of CD40 ligand, with naïve dendritic cells, resulted in generation of a tumor-specific immune response and suppression of tumor growth (36). Transgenic CD40 ligand expression by tumor cells was documented and clearly increased CD40 expression on dendritic cells, increasing their antitumor activity.

T cell gene modification is also a promising approach to immunomodulation of the host cancer defense. T lymphocytes from patients have been isolated and transduced with a new chimeric T cell receptor, which has an antigen specificity toward the targeted tumor (37–39). These cells are expanded ex vivo and then reinfused into the patient. These cells are fully functional with respect to activation through the transgenic T cell receptor. If in vivo stimulation continues, owing to the presence of the tumor peptide, the generation of a robust cell-mediated antitumor response can be expected.

Cytokine-Based Gene Transfer Strategies

Cytokine therapy has been examined as a way to modulate and enhance the immune response to tumors. A partial list of cytokines investigated includes IL-1β, IL-2, IL-4, IL-12, GM-CSF, and IFN-γ. Although the antitumor effects of systemic administration of recombinant cytokines can be substantial, the high doses required

TABLE 3   Cytokine gene therapy trials

Cytokine	Vector	Malignancy	Immune response	Clinical response	Reference
IL-12	Vaccinia	Mesothelioma	T cell infiltrate	0/6	78
GM-CSF	Retrovirus	Melanoma	Infiltrate at vaccine site	1/ 5 CR	79
IFN-γ	Retrovirus	Melanoma	Antibodies to tumor antigens	5/8 SD 3/8 CR/PR	80

CR, complete response; PR, partial response; SD, stable disease.

often result in severe systemic side effects. Therefore, gene therapy has been explored as a method to provide a local concentration of cytokine that would have minimal systemic effects, while enhancing the antitumor immune response. Cytokine gene-containing vectors have been injected intratumorally and tumor or dendritic cells have been transduced ex vivo and readministered to achieve the desired cytokine production. Several preclinical and clinical studies have been completed.

IL-12 has been delivered to tumor cells in a hepatocellular carcinoma mouse model (40). Electroporation into the tumor in vivo inhibited not only the electroporated tumor but also distant tumors. Lung metastases were inhibited and a greater influx of immune effector cells was observed in the IL-12–electroporated tumor. In another study, retroviral delivery of IFN-γ cDNA in a malignant glioma mouse model resulted in increased survival compared with controls (41). Interestingly, retroviral producer cells were implanted directly into the intracranial tumor, thus releasing virus for an extended period at the desired site. Inhibition of established tumors was also observed in a murine model after delivery of a combination of IL-2 and IL-12 genes using a vaccinia virus vector (42). At higher viral doses, however, some signs of cytokine toxicity were observed.

Clinical trials have been performed in patients with malignant mesotheliomas and melanomas, involving intratumoral injections of vectors or irradiated tumor cells transduced with cytokine genes. Such treatment has induced not only immune responses in the form of T cell infiltrates or antibodies to tumor antigens, but also clinical responses in a subset of patients, as summarized in Table 3.

DRUG RESISTANCE GENE THERAPY

Delivery of drug resistance genes to hematopoietic stem cells is aimed at attenuating the myelotoxicity of chemotherapy agents and linking the selective enrichment and protection of gene-transduced cells to dose-escalated inhibition of tumor growth. The pluripotent capacity of hematopoietic stem cells makes them ideal targets for gene transfer. However, their quiescent nature is a limiting factor in gene transfer efficiency, since the retroviral-based vectors currently in use require cell division for integration. More recently, lentiviral-based vectors have been shown to efficiently transduce nondividing cells. Although improved transduction is an encouraging development, a strong selection strategy remains crucial in the setting of stem cell–based cancer gene therapy. Several drug resistance genes have been investigated as agents for combining chemoprotection and stem cell selection, including the multidrug resistance 1 gene (MDR-1) and variants of the dihydrofolate reductase (DHFR) and O^6-methylguanine-DNA methyltransferase (MGMT) genes.

The MDR-1 gene encodes a transmembrane efflux pump, p-glycoprotein, which mediates drug resistance through its ability to expel a wide variety of lipophilic compounds from the cell, such as actinomycin D, the anthracylines, epipodophyllotoxins, taxanes, and the vinca alkaloids (43). Preclinical MDR-1 gene transfer studies in mice have demonstrated the ability to select for long-term repopulating cells in vivo with MDR-1 responsive agents (44–47). Clinical trials using MDR-1 gene transfer have focused on optimizing stem cell enrichment. Early trials resulted in low levels of MDR-1 marked cells (0.01%–1%) with no sign of enrichment after repeated cycles of paclitaxel or doxorubicin. Subsequent trials have demonstrated improved gene transfer efficiency through the use of the fibronectin fragment CH-296, with as many as 15% of cells in the bone marrow and 2% of cells in the peripheral blood being marked one year after continuous oral etoposide treatment (48).

Dihydrofolate reductase is a cytosolic enzyme involved in the formation of thymidylate, purines, and several other cellular constituents. Antifolate chemotherapeutic agents, such as methotrexate (MTX) and trimetrexate (TMTX), bind DHFR, disrupting DNA synthesis and arresting cell growth. DHFR variants that exhibit reduced affinity for folate analogs are currently being used in gene transfer experiments to mediate increased cellular resistance to these agents (49–53). Mice transplanted with hematopoietic cells expressing the L22R and L22Y human DHFR point mutants have been shown to prevent MTX- and TMTX-induced cytopenia, respectively (49, 50). Double mutant DHFR variants were subsequently generated that retain catalytic activity toward dihydrofolate but have a 10,000-fold reduction in antifolate affinity (54). Allay et al. (55) demonstrated the potential of using mutant DHFR for in vivo murine stem cell enrichment. Antifolate treatment was potentiated by cotreatment with the nucleoside transport inhibitor nitrobenzylmercapt-purine riboside 5′ monophosphate (NBMPR-P), and significantly increased vector-expressing cells in all lineages that persisted in secondary transplant recipients.

The O^6 alkylguanine–DNA alkyltransferase protein (AGT), encoded by the MGMT gene, removes cytotoxic alkyl lesions from the O^6 position of guanine residues, conferring protection from the cytotoxic effect of alkylating compounds such as the chloroethylating agent BCNU and the methylating agent temozolomide. Detoxification occurs in a stoichiometric reaction in which each AGT molecule transfers a single alkyl moiety to its active-site cysteine; this irreversible reaction inactivates the protein (56). The synthetic AGT inhibitor O^6-benzylguanine (BG) acts as a pseudosubstrate, inactivating the protein by a similar mechanism (57). Mutant forms of AGT have been identified that are resistant to BG inactivation and thus provide cellular protection from combined treatment with BG and alkylating agents (58–61). The low level of AGT expression in early hematopoietic stem cells and the ability to deplete endogenous AGT with BG gives mutant MGMT transduced stem cells a strong selective advantage in the setting of BG and alkylating agent treatment. Of several BG-resistant mutants identified, the G156A and P140K mutants of MGMT have been the most thoroughly characterized with respect to in vivo stem cell selection (62,63). Bone marrow and peripheral blood reconstitution has approached 100% following treatment in primary recipients, and secondary transplant experiments have demonstrated that selection occurs at the stem cell level. The potential of mutant MGMT–mediated enrichment was further established in G156A transduction experiments, in which nonmyeloablated mice receiving limiting numbers of transduced cells were protected from treatment with BG and BCNU, yielding a 1000-fold enrichment in transgene-positive cells (64). The strong evidence of stem cell selection using mutant MGMT has prompted the proposal of clinical trials using G156A MGMT gene transfer.

The proven potential of multiagent chemotherapy treatments has led to the development of vectors that deliver combinations of drug resistance genes for hematopoietic protection. Most strategies for expressing dual drug resistance include the use of gene fusions or bicistronic vectors. Double mutant DHFR-cytidine deaminase (CD) and MGMT-apurinic endonuclease fusions have been shown to provide dual resistance to antifolates and cytosine nucleotide analogs or combined alkylating agent treatments, respectively (65, 66). Several bicistronic drug resistance vectors have been evaluated, including MDR-1-DHFR, MDR-1-MGMT, and DHFR-CD combinations (67–69). Recently, Takebe et al. created a bicistronic vector containing an aldehyde dehydrogenase-1 and a double mutant DHFR expression cassette that protected human $CD34^+$ and murine hematopoietic progenitor cells from single or combined treatment with cyclophosphamide and MTX (70). Alternative genes may be transcriptionally linked for therapeutic efficacy of specific diseases if a single drug resistance gene can achieve substantial selection. Zhoa et al. (71) recently utilized this strategy in experiments aimed at conferring MTX resistance to hematopoietic progenitors and restoring a normal phenotype to chronic myelogenous leukemia (CML) progenitors. A vector containing the Y22-DHFR mutant and an antisense sequence directed against the b3a2 BCR/ABL breakpoint was shown to confer MTX resistance to normal and CML progenitors, suppress BCR/ABL expression, and restore a normal phenotype to CML cells in vivo. This dual-vector gene approach, using chemotherapy resistance genes to select for transduced hematopoietic progenitors, is not only applicable to cancer but is also being investigated in the setting of inherited somatic disorders such as chronic granulomatous disease.

SUMMARY

A wide variety of approaches use gene transfer to enhance antitumor activity. Some directly target tumor cells, whereas others alter the host defense by enhancing the immune response, protecting the marrow, or altering angiogenesis. In the coming years, one or more of these approaches will reach the critical point of affecting tumor response in humans in a consistent manner, but much needs to be learned in the process.

ACKNOWLEDGMENTS

This work was by Public Health Service Grants RO1CA84578, RO1ES06288, UO1CA75525, and P30CA43703.

Visit the Annual Reviews home page at www.AnnualReviews.org

LITERATURE CITED

1. el-Deiry WS, Tokino T, Velculescu VE, et al. 1993. WAF1, a potential mediator of p53 tumor suppression. *Cell* 75:817–25

2. Miyashita T, Reed JC. 1995. Tumor suppressor p53 is a direct transcriptional activator of the human bax gene. *Cell* 80:293–99

3. Sheard MA, Vojtesek B, Janakova L, et al. 1997. Up-regulation of Fas (CD95) in human p53 wild-type cancer cells treated with ionizing radiation. *Int. J. Cancer* 73:757–62

4. Spitz FR, Nguyen D, Skibber JM, et al. 1996. Adenoviral-mediated wild-type p53 gene expression sensitizes colorectal cancer cells to ionizing radiation. *Clin. Cancer Res.* 2:1665–71

5. Roth JA, Swisher SG, Meyn RE. 1999. p53 tumor suppressor gene therapy for cancer. *Oncol. (Huntingt.)* 13:148–54

6. Nielsen LL, Lipari P, Dell J, et al. 1998. Adenovirus-mediated p53 gene therapy and paclitaxel have synergistic efficacy in models of human head and neck, ovarian, prostate, and breast cancer. *Clin. Cancer Res.* 4:835–46

7. Nishizaki M, Fujiwara T, Tanida T, et al. 1999. Recombinant adenovirus expressing wild-type p53 is antiangiogenic: a proposed mechanism for bystander effect. *Clin. Cancer Res.* 5:1015–23

7a. Bischoff JR, Kirn DH, Williams A, et al. 1996. An adenovirus mutant that replicates selectively in p53-deficient human tumor cells. *Science* 274:373–76

7b. Khuri FR, Nemunaitis J, Ganly I, et al. 2000. A controlled trial of intratumoral ONYX-015, a selectively-replicating adenovirus, in combination with cisplatin and 5-fluorouracil in patients with recurrent head and neck cancer. *Nat. Med.* 6:879–85

7c. Rothmann T, Hengstermann A, Whitaker NJ, et al. 1998. Replication of ONYX-015, a potential anticancer adenovirus, is independent of p53 status in tumor cells. *J. Virol.* 72:9470–78

7d. Ilan Y, Prakash R, Davidson A, et al. 1997. Oral tolerization to adenoviral antigens permits long-term gene expression using recombinant adenoviral vectors. *J. Clin. Invest.* 99:1098–106

7e. Chillon M, Lee JH, Fasbender A, Welsh MJ. 1998. Adenovirus complexed with polyethylene glycol and cationic lipid is shielded from neutralizing antibodies in vitro. *Gene Ther.* 5:995–1002

7f. Stein CS, Pemberton JL, van Rooijen N, Davidson BL. 1998. Effects of macrophage depletion and anti-CD40 ligand on transgene expression and redosing with recombinant adenovirus. *Gene Ther.* 5:431–39

8. Mesnil M, Yamasaki H. 2000. Bystander effect in herpes simplex virus-thymidine kinase/ganciclovir cancer gene therapy: role of gap-junctional intercellular communication. *Cancer Res.* 60:3989–99

9. Springer CJ, Niculescu-Duvaz I. 2000. Prodrug-activating systems in suicide gene therapy. *J. Clin. Invest.* 105:1161–67

10. Ichikawa T, Tamiya T, Adachi Y, et al. 2000. In vivo efficacy and toxicity of 5-fluorocytosine/cytosine deaminase gene therapy for malignant gliomas mediated by adenovirus. *Cancer Gene Ther.* 7:74–82

11. Uckert W, Kammertons T, Haack K, et al. 1998. Double suicide gene (cytosine deaminase and herpes simplex virus thymidine kinase) but not single gene transfer allows reliable elimination of tumor cells in vivo. *Hum. Gene Ther.* 9:855–65

12. Block A, Freund CT, Chen SH, et al. 2000. Gene therapy of metastatic colon carcinoma: regression of multiple hepatic metastases by adenoviral expression of bacterial cytosine deaminase. *Cancer Gene Ther.* 7:438–45

13. Black ME, Newcomb TG, Wilson HM, et al. 1996. Creation of drug-specific herpes simplex virus type 1 thymidine kinase mutants for gene therapy. *Proc. Natl. Acad. Sci. USA* 93:3525–29

14. Qiao J, Black ME, Caruso M. 2000. Enhanced ganciclovir killing and bystander effect of human tumor cells transduced with a retroviral vector carrying a herpes simplex virus thymidine kinase gene mutant. *Hum. Gene Ther.* 11:1569–76

15. Folkman J. 1971. Tumor angiogenesis: therapeutic implications. *N. Engl. J. Med.* 285:1182–86

16. Liotta LA, Steeg PS, Stetler-Stevenson WG. 1991. Cancer metastasis and angiogenesis: an imbalance of positive and negative regulation. *Cell* 64:327–36

17. Holmgren L, O'Reilly MS, Folkman J. 1995. Dormancy of micrometastases: balanced proliferation and apoptosis in the presence of angiogenesis suppression. *Nat. Med.* 1:149–53

18. Hirschi KK, D'Amore PA. 1996. Pericytes in the microvasculature. *Cardiovasc. Res.* 32:687–98

19. Darland DC, D'Amore PA. 1999. Blood vessel maturation: vascular development comes of age. *J. Clin. Invest.* 103:157–58

20. Folkman J. 1998. Antiangiogenic gene therapy. *Proc. Natl. Acad. Sci. USA* 95:9064–66

21. Kong HL, Crystal RG. 1998. Gene therapy strategies for tumor antiangiogenesis. *J. Natl. Cancer Inst.* 90:273–86

22. Im SA, Gomez-Manzano C, Fueyo J, et al. 1999. Antiangiogenesis treatment for gliomas: transfer of antisense-vascular endothelial growth factor inhibits tumor growth in vivo. *Cancer Res.* 59:895–900

23. Davidoff AM, Leary MA, Ng CY, et al. 2001. Gene therapy–mediated expression by tumor cells of the angiogenesis inhibitor flk-1 results in inhibition of neuroblastoma growth in vivo. *J. Pediatr. Surg.* 36:30–36

24. Sauter BV, Martinet O, Zhang WJ, et al. 2000. Adenovirus-mediated gene transfer of endostatin in vivo results in high level of transgene expression and inhibition of tumor growth and metastases. *Proc. Natl. Acad. Sci. USA* 97:4802–7

25. Griscelli F, Li H, Cheong C, et al. 2000. Combined effects of radiotherapy and angiostatin gene therapy in glioma tumor model. *Proc. Natl. Acad. Sci. USA* 97:6698–703

26. Scappaticci FA, Smith R, Pathak A, et al. 2001. Combination angiostatin and endostatin gene transfer induces synergistic antiangiogenic activity in vitro and antitumor efficacy in leukemia and solid tumors in mice. *Mol. Ther.* 3:186–96

27. Carmeliet P, Jain RK. 2000. Angiogenesis in cancer and other diseases. *Nature* 407:249–57

28. Yu JS, Wheeler CJ, Zeltzer PM, et al.

2001. Vaccination of malignant glioma patients with peptide-pulsed dendritic cells elicits systemic cytotoxicity and intracranial T-cell infiltration. *Cancer Res.* 61:842–47

29. Wan Y, Emtage P, Zhu Q, et al. 1999. Enhanced immune response to the melanoma antigen gp100 using recombinant adenovirus-transduced dendritic cells. *Cell Immunol.* 198:131–38

30. Kaplan JM, Yu Q, Piraino ST, et al. 1999. Induction of antitumor immunity with dendritic cells transduced with adenovirus vector-encoding endogenous tumor-associated antigens. *J. Immunol.* 163:699–707

31. Ribas A, Butterfield LH, McBride WH, et al. 1999. Characterization of antitumor immunization to a defined melanoma antigen using genetically engineered murine dendritic cells. *Cancer Gene Ther.* 6:523–36

32. Tuting T, Steitz J, Bruck J, et al. 1999. Dendritic cell-based genetic immunization in mice with a recombinant adenovirus encoding murine TRP2 induces effective anti-melanoma immunity. *J. Gene Med.* 1:400–6

33. De Veerman M, Heirman C, Van Meirvenne S, et al. 1999. Retrovirally transduced bone marrow–derived dendritic cells require CD4$^+$ T cell help to elicit protective and therapeutic antitumor immunity. *J. Immunol.* 162:144–51

34. Li J, Holmes LM, Franek KJ, et al. 2000. Murine tyrosinase expressed by a T7 vector in bone marrow–derived dendritic progenitors effectively prevents and eradicates melanoma tumors in mice. *Cancer Gene Ther.* 7:1448–55

35. Kikuchi T, Miyazawa N, Moore MA, et al. 2000. Tumor regression induced by intratumor administration of adenovirus vector expressing CD40 ligand and naive dendritic cells. *Cancer Res.* 60:6391–95

36. Kikuchi T, Moore MA, Crystal RG. 2000. Dendritic cells modified to express CD40 ligand elicit therapeutic immunity against preexisting murine tumors. *Blood* 96:91–99

37. Jensen MC, Clarke P, Tan G, et al. 2000. Human T lymphocyte genetic modification with naked DNA. *Mol. Ther.* 1:49–55

38. Clay TM, Custer MC, Sachs J, et al. 1999. Efficient transfer of a tumor antigen-reactive TCR to human peripheral blood lymphocytes confers anti-tumor reactivity. *J. Immunol.* 163:507–13

39. Brocker T, Karjalainen K. 1998. Adoptive tumor immunity mediated by lymphocytes bearing modified antigen-specific receptors. *Adv. Immunol.* 68:257–69

40. Yamashita YI, Shimada M, Hasegawa H, et al. 2001. Electroporation-mediated interleukin-12 gene therapy for hepatocellular carcinoma in the mice model. *Cancer Res.* 61:1005–12

41. Saleh M, Jonas NK, Wiegmans A, et al. 2000. The treatment of established intracranial tumors by in situ retroviral IFN-gamma transfer. *Gene Ther.* 7:1715–24

42. Chen B, Timiryasova TM, Haghighat P, et al. 2001. Low-dose vaccinia virus-mediated cytokine gene therapy of glioma. *J. Immunother.* 24:46–57

43. Gottesman MM, Pastan I. 1993. Biochemistry of multidrug resistance mediated by the multidrug transporter. *Annu. Rev. Biochem.* 62:385–427

44. Podda S, Ward M, Himelstein A, et al. 1992. Transfer and expression of the human multiple drug resistance gene into live mice. *Proc. Natl. Acad. Sci. USA* 89:9676–80

45. Sorrentino BP, Brandt SJ, Bodine D, et al. 1992. Selection of drug-resistant bone marrow cells in vivo after retroviral transfer of human MDR1. *Science* 257:99–103

46. Hanania EG, Fu S, Roninson I, et al. 1995. Resistance to taxol chemotherapy produced in mouse marrow cells by safety-modified retroviruses containing a human MDR-1 transcription unit. *Gene Ther.* 2:279–84

47. Richardson C, Bank A. 1995. Preselection of transduced murine hematopoietic stem

cell populations leads to increased long-term stability and expression of the human multiple drug resistance gene. *Blood* 86:2579–89

48. Abonour R, Williams DA, Einhorn L, et al. 2000. Efficient retrovirus-mediated transfer of the multidrug resistance 1 gene into autologous human long-term repopulating hematopoietic stem cells. *Nat. Med.* 6:652–58

49. Williams DA, Hsieh K, DeSilva A, et al. 1987. Protection of bone marrow transplant recipients from lethal doses of methotrexate by the generation of methotrexate-resistant bone marrow. *J. Exp. Med.* 166:210–18

50. Spencer HT, Sleep SE, Rehg JE, et al. 1996. A gene transfer strategy for making bone marrow cells resistant to trimetrexate. *Blood* 87:2579–87

51. May C, Gunther R, McIvor RS. 1995. Protection of mice from lethal doses of methotrexate by transplantation with transgenic marrow expressing drug-resistant dihydrofolate reductase activity. *Blood* 86:2439–48

52. Li MX, Banerjee D, Zhao SC, et al. 1994. Development of a retroviral construct containing a human mutated dihydrofolate reductase cDNA for hematopoietic stem cell transduction. *Blood* 83:3403–8

53. Corey CA, DeSilva AD, Holland CA, et al. 1990. Serial transplantation of methotrexate-resistant bone marrow: protection of murine recipients from drug toxicity by progeny of transduced stem cells. *Blood* 75:337–43

54. Ercikan-Abali EA, Mineishi S, Tong Y, et al. 1996. Active site–directed double mutants of dihydrofolate reductase. *Cancer Res.* 56:4142–45

55. Allay JA, Persons DA, Galipeau J, et al. 1998. In vivo selection of retrovirally transduced hematopoietic stem cells. *Nat. Med.* 4:1136–43

56. Brent TP, Remack JS, Smith DG. 1987. Characterization of a novel reaction by human O6-alkylguanine-DNA alkyltransferase with 1,3-bis(2-chloroethyl)-1-nitrosourea-treated DNA. *Cancer Res.* 47:6185–88

57. Pegg AE, Boosalis M, Samson L, et al. 1993. Mechanism of inactivation of human O6-alkylguanine-DNA alkyltransferase by O6-benzylguanine. *Biochemistry* 32:11998–2006

58. Crone TM, Goodtzova K, Edara S, et al. 1994. Mutations in human O6-alkylguanine-DNA alkyltransferase imparting resistance to O6-benzylguanine. *Cancer Res.* 54:6221–27

59. Davis BM, Encell LP, Zielske SP, et al. 2001. Applied molecular evolution of O6-benzylguanine-resistant DNA alkyltransferases in human hematopoietic cells. *Proc. Natl. Acad. Sci. USA* 98:4950–54

60. Encell LP, Coates MM, Loeb LA. 1998. Engineering human DNA alkyltransferases for gene therapy using random sequence mutagenesis. *Cancer Res.* 58:1013–20

61. Xu-Welliver M, Kanugula S, Pegg AE. 1998. Isolation of human O6-alkylguanine-DNA alkyltransferase mutants highly resistant to inactivation by O6-benzylguanine. *Cancer Res.* 58:1936–45

62. Ragg S, Xu-Welliver M, Bailey J, et al. 2000. Direct reversal of DNA damage by mutant methyltransferase protein protects mice against dose-intensified chemotherapy and leads to in vivo selection of hematopoietic stem cells. *Cancer Res.* 60:5187–95

63. Sawai N, Zhou S, Vanin EF, et al. 2001. Protection and in vivo selection of hematopoietic stem cells using temozolomide, O6-benzylguanine, and an alkyltransferase-expressing retroviral vector. *Mol. Ther.* 3:78–87

64. Davis BM, Koc ON, Gerson SL. 2000. Limiting numbers of G156A O(6)-methylguanine-DNA methyltransferase-transduced marrow progenitors repopulate nonmyeloablated mice after drug selection. *Blood* 95:3078–84

65. Hansen WK, Deutsch WA, Yacoub A, et al. 1998. Creation of a fully functional

human chimeric DNA repair protein. Combining O6-methylguanine DNA methyltransferase (MGMT) and AP endonuclease (APE/redox effector factor 1 (Ref 1)) DNA repair proteins. *J. Biol. Chem.* 273:756–62

66. Sauerbrey A, McPherson JP, Zhao SC, et al. 1999. Expression of a novel double-mutant dihydrofolate reductase-cytidine deaminase fusion gene confers resistance to both methotrexate and cytosine arabinoside. *Hum. Gene Ther.* 10:2495–504

67. Galipeau J, Benaim E, Spencer HT, et al. 1997. A bicistronic retroviral vector for protecting hematopoietic cells against antifolates and P-glycoprotein effluxed drugs. *Hum. Gene Ther.* 8:1773–83

68. Beausejour CM, Le NL, Letourneau S, et al. 1998. Coexpression of cytidine deaminase and mutant dihydrofolate reductase by a bicistronic retroviral vector confers resistance to cytosine arabinoside and methotrexate. *Hum. Gene Ther.* 9:2537–44

69. Suzuki M, Sugimoto Y, Tsuruo T. 1998. Efficient protection of cells from the genotoxicity of nitrosoureas by the retrovirus-mediated transfer of human O6-methylguanine-DNA methyltransferase using bicistronic vectors with human multidrug resistance gene 1. *Mutat. Res.* 401:133–41

70. Takebe N, Zhao SC, Adhikari D, et al. 2001. Generation of dual resistance to 4-hydroperoxycyclophosphamide and methotrexate by retroviral transfer of the human aldehyde dehydrogenase class 1 gene and a mutated dihydrofolate reductase gene. *Mol. Ther.* 3:88–96

71. Zhao RC, McIvor RS, Griffin JD, et al. 1997. Gene therapy for chronic myelogenous leukemia (CML): a retroviral vector that renders hematopoietic progenitors methotrexate-resistant and CML progenitors functionally normal and nontumorigenic in vivo. *Blood* 90:4687–98

72. Roth JA, Nguyen D, Lawrence DD, et al. 1996. Retrovirus-mediated wild-type p53 gene transfer to tumors of patients with lung cancer. *Nat. Med.* 2:985–91

73. Swisher SG, Roth JA, Nemunaitis J, et al. 1999. Adenovirus-mediated p53 gene transfer in advanced non-small-cell lung cancer. *J. Natl. Cancer Inst.* 91:763–71

74. Clayman GL, el-Naggar AK, Lippman SM, et al. 1998. Adenovirus-mediated p53 gene transfer in patients with advanced recurrent head and neck squamous cell carcinoma. *J. Clin. Oncol.* 16:2221–32

75. Herman JR, Adler HL, Aguilar-Cordova E, et al. 1999. In situ gene therapy for adenocarcinoma of the prostate: a phase I clinical trial. *Hum. Gene Ther.* 10:1239–49

76. Sterman DH, Treat J, Litzky LA, et al. 1998. Adenovirus-mediated herpes simplex virus thymidine kinase/ganciclovir gene therapy in patients with localized malignancy: results of a phase I clinical trial in malignant mesothelioma. *Hum. Gene Ther.* 9:1083–92

77. Shand N, Weber F, Mariani L, et al. 1999. A phase 1–2 clinical trial of gene therapy for recurrent glioblastoma multiforme by tumor transduction with the herpes simplex thymidine kinase gene followed by ganciclovir. GLI328 European-Canadian Study Group. *Hum. Gene Ther.* 10:2325–35

78. Mukherjee S, Haenel T, Himbeck R, et al. 2000. Replication-restricted vaccinia as a cytokine gene therapy vector in cancer: persistent transgene expression despite antibody generation. *Cancer Gene Ther.* 7:663–70

79. Chang AE, Li Q, Bishop DK, et al. 2000. Immunogenetic therapy of human melanoma utilizing autologous tumor cells transduced to secrete granulocyte-macrophage colony-stimulating factor. *Hum. Gene Ther.* 11:839–50

80. Fujii S, Huang S, Fong TC, et al. 2000. Induction of melanoma-associated antigen systemic immunity upon intratumoral delivery of interferon-gamma retroviral vector in melanoma patients. *Cancer Gene Ther.* 7:1220–30

Annu. Rev. Med. 2002. 53:453–75

ISCHEMIC STROKE THERAPY

C. Stapf and J. P. Mohr

*The Neurological Institute, Columbia University College of Physicians and Surgeons,
710 West 168th Street, New York, New York 10032; e-mail: jpm10@columbia.edu*

Key Words   cerebral infarction, stroke management, hospitalization

■ **Abstract**   Stroke is the most common life-threatening neurologic disease and the
leading cause of serious long-term disability. The advent of new treatment options for
selected patients suffering ischemic stroke (such as systemic administration of tissue
plasminogen activator or catheter-guided intra-arterial thrombolysis), the structural
reorganization of patient care facilities into stroke units, and interdisciplinary cerebrovascular centers have broadened the scope of possible therapeutic interventions in
the acute and postacute phase after cerebral ischemia. This review summarizes currently available and recommended treatment modalities for acute ischemic stroke from
an interdisciplinary perspective, including medical, neurointerventional, and neurosurgical therapies.

INTRODUCTION

Current Statistics

Stroke is the most common life-threatening neurologic disease and ranks as the
third leading cause of death in the United States. It is also the leading cause of
serious long-term disability. Current estimates assume 500,000 to 700,000 incident
strokes in the United States every year, with an annual mortality of more than
150,000 and as many as 4.5 million stroke survivors, some having serious disabling deficits (1, 2). In 2001, the American Heart Association estimated the yearly
economic burden of stroke at approximately $50 billion of both direct and indirect
costs (1). Recent epidemiologic data suggest that the spectacular decline in both
stroke incidence and mortality reached a nadir in the early 1990s and is now rising
for the first time since 1915 (3, 4).

Primary Prevention

The best approach to reduce the burden of stroke remains primary prevention
(5). Nonmodifiable risk factors include age (relative stroke rates double for every decade of life after age 55), gender (stroke is more prevalent in men than in
women), race (blacks and Hispanic Americans have higher stroke incidence and

mortality rates than whites), and a family history of stroke or transient ischemic attacks (TIAs) on either the paternal or maternal side (6–9). Well-documented ischemic stroke risk factors whose modification is proven to have beneficial effects include arterial hypertension (10), smoking (11), diabetes (12), hyperlipidemia (13), atrial fibrillation (14), and sickle cell disease (15). Less well-documented risk factors whose treatment may reduce ischemic stroke risk include obesity (16, 17), physical inactivity (18), alcohol abuse (19), hyperhomocysteinemia (20), hypercoagulability (5), and oral contraceptive use (21). Preventive endarterectomy in patients with asymptomatic high-grade carotid stenosis may be considered only after careful patient selection (comorbidity, life expectancy) and when performed by a surgeon with documented <3% morbidity/mortality rate (22, 23).

CLINICAL MANIFESTATIONS OF ISCHEMIC STROKE

Among all strokes, roughly 20% are intracranial hemorrhages, such as subarachnoid, intracerebral, and/or intraventricular hemorrhage (24–28). The remaining 80% represent ischemic strokes, including the three most common patterns of cerebral infarction: "lacunar" (microvascular), territorial (arterial branch occlusion), and distal field (borderzone) infarcts. The three subtypes can be determined on clinical, morphologic, and etiologic grounds (Table 1). Early differentiation is

TABLE 1   Summary of morphologic infarct characteristics and associated pathogenic factors

		Lacunar/ small-vessel infarction	Territorial infarct (arterial branch/ stem occlusion)	Distal field/ borderzone infarction
Microangiopathy (a) (b) (h)		X	–	–
Large artery disease (a) (b) (c) (d) (e)	Local thrombosis (f)	–	X	X
	Artery-to-artery embolism	(X)	X	(X)
Heart disease (a) (b) (c) (d) (e)	Emboligenic (g)	(X)	X	–
	Pump failure, systemic hypotension	–	–	X

Associated risk factors: (a) arterial hypertension, (b) diabetes mellitus, (c) smoking, (d) hypercholesterolemia, (e) hyperhomocysteinemia, (f) hypercoagulability, (g) atrial fibrillation, intracardiac thrombus, valvular heart disease, cardiomyopathy, etc., (h) genetic disorders [e.g., CADASIL (cerebral autosomal dominant arteriopathy with subcortical infarcts and leucoencephalopathy), MELAS (mitochondrial encephalomyopathy with lactic acidosis and stroke-like episodes)].

important because, in the acute phase after stroke onset, some treatment options are potentially hazardous for certain stroke subtypes.

Lacunar Infarction

Lacunes represent up to one third of all ischemic strokes and are mainly associated with a history of arterial hypertension and diabetes mellitus (29). The lesions are caused by microvascular occlusions due to arteriolosclerotic changes. Lesions mainly involve the deep perforating arteries of the basal ganglia, the brainstem, and less often the deep vessels of the centrum semiovale, and they seldom exceed 1.5 mm^3 on computed tomography (CT) or magnetic resonance (MR) brain imaging (Figure 1). Clinical lacunar syndromes comprise pure motor, pure sensory, and sensorimotor strokes involving at least two of three parts of the body (i.e., face, arm, and/or leg), ataxic hemiparesis, dysarthria clumsy-hand syndrome, and acute hemiballismus. These syndromes have a high positive predictive value for the presence of lacunar infarcts on magnetic resonance imaging (MRI) (30, 31). Long-term morbidity and mortality are lower in lacunar stroke than in other stroke subtypes (32–37).

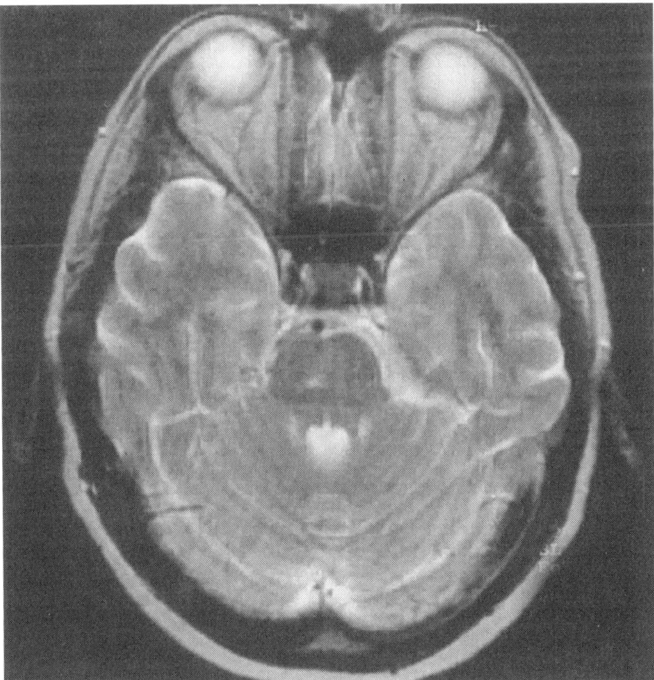

Figure 1   T2-weighted MRI shows a right paramedian pontine lacunar infarction involving a deep penetrator of the basilar artery that leads to a left pure motor hemiparesis. The patient is a 67-year-old diabetic with a history of arterial hypertension.

Territorial Infarction

Approximately two thirds of all ischemic strokes represent arterial branch or stem occlusions in the territory of the carotid or vertebrobasilar system. The causes comprise emboligenic heart disease, artery-to-artery embolism, or local thrombosis (38–40). In one third of cases, however, the source of the lesion remains undetermined or conflicting etiologic mechanisms are found. For supratentorial lesions, the clinical syndrome commonly includes (in addition to a sudden motor or sensory deficit) cortical symptoms, such as aphasia, apraxia, neglect, or homonymous visual disturbances, whereas in infratentorial lesions additional brainstem or cerebellar signs may be found. Prognosis becomes increasingly unfavorable with the size of the lesion and the severity of the initial syndrome, as well as with the patient's age and comorbidity (25–27).

Distal Field Infarction

Hemodynamic infarcts straddling the border zone (also known as the watershed) between two or three adjacent arterial territories represent only a small percentage of all ischemic strokes. They are commonly attributed to perfusion failure distal to the site of severe stenosis or occlusion of a major extra- or intracranial vessel (Figure 2). Bilateral borderzone infarcts may also occur in instances of prolonged systemic hypotension due to cardiac output failure or surgical procedures (41–44). The clinical presentation of distal field ischemia includes a wide range of symptoms from stereotypical TIAs to pseudoperipheral and other unusual patterns of limb paresis (e.g., man-in-the-barrel syndrome), complex neuropsychological syndromes (e.g., Balint's syndrome, Anton's syndrome), and larger hemispheric syndromes resembling those seen in large arterial territory infarctions (41, 45, 46). The prognosis is good if the underlying cause of the hemodynamic impairment can be treated (e.g., severe carotid artery stenosis) or if sufficient collateral flow through pial collaterals in the border zone may develop, whereas patients with further systemic hemodynamic disturbances do worse (43).

DIAGNOSIS

The diagnosis of acute ischemic stroke is mainly based on the patient's history (sudden onset of focal brain deficit), the neurologic exam (clinical syndrome), immediate brain imaging (cranial CT and/or MRI), and the exclusion of conditions

Figure 2   (*a*) T2-weighted MRI shows an area of subacute infarction in the border zone between the left middle and anterior cerebral artery. (*b*) Digital subtraction angiogram after injection into the left common carotid artery demonstrates the underlying filiform stenosis at the origin of the internal carotid artery.

(*a*)

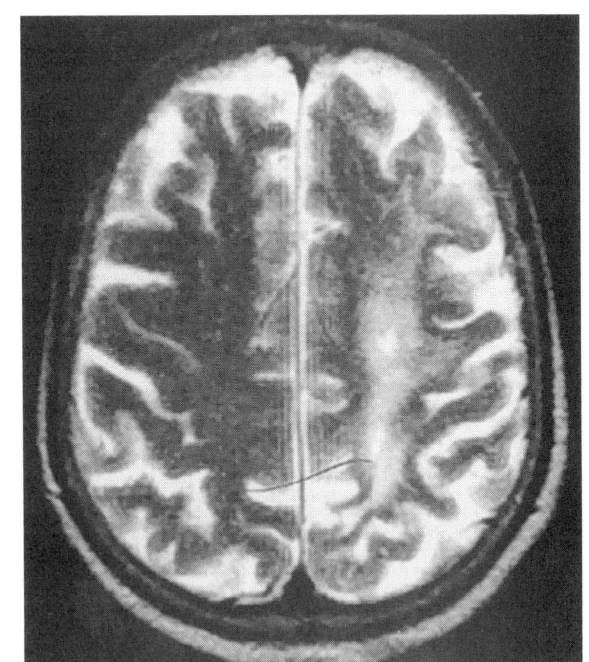

(*b*)

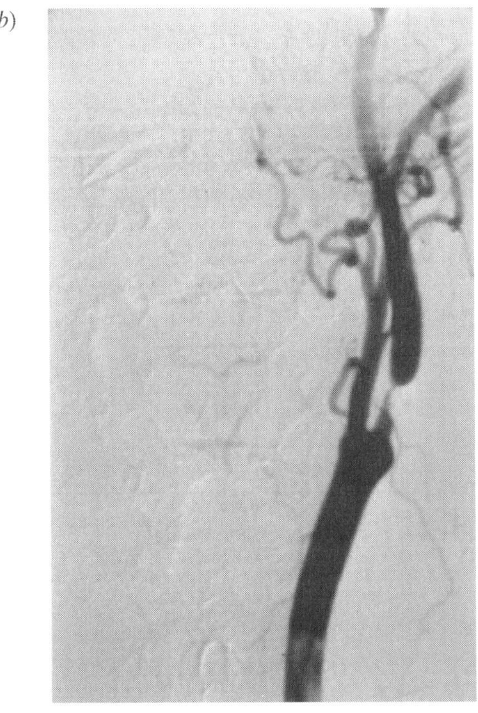

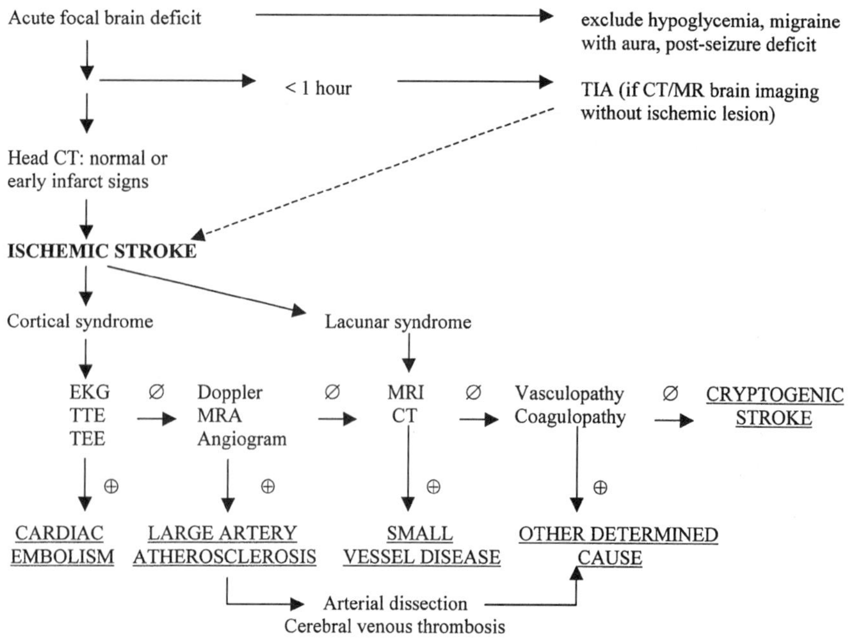

Figure 3 Ischemic stroke diagnostic algorithm. TIA, transient ischemic attack; EKG, electrocardiogram; TTE, transthoracic echocardiography; TEE, transesophageal echocardiography; MRA, magnetic resonance angiography. (Modified after 27.)

mimicking acute stroke syndromes such as hypoglycemia, migraine, or post-seizure. Vascular imaging (extracranial and transcranial Doppler ultrasonography, MR angiography, CT angiography, cerebral digital subtraction angiography) may help to elucidate the status of the arteries involved (arterial stenosis, occlusion, recanalization, etc.). Additional diagnostic findings (EKG, Holter-EKG, echocardiography, blood pressure profile, laboratory results) may further help to determine the actual etiology of the event, paving the way for more specific treatment of the underlying condition (Figure 3, Table 2).

TABLE 2 Cerebral ischemia: etiologic differential diagnosis

Etiologic group	Subtype	Specific source or condition
Embolism	Artery-to-artery	Aortic arch, common carotid, internal carotid
	Heart disease	Atrial brillation, intracardiac thrombus, valvular heart disease, cardiomyopathy, left ventricular aneurysm/hypokinesia after myocardial infarction, paradoxal embolism via patent cardiac

TABLE 2 (*Continued*)

Etiologic group	Subtype	Specific source or condition
		foramen ovale, atrial myxoma, endocarditis, Chagas disease
Atherosclerosis	Small-vessel disease	Arteriolosclerosis, lipohyalinosis
	Large-vessel disease	Extracranial and/or intracranial arteriosclerotic plaque or luminal narrowing
Vasculopathy	Inflammatory	Primary CNS vasculitis, systemic vasculitis with CNS involvement (giant cell arteritis, Takayasu arteritis, Wegener's granulomatosis, panarteritis nodosa, Churg-Strauss vasculitis), systemic collagenoses with CNS involvement (lupus erythematodes, Sneddon syndrome, sclerodermia, Behçet disease, mixed connective tissue disease), infectious vasculitis (luetic vasculitis, HIV, CMV, HBV, post-herpetic vasculitis, tuberculosis, borreliosis)
	Degenerative/genetic	Dolichoectasia, fibromuscular dysplasia, moya-moya, amyloid angiopathy, Ehlers-Danlos syndrome type IV, Marfan syndrome, Fabry's disease, CADASIL, MELAS
	Exogenous	Traumatic arterial dissection, radiation-induced vasculopathy, drug-induced vasculitis (cocaine, crack, i.v. drug abuse)
	Malignant	Neoplastic angioendotheliosis
Hematologic disorders	Coagulopathy	Antiphospholipid antibody syndrome, protein C deficiency, protein S deficiency, antithrombin III deficiency, activated protein C resistance, prothrombin 20210 mutation, factor V Leiden, paraneoplastic
	Hemoglobinopathy	Sickle cell disease, thalassemia
	Hyperviscosity syndrome	Polyglobulia, polycythemia vera, thrombocytosis, thrombophilia, myeloproliferative syndromes, macroglobulinemia, myeloma
Functional	Migraine	
	Vasospasm	Following subarachnoid hemorrhage, drug abuse (sympathomimetics)
	Pregnancy	Pre-eclampsia, eclampsia, hypercoagulability
Venous infarction	Venous thrombosis	Thrombosis of superficial (cortical) veins, deep cerebral veins and/or dural sinuses

Abbreviations: CNS, central nervous system; HIV, human immunodeficiency virus; CMV, cytomegalovirus; CADASIL, cerebral autosomal dominant arteriopathy with subcortical infarcts and leucoencephalopathy; MELAS, mitochondrial encephalomyopathy with lactic acidosis and stroke-like episodes.

TABLE 3   The 6 "Ds" of acute stroke management (modified after 51, 52)

Detection	Early recognition of stroke symptoms
Delivery	Rapid transport to hospital
Door	Emergency department arrival and triage to stroke unit, intensive care unit, or general ward
Data	History taking, physical exam, blood work, EKG, immediate head CT
Decision	Regarding drug, neuroradiological, or neurosurgical intervention
Drug	Initiation of drug treatment if appropriate

ACUTE STROKE PATIENT MANAGEMENT

The goal of any acute stroke treatment is to stabilize the patient's medical and neurologic condition and simultaneously to minimize or reverse the effect of any underlying arterial vessel occlusion, thereby reducing the amount of ischemic brain tissue in the hope of improving the patient's long-term outcome. Unfortunately, poor awareness of stroke symptoms among patients and/or their caregivers still tends to delay the time of presentation after onset (47–49). The mean time between stroke onset and hospital admission has been shown to be significantly shorter when the first medical contact was through emergency services rather than the personal physician (50). The concept of the "chain of survival" as established for patients with acute myocardial infarction has recently been translated into the 6 "Ds" (Table 3) of acute stroke management (51, 52).

Acute stroke assessment on arrival in the emergency department includes documentation of the patient's level of consciousness, history taking, a neurologic exam, and a medical exam focusing on arterial blood pressure, respiration (disturbed breathing, low PO_2, aspiration), cardiac function (arrhythmia, murmur, heart failure), body temperature, and signs of dehydration. After EKG is performed and blood drawn for basic metabolic (blood glucose level, electrolytes, renal/hepatic function) and hematologic parameters (complete blood and platelet count, coagulation profile), immediate CT (or MR) brain imaging is mandatory because it effectively discriminates between hemorrhagic and ischemic stroke, as well as distinguishing stroke from nonvascular lesions such as brain tumors that can produce focal neurologic signs (53). MR scanning more precisely documents smaller areas of stroke compared with CT but is more expensive in many places.

Any further stroke-specific treatment decisions (medical, neurointerventional, neurosurgical therapy; see below) depend heavily on the completeness and results of the initial emergent evaluation. Following current recommendations, any acute stroke patient is ideally treated in a dedicated stroke care facility such as a stroke unit, intensive care unit, or cerebrovascular service (depending on individual needs for monitoring and intervention). Dedicated stroke care has been proven to reduce stroke-related morbidity and mortality (54, 55). A stroke unit–type monitoring facility provides the ideal setting for awake or somnolent stroke patients, particularly those with fluctuating or progressive symptoms or those who require monitoring during and after thrombolytic therapy. Stuporous or comatose stroke patients requiring intubation need to be treated in a medical or neurologic intensive care unit, along with those showing signs of elevated intracranial pressure and those with high comorbidity (cardiopulmonary, renal, metabolic, or septic complications).

SPECIFIC TREATMENT OPTIONS FOR ACUTE ISCHEMIC STROKE

Medical Treatment

SYSTEMIC THROMBOLYSIS   Based on the results from the NINDS (National Institute of Neurological Disorders and Stroke) trial in 1995 (56), intravenous recombinant tissue plasminogen activator (rt-PA; 0.9 mg/kg, maximum 90 mg with 10% of total dose given as a bolus followed by an infusion lasting 60 min) is recommended for selected patients within 3 h of ischemic stroke (57). Beyond this time window, systemic rt-PA does not appear to be as beneficial and increases the risk of serious side effects (symptomatic and/or fatal intracranial hemorrhage) (58–60). Owing to the hazard of treatment-related symptomatic brain hemorrhage (in the NINDS study: 6.4% versus 0.6% in the placebo group), only selected patients meeting the established treatment criteria (Table 4) should be made eligible for rt-PA therapy (56, 61, 62).

From a clinical standpoint, the effect of rt-PA remains poorly understood. Rarely is an acute response observed. Instead, the NINDS study found differences favoring therapy on clinical follow-up performed three months after the therapy (57). Moreover, the biomolecular mechanism of clot-resolving fibrinolytics would suggest better results for freshly occluded large arteries, but rt-PA is effective across all ischemic stroke subtypes (i.e., small-vessel, atherosclerotic, and embolic stroke) and different grades of stroke severity. In one documented case of acute right middle cerebral artery (MCA) stroke, the initial large-hemisphere syndrome resolved after rt-PA treatment with autopsy data showing the blood clot still in place (63). Early infarct signs on CT brain imaging and high NIH Stroke Scale scores have been shown to be predictors of post-treatment intracerebral hemorrhage, although in the NINDS study even these subgroups benefited from rt-PA treatment (64).

Ancrod, a purified fraction of venom from the Malaysian pit viper, induces rapid defibrogenation and stimulates the release of plasminogen activator from the endothelium. After promising data from smaller series, one larger randomized controlled trial recently demonstrated a favorable benefit-risk profile for patients treated within 3 h after stroke onset when compared with placebo (65). Ancrod may therefore be a candidate as a future alternative to rt-PA treatment of ischemic stroke.

PLATELET ANTIAGGREGATION   Based on data from >40,000 patients, the International Stroke Trial and the Chinese Acute Stroke Trial demonstrated a reduction of 10 deaths or recurrent strokes per 1000 cases when ischemic stroke patients were

TABLE 4   Patient eligibility criteria for systemic rt-PA treatment of acute ischemic stroke

Age ≥ 18 years

Diagnosis of ischemic stroke causing a potentially disabling neurological deficit

Reliable onset of symptoms less than 3 h prior to i.v. administration of rt-PA

Initial CT brain imaging showing no signs of recent ischemia or early infarct
  signs no larger than 1/3 of the middle cerebral artery territory

No rapidly improving neurological deficits

No seizures at onset of stroke

No stroke or serious head injury in the previous 3 months

No major surgical procedure within the preceding 14 days

No gastrointestinal or urinary bleeding within the preceding 21 days

No recent myocardial infarction

No history or current signs of intracranial hemorrhage

Pretreatment blood pressure: systolic ≤ 185 mmHg, diastolic ≤ 110 mmHg[a]

Normal coagulation profile: INR ≤ 1.7, PTT in normal range, platelet count $\geq 100,000/mm^3$

Blood glucose ≥ 50 mg/dL and ≤ 400 mg/dL

Emergent ancillary care and facilities available during patient monitoring[b]
  to handle possible bleeding complication[c]

Potential treatment risk and benefit discussed with patient and/or family

[a]Recommended management (data based on References 56, 57): i.v. labetalol (10 mg over 1–2 min repeated every 10 min up to total dose of 150 mg); i.v. sodium nitroprusside (0.5–10 μg/kg/min).

[b]Monitoring in a dedicated stroke care facility (stroke unit) or intensive care unit recommended. Avoid placement of indwelling bladder catheter until 30 min after drug infusion. Avoid administration of antithrombotic or antiplatelet aggregating drugs, nasogastric tube, central venous access, and arterial punctures during the first 24 h.

[c]Bleeding should be considered as the likely cause of neurological worsening until CT is obtained. If signs of life-threatening bleeding occur, discontinue ongoing rt-PA infusion; obtain blood sample for coagulation tests (hematocrit, hemoglobin, PTT, INR, platelet count, fibrinogen); obtain surgical consultation as necessary; consider transfusion, cryoprecipitate, fresh frozen plasma, donor platelets.

treated with daily doses of aspirin (160–300 mg) starting within 48 h after stroke onset (66, 67). In the acute phase, prior aspirin treatment is no contraindication against the use of rt-PA, but no anti–platelet aggregation compound should be administered during the first 24 h following thrombolytic therapy.

The combination of 25 mg aspirin and 200 mg extended-release dipyridamole (each twice daily) has been found superior to aspirin alone in the secondary prevention of ischemic stroke (68). Whether the combined therapy is also superior to aspirin alone in a setting of acute ischemic stroke remains to be investigated. Though not tested in a setting of acute cerebral ischemia alone, clopidogrel may be used for patients with medical (gastrointestinal or respiratory) contraindications against aspirin. Clopidogrel (75 mg/day) has been shown to carry the same potential for reducing the relative risk of ischemic stroke as aspirin (325 mg/day) and to be superior in reducing the relative risk of ischemic stroke, myocardial infarction, or vascular death taken together (if not for reducing the risk of ischemic stroke alone) (69). Several trials comparing clopidogrel plus aspirin versus aspirin alone for recurrent ischemic stroke are currently being organized (SPS3, MATCH), given the favorable results in the recently completed, as-yet-unpublished CURE trial.

ANTICOAGULATION   Prophylactic administration of low-dose subcutaneous heparin [5000–7500 international units (I.U.) twice daily], low-molecular-weight heparins, or heparinoids is strongly recommended in immobilized stroke patients to prevent deep vein thrombosis (53, 70–73). In the International Stroke Trial, subcutaneous administration of higher (unadjusted) doses of heparin after acute ischemic stroke provided no benefit in the treatment of acute ischemic stroke (66). Instead, the benefit of doses of >5000 I.U. twice a day was offset by the incidence of hemorrhage associated with the therapy.

Although one randomized study showed dose-dependent outcome improvement in patients treated with nadroparin, a low-molecular-weight heparin, within 48 h after stroke (74), subsequent trials using similar compounds failed to reproduce a similar effect (75, 76). The benefit of early treatment with dose-adjusted intravenous (i.v.) heparin in ischemic stroke remains unresolved. One randomized trial, RAPID (Rapid Anticoagulation Prevents Ischemic Damage), is under way and awaits completion in 2002 (77). Until better data are available, dose-adjusted i.v. heparin [target partial thromboplastin test (PTT): 50–60 s] may be given after ischemic stroke in a setting of atrial fibrillation (especially new-onset, intermittent, or in association with fresh thrombotic material in left atrium or mitral valve stenosis), high-risk cardiac embolic sources (i.e., acute or subacute myocardial infarction, artificial valve), coagulopathies, arterial dissection (78), and symptomatic high-grade carotid stenosis awaiting surgical therapy. Within the first 24 h after systemic rt-PA treatment, however, i.v. heparin should not be given (79).

Neurointerventional Treatment

INTRA-ARTERIAL THROMBOLYSIS   To accomplish intra-arterial thrombolysis, cerebral angiography is used to visualize the occluded vessel, and a microcatheter is navigated to the site of the clot in the hope of dislodging the occlusion and achieving restoration of brain blood flow. Thrombolytic agents administered proximally and distally as well as into the core of the obstruction provide high local concentrations at the site of the actual occlusion and reduce systemic effects. Prior findings from uncontrolled case series suggested the possibility of safe and effective intra-arterial treatment even beyond a three-hour time window (80, 81), but a randomized placebo-controlled trial failed to demonstrate significant differences between treated patients and controls (82).

In the following PROACT II study, 180 patients with acute ischemic stroke (without hemorrhage or major early infarct signs on initial CT scan) caused by angiographically proven MCA occlusion were randomized within 6 h after symptom onset to receive intra-arterial prourokinase (r-proUK) plus heparin or heparin alone (83). The r-proUK group received a total of 9 mg over 2 h and all patients received an initial 2000 I.U. bolus of i.v. heparin followed by a 500 I.U./h infusion of i.v. heparin beginning at the time of angiography. The results showed significantly better outcome at 90 days for the prourokinase + heparin treated group (40% with Rankin score ≤2 versus 25% of controls), despite an increased frequency of early symptomatic intracranial hemorrhage (10% versus 2% of controls). Though not approved as a standard therapy, the PROACT II design may provide a guideline for intra-arterial thrombolysis for patients past the three-hour time window whose clinical syndrome and transcranial Doppler suggest acute MCA occlusion.

BALLOON ANGIOPLASTY AND STENTING   Percutaneous transluminal angioplasty and intravascular stenting of affected arteries in acute stroke patients represent a promising approach, but in the absence of controlled studies, this must be considered an experimental procedure carrying an unknown risk (84). Several uncontrolled series including both symptomatic and asymptomatic carotid stenosis patients suggested both technical feasibility and safety of this procedure (85, 86). Therefore, carotid angioplasty and stenting may be currently performed in symptomatic patients with contraindications (e.g., neck-radiation–induced carotid stenosis, local tumor mass) against surgical treatment, but should otherwise be limited to well-designed randomized studies.

Results from the larger Carotid and Vertebral Artery Transluminal Angioplasty Study (CAVATAS) trial in 504 patients with carotid stenosis randomized to carotid stenting or endarterectomy suggest that both treatments are equally effective at preventing stroke recurrence for up to three years (87). During the course of the trial, however, techniques of carotid angioplasty and stenting improved immensely as new designs of carotid stents and protection devices were developed. Further large, randomized, multicenter trials based on novel technology are therefore needed. Several are under way, each independently evaluating the benefit of percutaneous transluminal angioplasty and intravascular stenting in patients with symptomatic and/or asymptomatic carotid stenosis versus conventional endarterectomy (88, 89).

Intracranial angioplasty has also been reported to be technically feasible in patients with symptomatic intracranial atherosclerotic narrowing who failed maximal (antiplatelet aggregation drugs, anticoagulation, blood pressure control) medical treatment (90). Lack of response to conservative treatment is often seen in instances of subacute or chronic perfusion failure in which, for anatomic reasons, the endovascular approach may be the only way to access the actual stenosis (91, 92). Vessels technically accessible for treatment include the intracranial segments of the internal carotid artery, the MCA stem, and the basilar and vertebral arteries (90, 93, 94). Data from larger controlled series, however, are still lacking, in expectation of progress in the development of dedicated treatment devices for intracranial arteries.

Neurosurgical Treatment

DECOMPRESSIVE SURGERY   Large-hemispheric stroke syndromes due to space-occupying MCA (also called malignant MCA infarction) or other territorial infarcts have been associated with up to 80% mortality rates despite optimal conservative treatment (95, 96). Data from well-documented uncontrolled series suggest that early hemicraniectomy may be life-saving, but its potential of improving outcome remains subject to debate (96–100). Several independent, prospective, randomized trials evaluating safety and outcome after hemicraniectomy versus best medical treatment alone are under way (101, 102). Current treatment approaches favor patients $\leq$70 years of age with initial Glasgow Coma Scale scores of 7 or better, who develop clinical and CT-morphologic signs of severe intracranial pressure and midline shift due to growing hemispheric infarct edema within the affected vascular territory (103). The surgical intervention consists of a sufficiently large osteoclastic trepanation ($\geq$10 cm in diameter) and duraplasty (Figure 4) to allow "extracranial herniation" of the infarcted brain tissue, reduction of intracranial pressure, and increased perfusion pressure in peri-infarct areas at risk (104).

Although their prognosis is generally good, larger cerebellar territorial infarcts (especially those involving the superior cerebellar artery or more than one arterial territory) may develop space-occupying infarct edema, causing brainstem compression and/or occlusive hydrocephalus with the hazard of rapid clinical deterioration (105). Timely osteoclastic trepanation with a sufficiently large occipital bone flap should be performed early, before clinical signs of secondary brainstem injury or hydrocephalus occur (106).

CAROTID ENDARTERECTOMY   Based on data from >1400 patients, the large randomized trials in North America [North American Symptomatic Carotid Endarterectomy Trial (NASCET)] and Europe [European Carotid Surgery Trial (ECST)] independently showed that for patients with symptomatic high-grade carotid artery stenoses, endarterectomy had a beneficial effect on the risk of recurrent stroke and death (107–109). Emergency endarterectomy early after ipsilateral cerebral infarction remains controversial for fear of reperfusion injury and hemorrhagic transformation of fresh ischemic lesions (110). Therefore, early endarterectomy <4 weeks after infarction has been recommended for patients presenting with TIA or minor strokes only (111, 112). This reasoning is now supported by secondary analyses from the NASCET dataset that suggest no difference in outcome after surgery between those patients operated on within 30 days after a minor index stroke when compared to those operated on later (113). Moreover, 4.9% of the medically treated symptomatic patients had a recurrent ipsilateral stroke within 30 days of randomization. Until better data are available, early carotid endarterectomy may therefore be considered in patients with symptomatic high-grade stenosis presenting with TIA or minor stroke.

REVASCULARIZATION PROCEDURES   In instances of distal perfusion failure due to proximal large-artery occlusion or moya-moya disease, direct or indirect surgical bypass procedures have been proposed to provide additional collateral flow to brain areas at risk for hemodynamic stroke (114, 115). Direct superficial

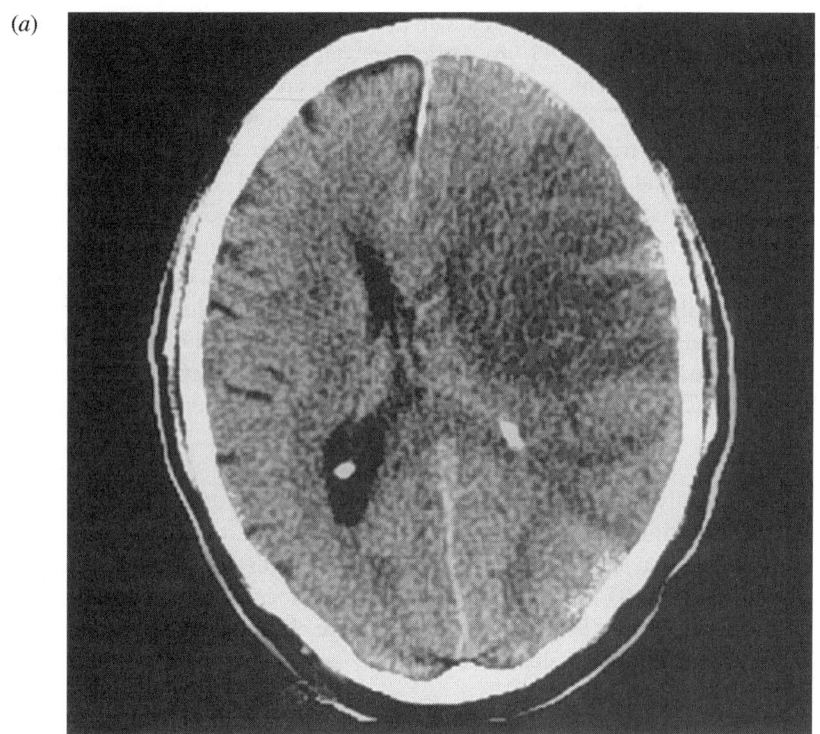

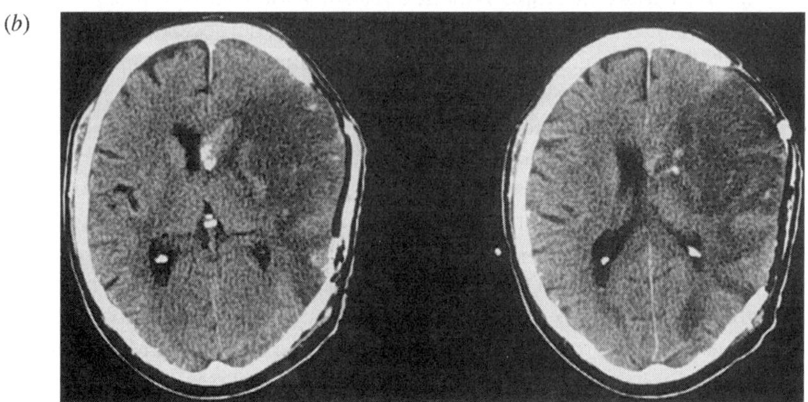

Figure 4   (*a*) Cranial CT showing a large subacute infarct of the left middle cerebral artery (MCA) with space-occupying edema leading to compression of the ipsilateral ventricular system, midline shift, and beginning subfalcial herniation. (*b*) Cranial CT after cranioclastic decompression surgery showing normal midline structures and extension of the edematous infarct tissue extending over the former bone limits.

temporal artery–to–middle cerebral artery (STA/MCA) bypass surgery requires special microsurgical skills, is often impossible owing to lack of a suitably large recipient vessel, and carries the risk of flow reversal in the successfully treated arterial branches (116, 117). Indirect encephaloduroarteriosynangiosis (EDASS) or encephalomyosynangiosis (EMS) through simple burr-holes are less challenging to the neurosurgeon, and may provide more physiologic ingrowth of extracranial vessels into hypoperfused vascular territories (118, 119).

Monitoring, Prevention, and Therapy of Common Complications

Continuous monitoring of EKG, blood pressure, oxygen saturation, and body temperature during the first 24 h after stroke onset is recommended, as well as intermittent monitoring of the neurologic status, level of consciousness, blood glucose level, and fluid balance (52, 53). Follow-up CT or MRI evaluation may be indicated if clinical deterioration suggests growing infarct edema, elevated intracranial pressure, secondary hemorrhagic transformation, or recurrent ischemic stroke.

EKG monitoring during the acute phase after ischemic stroke may help to identify emboligenic cardiac arrythmias or other hazardous conditions requiring immediate intervention (e.g., atrial fibrillation, atrioventricular block, bradycardia, tachycardia, other significant arrhythmia, or myocardial ischemia).

Monitoring of respiration rate and sufficient oxygen saturation ($PO_2 \geq 95\%$) should keep physicians alert to hypoventilation, disturbed pulmonary gas exchange, and the need for supplemental oxygen.

Elevated body temperature should be controlled by generous use of antipyretics, since the relative risk of poor outcome after stroke has been shown to double for each 1°C increase in body temperature (120). Clinical data on the use of hypothermia are still insufficient to recommend this therapy.

Any fever source should be ascertained and infection immediately treated. Particular attention should be given to preventing aspiration.

Arterial blood pressures in the acute phase after ischemic stroke should be kept within higher normal limits. If hypotension occurs, volume depletion is the most common cause, but other serious (cardiac or septic) conditions should be considered and treated. Markedly elevated blood pressure (>130 mmHg mean arterial pressure; >220 mmHg systolic blood pressure; >110 mmHg diastolic blood pressure) may be acutely treated with quick-acting oral or parenteral antihypertensive drugs such as nitroglycerin (10 mg orally or 5 mg i.v.), clonidine (0.075 mg subcutaneously), uripidil (12.5 mg i.v.), labetalol (10 mg i.v. over 1–2 min repeated every 10 min up to total dose of 150 mg), or sodium nitroprusside (continuous i.v. 0.5–10 μg/kg/min). It has been inferred that overzealous reduction in acute blood pressure could precipitate perfusion failure in the territory suffering occlusion or high-grade stenosis.

Blood glucose should be kept at physiologic levels using oral or i.v. glucose sources in cases with hypoglycemia, as well as subcutaneous or i.v. insulin administration in those showing hyperglycemia after stroke.

Patients showing signs of elevated intracranial pressure may be acutely treated using osmotherapy (glycerol 10%, 4 × 125–250 ml/24 h; mannitol 15%, 4–6 × 100 ml/24 h for ≤2 days), controlled hyperventilation ($PaCO_2$: 30–35 mmHg), barbiturates (thiopental bolus application of 0.25–0.5 g, up to 0.1 g/kg body weight), or THAM [tris-(hydroxymethyl)-aminomethane] buffer solution (blood gas base excess <+6 mEq, pH ≤ 7.55), before surgical intervention is considered. However, none of these treatments have yet been tested in a clinical trial large enough to determine their clinically important benefit.

Stroke-related symptomatic seizures are best treated with carbamazepine or phenytoin. Lorazepam (1 to 2 mg i.v.), diazepam (5–10 mg i.v.,) or phenytoin (20 mg/kg body weight loading dose) can be used to treat status epilepticus.

Early mobilization and measures to prevent further subacute complications of stroke (e.g., malnutrition, deep vein thrombosis, pulmonary embolism, decubitus ulcers, contractures, or joint abnormalities) are strongly recommended with special emphasis on the use of heparin or low-molecular-weight heparins (heparinoids) for prevention of deep vein thrombosis.

SECONDARY STROKE PREVENTION

Reported five-year cumulative recurrence rates after prior cerebral ischemia range from 24% to 42% (121–123), with one third of recurrences occurring within the first 30 days after the initial event (124). Therapeutic control of modifiable vascular risk factors is highly recommended (125). Stroke patients with atrial fibrillation require dose-adjusted oral anticoagulation (target INR: 2.5 ± 0.5) unless there is a specific contraindication, in which case the patient may be treated with aspirin (14, 126). Patients presenting with symptomatic high-grade (≥75%) carotid artery stenosis are eligible for endarterectomy by a surgeon with a low complication rate (morbidity and mortality <6%) (108–110). For stroke patients with no atrial fibrillation or symptomatic carotid stenosis, treatment with oral platelet aggregation inhibitors is indicated, using aspirin (50–325 mg/day), clopidogrel (75 mg/day), aspirin plus clopidogrel, or extended-release dipyridamole (2 × 200 mg/day) plus aspirin (2 × 25 mg/day). Initial results from the recent warfarin-aspirin recurrent stroke study (WARSS) found no additional benefit for oral anticoagulation (mean INR 2.1 in the warfarin group) compared with 325 mg/day of aspirin for secondary prevention after lacunar, atherosclerotic, or cryptogenic stroke (127). WARSS also showed no statistically significant difference in the low (<2%) hemorrhagic adverse event rates in the two treatment arms. Physicians now face a decision whether to use aspirin or warfarin, recognizing similarity in two-year rates of stroke and death and of hemorrhagic complications.

Distinct etiologic causes (vasculitis, endocarditis, prothrombotic states, etc.; Table 2) may require more specific therapy.

Visit the Annual Reviews home page at www.AnnualReviews.org

LITERATURE CITED

1. American Heart Association. 2001. *2001 Heart and Stroke Statistical Update.* http://www.americanheart.org/statistics/stroke.html
2. Broderick J, Brott T, Kothari R, et al. 1998. The Greater Cincinnati/Northern Kentucky Stroke Study: preliminary first-ever and total incidence rates of stroke among blacks. *Stroke* 29:415–21
3. Wolf PA, D'Agostino RB. 1998. Epidemiology of stroke. See Ref. 3a, 1:3–28
3a. Barnett HJM, Mohr JP, Stein BM, Yatsu FM. 1998. *Stroke. Pathophysiology, Diagnosis, and Management.* New York: Churchill Livingstone. 1459 pp.
4. Gillum RF, Sempos CT. 1997. The end of the long-term decline in stroke mortality in the United States? *Stroke* 28:1507–17
5. Goldstein LB, Adams R, Becker K, et al. 2001. Primary prevention of stroke. A statement for healthcare professionals from the Stroke Council of the American Heart Association. *Stroke* 32:280–99
6. Brown RD, Whisnant JP, Sicks JD, et al. 1996. Stroke incidence, prevalence, and survival: secular trends in Rochester, Minnesota, through 1989. *Stroke* 27:373–80
7. Wolf PA, D'Agostino RB, O'Neil MA, et al. 1992. Secular trends in stroke incidence and mortality: the Framingham study. *Stroke* 23:1551–55
8. Sacco RL, Boden-Albala B, Gan R, et al. 1998. Stroke incidence among white, black, and Hispanic residents of an urban community. *Am. J. Epidemiol.* 147:259–68
9. Kiely DK, Wolf PA, Cupples LA, et al. 1993. Familial aggregation of stroke: the Framingham study. *Stroke* 24:1366–71
10. Whisnant JP. 1996. Effectiveness versus efficacy of treatment of hypertension for stroke prevention. *Neurology* 46:301–7
11. Wolf PA, D'Agostino RB, Kannel WB, et al. 1988. Cigarette smoking as a risk factor for stroke: the Framingham study. *JAMA* 259:1025–29
12. UK Prospective Diabetes Study Group. 1998. Effect of intensive blood glucose control with metformin on complications in overweight patients with type 2 diabetes (UKPDS 34). *Lancet* 352:854–65
13. Atkins D, Psaty BM, Koepsell TD, et al. 1993. Cholesterol reduction and the risk for stroke in men: a meta-analysis of randomized, controlled trials. *Ann. Intern. Med.* 119:136–45
14. The Atrial Fibrillation Investigators. 1994. Risk factors for stroke and efficacy of antithrombotic therapy in atrial fibrillation: analysis of pooled data from five randomized controlled trials. *Arch. Intern. Med.* 154:1449–57
15. Adams RJ, McKie VC, Hsu L, et al. 1998. Prevention of a first stroke by transfusion in children with sickle cell anemia and abnormal results on transcranial Doppler ultrasonography. *N. Engl. J. Med.* 339:5–11
16. Walker SP, Rimm EB, Ascherio A, et al. 1996. Body size and fat distribution as predictors of stroke among US men. *Am. J. Epidemiol.* 144:1143–50
17. Rexrode KM, Hennekens CH, Willett WC, et al. 1997. A prospective study of body mass index, weight change, and the risk of stroke in women. *JAMA* 277:1539–45
18. Sacco RL, Gan R, Boden-Albala B, et al. 1998. Leisure-time physical activity and ischemic stroke risk: the Northern Manhattan Stroke Study. *Stroke* 29:380–87
19. Sacco RL, Elkind M, Boden-Albala B, et al. 1999. The protective effect of moderate alcohol consumption on ischemic stroke. *JAMA* 281:53–60
20. Boushey CJ, Beresford SA, Omenn GS, et al. 1995. A quantitative assessment of plasma homocysteine as a risk factor for vascular disease: probable benefits of

increasing folic acid intakes. *JAMA* 274: 1049–57

21. Gillum LA, Mamidipudi SK, Johnston SC. 2000. Ischemic stroke risk with oral contraceptives: a meta-analysis. *JAMA* 284:72–78

22. Executive Committee for the Asymptomatic Carotid Atherosclerosis Study. 1995. Endarterectomy for asymptomatic carotid artery stenosis. *JAMA* 273:1421–28

23. Hartmann A, Hupp T, Koch HC, et al. 1999. Prospective study on the complication rate of carotid surgery. *Cerebrovasc. Dis.* 9:152–56

24. Foulkes MA, Wolf PA, Price TR, et al. 1988. The Stroke Data Bank: design, methods, and baseline characteristics. *Stroke* 19:547–54

25. Bogousslavsky J, Van Melle G, Regli F. 1988. The Lausanne stroke registry: analysis of 1000 consecutive patients with first stroke. *Stroke* 19:1083–92

26. Bamford J, Sandercock P, Dennis M, et al. 1991. Classification and natural history of clinically indentifiable subtypes of cerebral infarction. *Lancet* 337:1521–26

27. Sacco RL, Toni D, Mohr JP. 1998. Classification of ischemic stroke. See Ref. 3a, 16:341–54

28. Rosamond WD, Folsom AR, Chambless LE, et al. 1999. Stroke incidence and survival among middle-aged adults: 9-year follow-up of the Atherosclerosis Risk in Communities (ARIC) cohort. *Stroke* 30:736–43

29. Mast H, Thompson JLP, Lee SH, et al. 1995. Hypertension and diabetes mellitus as determinants of multiple lacunar infarcts. *Stroke* 26:30–33

30. Gan R, Sacco RL, Kargman DE, et al. 1987. Testing the validity of the lacunar hypothesis: the Northern Manhattan Stroke Study experience. *Neurology* 48:1204–11

31. Stapf C, Hofmeister C, Hartmann A, et al. 2000. Predictive value of lacunar syndromes for lacunar lesions on magnetic resonance brain imaging. *Acta Neurol. Scand.* 101:13–18

32. Bamford J, Sandercock P, Jones L, Warlow C. 1987. The natural history of lacunar infarction: the Oxfordshire Community Stroke Project. *Stroke* 18:545–51

33. Arboix A, Martí-Vilalta JL, García JH. 1990. Clinical study of 227 patients with lacunar infarcts. *Stroke* 21:842–47

34. Sacco SE, Whisnant JP, Broderick JP, et al. 1991. Epidemiological characteristics of lacunar infarcts in a population. *Stroke* 22:1236–41

35. Sacco RL, Shi T, Zamanillo MC, Kargman DE. 1994. Predictors of mortality and recurrence after hospitalized cerebral infarction in an urban community: the Northern Manhattan Stroke Study. *Neurology* 44:626–34

36. Clavier I, Hommel M, Besson G, et al. 1994. Long-term prognosis of symptomatic lacunar infarcts. A hospital-based study. *Stroke* 25:2005–9

37. Salgado AV, Ferro JM, Gouveia-Oliveira A. 1996. Long-term prognosis of first-ever lacunar strokes. A hospital-based study. *Stroke* 7:661–66

38. Bogousslavsky J, van Melle G, Regli F. 1988. The Lausanne Stroke Registry: analysis of 1,000 consecutive patients with first stroke. *Stroke* 19:1083–92

39. Sandercock PAG, Warlow CP, Jones LN, Starkey IR. 1989. Predisposing factors for cerebral infarction: the Oxfordshire Community Stroke Project. *BMJ* 298:75–80

40. Mast H, Thompson JLP, Völler H, et al. 1994. Cardiac sources of embolism in patients with pial artery infarcts and lacunar strokes. *Stroke* 25:776–81

41. Mohr JP. 1979. Neurological complications of cardiac valvular disease and cardiac surgery including systemic hypotension. In *Handbook of Clinical Neurology, Vol. 38. Neurological Manifestations of Systemic Diseases*, ed. PJ Vincken, GW Bruyn, pp. 143–71. Amsterdam: North-Holland

42. Torvik A. 1984. The pathogenesis of watershed infarcts in the brain. *Stroke* 15:221–23

43. Bogousslavsky J, Regli F. 1986. Border-zone infarctions distal to carotid artery occlusion: prognostic implications. *Ann. Neurol.* 20:346–50

44. Angeloni U, Bozzao L, Fantozzi L, et al. 1990. Internal borderzone infarction following acute middle cerebral artery occlusion. *Neurology* 40:1196–98

45. Mohr JP. 1969. Distal field infarction. *Neurology* 19:279 (Abstr.)

46. Sage JI, van Uitert RL. 1986. Man-in-the-barrel syndrome. *Neurology* 36:1102–3

47. Alberts MJ, Bertels CD, Dawson DV. 1990. An analysis of the time of presentation after stroke. *JAMA* 263:65–68

48. Wellwood I, Dennis MS, Warlow CP. 1994. Perceptions and knowledge of stroke among surviving patients with stroke and their carers. *Age Ageing* 23:293–98

49. Fogelholm R, Murros K, Rissanen A, Ilmavirta M. 1996. Factors delaying hospital admission after acute stroke. *Stroke* 27:398–400

50. Barsan WG, Brott TG, Broderick JP, et al. 1993. Time of hospital presentation in patients with acute stroke. *Arch. Intern. Med.* 153:2558–61

51. Hazinski MF. 1996. De-mystifying recognition and management of stroke. *Curr. Emerg. Cardiac Care* 7:9

52. The European Ad Hoc Consensus Group. 1997. Optimizing intensive care in stroke: a European perspective. *Cerebrovasc. Dis.* 7:113–28

53. Adams HP, Brott TG, Crowell RM, et al. 1994. Guidelines for the managemant of patients with acute ischemic stroke. A statement for healthcare professionals from a special writing group of the Stroke Council, American Heart Association. *Stroke* 25:1901–14

54. Langhorne P, Williams BO, Gilchrist W, Howle K. 1993. Do stroke units save lives? *Lancet* 342:395–98

55. Jørgensen HS, Nakayama H, Raaschou HO, et al. 1995. The effect of a stroke unit: reductions in mortality, discharge rate to nursing home, length of hospital stay, and cost. A community-based study. *Stroke* 26:1178–82

56. The National Institute of Neurological Disorders and Stroke rt-PA Stroke Study Group. 1995. Tissue plasminogen activator for acute ischemic stroke. *N. Engl. J. Med.* 333:1581–87

57. Adams HP, Brott TG, Furlan AJ, et al. 1996. Guidelines for thrombolytic therapy for acute ischemic stroke: a supplement to the guidelines for the management of patients with acute ischemic stroke. A statement for healthcare professionals from a special writing group of the Stroke Council, American Heart Association. *Circulation* 94:1167–74

58. Hacke W, Kaste M, Fieschi C, et al. for the ECASS study group. 1995. Intravenous thrombolysis with recombinant tissue plasminogen activator for acute hemispheric stroke. *JAMA* 274:1017–25

59. Hacke W, Kaste M, Fieschi C, et al. for the Second European-Australasian Acute Stroke Study investigators. 1998. Randomized double-blind placebo-controlled trial of thrombolytic therapy with intravenous Alteplase in acute ischemic stroke (ECASS II). *Lancet* 352:1245–51

60. Clark WM, Wissman S, Albers GW, et al. for the ATLANTIS study investigators. 1999. Recombinant tissue-type plasminogen activator (Alteplase) for ischemic stroke 3 to 5 hours after symptom onset. *JAMA* 282:2019–26

61. The NINDS rt-PA Stroke Study Group. 1997. Intracerebral hemorrhage after rt-PA therapy for ischemic stroke. *Stroke* 28:2109–18

62. Lopez-Yunez AM, Bruno A, Williams LS, et al. 2001. Protocol violations in community-based rTPA stroke treatment are associated with symptomatic intracerebral hemorrhage. *Stroke* 32:12–16

63. Stapf C, Mohr JP, Théallier-Jankó A, Mast H. 1999. Cerebral hemorrhage after systemic fibrinolysis in a patient with severe

carotid artery stenosis. *Acta Neurol. Scand.* 100:407–10

64. The NINDS rt-PA Stroke Study Group. 1997. Generalized efficacy of t-PA for acute stroke: subgroup analysis of the NINDS rt-PA stroke trial. *Stroke* 28:2119–25

65. Sherman D, Atkinson R, Chippendale T, et al. for the STAT participants. 2000. Intravenous ancrod for treatment of acute ischemic stroke. The STAT study: a randomized controlled trial. *JAMA* 283:2395–403

66. International Stroke Trial Collaborative Group. 1997. The International Stroke Trial (IST): a randomized trial of aspirine, subcutaneous heparin, both, or neither among 10435 patients with acute ischemic stroke. *Lancet* 349:1569–81

67. CAST (Chinese Acute Stroke Trial) Collaborative Group. 1997. CAST: randomized placebo-controlled trial of early aspirin use in 20000 patients with acute stroke. *Lancet* 349:1641–49

68. Diener HC, Cunha L, Forbes C, et al. 1996. European Stroke Prevention Study 2. Dipyridamole and acetylsalicylic acid in the secondary prevention of stroke. *J. Neurol. Sci.* 143:1–13

69. CAPRIE Steering Committee. 1996. A randomized, blinded, trial of clopidogrel versus aspirin in patients at risk for ischemic events (CAPRIE). *Lancet* 348: 1329–39

70. McCarthy ST, Turner JJ, Robertson D, Hawkey CJ. 1977. Low dose heparin as a prophylaxis against deep vein thrombosis after acute stroke. *Lancet* 2:800–1

71. Turpie AGG, Levin MN, Hirsh J, et al. 1987. A double-blind randomized trial of Org 10172 low molecular weight heparinoid in prevention of deep vein thrombosis in thrombotic stroke. *Lancet* 1:523–26

72. Prins MH, Gelsema R, Sing AK, et al. 1989. Prophylaxis of deep venous thrombosis with a low molecular weight heparin (Kabi 2165/Fragmin) in stroke patients. *Haemostasis* 19:245–50

73. Turpie AGG, Gent M, Cote R, et al. 1992. A low-molecular-weight heparinoid compared with unfractionated heparin in the prevention of deep venous thrombosis in patients with acute ischemic stroke. A randomized, double-blind study. *Ann. Intern. Med.* 117:353–57

74. Kay R, Wong KS, Yu YL, et al. 1995. Low-molecular-weight heparin for the treatment of acute ischemic stroke. *N. Engl. J. Med.* 333:1588–93

75. The Publication Committee for the Trial of ORG 10172 in Acute Stroke Treatment (TOAST) Investigators. 1998. Low molecular weight heparinoid, ORG 10172 (danaparoid), and outcome after acute ischemic stroke: a randomized controlled trial. *JAMA* 279:1265–72

76. Berge E, Abdelnoor M, Nakstad PH, Sandset PM. 2000. Low molecular-weight heparin versus aspirin in patients with acute ischemc stroke and atrial fibrillation: a double blind randomised study. HAEST Study Group. Heparin in Acute Embolic Stroke Trial. *Lancet* 355:1205–10

77. Chamorro A. 2001. Immediate anticoagulation in acute focal brain ischemia revisited. Gathering the evidence. *Stroke* 32: 577–78

78. Stapf C, Elkind MSV, Mohr JP. 2000. Carotid artery dissection. *Annu. Rev. Med.* 51:329–47

79. Adams HP, Brott TG, Furlan AJ, et al. 1996. Guidelines for thrombolytic therapy for acute ischemic stroke: a supplement to the guidelines for the management of patients with acute ischemic stroke. A statement for healthcare professionals from a special writing group of the Stroke Council, American Heart Association. *Circulation* 94:1167–74

80. Brott TG, Hacke W. 1998. Thrombolytic and defibrogenating agents for ischemic and hemorrhagic stroke. See Ref. 3a, 51: 1155–76

81. Stapf C, Marshall RS, Mohr JP, et al. 2000. Late intra-arterial thrombolysis. *Eur. J. Med. Res.* 5:303–6

82. del Zoppo GJ, Higashida RT, Furlan AJ, et al. 1998. PROACT: a phase II randomized trial of recombinant pro-urokinase by direct arterial delivery in acute middle cerebral artery stroke. *Stroke* 29:4–11

83. Furlan A, Higashida R, Wechsler L, et al. for the PROACT Investigators. 1999. Intra-arterial prourokinase for acute ischemic stroke. The PROACT II study: a randomized controlled trial. *JAMA* 282:2003–11

84. Bettmann MA, Katzen BT, Whisnant J, et al. 1998. Carotid stenting and angioplasty. A statement for healthcare professionals from the Councils on Cardiovascular Radiology, Stroke, Cardio-Thoracic and Vascular Surgery, Epidemiology and Prevention, and Clinical Cardiology, American Heart Association. *Circulation* 97:121–23

85. Theron JG, Payelle GG, Coskun O, et al. 1996. Carotid artery stenosis: treatment with protected balloon angioplasty and stent placement. *Radiology* 201:627–36

86. Yadav JS, Roubin GS, Iyer S, et al. 1997. Elective stenting of the extracranial carotid arteries. *Circulation* 95:376–81

87. Brown MM. 2001. Carotid angioplasty and stenting: Are they therapeutic alternatives? *Cerebrovasc. Dis.* 11(Suppl. 1):112–18

88. Hobson RW 2nd. 2000. CREST (Carotid Revascularization Endarterectomy versus Stent Trial): background, design, and current status. *Semin. Vasc. Surg.* 13:139–43

89. Brown MM, Silver L. 2001. Protocol for the International Carotid Stenting Study (ICSS). *Cerebrovasc. Dis.* 11(Suppl. 4):29 (Abstr.)

90. Alazzaz A, Thornton J, Aletich VA, et al. 2000. Intracranial percutaneous transluminal angioplasty for arteriosclerotic stenosis. *Arch. Neurol.* 57:1625–30

91. Ramee SR, Dawson R, McKinley KL, et al. 2001. Provisional stenting for symptomatic intracranial stenosis using a multidisciplinary approach: acute results, unexpected benefit, and one-year outcome. *Catheter Cardiovasc. Interv.* 52:457–67

92. Stapf C, Marshall RS, Elkind M, et al. 2000. Symptomatic middle cerebral artery stenosis: Should angioplasty be attempted? *Stroke* 31:325 (Abstr.)

93. Clark WM, Barnwell SL, Nesbit G, et al. 1995. Safety and efficacy of percutaneous transluminal angioplasty for intracranial atherosclerotic disease. *Stroke* 26:1200–4

94. Higashida RT, Tsai FY, Halbach VV, et al. 1993. Transluminal angioplasty for atherosclerotic disease of vertebral and basilar arteries. *J. Neurosurg.* 78:192–98

95. Hacke W, Schwab S, Horn M, et al. 1996. The "malignant" middle cerebral artery infarction: clinical course and neuroradiological signs. *Arch. Neurol.* 53:309–15

96. Rieke K, Schwab S, Krieger D, et al. 1995. Decompressive surgery in space-occupying hemispheric infarction: results of an open prospective trial. *Crit. Care Med.* 23:1576–87

97. Delashaw JB, Broaddus WC, Kassell NF, et al. 1990. Treatment of right hemispheric cerebral infarction by hemicraniectomy. *Stroke* 21:874–81

98. Schwab S, Rieke K, Aschoff A, et al. 1996. Hemicraniectomy in space-occupying hemispheric infarction: useful early intervention or desperate activism? *Cerebrovasc. Dis.* 325–29

99. Holtkamp M, Buchheim K, Unterberg A, et al. 2001. Hemicraniectomy in elderly patients with space occupying media infarction: improved survival but poor functional outcome. *J. Neurol. Neurosurg. Psychiatr.* 70:226–28

100. Leistner S, Boegner F, Marx P, Koennecke HC. 2001. Transtentorial herniation after unilateral infarction of the anterior cerebral artery. *Stroke* 32:649–51

101. HeADDFIRST Data Coordinating Center Home Page. 2001. http://hf.bsd.uchicago.edu

102. Hofmeijer J, van der Worp HB, Amelink GJ, et al. 2001. Decompressive surgery

in space-occupying hemispheric infarction. A randomized controlled trial. *Cerebrovasc. Dis.* 11(Suppl. 4):34 (Abstr.)

103. Hacke W. 1997. Intensive care in acute stroke. *Cerebrovasc. Dis.* 7(Suppl. 3):18–23

104. Krieger D, Hacke W. 1998. The intensive care of the stroke patient. See Ref. 3a, 50:1133–54

105. Rieke K, Krieger D, Adams HP, et al. 1993. Therapeutic strategies in space-occupying cerebellar infarction based on clinical, neuroradiological, and neurophysiological data. *Cerebrovasc. Dis.* 3: 45–55

106. Heros RC. 1992. Surgical treatment of cerebellar infarction. *Stroke* 23:937–38

107. North American Symptomatic Carotid Endarterectomy Trial Collaborators. 1991. Beneficial effect of carotid endarterectomy in symptomatic patients with high grade carotid stenosis. *N. Engl. J. Med.* 325:445–53

108. North American Symptomatic Carotid Endarterectomy Trial Collaborators. 1998. Benefit of carotid endarterectomy in patients with symptomatic moderate or severe stenosis. *N. Engl. J. Med.* 339: 1415–25

109. European Carotid Surgery Trialists' Collaborative Group. 1991. MRC European Carotid Surgery Trial: iterim results for symptomatic patients with severe (70–90%) or with mild (0–29%) carotid stenosis. *Lancet* 337:1235–43

110. Bruetman ME. 1979. Hemorrhage complication in carotid endarterectomy. *Stroke* 10:214

111. Whittemore AD, Ruby ST, Couch NP, Mannick JA. 1984. Early carotid endarterectomy in patients with small, fixed neurologic deficits. *J. Vasc. Surg.* 1:795–99

112. Piotrowski JJ, Bernhard VM, Rubin JR, et al. 1990. Timing of endarterectomy after acute stroke. *J. Vasc. Surg.* 11:45–51

113. Gasecki AP, Ferguson GG, Eliasziw M, et al. 1994. Early endarterectomy for severe carotid artery stenosis after a nondisabling stroke: results from the North American Symptomatic Carotid Endarterectomy Trial. *J. Vasc. Surg.* 20: 288–95

114. Masuda J, Ogata J, Yamaguchi T. 1998. Moyamoya disease. See Ref. 3a, 31:815–32

115. Chiu D, Shedden P, Bratina P, Grotta J. 1998. Clinical features of moyamoya disease in the United States. *Stroke* 29:1347–51

116. Nakashima H, Meguro T, Kawada S, et al. 1997. Long-term results of surgically treated moyamoya disease. *Clin. Neurol. Neurosurg.* 99(Suppl. 2):S156–61

117. Wang MY, Steinberg GK. 1996. Rapid and near-complete resolution of moyamoya vessels in a patient with superficial temporal artery–to–middle cerebral artery bypass. *Pediatr. Neurosurg.* 24:145–50

118. Ross IB, Shevell MI, Montes JL, et al. 1994. Encephaloduroarteriosynangiosis (EDASS) for the treatment of childhood moyamoya disease. *Pediatr. Neurol.* 10: 199–204

119. Yoon HK, Shin HJ, Lee M, et al. 2000. MR angiography of moyamoya disease before and after encephaloduroarteriosynangiosis. *Am. J. Roentgenol.* 174:195–200

120. Reith J, Jørgensen HS, Pedersen PM, et al. 1996. Body temperature in acute stroke: relation to stroke severity, infact size, mortality, and outcome. *Lancet* 347:422–25

121. Sacco RL, Wolf PA, Kannel WB, McNamara PM. 1982. Survival and recurrence following stroke: the Framingham Study. *Stroke* 13:290–95

122. Petty GW, Brown RD Jr, Whisnant JP, et al. 1998. Survival and recurrence after first cerebral infarction: a population-based study in Rochester, Minnesota, 1975 through 1989. *Neurology* 50:208–16

123. Sacco RL, Shi T, Zamanillo MC,

Kargman DE. 1994. Predictors of mortality and recurrence after hospitalized cerebral infarction in an urban community: the Northern Manhattan Stroke Study. *Neurology* 44:626–34

124. Hier DB, Foulkes MA, Swiontoniowski M, et al. 1991. Stroke recurrence within 2 years after ischemic infarction. *Stroke* 22:155–61

125. Wolf PA, Clagett GP, Easton JD, et al. 1999. Preventing ischemic stroke in patients with prior stroke and transient ischemic attack. A statement for healthcare professionals from the Stroke Council American Heart Association. *Stroke* 30:1991–94

126. EAFT Study Group. 1993. Secondary prevention in non-rheumatic atrial fibrillation after transient ischemic attack or minor stroke. *Lancet* 342:1255–62

127. Mohr JP. 2001. The Warfarin-Aspirin Recurrent Stroke Study (WARSS): initial results. *Cerebrovasc. Dis.* 11(Suppl. 4):127 (Abstr.)

Annu. Rev. Med. 2002. 53:477–98

THE PATHOPHYSIOLOGY OF ASTHMA

Lee Maddox and David A. Schwartz

Pulmonary and Critical Care Division, Duke University Medical Center, Research Drive, Durham, North Carolina 27710; e-mail: david.schwartz@duke.edu

Key Words   atopy, cytokines, Th-2 cells, airway obstruction, bronchial hyperreactivity, lungs

■ **Abstract**   Asthma is a chronic disorder of the airways that is characterized by reversible airflow obstruction and airway inflammation, persistent airway hyperreactivity, and airway remodeling. The etiology of asthma is complex and multifactorial. Recent advances have demonstrated the importance of genetics in the development of asthma, particularly atopic asthma. Environmental stimuli, particularly early childhood infections, have also been associated with the development of asthma. Most current data seem to suggest that these factors drive the development of a Th-2 lymphocyte–predominant immune response, which has been associated with atopy and IgE-mediated inflammation. The concept of reversible airflow obstruction has also recently been challenged. It is now clear that chronic airway changes occur, which may contribute to progressive airflow obstruction. We discuss the important influence of genetic and environmental factors on the emergence of the asthmatic phenotype. The significance of Th-1 and Th-2 lymphocyte–mediated immunity are discussed, and the inflammatory processes leading to chronic airway inflammation are detailed.

INTRODUCTION

Asthma is a chronic disorder of the airways that is characterized by reversible airflow obstruction and airway inflammation, persistent airway hyperreactivity (AHR), and airway remodeling (1). An estimated 15 million Americans are affected by asthma and the morbidity and mortality associated with it is increasing in industrialized nations (2, 3). Morbidity is disproportionately high among inner-city residents (4). The annual cost of caring for asthmatics exceeds six billion dollars per year in the United States, and the worldwide market for asthma medication is currently valued at 5.5 billion dollars each year (5).

ETIOLOGY

The etiology of asthma is complex and multifactorial. It involves the interaction between genetic factors and environmental stimuli. The vast majority of the data regarding the pathogenesis of asthma concentrates on atopic asthma and the imbalance between the Th-1 (cell-mediated immunity) and Th-2 (humorally mediated immunity) phenotypes. However, asthma (reversible airflow obstruction, persistent AHR, and airway remodeling) may also occur through nonallergic mechanisms of inflammation. Genetics, the uterine environment, maternal and infant diet, respiratory infections, and occupational and environmental exposures all contribute to this delicate balance. The manner in which all these factors converge will determine whether the reaction of a particular subject's immune system results in airway inflammation and airway remodeling. An overabundance of factors that favor a Th-2 phenotype may ultimately lead to atopy. Although the Th-1/Th-2 balance provides a framework within which to understand the immune events that promote airway inflammation and bronchial hyperreactivity, this construct is clearly over simplified. In fact, Th-1 responses alone have been shown to induce reversible airway inflammation and AHR (6, 7). Asthma is best thought of as a syndrome, a common pathway of injury and repair from a variety of insults, and can be mediated through multiple mechanisms of inflammation and repair (Figure 1).

Genetics

Although classical Mendelian patterns of inheritance do not apply to asthma, there is little doubt that inheritance plays a role in this disease (8–11). Familial aggregation of asthma was recognized historically by 1860 (12). More recently, it has been demonstrated that methacholine responsiveness is bimodally distributed in families of asthmatics (compared with control families). However, a segregation analysis strongly rejected a single-major-locus model (13), and the heritability (proportion of the variance in asthma due to genetic factors) of nonspecific bronchial

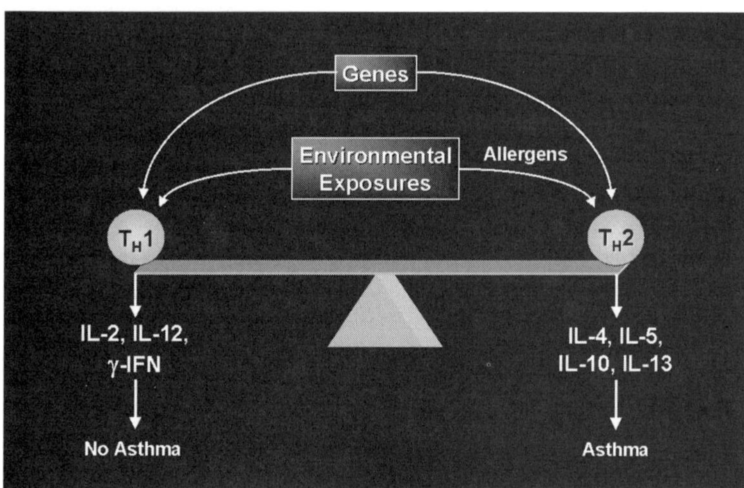

Figure 1   Role of Th-1 and Th-2 cells in asthma.

responsiveness has been estimated at 27% (14). Community-based twin studies of asthma estimate the heritability of asthma at 35% to 75% (15–20). A recent twin-family study estimated that in families with one asthmatic parent, as much as 87% of the variation in susceptibility to asthma in twins was explained by genetic factors; however, among twins whose parents were unaffected, environmental factors alone were sufficient to explain the development of asthma (21). Although strong familial aggregation of asthma has been observed in segregation studies (14, 22, 23), variable conclusions have been reached regarding the pattern of inheritance (autosomal recessive, dominant, codominant, and polygenic). An extensive segregation analysis on a random cohort of families using multiple asthma traits [immunoglobulin E (IgE), bronchial hyperreactivity, atopy, wheeze, and asthma] has demonstrated that the inheritance of these traits is likely to be polygenic (14). Although these twin studies and segregation analyses clearly indicate the importance of genetic factors, these studies also serve to demonstrate that a substantial portion of the variability of asthma is caused by factors unique to the individual, such as environmental exposures.

Although genetic loci and candidate genes within and outside of these loci have been associated with asthma phenotypes (serum IgE levels, atopy, bronchial hyperreactivity, and asthma), major susceptibility genes for asthma have not been definitively identified (8, 24). Candidate gene/loci studies have reported linkage of atopy and nonspecific AHR to chromosomes 5q (25, 26), 6p (27), 11q (28, 29), 12q (30), and 14q (31). Among atopic sibling pairs with only a 12% prevalence of asthma, a genome-wide screen identified linkage to 4q, 6p, 7p, 11q, 13q, and 16q (32). A genome-wide screen for linkage with asthma in three racial groups (African Americans, Caucasians, and Hispanics) yielded six novel regions (2q33, 5p15, 11p15, 17p11, 19q13, and 21q21) and confirmed several previously identified loci (5q23–31, 6p21–23, 12q14–24, 13q21–qter, and 14q11–13) (33). A recent genomic screen in a series of 156 asthmatic sibling pairs from Germany identified regions of interest on chromosomes 2, 6, 9, and 12 (34), and several of these regions were replicated within the same sample using varied asthma-related phenotypes. Finally, a genome-wide search in a founder population (Hutterites) identified linkage to five regions—5q23–31, 12q15–24.1, 16p, 19q13, and 21q21 (35). Selected genes within these loci that are potentially involved in the susceptibility to asthma include:

- 5q31–32: interleukin (IL)-3, IL-4, IL-5, IL-6, IL-9, IL-12, IL-13, transforming growth factor (TGF)-β1, CD14, granulocyte macrophage colony-stimulating factor (GM-CSF), catenin, fibroblast growth factor-1, glucocorticoid receptor, and β_2-adrenergic receptor;
- 6p21–22: HLA complex and tumor necrosis factor (TNF)-α;
- 11q13: FcεR1 and Clara cell secretory protein (CC16);
- 12q: interferon (IFN)-γ, IGF1, glutathione-S-transferase, nitric oxide synthetase (NOS1), leukotriene A4 hydrolase, selectin P ligand, and mast cell growth factor;
- 13q: esterase D;

- 14q: TCR α/δ complex;
- 16p: α chain of the IL-4 receptor.

In fact, many studies have demonstrated a relationship between asthma and several of these positional candidate genes. For instance, the Gly16 polymorphism of the β_2-adrenergic receptor appears to be overrepresented in nocturnal (36) or more severe cases (37) of asthma, and the Glu27 polymorphism of the β_2-adrenergic receptor is associated with less AHR (38); however, these associations remain controversial (39, 40). Polymorphisms of the β_2-adrenergic receptor are thought to act as disease modifiers in asthma (41, 42). Although the relationship between the $-$C589T IL-4 polymorphism and atopy is controversial (43), linkage analysis suggests that this gene may regulate IgE production in a non–antigen-specific fashion (26), that FEV_1 in asthma is, in part, determined by this polymorphism (44), and that this polymorphism may play a role in asthma susceptibility in children (45, 46). A polymorphism of IL-13 (Gln110Arg) has been associated with asthma in study populations from Britain and Japan (47). Polymorphisms in the promoter regions of TGF-β1 (48) and CD14 (49) were found to be associated with total IgE levels in atopic subjects. Polymorphisms of TNF-α (LTα*Nco*I and TNF-308) appear to be associated with asthma (50–53), but not atopy or IgE levels, suggesting that asthma is not simply the result of allergic mechanisms. Polymorphisms of the high-affinity IgE receptor (FcεRIβ) appear to be related to the level of IgE (29, 54) but are inconsistently associated with other asthma phenotypes (45, 54–57). An association study has shown that a polymorphism of the glutathione-S-transferase gene was strongly related to asthma and bronchial hyperreactivity (58). NOS1 variants were associated (odds ratio $= 2.08$; $p = 0.008$) with asthma in a British population (59), and the α chain of the IL-4 receptor appears to further define an atopy/asthma susceptibility locus (60, 61). Genes outside these regions that have demonstrated a relationship with asthma susceptibility, severity, or pharmacologic responsiveness include 5-lipoxygenase (62), α-1 antitrypsin (63), IL-10 (48), CFTR (64), and platelet-activating factor (65).

Importance of Gene-Environment Interactions in Asthma

The dramatic increase in the prevalence of asthma in the past 20 years provides further evidence that exposures play an important role in the development of this disease. Asthma occurs more frequently in low-income populations and developed countries (10, 66–68). Although demographic factors, such as age, race, and socioeconomic status, appear to be risk factors for the development and progression of asthma (66, 69, 70), its increasing prevalence and severity suggest that aeroallergens (71), smoking behavior (72), agents in the workplace (73), indoor and outdoor air pollution (74, 75), viruses (76), domestic (77–80) and occupational (81–88) exposure to endotoxin, or immunization against certain infectious diseases (89) are particularly important in the etiology and pathogenesis of this condition. Moreover, avoidance of allergens and cigarette smoke appears to decrease the risk of childhood asthma (10, 90, 91).

In Utero Events

Although the contribution of genetics to the asthmatic phenotype is substantial, the penetrance of genetic traits is highly dependent on interactions with the environment. Environmental exposure begins at conception. Because the fetus contains a non-self paternal antigen, it would be expected to be rejected by the mother's immune system as a transplanted allograft might. In transplantation models, it is thought that Th-1 lymphocytes are responsible for acute rejection and that Th-2 cells work to maintain tolerance. Although it is not a universal observation, some animal data demonstrate a strong Th-2 cytokine response in grafts of tolerant animals (92). During pregnancy, the maternal-fetal interface is an immunologically active site producing many cytokines. Numerous lines of evidence point to a dominance of Th-2–type cytokines in the uterine environment. Fetal cord blood lymphocytes are skewed toward the Th-2 type. Neonatal T cells produce low levels of IFN-γ and overproduce Th-2 cytokines (93). Maternal lymphocytes produce IL-5 in response to normal allogenic placenta, whereas placentas from abortion-prone pregnancies cause lymphocytes to secrete IL-2 and IFN-γ. In mouse models, injection of GM-CSF or IL-3 into mice prone to fetal loss will enhance fetal survival. Injection of IL-2, TNF, and IFN-γ causes fetal loss in normal pregnancies (94, 95). At birth, the immune system of the fetus has been strongly shifted toward a Th-2 lymphocyte profile. In mothers with atopic disease, this effect may be exaggerated. If this skewed fetal immune response is not rebalanced by stimuli that restore the normal Th-1/Th-2 balance, the child may become predisposed to asthma and atopy.

Respiratory Infections

One of the major influences on the Th-1/Th-2 balance is exposure to infectious agents. Measles, hepatitis A, and tuberculosis have all been associated with a decrease in the rate of atopy. Respiratory syncytial virus (RSV) and viruses that cause lower respiratory tract infections (LRTIs) appear to increase rates of wheezing and atopy (96). Viral bronchiolitis in children closely mimics the asthmatic state in that it causes AHR and wheezing and responds to bronchodilator therapy. In children, bronchiolitis is caused by a number of viruses: RSV, parainfluenza virus, coronavirus, influenza virus, and rhinovirus. Over 70% of LRTIs are caused by RSV (93). Almost 100% of children are infected with RSV in the first few years of life, 66% in the first year. Twelve to 40 percent of RSV cases result in LRTI, pneumonia, or bronchiolitis, and 1%–2% of previously healthy infants require hospitalization (97). Epidemiologic studies have long linked RSV and asthma, but many are plagued by inadequate control groups, lack of knowledge whether the infants wheezed prior to the study, poor documentation of the agent causing the bronchiolitis, and short follow-up times. Taken as a whole, they seem to suggest that severe RSV infections necessitating hospitalization are associated with wheezing and AHR. Seventy-five percent of hospitalized patients wheeze at 2 years, 50% at 3 years, and 40% at 5 years after the initial episode (93). In one prospective trial by Sigurs et al. of 47 infants hospitalized with RSV bronchiolitis over one RSV season and 93 control subjects, physician-verified asthma (three or more episodes of bronchial obstruction verified by a physician) was present in 23% of the RSV group and 1% of the control group at 3 years. At 7.5 years of follow-up, 30% in the RSV group versus 3% in the control group cumulatively had been diagnosed with asthma, though only 23% versus 2% were currently asthmatic. Current atopic asthma (as determined by the presence of IgE antibodies on skin-prick and/or serum test) was present in 14.9% of the RSV group and only 1% of the control group (97). Although multiple studies have demonstrated that LRTI may cause wheezing, the long-term relationship of wheezing to the development of asthma is not entirely clear. The data by Sigurs et al. do suggest that RSV bronchiolitis in infancy severe enough to require hospitalization could drive the development of asthma.

Although some respiratory viruses may produce long-term sequelae that mimic asthma, a rapidly growing body of evidence also suggests that childhood infections are protective against the development of asthma. The reported frequency of asthma in children varies substantially worldwide, from 2% in China up to 30% in Great Britain and Australia (98). Some of this variation has been attributed to varying exposure to infectious agents.

Alm et al. looked at Swedish children who belonged to families leading anthroposophic lifestyles (restricted use of antibiotics, antipyretics, and vaccinations) and who attended schools that applied these principles. Only 50% of the study children had used antibiotics versus 90% of the controls. Most of the anthroposophic children had been vaccinated only against tetanus and polio. Alm et al. found that among the anthroposophic children, only 13% were diagnosed with atopy, versus 25% of the control children. Asthma, as diagnosed by a physician, occurred in only 2.7% versus 9.5% of control children (96). This and similar studies have suggested a protective effect of the "traditional" lifestyle. Vaccination and the implied reduction in exposure to many childhood diseases may deny the child's immune system exposure to agents that promote a Th-1 phenotype. During one year of the study, 71% of the anthroposophic group contracted measles during an epidemic. Measles has been associated with the Th-1 phenotype (96). Similarly, alterations in the intestinal flora by frequent antibiotic use may decrease or alter bacterial counts, possibly diminishing the usual antigenic stimuli that prompt a Th-1 response.

A recently published American study also supports a role for childhood infection in preventing the asthmatic phenotype. Daycare centers are notorious for spreading disease, and the spread of colds from one sibling to the next is familiar to most parents. Ball et al., in a large prospective trial involving 1035 children followed since birth as part of the Tucson Children's Respiratory Study, examined the risk of developing asthma in relation to both the total number of siblings and enrollment in daycare (99). Despite a higher prevalence of wheezing in those with multiple siblings or early exposure to daycare, relative risk 1.4, daycare attendance during the first six months of life and the presence of one or more older siblings at home

TABLE 1   Relative risk of asthma by sibling count and age at daycare entry (99)

Number of older siblings	% With asthma	Relative risk (95% CI)
0	21%	1.0
1	19%	0.9 (0.7–1.0)
2	14%	0.7 (0.5–1.0)
>3	13%	0.6 (0.4–1.0)
Age at daycare entry		
>12 months	19%	1.0
7–12 months	18%	0.9 (0.4–2.1)
Birth to 6 months	9%	0.4 (0.2–1.0)

protected against the development of asthma, relative risk 0.4 (95% CI 0.2–1) and 0.8 (95% CI 0.7–1.0) respectively (Table 1).

Although more children wheezed in the preschool years, this was actually protective by the age of 13, relative risk 0.3 (95% CI 0.2–0.5). Epidemiologic studies like these, combined with an attempt to give clinical relevance to the different populations of T cells, have given birth to the "hygiene hypothesis." The hygiene hypothesis suggests that at birth the immune system is skewed toward a Th-2 T cell profile. As the child is sequentially exposed to infectious, endogenous, and environmental antigens, its immune system shifts back toward a Th-1/Th-2 balance. Failure to expose the child to these antigens by vaccination, frequent antibiotic use, increased indoor activity, and less antigenic food may prevent the necessary shift and lead to a progressive Th-2 state and atopy (100). It is interesting that the prevalence of atopy is greatest in industrialized nations with excellent vaccination programs and increased antibiotic use. If this hypothesis is true, it may also help explain the increase in asthma morbidity and mortality among low-income urban children. Daycare attendance is lowest among children of low-income families (99).

PATHOGENESIS

The development of clinical asthma results from a complex biologic interaction between multiple gene products (one or more containing genetic variations that enhance susceptibility) and at least one environmental toxin (10, 91). An individual may be predisposed to the effect of an irritant or allergen through any of several potential mechanisms:

1. Major histocompatibility complex (MHC) class II antigens may allow specific inhaled allergens to be presented more effectively to T lymphocytes by monocytes or dendritic cells.

2. Specific T cell receptor types may allow more effective T cell response to specific combinations of MHC II antigens and allergens.

3. More, or more active, IL-4 may cause an exaggerated production of IgE.

4. More effective high-affinity IgE receptors on mast cells, basophils, or other effector cells may cause an exaggerated response to allergen-IgE interaction, releasing more inflammatory mediators, which may then further increase IgE levels in a positive feedback loop.

5. The smooth muscle response to contractile agonists released from effector cells may be enhanced by defective or downregulated β_2-adrenergic receptors.

6. Because of changes in the specific receptors, the individual may respond more efficiently to an inhaled toxin.

Each of these mechanisms of susceptibility will prove relevant to a limited number of inhaled agents.

Acquired Immunity in Asthma

Acquired immunity is particularly important in allergic asthma. Epidemiologic studies demonstrate that atopy is associated with AHR (101), as well as asthma incidence (102, 103), persistence (104), and severity (105). In a large population-based study, atopy was the most important risk factor for developing AHR (106). Allergen sensitization (predominantly to indoor allergens) confers an odds ratio of 1:6–1:20 for symptomatic AHR (107, 108).

Both in vitro and in vivo data suggest that the atopic condition results from a disequilibrium in the acquired immune system. The immune system may polarize its response in one of two very different directions: a delayed-type hypersensitivity (DTH) reaction with relatively low levels of humoral response or a response characterized by high levels of antibody and little DTH. This marked dichotomy exists even though both antibody-mediated and DTH responses depend on a common CD4+ lymphocyte. To some degree, this paradox has been explained by technologies that measure T cell cytokines. In 1986, Mosmann et al. described two populations of T cells in mice based on their cytokine profiles (109). Lymphocytes termed Th-1 cells produced primarily IL-2, IFN-γ, and TNF-α. In contrast, the Th-2 cells produced IL-4, IL-5, IL-6, and IL-13 (109, 110). The cytokines produced by each subset function in an autocrine fashion to promote the growth of its own phenotype. Feedback of IL-4 onto a Th-2 cell will further activate it. In addition to the positive regulation of IL-4 on Th-2 cells and IFN-γ on Th-1 cells, these cytokines will downregulate T cells of the opposite type. IL-2 and IFN-γ produced by Th-1 cells will amplify Th-1 development while inhibiting the Th-2 response. IL-4–producing Th-2 cells induce Th-2 phenotype amplification and inhibit the Th-1 response. Thus, once a particular pathway is entered, the response will be skewed toward that cell line (110, 111).

Th-1 and Th-2 lymphocytes are derived from the same T cell precursor. Their differentiation into Th-1 or Th-2 cells depends on interactions with the microenvironment. If antigen-presenting cells present allergen to the naïve T cell precursor in the presence of IL-12, a Th-1 cell line will be created (112, 113). Development of the Th-2 phenotype is regulated by IL-4 (114). It is not clear what determines whether IL-12 or IL-4 will predominate in an immune response. Endotoxin, viral wall components, and intracellular bacteria (Legionella and Mycoplasma) all stimulate IL-12 production and push the immune system toward a Th-1 phenotype. However, if IL-4 is present in the cytokine milieu, it seems to take precedence over other cytokines (110). The concentration of the antigen also seems to be important. With low-dose antigen exposure, a Th-1 response is produced. Higher doses of antigen, which are often seen in aerosol and food exposures, tend to increase IL-4 and produce a Th-2–type reaction (110).

Although most of the above data were derived from murine models, it is clear that Th-1– and Th-2–type immune responses occur in human disease. This is particularly apparent in atopic diseases and asthma. Cells in bronchoalveolar lavage samples from patients with atopic asthma contained more cells producing IL-4, IL-5, and GM-CSF messenger RNA (mRNA) than cells obtained from control patients (111). In bronchial biopsies from patients with both "extrinsic" and "intrinsic" asthma, levels of IL-4 and IL-5 mRNA were elevated (115). GATA-3, a transcription factor necessary for the production of IL-5, is confined to Th-2 cells. GATA-3 mRNA expression is significantly higher in the airways of asthmatic subjects than in controls (116). These findings suggest that the human immune system, like that of the mouse, is also divided into subsets of T cells that produce a discrete set of cytokines.

The cardinal manifestation of asthma is inflammation. Bronchial inflammation and AHR begin with the inhalation of environmental antigen. The majority of antigen is cleared by the mucocilliary escalator. Inhaled antigen that avoids clearance and penetrates the underlying epithelial layer is intercepted by dendritic cells. The alveolar surfaces are policed by alveolar macrophages as well as dendritic cells lining the subepithelial spaces (117). The dendritic cells then move to the regional lymph nodes, where they act as antigen-presenting cells to the B and T cells. In the presence of IL-4 and IL-13, the B cell undergoes class switching to produce IgE (100). IL-4 and IL-13 appear to be the quintessential cytokines responsible for initiating the Th-2 response. In vitro, IL-4 and IL-13 can induce the release of proinflammatory cytokines and the expression of adhesion molecules (118). Inhaled IL-4 causes increased AHR to methacholine and increased sputum eosinophilia in asthmatic subjects (119), and transgenic mice overexpressing IL-13 (120) develop increased AHR and airway eosinophilia. Moreover, lung tissue from allergic asthmatics is infiltrated with activated, cytokine-secreting Th-2 cells (121, 122) that produce IL-4 (123). Blockade of IL-4 during antigen sensitization abolishes the development of allergic asthma. However, blockade of IL-4 before or during an antigen challenge does not inhibit inflammation or AHR (124). IL-13 binds to the alpha chain of the IL-4 receptor. Blockade of IL-13 resulted in a complete reversal of allergen-induced AHR and mucus production. The administration of recombinant IL-13 induced an increase in airway mucus production (125).

After being primed by the T cell and antigen-presenting cell, the B cell is directed to produce allergen-specific IgE. This IgE is released into the blood and quickly binds to high-affinity IgE receptors (FcεRI) on the surface of mast cells and peripheral blood basophils and to the low-affinity IgE receptors (FCεRII or CD23) on the surface of lymphocytes, eosinophils, platelets, and macrophages (100). Once mast cells are coated with antigen-specific IgE, future exposure to the antigen will lead to mast cell activation.

Mast cells are bone marrow–derived CD34+ mononuclear cells that express the FcεRI receptor. When allergen-specific IgE molecules on the surface of the mast cells interact with allergen, a cross linking of the IgE occurs. This cross linking induces the activation of signaling cascades and causes the release of preformed granules containing histamine, tryptase, chymase, eicosanoids, free radicals, and preformed Th-2–like cytokines (100). This exocytosis of preformed mediators constitutes the "early phase reaction." These substances are quite toxic and are responsible for acute asthmatic symptoms. Histamine induces the contraction of airway smooth muscle, mucus secretion, and vasodilatation. A loss of microvascular integrity follows and plasma proteins and plasma leak into the airway walls, causing lumen narrowing (126). Tryptase potentiates histamine-induced smooth muscle contraction, whereas chymase has a procollagen proteinase activity and is probably directly toxic to the airway cells (126). The release of the cysteinyl leukotrienes as well as other inflammatory cytokines leads to the "late phase reaction," which primarily involves the recruitment and activation of eosinophils, Th-2–type CD4+ cells, macrophages, and neutrophils (127). Once the inflammatory reaction or late phase is initiated, eosinophils become one of the major mediators of chronic inflammation in allergic asthma.

Eosinophils are bone marrow–derived from pluripotent stem cells. IL-5 is the cytokine primarily responsible for selective differentiation of the eosinophil. Overproduction of IL-5 in transgenic mice results in profound eosinophilia, whereas deletion of the IL-5 gene substantially reduces pulmonary eosinophilia after antigen challenge (127). Eosinophils are recruited to the lung by chemoattractant molecules released by mast cells and T cells. Four substances attract eosinophils into inflamed tissue: leukotriene B4, IL-16, and eotaxin 1 and 2 (126, 127). Once in the airways, eosinophils can release a cornucopia of toxic granules (Table 2) that cause direct tissue damage, smooth muscle contraction, and increased vascular permeability, ultimately leading to the recruitment of more eosinophils and Th-2–type cells to the airway.

Once established, the repetitive cycle of tissue damage and inflammatory cell recruitment becomes chronic. Even in the absence of sustained allergen, the chronic inflammation persists. This is evident from studies that have looked at free radical formation as a measure of ongoing inflammation. Neutrophils, eosinophils, and other cells involved in the inflammatory response produce large amounts of

TABLE 2   Eosinophil-derived proteins

Toxic granule protein	Function
Major basic protein	Cytotoxic to respiratory epithelium Degranulation of mast cells Increased smooth muscle activity
Eosinophil cationic protein	Cytotoxic to respiratory epithelium
Eosinophil-derived neurotoxin	Ribonuclease activity
Cysteinyl leukotrienes	Increase vascular permeability Smooth muscle contraction Increase mucus secretion
RANTES	Eosinophil chemoattractant
Eotaxin 1 and 2	Eosinophil chemoattractant
Th-2–type cytokines	Perpetuation of Th-2 inflammation Eosinophil chemoattractant

free radicals such as superoxide and peroxynitrite. These can be measured in exhaled gas. Studies of free radical production in patients with asthma that is well controlled without steroids (symptoms <2 times per week and an FEV_1 > 80% of predicted) demonstrated significantly elevated levels of exhaled free radical metabolites compared with controls (128). Whether this ongoing inflammation in a minimally symptomatic patient is enough to lead to progressive chronic airway changes is not yet clear.

Innate Immunity in Asthma

Innate immunity acts as the first line of host defense against microbial pathogens. It is conserved over a wide variety of species from flies to mammals (129). Innate immunity uses germline-encoded receptors to aid in antimicrobial host defense (130, 131). These receptors recognize certain patterns rather than particular structures, and a limited number of pattern recognition receptors (PRRs) can recognize a wide variety of microbes. In the case of endotoxin or lipopolysaccharide (LPS), the PRR is directed against the highly conserved portion of lipid A, which acts as the pathogen-associated molecular pattern (PAMP) against which the PRR developed in defense against gram-negative bacterial infection. Some PRRs bind directly to PAMPs (e.g., CD14 recognizes and binds LPS), whereas others, such as the TLR4 receptor, are thought to recognize complexes generated by PAMP recognition, e.g., the CD14/LBP/LPS complex (130, 132). Endotoxin or LPS is ubiquitous in the environment and is often present in high concentrations in organic dusts (86), as well as in air pollution (133) and household dusts (78).

There is convincing evidence that endotoxin exacerbates airflow obstruction and airway inflammation in allergic asthmatics. Among allergic asthmatics who are sensitive to house dust-mite allergen, the concentration of endotoxin in the home environment, but not the concentration of mite allergen (Der p1), was significantly associated with the severity of asthma (78). Experimentally, allergic asthmatics are more sensitive to the bronchoconstrictive effects of inhaled endotoxin than non-asthmatics (134). Moreover, among allergic asthmatics, prior allergen challenge significantly augments the inflammatory response to inhaled endotoxin (135). The enhanced response to inhaled endotoxin among allergic asthmatics may simply reflect the additive effect of preexisting airway inflammation but could also be caused by release of LPS-binding protein (LBP) when allergic asthmatics are challenged with allergen (136). In mice sensitized to ovalbumin, inhalation of LPS exacerbates the inflammatory response to ovalbumin (137). In aggregate, these findings indicate that allergic airways can enhance the response to inhaled endotoxin and that endotoxin can enhance the airway response to allergens.

However, the timing of the exposure appears to be critical to the interaction between endotoxin and allergens. Emerging evidence suggests that early exposure to endotoxin, a potent inducer of Th-1–type cytokines (IFN-γ and IL-12), may minimize the risk of allergen sensitization (80, 137), which could have profound effects on the development of allergic asthma. Although this seems to support the importance of a Th-2 phenotype in the development of allergic asthma (89, 99, 125, 138), these recent findings should be interpreted with caution. Th-1 responses alone have been shown to induce reversible airway inflammation and AHR (6, 7), and recent findings (79) clearly demonstrate an independent relationship between endotoxin exposure and repeated wheezing during infancy.

Independent of its effect in allergic asthma, several studies demonstrate that inhalation of air contaminated with endotoxin is associated with the classical features of asthma (reversible airflow obstruction and airway inflammation, AHR, and airway remodeling). Epidemiologic studies show that the concentration of inhaled endotoxin in the bioaerosol is strongly and consistently associated with reversible airflow obstruction among cotton workers (84), agricultural workers (82), and fiberglass workers (139). In fact, the concentration of endotoxin in the bioaerosol is the most important occupational exposure associated with the development (83) and progression (82) of airway disease in agricultural workers. Experimentally, inhalation of endotoxin can cause reversible airflow obstruction and airway inflammation in previously unexposed healthy study subjects (81, 140). In fact, healthy study subjects challenged with dust from animal confinement buildings develop airflow obstruction and an increase in the serum concentration of neutrophils and IL-6, all of which are most strongly associated with the concentration of endotoxin (not dust) in the bioaerosol (141). Finally, following subchronic inhalation of grain dust, endotoxin-sensitive (C3H/BFeJ), but not endotoxin-resistant (C3H/HeJ), mice develop persistent AHR and airway remodeling, which suggests that endotoxin is one of the principal components of grain dust that causes the development of chronic airway disease (142).

Innate immunity may also be involved in airway disease caused by air pollution. Recent studies have shown that particulate matter, which is strongly associated with the progression of airway disease (143), is contaminated with endotoxin

(133, 144). The concentration of endotoxin in particulate matter is directly related to the induction of growth factors (133) and the release of IL-6 (144) by monocytes in vitro. Moreover, in murine models, TLR4 appears to play a role in ozone-induced asthma (145).

AIRWAY REMODELING

Traditional definitions of asthma have included the concept of reversible airflow obstruction. Recently however, the absolute reversibility of the asthmatic state by steroids and beta-agonist has met with skepticism. Several studies have demonstrated that asthmatics experience an accelerated rate of respiratory functional decline. In data derived from the Copenhagen City Heart Study, a group of 1095 self-reported asthmatics had a higher rate of decline in their FEV_1 than nonasthmatic patients, 38 ml/year versus 22 ml/year. Smoking significantly accelerated this functional decline (146). Such studies suggest a fixed component of asthma and have given birth to the complex concept of airway remodeling, which involves changes in most airway components. Presumably, this results from protracted inflammation, although this relationship is not absolutely clear.

Remodeling is perhaps best considered in the context of injury and wound healing (3). Repair of injured tissue may involve two general processes: (*a*) the regeneration of parencymal components that restore normal structure and function and (*b*) the replacement of damaged airway tissues by connective tissue that may or may not be normal (126). Airway changes include wall thickening, subepithelial fibrosis, increased mucus production and goblet cell mass, myofibroblast hyperplasia, myocyte hyperplasia and hypertrophy, and epithelial cell hypertrophy.

The airway mass is 50%–300% greater in fatal asthma, and 10%–100% greater in nonfatal asthma, than in nonasthmatic controls (3). All layers of the airway wall are believed to contribute to this thickening. Early postmortem studies noted thickening of the epithelial basement membrane in asthmatics. The true basement membrane, the lamina densa, and the lamina rara appear normal. Thickening or subepithelial fibrosis is found within the lamina reticularis. Asthmatics, as well as patients with chronic rhinitis, have basement membrane thickening, but patients with chronic obstructive pulmonary disease do not. Increased amounts of type I, III, and V collagens make up the subepithelial fibrosis. This significance of the thickened lamina reticularis is not entirely clear, but in some studies, increasing degrees of fibrosis have been positively correlated with the asthma severity score and the response to methacholine (147).

Further increases in airway thickness result from both hypertrophy and hyperplasia of the airway myocytes. In fatal asthma, there is a marked increase in myocyte mass in the large central airways. The large, membranous bronchioles have a greater myocyte mass in nonfatal asthma (3). Whether hypertrophy or hyperplasia contributes to the majority of wall thickening is not firmly established. Two patterns have been demonstrated. Type I asthma features hyperplasia restricted to the central airways. In Type II asthma, fairly mild hyperplasia is seen in the central airways but hypertrophy is found peripherally (3, 148). Functionally, a thickened airway wall may cause more narrowing than a thin wall. This has been confirmed by computer modeling in a symmetrical dichotomous branching model of the tracheobronchial tree (126).

Mucus hypersecretion and airway obstruction due to mucus impaction are well-documented features of both fatal and nonfatal asthma. In the nonasthmatic airways, subepithelial mucous glands are distributed only in the cartilaginous airways. In asthma, they may also be present in the peripheral bronchioles (3). Hypersecretion of mucus reduces surface tension and increases the likelihood of airway collapse. Death from fatal asthma is most often due to endobronchial mucus plugging (126).

The events that lead to chronic airway remodeling are poorly understood. What limited data exist suggest that fibrogenic cytokines may play an essential role. Proteins of the TGF-B family are found in increased quantities in the BAL fluid of asthmatics and are produced in higher concentrations by eosinophils and fibroblasts from patients with severe and mild asthma (3). Matrix metalloproteinase–9 (MMP-9) is the major MMP found at sites of healing wounds. MMP-9 has been recovered in exaggerated quantities from sputum and biopsy samples of asthmatics (149). Some of the airway changes, particularly the subepithelial fibrosis, may correlate with attempts by the immune system to stop inflammation rather than direct toxic effects of inflammatory cells and cytokines.

IL-6 and IL-11 are involved in diminishing antigen-induced tissue inflammation and resulting injury. Both IL-6 and IL-11 have been found in exaggerated quantities in tissues and BAL fluids of patients with the asthmatic phenotype. Transgenic animal models that overexpress IL-6 and IL-11 develop impressive subepithelial fibrosis (148). It may be that IL-6 and IL-11, while diminishing tissue inflammation, promote subepithelial fibrosis and myocyte mitogenesis.

The significance of many of these chronic airway changes has yet to be fully explained. How these changes relate to the morbidity and mortality associated with asthma remains murky. Future investigation seems critical. New targets of therapy to prevent the long-term sequelae will probably be elucidated as these airway changes are better understood. It is clear, however, that asthma is no longer a disease of purely reversible airflow obstruction.

CONCLUDING REMARKS

In recent decades a vast amount of information has accumulated on the pathogenesis of asthma. The paradigm has shifted from one of primary smooth muscle dysfunction to reversible airway inflammation and now includes irreversible airway remodeling. Much of this article has focused on proposed imbalances between Th-1 and Th-2 lymphocytes, which favor a Th-2 predominance. However, even these data have recently been called into question by studies showing that Th-1 cells fail to ameliorate the asthmatic response and may even promote acute airway pathology (6, 7, 150). The jury is still out on the Th-2 phenomenon, and the paradigm may shift yet again.

Future investigations should continue to explore the relationship between Th-1 and Th-2 responses, what genetic and environmental factors determine, why Th-2 responses develop, and what role the Th-1 cell may have in perpetuating this inflammatory response. Research should also be directed to further delineate (*a*) the role of genetics in atopy and the individual response to environmental antigen, (*b*) airway smooth muscle mechanisms, and (*c*) the fundamental mechanisms of airway remodeling. Given the enormous amount of divergent information accumulated to date, it seems unlikely that a grand unification theory for asthma lurks on the horizon. Rather than defining a specific disease, the term asthma will probably turn out to describe a syndrome of reversible airflow obstruction, airway inflammation, persistent AHR, and airway remodeling mediated by pathogenic mechanisms that are restricted to specific gene/environment interactions.

ACKNOWLEDGMENT

This study was supported by grants from the National Institutes of Health (ES07498, ES06537, ES09607, and HL62628) and the Department of Veterans' Affairs (Merit Review).

Visit the Annual Reviews home page at www.AnnualReviews.org

LITERATURE CITED

1. National Institutes of Health. 1997. *Guidelines for the diagnosis and management of asthma. Rep. No. 97-4051.* Washington, DC: U.S. Dep. Health Hum. Serv., Natl. Heart Lung Blood Inst.
2. American Thoracic Society. 2000. Proceedings of the ATS workshop on refractory asthma: current understanding, recommendations, and unanswered questions. *Am. J. Respir. Crit. Care Med.* 162 (6):2341–51
3. Elias J, Zhum A, Chupp G, Homer R. 1999. Airway remodeling in asthma. *J. Clin. Invest.* 104(8):1001–6
4. Rosenstreich DL, Eggleston P, Kattan M, et al. 1997. The role of cockroach allergy and exposure to cockroach allergen in causing morbidity among inner-city children with asthma. *N. Engl. J. Med.* 336:1356–63
5. Palmer LJ, Cookson WO. 2000. Genomic approaches to understanding asthma. *Genome Res.* 10(9):1280–87
6. Castro M, Chaplin D, Walter M, Holtzman M. 2000. Could asthma be worsened by stimulating the T-helper type 1 immune response? *Am. J. Respir. Cell. Mol. Biol.* 22:143–46
7. Hansen G, Berry G, DeKruyff RH, Umetsu DT. 1999. Allergen-specific Th1 cells fail to counterbalance Th2 cell-induced airway hyperreactivity but cause severe airway inflammation. *J. Clin. Invest.* 103:175–83
8. Sandford A, Weir T, Pare P. 1996. The genetics of asthma. *Am. J. Respir. Crit. Care Med.* 153:1749–65
9. Holberg CJ, Halonen M, Wright AL, Martinez FD. 1999. Familial aggregation and segregation analysis of eosinophil levels. *Am. J. Respir. Crit. Care Med.* 160: 1604–10

10. Los H, Koppelman G, Postma D. 1999. The importance of genetic influences in asthma. *Eur. Respir. J.* 14:1210–27

11. Gray L, Peat J, Belousova E, et al. 2000. Family patterns of asthma, atopy and airway hyperresponsiveness: an epidemiological study. *Clin. Exp. Allergy* 30:393–99

12. Wiener A, Zieve I, Fries J. 1936. The inheritance of allergic disease. *Ann. Hum. Genet.* 7:141–62

13. Townley R, Bewtra A, Wilson A, et al. 1986. Segregation analysis of bronchial response to methacholine inhalation challenge in families with and without asthma. *J. Allergy Clin. Immunol.* 77:101–7

14. Lawrence S, Beasley R, Doull I, et al. 1994. Genetic analysis of atopy and asthma as quantitative traits and ordered polychotomies. *Ann. Hum. Genet.* 58:359–68

15. Edfors-Lubs M-L. 1971. Allergy in 7000 twin pairs. *Acta Allergologica* 26:249–85

16. Duffy DL, Martin NG, Battistutta D, et al. 1990. Genetics of asthma and hay fever in Australian twins. *Am. Rev. Respir. Dis.* 142:1351–58

17. Nieminen MM, Kaprio J, Koskenvuo M. 1991. A population-based study of bronchial ashthma in adult twin pairs. *Chest* 100:70–75

18. Skadhauge L, Christensen K, Kyvik K, Sigsgaard T. 1999. Genetic and environmental influence on asthma: a population-based study of 11,688 Danish twin pairs. *Eur. Respir. J.* 13:8–14

19. Harris JR, Magnus P, Samuelsen SO, Tambs K. 1997. No evidence for effects of family environment on asthma: a retrospective study of Norwegian twins. *Am. J. Respir. Crit. Care Med.* 156:43–49

20. Koppelman G, Los H, Postma D. 1999. Genetic and environment in asthma: the answer of twin studies. *Eur. Respir. J.* 13:2–4

21. Laitinen T, Rasanen M, Kaprio J, et al. 1998. Importance of genetic factors in adolescent asthma: a population-based twin-family study. *Am. J. Respir. Crit. Care Med.* 157:1073–78

22. Mrazek D, Pauls D, Anderson I, et al. 1989. Segregation analysis of 145 asthmatic families. *Am. J. Hum. Genet.* 45 (Suppl.):A245

23. Holberg CJ, Elston RC, Halonen M, et al. 1996. Segregation analysis of physician-diagnosed asthma in Hispanic and non-Hispanic white families. *Am. J. Respir. Crit. Care Med.* 154:144–50

24. Holgate ST. 1997. Asthma genetics: waiting to exhale. *Nat. Genet.* 15:227–29

25. Postma DS, Bleecker ER, Amelung PJ, et al. 1995. Genetic susceptibility to asthma-bronchial hyperresponsiveness coinherited with a major gene for atopy. *N. Engl. J. Med.* 333:894–900

26. Marsh DG, Neely JD, Breazeale DR, et al. 1994. Linkage analysis of IL4 and other chromosome 5q31.1 markers and total serum immunoglobulin E concentrations. *Science* 264:1152–56

27. Blumenthal M, Marcus-Bagley D, Awdeh Z, et al. 1992. HLA-DR2, [HLA-B7, SC31, DR2], and [HLA-B8, SC01, DR3] haplotypes distinguish subjects with asthma from those with rhinitis only in ragweed pollen allergy. *J. Immunol.* 148(2):411–16

28. Cookson WOC, Sharp PA, Faux J, et al. 1989. Linkage between immunologloblulin responses underlying asthma and rhinitis and chromosome 11q. *Lancet* June:1292–94

29. Shirakawa T, Li A, Dubowitz M, et al. 1994. Association between atopy and variants of the b subunit of the high-affinity immunoglobulin E receptor. *Nat. Genet.* 7:125–30

30. Barnes KC, Neely JD, Duffy DL, et al. 1996. Linkage of asthma and total serum IgE concentration to markers on chromosome 12q: evidence from Afro-Caribbean and Caucasian populations. *Genomics* 37:41–50

31. Moffatt MF, Hill MR, Cornelis F, et al. 1994. Genetic linkage of T-cell receptor

a/b complex to specific IgE responses. *Lancet* 343:1597–600

32. Daniels SE, Bhattacharrya S, James A, et al. 1996. A genome-wide search for quantitative trait loci underlying asthma. *Nature* 383:247–50

33. CSGA CSotGoA. 1997. A genome-wide search for asthma susceptibility loci in ethnically diverse populations. *Nat. Genet.* 15:389–92

34. Wjst M, Fischer G, Immervoll T, et al. 1999. A genome-wide search for linkage to asthma. *Genomics* 58:1–8

35. Ober C, Cox N, Abney M, et al. 1998. Genome-wide search for asthma susceptibility loci in a founder population. *Hum. Mol. Genet.* 7(9):1393–98

36. Turki J, Pak J, Green SA, et al. 1995. Genetic polymorphisms of the b2-adrenergic receptor in nocturnal and nonnocturnal asthma. *J. Clin. Invest.* 95:1635–41

37. Reihsaus Innis M, MacIntyre N, Liggett SB. 1993. Mutations in the gene encoding for the b2-adrenergic receptor in normal and asthmatic subjects. *Am. J. Respir. Cell Mol. Biol.* 8:334–39

38. Hall IP. 1996. b2 adrenoceptor polymorphisms: Are they clinically important? *Thorax* 51:351–53

39. Weir T, Mallek N, Sandford A, et al. 1998. b2-adrenergic receptor haplotypes in mild, moderate and fatal/near fatal asthma. *Am. J. Respir. Crit. Care Med.* 158:787–91

40. Israel E, Drazen J, Liffett S, et al. 2000. The effect of polymorphisms of the b2-adrenergic receptor on the response to regular use of albuterol in asthma. *Am. J. Respir. Crit. Care Med.* 162:75–80

41. Liggett S. 1997. Polymorphisms of the b2-adrenergic receptor and asthma. *Am. J. Respir. Crit. Care Med.* 156:S156–S162

42. Martinez FD, Graves PE, Baldini M, et al. 1997. Assoociation between genetic polymorphisms of the b2-adrenoceptor and response to albuterol in children with and without a history of wheezing. *J. Clin. Invest.* 100(12):3184–88

43. Walley A, Cookson W. 1996. Investigation of an interleukin-4 promoter polymorphism for associations with asthma and atopy. *J. Med. Genet.* 33:689–92

44. Burchard E, Silverman E, Rosenwasser L, et al. 1999. Association between a sequence variant in the IL-4 gene promoter and FEV$_1$ in asthma. *Am. J. Respir. Crit. Care Med.* 160:919–22

45. Zhu S, Chan-Yeung M, Becker A, et al. 2000. Polymorphisms of the IL-4, TNF-α, and FcεRIβ genes and the risk of allergic disorders in at-risk infants. *Am. J. Respir. Crit. Care Med.* 161:1655–59

46. Noguchi E, Shibasaki M, Arinami T, et al. 1998. Association of asthma and the interleukin-4 promoter gene in Japanese. *Clin. Exp. Allergy* 28:449–53

47. Heinzmann A, Mao X, Akaiwa M, et al. 2000. Genetic variants of IL-13 signalling and human asthma and atopy. *Hum. Mol. Genet.* 9(4):549–59

48. Hobbs K, Negri J, Klinnert M, et al. 1998. Interleukin-10 and transforming growth factor-β promoter polymorphisms in allergies and asthma. *Am. J. Respir. Crit. Care Med.* 158:1958–62

49. Baldini M, Lohman IC, Halonen M, et al. 1999. A polymorphism in the 5′ flanking region of the CD-14 gene is associated with circulating soluble CD14 levels and with total serum immunoglobulin E. *Am. J. Respir. Cell Mol. Biol.* 20:976–83

50. Moffatt M, Cookson W. 1997. Tumour necrosis factor haplotypes and asthma. *Hum. Mol. Genet.* 6:551–54

51. Trabetti E, Patuzzo C, Malerba G, et al. 1999. Association of a lymphotoxin (alpha) gene polymorphism and atopy in Italian families. *J. Med. Genet.* 36:323–25

52. Albuquerque R, Hayden C, Palmer L, et al. 1998. Association of polymorphisms within the tumour necrosis factor (TNF) genes and childhood asthma. *Clin. Exp. Allergy* 28:578–84

53. Wa T, Mansur A, Britton J, et al. 1999. Association between −308 tumour necrosis factor promoter polymorphism and

bronchial hyperreactivity in asthma. *Clin. Exp. Allergy* 29:1204–8

54. Hill MR, James AL, Faux JA, et al. 1995. FcεRIβ polymorphism and risk of atopy in a general population sample. *BMJ* 311:776–79

55. Trabetti E, Cusin V, Malerba G, et al. 1998. Association of the FcεRIβ gene with bronchial hyper-responsiveness in an Italian population. *J. Med. Genet.* 35:680–81

56. Hill M, Cookson W. 1996. A new variant of the β subunit of the high-affinity receptor for immunoglobulin E (FcεRI-β Ed237G): associations with measures of atopy and bronchial hyper-responsiveness. *Hum. Mol. Genet.* 5(7):959–62

57. Amelung P, Postma D, Xu J, et al. 1998. Exclusion of chromosome 11q and the FcεRI-β gene as aetiological factors in allergy and asthma in a population of Dutch asthmatic families. *Clin. Exp. Allergy* 28:397–403

58. Fryer A, Bianco A, Hepple M, et al. 2000. Polymorphism at the glutathione S-transferase GSTP1 locus. *Am. J. Respir. Crit. Care Med.* 161:1437–42

59. Gao P, Kawada H, Kasamatsu T, et al. 2000. Variants of NOS1, NOS2, and NOS3 genes in asthmatics. *Biochem. Biophys. Res. Comm.* 267:761–63

60. Hershey GK, Friedrich MF, Esswein LA, et al. 1997. The association of atopy with a gain-of-function mutation in the alpha subunit of the interleukin-4 receptor. *N. Engl. J. Med.* 337:1720–25

61. Ober C, Leavitt S, Tsalenko A, et al. 2000. Variation in the interleukin 4-receptor alpha gene confers susceptibility to asthma and atopy in ethnically diverse populations. *Am. J. Hum. Genet.* 66:517–26

62. In KH, Asano K, Beier D, et al. 1997. Naturally occurring mutations in the human 5-lipoxygenase gene promoter that modify transcription factor binding and reporter gene transcription. *J. Clin. Invest.* 99(5):1130–37

63. Katz RM, Lieberman J, Siegel SC. 1976. Alpha-1 antitrypsin levels and prevalence of Pi variant phenotypes in asthmatic children. *J. Allergy Clin. Immunol.* 57:41–45

64. Lazaro C, de Cid R, Sunyer J, et al. 1999. Missense mutations in the cystic fibrosis gene in adult patients with asthma. *Hum. Mutat.* 14:510–19

65. Stafforini DM, Satoh K, Atkinson DL, et al. 1996. Platelet-activating factor acetylhydrolase deficiency: a missense mutation near the active site of an anti-inflammatory phospholipase. *J. Clin. Invest.* 97:2784–91

66. MMWR. 1995. Current trends asthma—United States 1982–1992. *Morbid. Mortal. Wkly. Rep.* 43:952–55

67. Weiss KB, Wagener DK. 1990. Changing patterns of asthma mortality: identifying target populations at high risk. *JAMA* 264:1683–87

68. Weiss KB, Wagener DK. 1990. Geographic variations in US asthma mortality: small-area analyses of excess mortality, 1981–1985. *Am. J. Epidemiol.* 132(Suppl. 1):S107–S115

69. National Institutes of Health. 1991. *Executive summary: guidelines for the diagnosis and management of asthma. Rep. No. 91-3042.* Washington, DC: U.S. Dep. Health Hum. Serv., Natl. Heart Lung Blood Inst.

70. Evans R, Mulally DI, Wilson RW, et al. 1987. National trends in the morbidity and mortality of asthma in the United States. *Chest* 91(Suppl.):65S–74S

71. Sporik R, Holgate ST, Platts-Mills TA, Cogswell JJ. 1990. Exposure to house-dust mite allergen (Der p I) and the development of asthma in childhood. A prospective study. *N. Engl. J. Med.* 323(8):502–7

72. Young S, Le Souef PN, Geelhoed GC, et al. 1991. The influence of a family history of asthma and parental smoking on airway responsiveness in early infancy. *N. Engl. J. Med.* 324(17):1168–73. Erratum. 1991. *N. Engl. J. Med.* 325(10):747

73. Chan-Yeung M, Malo JL. 1995. Occupational asthma. *N. Engl. J. Med.* 333 (2):107–12

74. Samet JM, Lambert WE. 1991. Epidemiologic approaches for assessing health risks from complex mixtures in indoor air. *Environ. Health Perspect.* 95:71–74

75. Speizer FE. 1990. Asthma and persistent wheeze in the Harvard six cities study. *Chest* 98:191S–195S

76. Folkerts G, Busse W, Nijkamp F, et al. 1998. State of the art: virus-induced airway hyperresponsiveness and asthma. *Am. J. Respir. Crit. Care Med.* 157:1708–20

77. Michel O, Ginanni R, Duchateau J, et al. 1991. Domestic endotoxin exposure and clinical severity of asthma. *Clin. Exp. Allergy* 21:441–48

78. Michel O, Kips J, Duchateua J, et al. 1996. Severity of asthma is related to endotoxin in house dust. *Am. J. Respir. Crit. Care Med.* 154:1641–46

79. Park JH, Gold DR, Spiegelman DL, et al. 2001. House dust endotoxin and wheeze in the first year of life. *Am. J. Respir. Crit. Care Med.* 163(2):322–28

80. Gereda J, Leung D, Thatayatikom A, et al. 2000. Relation between house-dust endotoxin exposure, type 1 T-cell development, and allergen sensitisation in infants at high risk of asthma. *Lancet* 355:1680–83

81. Rylander R, Bake B, Fischer JJ, Helander IM. 1989. Pulmonary function and symptoms after inhalation of endotoxin. *Am. Rev. Respir. Dis.* 140:981–86

82. Schwartz DA, Thorne PS, Yagla SJ, et al. 1995. The role of endotoxin in grain dust-induced lung disease. *Am. J. Respir. Crit. Care Med.* 152:603–8

83. Schwartz DA, Donham KJ, Olenchock SA, et al. 1995. Determinants of longitudinal changes in spirometric functions among swine confinement operators and farmers. *Am. J. Res. Crit. Care Med.* 151: 47–53

84. Kennedy SM, Christiani DC, Eisen EA, et al. 1987. Cotton dust and endotoxin exposure-response relationships in cotton textile workers. *Am. Rev. Respir. Dis.* 135:194–200

85. Haglind P, Rylander R. 1984. Exposure to cotton dust in an experimental cardroom. *Br. J. Ind. Med.* 41:340–45

86. Rylander R, Haglind P, Lundholm M. 1985. Endotoxin in cotton dust and respiratory function decrement among cotton workers in an experimental cardroom. *Am. Rev. Respir. Dis.* 131:209–13

87. Donham K, Haglind P, Peterson Y, 1989. Environmental and health studies of farm workers in Swedish swine confinement buildings. *Br. J. Ind. Med.* 46:31–37

88. Thelin A, Tegler O, Rylander R. 1984. Lung reactions during poultry handling related to dust and bacterial endotoxin levels. *Eur. J. Respir. Dis.* 65:266–71

89. Shirakawa T, Enomoto T, Shimazu SI, Hopkin JM. 1997. The inverse association between tuberculin responses and atopic disorder. *Science* 275:77–79

90. Chan-Yeung M, Manfreda J, Dimich-Ward H. 2000. A randomized controlled study on the effectiveness of a multifaceted intervention program in the primary prevention of asthma in high-risk infants. *Arch. Pediatr. Adolesc. Med.* 154:657–63

91. Cookson W. 1999. The alliance of genes and environment in asthma and allergy. *Nature* 402(Suppl.):B5–B11

92. Kishimoto K, Dong VM, Issazadeh S, et al. 2000. The role of CD154-CD40 versus CD28-B7 costimulatory pathways in regulating allogeneic Th1 and Th2 responses in vivo. *J. Clin. Invest.* 106(1):63–72

93. Gern J, Lemanske RF Jr, Busse W. 1999. Early life origins of asthma. *J. Clin. Invest.* 104(7):837–43

94. Wegmann T, Lin H, Guilbert L, Mosmann T. 1993. Bidirectional cytokine interactions in the maternal-fetal relationship: Is successful pregnancy a Th2 phenomenon? *Immunol. Today* 14(7):353–56

95. Mellor AL, Munn DH. 2000. Immunology at the maternal-fetal interface: lessons for T cell tolerance and suppression. *Annu. Rev. Immunol.* 18:367–91

96. Alm JS, Swartz J, Lilja G, et al. 1999. Atopy in children of families with an anthroposophic lifestyle. *Lancet* 353 (9163):1485–88

97. Sigurs N. 2001. Epidemiologic and clinical evidence of a respiratory syncytial virus-reactive airway disease link. *Am. J. Respir. Crit. Care Med.* 163:S2–6

98. Christiansen S. 2000. Day care, siblings, and asthma—please, sneeze on my child. *N. Engl. J. Med.* 343(8):574–75

99. Ball T, Castro-Rodriguez J, Griffith K, et al. 2000. Siblings, day-care attendance, and the risk of asthma and wheezing during childhood. *N. Engl. J. Med.* 343:538–43

100. Busse WW, Lemanske RF. 2001. Asthma. *N. Engl. J. Med.* 344(5):350–62

101. Peat JK, Britton WJ, Salome CM, Woolcock AJ. 1987. Bronchial hyperresponsiveness in two populations of Australian schoolchildren. III. Effect of exposure to environmental allergens. *Clin. Allergy* 17(4):291–300

102. Zimmerman B, Feanny S, Reisman J, et al. 1988. Allergy in asthma. I. The dose relationship of allergy to severity of childhood asthma. *J. Allergy Clin. Immunol.* 81(1):63–70

103. Stempel DA, Clyde WA Jr., Henderson FW, Collier AM. 1980. Serum IgE levels and the clinical expression of respiratory illnesses. *J. Pediatr.* 97(2):185–90

104. Giles GG, Lickiss N, Gibson HB, Shaw K. 1984. Respiratory symptoms in Tasmanian adolescents: a follow up of the 1961 birth cohort. *Aust. NZ J. Med.* 14(5):631–37

105. Peat JK, Britton WJ, Salome CM, Woolcock AJ. 1987. Bronchial hyperresponsiveness in two populations of Australian schoolchildren. II. Relative importance of associated factors. *Clin. Allergy* 17(4):283–90

106. Peat JK, Salome CM, Woolcock AJ. 1992. Factors associated with bronchial hyperresponsiveness in Australian adults and children. *Eur. Respir. J.* 5(8):921–29

107. Platts-Mills TAE, Carter MC. 1997. Asthma and indoor exposure to allergies. *N. Engl. J. Med.* 336(19):1382–84

108. Platts-Mills T, Rakes G, Heymann P. 2000. The relevance of allergen exposure to the development of asthma in childhood. *J. Allergy Clin. Immunol.* 105: S503–S8

109. Mosmann TR, Cherwinski H, Bond MW, et al. 1986. Two types of murine helper T cell clone. I. Definition according to profiles of lymphokine activities and secreted proteins. *J. Immunol.* 136(7):2348–57

110. Abbas AK, Murphy KM, Sher A. 1996. Functional diversity of helper T lymphocytes. *Nature* 383(6603):787–93

111. Robinson D, Hamid Q, Ying S, et al. 1992. Predominant TH2-like bronchoalveolar T-lymphocyte population in atopic asthma. *N. Engl. J. Med.* 326(5):298–304

112. Hsieh CS, Macatonia SE, Tripp CS, et al. 1993. Development of TH1 CD4+ T cells through IL-12 produced by Listeria-induced macrophages. *Science* 260(5107):547–49

113. Gazzinelli RT, Hieny S, Wynn TA, et al. 1993. Interleukin 12 is required for the T-lymphocyte-independent induction of interferon gamma by an intracellular parasite and induces resistance in T-cell-deficient hosts. *Proc. Natl. Acad. Sci. USA* 90(13):6115–19

114. Hou J, Schindler U, Henzel WJ, et al. 1994. An interleukin-4-induced transcription factor: IL-4 Stat. *Science* 265 (5179):1701–6

115. Humbert M, Durham SR, Ying S, et al. 1996. IL-4 and IL-5 mRNA and protein in bronchial biopsies from patients with atopic and nonatopic asthma: evidence against "intrinsic" asthma being a distinct immunopathologic entity. *Am. J. Respir. Crit. Care Med.* 154:1497–504

116. Nakamura Y, Ghaffar O, Olivenstein R, et al. 1999. Gene expression of the GATA-3 transcription factor is increased in atopic asthma. *J. Allergy Clin. Immunol.* 103:215–22

117. Holt PG. 2000. Antigen presentation in the lung. *Am. J. Respir. Crit. Care Med.* 162:S151–56

118. Doucet C, Brouty-Boye D, Pottin-Clemenceau C, et al. 1998. IL-4 and IL-13 specifically increase adhesion molecule and inflammatory cytokine expression in human lung fibroblasts. *Int. Immunol.* 10(10):1421–33

119. Shi HZ, Deng JM, Xu H, et al. 1998. Effect of inhaled interleukin-4 on airway hyperreactivity in asthmatics. *Am. J. Respir. Crit. Care Med.* 157:1818–21

120. Zhu Z, Homer R, Wang Z, et al. 1999. Pulmonary expression of interleukin-13 causes inflammation, mucas hypersecretion, subepithelial fibrosis, physiologic abnormalities, and eotaxin production. *J. Clin. Invest.* 103:779–88

121. Azzawi M, Bradley B, Jeffrey PK, et al. 1990. Identification of activated T lymphocytes and eosinophils in bronchial biopsies in stable atopic asthma. *Am. Rev. Respir. Dis.* 142:1407–13

122. Jeffery PK, Wardlaw AJ, Nelson FC, et al. 1989. Bronchial biopsies in asthma: an ultrastructural, quantitative study and correlation with hyperreactivity. *Am. Rev. Respir. Dis.* 140:1745–53

123. Maestrelli P, Occari P, Turato G, et al. 1997. Expression of interleukin (IL)-4 and IL-5 proteins in asthma induced by toluene diisocyanate (TDI). *Clin. Exp. Allergy* 27(11):1292–98

124. Coyle AJ, Le Gros G, Bertrand C, et al. 1995. Interleukin-4 is required for the induction of lung Th2 mucosal immunity. *Am. J. Respir. Cell Mol. Biol.* 13(1):54–59

125. Wills-Karp M, Luyimbazi J, Xu X, et al. 1998. Interleukin-13: central mediator of allergic asthma. *Science* 282:2258–61

126. Bousquet J, Jeffery P, Busse W, et al. 2000. Asthma: from bronchoconstriction to airways inflammation and remodeling. *Am. J. Respir. Crit. Care Med.* 161:1720–45

127. Rothenberg ME. 1998. Eosinophilia. *N. Engl. J. Med.* 338(22):1592–600

128. Hanazawa T, Kharitonov SA, Barnes PJ. 2000. Increased nitrotyrosine in exhaled breath condensate of patients with asthma. *Am. J. Respir. Crit. Care Med.* 162:1273–76

129. Hoffmann J, Kafatos F, Janeway CJ, Ezekowitz R. 1999. Phylogenetic perspectives in innate immunity. *Science* 284:1313–18

130. Medzhitov R, Janeway CA. 1997. Innate immunity: the virtues of a nonclonal system of recognition. *Cell* 91:295–98

131. Wright SD. 1999. Toll, a new piece in the puzzle of innate immunity. *J. Exp. Med.* 189(4):605–9

132. Medzhitov R, Janeway CA. 1997. Innate immunity: impact on the adaptive immune response. *Curr. Opin. Immunol.* 9:4–9

133. Bonner JC, Rice AB, Lindroos PM, et al. 1998. Induction of the lung myofibroblast PDGF receptor system by urban ambient particles from Mexico City. *Am. J. Respir. Cell Mol. Biol.* 19:672–80

134. Michel O, Duchateau J, Sergysels R. 1989. Effect of inhaled endotoxin on bronchial reactivity in asthmatic and normal subjects. *J. Appl. Physiol.* 66:1059–64

135. Eldridge M, Peden D. 2000. Allergen provocation augments endotoxin-induced nasal inflammation in subjects with atopic asthma. *J. Allergy Clin. Immunol.* 105:475–81

136. Dubin W, Martin TR, Swoveland P, et al. 1996. Asthma and endotoxin: lipopolysaccharide-binding protein and soluble CD14 in bronchoalveolar compartment. *Am. J. Physiol. Lung Cell Mol. Physiol.* 270:L736–L744

137. Tulic M, Wale J, Holt P, Sly P. 2000. Modification of the inflammatory

response to allergen challenge after exposure to bacterial lipopolysaccharide. *Am. J. Respir. Cell Mol. Biol.* 22:604–12

138. Grunig G, Warnock M, Wakil AE, et al. 1998. Requirement for IL-13 independently of IL-4 in experimental asthma. *Science* 282:2261–63

139. Milton D, Wypij D, Kriebel D, et al. 1996. Endotoxin exposure-response in a fiberglass manufacturing facility. *Am. J. Ind. Med.* 29:3–13

140. Michel O, Ginanni R, Le Bon B, et al. 1992. Inflammatory response to acute inhalation of endotoxin in asthmatic patients. *Am. Rev. Respir. Dis.* 146:352–57

141. Zhiping W, Malmberg P, Larsson B-M, et al. 1996. Exposure to bacteria in swinehouse dust and acute inflammatory reactions in humans. *Am. J. Respir. Crit. Care Med.* 154:1261–66

142. George C, Jin H, Wohlford-Lenane C, et al. 2001. Endotoxin responsiveness and subchronic grain dust-induced airway disease. *Am. J. Physiol. Lung Cell Mol. Physiol.* 280:L203–L213

143. Dockery DW, Pope CA, Xu X, et al. 1993. An association between air pollution and mortality in six U.S. cities. *N. Engl. J. Med.* 329(24):1754–59

144. Becker S, Soukup JM, Gilmour MI, Devlin RB. 1996. Stimulation of human and rat alveolar macrophages by urban air particulates: effects on oxidant radical generation and cytokine production. *Toxicol. Appl. Pharmacol.* 141:637–48

145. Kleeberger S, Reddy S, Zhang L, Jedlicka A. 2000. Genetic susceptibility to ozone-induced lung hyperpermeability. Role of toll-like receptor 4. *Am. J. Respir. Cell Mol. Biol.* 22:620–27

146. Lange P, Parner J, Vestbo J, et al. 1998. A 15-year follow-up study of ventilatory function in adults with asthma. *N. Engl. J. Med.* 339:1194–200

147. Chetta A, Forest A, Del Donno M, et al. 1997. Airways remodeling is a distinctive feature of asthma and is related to severity of disease. *Chest* 111:852–57

148. Elias JA. 2000. Airway remodeling in asthma. Unanswered questions. *Am. J. Respir. Crit. Care Med.* 161:S168–71

149. Vignola A, Riccobono L, Mirabella A, et al. 1998. Sputum metalloproteinase-9/tissue inhibitor of metalloproteinase-1 ratio correlates with airflow obstruction in asthma and chronic bronchitis. *Am. J. Respir. Crit. Care Med.* 158:1945–50

150. Randolph DA, Carruthers CJ, Szabo SJ, et al. 1999. Modulation of airway inflammation by passive transfer of allergen-specific Th1 and Th2 cells in a mouse model of asthma. *J. Immunol.* 162(4):2375–83

Annu. Rev. Med. 2002. 53:499–518

VIRAL PERSISTENCE: HIV's Strategies of Immune System Evasion

Welkin E. Johnson and Ronald C. Desrosiers
*New England Regional Primate Research Center, One Pine Hill Drive, Southborough,
Massachusetts 01772-9102; e-mail: ronald_desrosiers@hms.harvard.edu*

Key Words   SIV, AIDS vaccine, antigenic escape, neutralizing antibody, lentivirus

■ **Abstract**   In contrast to most animal viruses, infection with the human and simian immunodeficiency viruses results in prolonged, continuous viral replication in the infected host. Remarkably, viral persistence is not thwarted by the presence of apparently vigorous, virus-specific immune responses. Several factors are thought to contribute to persistent viral replication, most notably the destruction of virus-specific T helper cells, the emergence of antigenic escape variants, and the expression of an envelope complex that structurally minimizes antibody access to conserved epitopes. Not as well understood, though potentially important, is the ability of at least one viral encoded protein (Nef) to prevent presentation of viral antigens in the context of major histocompatibility complex. The future success of antiviral therapies and vaccination strategies may depend largely on understanding how and to what degree each of these factors (and presumably others) contributes to immune evasion.

INTRODUCTION

All viruses are obligate, intracellular parasites, and as such depend on an unbroken chain of transmission for survival. For animal viruses, a major obstacle to forging every link in this chain is the encounter with the unique, adaptive immune response of each newly infected individual. In fact, spread of many viruses depends on frequent and rapid transmission during the acute phase of infection, in the days before the immune response clears the infection, or before the virus kills its host. It is not surprising that acutely infectious viruses, such as measles virus and influenza virus, are considered highly contagious.

A few viruses, including the herpes simplex viruses (HSV), can establish life-long, persistent infections. Transmission of HSV can occur during the initial, acute phase of infection and during intermittent periods of reactivation from a latent state. In between bouts of replication, the HSV genome is either silent or only minimally expressed, and the "infected" cell remains invisible to immune recognition. When they are expressed, such viruses are also subject to effective immune control; thus, persistence depends on establishing and maintaining latently infected cells.

In contrast, the human and simian immunodeficiency viruses (HIV and SIV) establish persistent infections distinguished by continuous, unrelenting viral replication. It is now clear that these viruses represent a unique mode of viral persistence (1). The challenge of understanding (and possibly controlling) HIV- and SIV-induced disease is to account for the unprecedented ability of these viruses to continue replicating even when the host has mounted apparently vigorous, virus-specific immune responses. In the following pages we discuss five features of HIV infection that are thought to contribute to this amazing capacity for immune evasion: (*a*) antigenic escape, (*b*) accessibility of antibody epitopes on the viral envelope complex, (*c*) downregulation of major histocompatibility complex (MHC), (*d*) destruction of CD4+ T helper cells, and (*e*) integration.

ANTIGENIC ESCAPE

The defining property of all retroviruses, including HIV and SIV, is conversion of the viral RNA genome into a double-stranded DNA molecule (2). This process is mediated by the viral reverse transcriptase (RT), an enzyme that is incorporated into the virion during viral assembly. Reverse transcription is completed during the early phase of infection, after entry of the viral nucleoprotein complex into the target cell cytoplasm. Expression of viral-encoded gene products occurs only after reverse transcription is complete and the resulting DNA provirus has been inserted into a host cell chromosome.

The extreme adaptability of retroviruses is an advantage conferred in part by RT, which determines the spectrum of mutations that will be generated during each round of viral replication. Because RTs have no proofreading activity, their error rates are several orders of magnitude higher than those of cellular DNA polymerases (3). Furthermore, RT has an intrinsic ability to "jump" between templates during DNA synthesis, leading to high rates of recombination between copackaged genomes, between viral and cellular RNAs, and between different regions of the viral genome (2). Finally, upon integration into the host cell, the provirus becomes a stable component of the host cell chromosome. As such, the provirus is subject to the same mutagenic processes that affect cellular genes, although their contribution to viral diversity is probably minimal compared to the effects of RT.

As a consequence of these properties, all manner of errors occur during retroviral replication, including transitions, transversions, insertions, deletions, and duplications of viral sequence. There may be biochemical biases toward particular types of substitutions (for example, some viral RTs demonstrate a propensity for G to A hypermutation), and sequence context can strongly influence the frequency of certain types of errors (2). Error rates for RT in vitro have been measured to be as high as 5×10^{-3} (errors per base pair) in some systems, and current estimates for the error rate of HIV-1 RT are as high as 10^{-4} (4, 5). Given that the genomes of HIV and SIV are approximately 10^4 nucleotides long, this predicts the occurrence of at least one error per viral genome per replication cycle. Put another way, most newly infected cells will, on average, contain a provirus that differs from the previous cell by about one mutation. Given that billions of cells are newly infected each day during chronic HIV infection, the potential exists for every possible point-mutant to be generated thousands of times each day in an infected individual (6). Such diversity is the fodder upon which selection feeds, and the consequences have been observed in HIV-infected patients as well as in animals experimentally infected with SIV. Viral escape from adaptive immune responses, including virus-specific cytotoxic T lymphocytes (CTLs), and antibody-mediated neutralization, are of particular relevance to vaccine development. Little information is available on escape from CD4 T helper cell recognition, but it is possible, perhaps even likely, that this also occurs (7).

Escape from Cytotoxic T Lymphocytes

Virally infected cells process short peptides from viral proteins and display them on the cell surface in conjunction with MHC class 1. The host's CTLs, which interact with specific combinations of peptide and MHC, can then recognize and destroy the infected cells. Because CTL responses in infected individuals appear early in infection and coincide with resolution of the acute phase of viral replication, it is reasonable to hypothesize that CTL activity will select for viral variants that can escape CTL recognition. The ability of altered peptide sequences to facilitate escape has been observed in studies on simple retroviruses (8, 9) and demonstrated definitively during experimental lymphocytic choriomeningitis virus (LCMV) infection of mice (10). Strong evidence for escape has been harder to obtain in HIV-1–infected individuals, but several cases have now been reported in which epitope alteration appeared to be strongly selected and reduced recognition of the altered peptides was demonstrated biochemically (11). One of the earliest examples of CTL escape was observed after adoptive transfer of cloned CTL to an HIV-infected patient. The transfused CTLs effectively mimicked an immunodominant CTL response and quickly selected for viral variants that had deleted a peptide epitope in the viral Nef protein (12). One of the more definitive studies demonstrating escape involved a single patient with a strong, immunodominant CTL response against the viral envelope protein (Env) (13). Because the patient was identified within weeks of initial infection, Borrow and coworkers were able to bank frequent blood samples and look for a temporal correlation between the onset of the highly immunodominant CTL response and the appearance of selected changes in the target epitope. Extensive analysis of sequences obtained at multiple time points by RT-PCR demonstrated the rapid appearance and fixation of a substitution in the second residue of the epitope; in vitro analysis suggested that substitutions at this residue reduced binding of the peptide to MHC, providing a mechanistic explanation for escape. Similar results have been reported for another patient (14), as well as for two patients in later stages of infection (15).

Definitive proof of CTL escape comes primarily from studies that took advantage of the SIV animal model for AIDS pathogenesis. Experimental infection of macaques with SIV results in patterns of viral replication and pathogenesis remarkably similar to those seen in HIV-1–infected patients, including an acute phase characterized by high levels of viremia, reduction of viremia coincident with the appearance of virus-specific CTL and antibodies, and a prolonged asymptomatic phase that eventually culminates in reduction in the numbers of CD4+ T cells, an increase in viral load, and development of opportunistic infections. One obvious advantage of studying the SIV-infected macaque is the much shorter duration of the asymptomatic stage. Other advantages of the SIV system bearing directly on studies of CTL escape are that (*a*) the viral inoculum is typically a genetically defined, clonal stock; (*b*) the exact time of infection is known; (*c*) multiple animals can be injected in parallel with the same virus stock; and (*d*) animals can be chosen whose MHC haplotypes (and any corresponding viral epitopes) are known.

In one study, immunization of two macaques with pooled peptides corresponding to CTL eptitopes in the SIV Nef and Gag proteins led to CTL responses directed toward a single epitope in Nef (16). Challenge of the vaccinated animals with SIV led to the selection of a viral variant containing a difference of one amino acid in the Nef epitope (A136T). In one animal, an additional escape variant eventually emerged that contained a second substitution in the same peptide (G131E + A136T). Chromium release assays revealed strong, specific lysis of cells pulsed with the parental peptide, diminished lysis of cells pulsed with the singly substituted peptide (A136T), and no significant lysis of cells pulsed with the doubly substituted peptide (G131E + A136T). Retrospective sequence analysis revealed that the first variant virus (A136T) was present in the original SIV challenge stock. The second variant (G131E + A136T) was not detectable in the stock and probably represents a mutation that emerged during viral replication in the animal.

One convincing demonstration of selection for CTL escape came from a well-controlled study in which five closely related, MHC-defined rhesus monkeys were experimentally infected in parallel with identical doses of the same SIV stock (17). The investigators concentrated on five well-defined viral epitopes, including three epitopes in *nef* and two epitopes in *env* (18). Two animals whose MHC did not restrict any of the five epitopes progressed rapidly to disease. In the remaining three animals, progression to disease was delayed and may have correlated with the number of epitopes recognized. Importantly, each of these three animals recognized different but overlapping subsets of the five epitopes, providing important internal controls. Sequence analysis revealed evidence for selection at each CTL epitope only in those animals genetically predisposed to recognize that particular epitope, whereas there was no obvious selection operating on epitopes in those animals whose haplotypes excluded recognition (17).

One of the first viral proteins synthesized after infection of a cell is the regulatory Tat protein, and interestingly, Allen et al. found that one of the earliest and strongest CTL responses to SIV in experimentally infected monkeys was directed to Tat (19). There was strong evidence of selection for escape at an epitope in Tat, with escape variants emerging during acute infection and reaching fixation within the first two months of infection. In the same time frame, escape from CTL recognizing the viral Gag protein was not apparent in the same animals. It has been proposed that for CTL-mediated killing of infected cells to be most effective, cells should be lysed before the emergence of progeny virions (20). Hypothetically, CTLs that recognize viral peptides presented early after infection of a cell have a better chance of destroying the cell before virus production ensues. It is interesting to speculate that because Tat is synthesized earlier than Gag in the course of infection of a cell, CTL-mediated selection against the Tat epitope may be stronger than selection operating on the Gag epitope. However, it is also possible that there is less cost associated with changes in the Tat epitope; that is, substitutions in the Gag epitope may have been more severely counterselected (21).

At what level do mutations that result in escape from CTL operate? In vitro experiments with peptide-pulsed cells reveal that, in most cases, the selected changes in the epitope interfere with the binding of peptide to MHC or weaken the stability of the peptide-MHC interaction. Alternative mechanisms have been observed, including loss of recognition by the corresponding T cell receptor, inefficient or incorrect processing of peptide, and antagonism (11, 20).

Escape from Antibody-Mediated Neutralization

Although the exact mechanisms by which antibodies control HIV and SIV in vivo are difficult to ascertain, a correlation between protection in vivo and the ability of an antibody (or antibody-containing serum) to block infection of cultured target cells in vitro has been observed in passive transfer experiments (22–26). Neutralization assays typically involve preincubating virus with serial dilutions of serum, then adding the virus/serum mixture to target cells in culture. Neutralization is then quantified as the maximum dilution that will effectively reduce infectivity by a given percentage (typically reported as 50% or 90% neutralizing-antibody titer). If antibody-mediated mechanisms contribute to the immunologic control of viral replication, then it is reasonable to expect that the antibody response will select for viral variants that escape antibody recognition.

The simplest demonstrations of viral escape from neutralizing antibody involved selection of virus growing in culture in the presence of a neutralizing antibody or serum sample of known specificity (27–33). Growth of HIV-1 in the presence of the neutralizing antibody G3-4, which recognizes a linear epitope in the V2 domain of gp120, selected for escape variants with single-amino-acid changes that altered recognition of the antibody binding site (33). When selection operates at multiple sites, as might be expected in a polyclonal antibody response, global alterations in the envelope complex affecting multiple sites may be preferentially selected. For example, when Reitz et al. selected for escape in the presence of neutralizing antiserum, a single-amino-acid change in gp41 altered the exposure of multiple antibody-binding sites in gp120 (30, 32, 34). Similarly, Park et al. demonstrated that changes in different regions of the envelope complex can cooperate to influence overall neutralization sensitivity (35).

But is escape an immune evasion strategy in vivo? Traditionally, a case can be made for escape when a temporal correlation is observed between the emergence of a neutralizing antibody response and the subsequent appearance of neutralization-resistant viral variants. Evidence for escape from neutralizing antibodies has been observed for nonprimate lentiviruses such as equine infectious anemia virus (EIAV) (36, 37), the Visna-viruses of sheep (38), and feline immunodeficiency virus (FIV) (39–41). HIV-1 escape from passively transferred antibody has been observed in SCID-Hu mice (42). Escape has also been noted in chimpanzees experimentally infected with HIV-1 (43), and in a laboratory worker accidentally infected with a laboratory isolate of HIV-1 (44–46). There are also numerous reports of escape in HIV-1 patients (47–51). However, signs of escape in naturally infected AIDS patients are often difficult to corroborate at the genetic level. In most cases, the viral sequence(s) that initiated infection are not precisely known, and may have been a complex mixture of variants; the elapsed time since infection, which is relevant to maturation of neutralizing antibodies, is not always known; and analysis may be complicated by therapeutic interventions on behalf of the patient, such as treatment with antiviral drugs. In this regard, experimental infections of animals with SIV or chimeric simian-human immunodeficiency viruses (SHIV) are especially useful, because the sequence of putative escape variants can be directly compared to the viral sequences used to initiate infection. Cloned virus of defined sequence may be used to initiate these experimental monkey infections. Furthermore, in experimental animal systems, evidence can be obtained from multiple animals, and putative "escape" mutants can also be cloned and passaged in naive animals for further assessment.

Convincing experimental demonstration of escape in SIV-infected animals was first reported by Burns et al. (52). Rhesus monkeys were infected with SIVmac239, a molecularly cloned virus for which the entire genomic sequence was already known (53). Careful comparison of viral envelope sequences obtained from the original inoculum and at several time points during the course of infection revealed strong selective pressure working on the envelope sequences, as evidenced by an extraordinarily high ratio of nonsynonomous to synonomous substitutions within the variable regions of the envelope protein (54). Specifically, more than 95% of all the nucleotide changes in the gp120 envelope protein resulted in an amino acid change (in the absence of selection, random substitutions are expected to lead to nonsynonomous changes only about 70% of the time) (54). Furthermore, it was demonstrated that sequential plasma samples recovered from infected animals could neutralize virus from the starting inoculum but were ineffective against variants that emerged during infection (52, 55).

EPITOPE ACCESSIBILITY

The HIV envelope complex is expressed on the surface of virions and infected cells and is therefore the most likely target for antibody-mediated immune mechanisms. The complex contains two subunits, the gp120 surface (SU) subunit and the gp41 transmembrane (TM) subunit. The subunit heterodimers are arranged as a multimer (likely to be a trimer), with the membrane-spanning domains of the gp41 subunits serving to anchor the complex in the lipid bilayer. Sequential interactions between specific residues in gp120 and the cellular receptor (CD4) and coreceptor (typically CCR5 or CXCR4) induce conformational changes that allow the gp41 protein to unfurl its hydrophobic N terminus and insert it into the target cell membrane. Refolding of gp41 then drives the fusion of the viral and cellular membranes, and the viral nucleoprotein core is released into the target cell cytoplasm (56, 57).

The HIV envelope complex is "exposed" on the surface of virions and infected cells, where selective forces have molded the complex in such a way as to reduce its overall immunogenicity while still maintaining its capacity to function during attachment and entry into target cells. In fact, the physical state of the envelope complex probably represents a compromise between replicative function and immune evasion. When the selective forces imposed by an immune response are removed, for example by growing viral isolates in cultured T cell lines, the envelope complex often acquires changes that increase the efficiency of viral replication but leave the virus sensitive to antibody-mediated neutralization. Viral strains that have been passaged extensively in culture are often referred to as T cell line adapted (TCLA) viruses, to distinguish them from primary, patient-derived viral isolates. In general, primary viral isolates are much less sensitive to antibody-mediated neutralization than their TCLA counterparts (58, 59).

Unlike HIV and SIV, acutely infectious viral agents are quite uniformly neutralization-sensitive. This is a direct reflection of the differences in propagation strategies. Acutely infectious agents work around the immune response by being highly contagious, relying on high levels of replication and transmission before the host mounts an immune attack. The replication strategy of HIV and SIV, involving a prolonged period of continuous replication in each infected individual, requires an envelope complex structure that sacrifices some efficiency in inherent infectivity in order to achieve a level of neutralization resistance not seen with the acute viruses.

HIV-infected patients and monkeys experimentally infected with SIV typically generate high levels of circulating antibodies that recognize both linear and conformational epitopes in gp120 and gp41. These antibodies generally react well with envelope monomers by ELISA and with gp120 and gp41 proteins in western blots. However, they react poorly, if at all, with the fully assembled complex on virions and the surface of infected cells. Recent advances in our understanding of the physical and immunogenic structure of the HIV-1 envelope proteins have led to the conclusion that the complex, as it exists on the surfaces of cells and virions, is highly resistant to recognition by the very antibodies its proteins invoke.

So what is the stimulus for the high levels of envelope-specific antibodies seen in infected patients? One popular theory is that monomeric gp120 and gp41, from spontaneously disassociated complexes or in the form of viral debris released from lysed cells, are largely responsible for the anti-Env antibody response (60). When antibodies do arise that recognize the envelope complex and neutralize viral infectivity, the relevant epitope(s) often fall within one of several highly variable regions of gp120 and result in a very strain-restricted pattern of reactivity. In addition to antigenic variation, structural features that make the HIV envelope complex resistant to antibodies include (*a*) transient exposure of epitopes only at critical moments during the entry process, (*b*) occlusion of conserved domains within the oligomer, (*c*) extrusion of variable domains from the exposed surfaces of the complex, and (*d*) extensive glycosylation of the envelope proteins. As a consequence of these features, discussed in more detail below, broadly effective, potent neutralizing antibodies against HIV and SIV are exceedingly rare.

Structural Features That Reduce Antibody Access to Envelope

THE ENVELOPE COMPLEX AND ENTRY   The two-receptor entry mechanism of HIV and SIV has not been observed among nonlentiviral members of the *retroviridae*. CD4 is referred to as the primary receptor, but in some ways the role of the coreceptor more closely resembles that of a traditional retroviral receptor (61). For example, interactions with the coreceptor facilitate completion of the fusion reaction (62), and there are variants of HIV-1, HIV-2, and SIV that can utilize the coreceptor directly, without prior interactions with CD4 (63–69). The converse, variants that utilize solely CD4, has not been observed. One attractive hypothesis is that the coreceptor resembles the original, ancestral receptor, and that the interaction with CD4 evolved later—possibly as a mechanism for concealing functionally conserved elements within the core of the envelope complex until an appropriate target cell is encountered (61).

The suggestion that the two-receptor mechanism functions as an immune evasion strategy is supported by the existence of CD4-induced (CD4i) epitopes. These conserved epitopes overlap the coreceptor binding elements of gp120 and are targeted by several potently neutralizing antibodies. In the native envelope complex, the CD4i epitopes are only weakly reactive with these antibodies. However, accessibility of the CD4i epitopes is greatly enhanced by the interaction of gp120 with CD4. Similar mechanisms may also limit the exposure of other conserved, functional residues in the envelope oligomer (70, 71). For example, conserved features of gp41 are exposed to the actions of inhibitors only during the fusion process (56, 72); antibody epitopes in this same region of gp41 may similarly be inaccessible in the prefusion state (73).

Also consistent with the hypothesis that the two-receptor entry mechanism is an immune evasion strategy is emerging evidence that CD4-independent viruses are extremely sensitive to antibody-mediated neutralization (74–76).

OCCLUSION   Mapping of antibody epitopes on gp120 identified two "faces" of the protein (77). Epitopes that mapped to the "neutralizing face" were characterized by antibodies that can also react with envelope oligomers and prevent viral replication in neutralization assays. In contrast, antibodies that recognized epitopes on the "non-neutralizing face" of gp120 were not effective in neutralization assays. The proposed explanation, borne out by mutagenesis, antibody mapping, and structural studies, is that the non-neutralizing face of gp120 is buried within the trimeric Env complex on the virion (58, 78). Similarly, a great many antibodies that react with the gp41 subunit do not interact with the envelope complex, most likely because the relevant epitopes are largely occluded by oligomeric interactions and overlapping domains of gp120.

VARIABLE LOOPS   Comparison of gp120 sequences from different HIV-1 isolates reveals the presence of discrete, highly variable domains interspersed among-more conserved regions (79). A similar pattern has also been noted for the gp120 molecules of SIV isolates. Most of these variable regions are flanked by conserved cysteine residues, which in turn form intrachain disulfide bonds (80–82). Thus, the variable regions came to be known as the variable loops. Antibody mapping and structural data indicate that the mature envelope oligomer folds in such a way that the variable loops lie on the exposed outer surface of the complex (71, 83, 84). Thus, the variable loops may serve as an antigenically variable shield covering the more conserved, functional elements within the core of the complex. Although not all of the loops can be deleted without abrogating viral replication, at least two groups have reported replication-competent isolates of HIV-1 lacking the V1 and/or V2 variable loops (85, 86). In both cases, the variable-loop deletion mutants were extremely sensitive to neutralization by antibodies and HIV-1 positive sera, supporting the variable-loop shield hypothesis. Although the hypothesis has not been directly confirmed in an animal model, experimentally infected monkeys quickly control replication of an SIV variant lacking the V1 and V2 variable loops, in a timeframe coincident with the onset of the antiviral antibody response (W.E. Johnson, R.C. Desrosiers, unpublished observations). Characterization of the specificity of the immune response in such animals should help to confirm the hypothesis.

GLYCOSYLATION   Oligosaccharides can be attached cotranslationally to proteins via an N-glycosidic linkage between the carbohydrate precursor and asparagine residues found within the motif asp-X-ser/thr. Evidence from HIV, SIV, and other viral systems has demonstrated that glycosylation can modulate the immunogenicity and antigenicity of viral surface proteins. The HIV and SIV envelope precursor protein (gp160) contains an average of 28 sites for N-linked glycosylation, including 24 sites in gp120 and 3–4 sites in gp41. Collectively, the N-glycans make up 50% of the mass of the extracellular portion of envelope (gp120 + the gp41 ectodomain), making these among the most densely glycosylated proteins known. Alterations in the number and placement of N-glycans in gp120 can modulate the exposure of antibody epitopes on the surface of the Env complex (87). For example, removal of an N-glycan attachment site from the V3 loop of HIV-1 markedly increased the virus' sensitivity to neutralizing antibodies (88, 89). Moreover, growth of a virus lacking an N-glycan in V3 in the presence of a V3-directed neutralizing antibody selected for rapid reversion of the N-glycan attachment site (31). SIV envelope genes cloned from experimentally infected animals during various stages of infection evolved new N-glycan attachment sites in the V1 loop (87, 90), and similar results have been observed with SHIV (91). N-glycan–deficient variants of SIV were used to demonstrate that specific N-glycans in the V1 loop of gp120 directly shield antibody epitopes in vivo (92). Sera from the monkeys infected with the N-glycan–deficient viruses could neutralize not only the homologous viruses but also the fully glycosylated parental virus, providing direct evidence that carbohydrate removal can increase the immunogenicity of an existing epitope. Another SIV mutant, lacking five glycans in the V1–V2 region of gp120, replicates to normal levels during acute infection but rapidly falls to low or undetectable levels concomitant with the onset of virus-specific immune responses (92).

DOWNREGULATION OF MAJOR HISTOCOMPATIBILITY COMPLEX

In addition to the four genes common to all retroviruses (*gag, pro, pol*, and *env*), primate lentiviruses contain several additional genes that encode the regulatory factors Tat and Rev and the accessory gene products Vif, Vpu, Vpr, Vpx, and Nef (93). Although the accessory genes are generally not required for viral replication in immortalized T cell lines, deletions of various subsets of these genes from SIV have measurable effects on viral replication and pathogenesis in experimentally infected animals (94). The *nef* gene, which is unique to the primate lentiviruses, contributes importantly to the virus' capacity to achieve high viral loads and to cause disease progression (95–98). *Nef* codes for a small (27–34 kDa) myristoylated protein and is among the first genes expressed after infection of a cell by HIV or SIV. This multifunctional protein interacts with components of several cellular signaling pathways (99, 100) and with the endocytic sorting machinery (101–104) of the newly infected cell. Among the numerous functions attributed to *nef*, one in particular has the potential to interfere with the antiviral immune response— downregulation of MHC class 1 from the surface of the infected cell.

The list of viral genes known to interfere with the antigen processing-and-presentation machinery of the cell is now quite extensive (105). Certain strains of adenovirus encode a protein (E3) that prevents MHC class I expression on the cell surface (106, 107). The ICP47 protein of herpes simplex virus inhibits the transporter associated with antigen processing (TAP), which transports processed peptides to the MHC complexes for presentation (108), and the K3 and K5 gene products of Kaposi's sarcoma–associated herpesvirus reroute MHCs from the cell surface (109, 110). The *nef* genes of HIV and SIV can now be added to this list. Nef has been shown to interfere with the expression of MHC class I proteins on the cell surface, and infected cells expressing high levels of Nef become resistant to destruction by MHC-restricted CTLs (111–113).

It is tempting to speculate that Nef-mediated downregulation of MHC in the infected host helps to protect infected cells from CTL-mediated destruction. However, downregulation in vitro is seen only at the highest levels of Nef expression, and the physiological relevance of this activity, or its relative importance to the total functional contribution of Nef, is yet to be demonstrated. Clearly, Nef expression is not sufficient to prevent the MHC-dependent induction of the vigorous, virus-specific CTL responses observed in most HIV-infected patients and experimentally infected rhesus monkeys. Of course, the effect of Nef could be subtle. In order for virus-specific CTL to be most effective, infected cells must be destroyed before they release infectious progeny virions (20). A small delay in the kinetics of CTL-mediated destruction of virus-producing cells could conceivably translate into a significant fitness advantage for the virus, simply by increasing the length of time during which progeny virions can be produced and released (20). Even if Nef expression does not completely block CTL, it may serve to delay cytolysis of the infected cell.

Besides being involved in recognition by CTL, MHC complexes are important in inhibiting destruction of healthy cells by natural killer (NK) cells. Nef-mediated downregulation of MHC, it turns out, is specific for certain classes of MHC but not others (102, 111, 114). Although this effect has only been observed in vitro, it suggests that selective downregulation of MHC by Nef has been fine-tuned to minimize antigen presentation by MHC as much as possible while still inhibiting NK-mediated cytolysis of infected cells (114). Specific motifs in the HIV and SIV Nef proteins that are required for MHC downregulation have been identified, and mutations in these motifs do not appear to interefere with other well-established functions of Nef (114–117). SIV variants containing such mutations in *nef* should be useful for determining the extent to which MHC downregulation contributes to viral replication and pathogenesis in vivo.

DESTRUCTION OF CD4+ T HELPER CELLS

The principal targets of HIV and SIV infection are cells expressing the cell-surface protein CD4 in conjunction with an appropriate coreceptor (e.g., the chemokine receptors CXCR4 or CCR5). Such targets include macrophages and CD4-positive subpopulations of T lymphocytes (118). Kinetic studies have shown that the vast majority of infected cells in HIV-infected patients and experimentally infected animals are CD4+ T cells, which are very rapidly destroyed by infection (119, 120). Infection of cultured cells is cytolytic, and infected cells in vivo may also be destroyed by immune-mediated mechanisms such as virus-specific CTL and antibody-dependent cellular cytotoxicity. Mechanisms have also been proposed by which ongoing HIV infection can lead to apoptosis of large numbers of uninfected "bystander" cells (121).

CD4+ T helper cells recognize infected cells and respond to sites of infection through interactions between the T cell receptor and antigen presented in the context of MHC class II on the surface of infected cells. Encounter with antigen activates T helper cells, which then orchestrate the activities of the CTL and B cell responses through the release of various lymphokines. Unfortunately for the infected host, activated CD4+ T cells are ideally suited for supporting the propagation of HIV-1. Although it typically takes several years for an infected individual to progress to AIDS, the scales may be tipped in favor of the virus during the first few weeks of infection by limiting the virus-specific CD4 helper cell response. In the absence of therapeutic intervention, patients in the early weeks of infection display significant defects in CD4+ T helper cell activity. T helper responses become difficult to detect using traditional proliferative assays (122, 123), and quantitative measurement of virus-specific CD4+ T helper cells in typical patients often requires sensitive, rapid assays of cytokine/chemokine production (124, 125). When acutely infected patients receive highly active antiretroviral therapy (HAART), virus-specific CD4+ T helper responses can be recovered (126), but in chronically infected patients this may become increasingly difficult to achieve as time passes (124). Early, viral-mediated destruction of CD4+ T cells appears to prevent coordination and maturation of the immune response sufficient to control or clear infection. During the long asymptomatic period of infection, virus replication not only leads to destruction of virus-specific memory T cells but slowly depletes the pool of naive T cells as they become activated in response to antigens (118). Eventually, homeostatic mechanisms fail to maintain normal CD4+ T cell levels and opportunistic infections take hold.

INTEGRATION AND REACTIVATION ("LATENCY")

After reverse transcription, the double-stranded DNA genomes of retroviruses are inserted irreversibly into the host cell's chromosomal DNA in a reaction directed by the viral integrase enzyme. HIV and SIV do not have a demonstrable mechanism for instituting programmed latency in an infected cell; instead, infection typically leads to the rapid production of progeny virions and death of the cell. However, it has recently been demonstrated that cells "latently" infected with HIV—that is, cells harboring an integrated viral genome but not expressing viral proteins—can arise at low frequency and persist for months or years in infected individuals (127–130). It is currently believed that the generation of such cells is a stochastic event and not specifically directed by any viral protein(s). In some instances, the degree of activation may determine the likelihood of latency versus productive infection in a given cell. The specific mechanisms by which such cells are thought to arise have been reviewed previously (129, 131) and are described elsewhere in this volume (132).

Unlike true latency (for example, as seen in HSV infection), the appearance of cells latently infected with HIV does not herald a cessation of viral replication elsewhere in the infected host. In fact, given the enormous rate of ongoing viral replication and turnover of CD4+ T cells in most HIV-infected individuals, it seems unlikely that the presence of latently infected cells is essential for viral persistence. However, this pool of cells has clinical significance for patients who are being treated with antiretroviral drugs. Because the genomes in these infected cells may persist for years, they can give rise to residual levels of viral replication during therapy, or reignite viremia if drug therapy is interrupted. Patients who have low or undetectable viral loads owing to successful drug therapy also display declines in their virus-specific T helper responses, probably due to the prolonged absence of antigen (124). For the many individuals who cannot stay on HAART indefinitely, therapeutic vaccination may be one way to maintain immune readiness and control the reemergence of replicating virus.

CONCLUSIONS

Traditionally, successful vaccines have targeted acutely infectious viral agents— that is, viruses that are typically well-controlled by the host's immune system (133). Such vaccines prevent progression to disease and limit transmission within a population. Viral agents that are controlled by vaccination also tend to be antigenically stable or, like influenza, vary little enough from cycle to cycle that a vaccine can be tailored to the predominant serotype on a seasonal basis. HIV does not have these qualifications; the virus replicates perfectly well in otherwise healthy individuals, despite strong, virus-specific immune responses, and can generate extreme viral diversity in just a few rounds of replication.

Improvements to current therapeutic interventions and progress in vaccine development for AIDS must preempt or circumvent the virus' strategies of immune evasion. Problems of the current drug treatment regimens include continuous drug intake for prolonged periods, side effects, antiviral drug resistance, rebounds in viral loads to pretreatment levels upon drug removal, and the failure of the antiviral immune responses to contain virus replication upon drug removal. Current efforts are largely directed to defining treatment regimens that allow the immune system to contain virus replication during prolonged periods in the absence of antiviral drugs.

Development of an effective vaccine for HIV-1 must similarly preempt or circumvent the immune evasion strategies of the virus. The severe difficulty in achieving vaccine protection against some SIV strains in monkey trials and the failure of many vaccine tests in monkeys attest to the overwhelming power of these immune evasion strategies. Breakthrough discoveries that will lead to an effective vaccine have probably not yet been made. Better understanding of the reasons why some vaccine tests in animals have been successful and why some rare individuals do manage to control their HIV-1 infections are promising avenues of continued investigation.

Visit the Annual Reviews home page at www.AnnualReviews.org

LITERATURE CITED

1. Ahmed R, Morrison LA, Knipe DM. 1996. Persistence of viruses. In *Fields Virology*, ed. BN Fields, DM Knipe, PM Howley, pp. 219–49. Philadelphia: Lippincott-Raven

2. Telesnitsky A, Goff SP. 1997. Reverse transcriptase and the generation of retroviral DNA. In *Retroviruses*, ed. JM Coffin, SH Hughes, HE Varmus, pp. 121–60. Plainview, NY: Cold Spring Harbor Lab. Press

3. Bebenek K, Kunkel TA. 1993. The

fidelity of retroviral reverse transcriptases. In *Reverse Transcriptase*, ed. AM Skalka, SP Goff, pp. 85–102. Plainview, NY: Cold Spring Harbor Lab. Press

4. Dougherty JP, Temin HM. 1986. High mutation rate of a spleen necrosis virus-based retrovirus vector. *Mol. Cell Biol.* 6:4387–95

5. Mansky LM, Temin HM. 1995. Lower in vivo mutation rate of human immunodeficiency virus type 1 than that predicted from the fidelity of purified reverse transcriptase. *J. Virol.* 69:5087–94

6. Coffin JM. 1995. HIV population dynamics in vivo: implications for genetic variation, pathogenesis, and therapy. *Science* 267:483–89

7. Harcourt GC, Garrard S, Davenport MP, et al. 1998. HIV-1 variation diminishes CD4 T lymphocyte recognition. *J. Exp. Med.* 188:1785–93

8. Green WR, Smith PM. 1996. Endogenous ecotropic and recombinant MCF mouse retroviral variation and escape from antiviral CTL. *Semin. Virol.* 7:49–60

9. Ossendorp F, Eggers M, Neisig A, et al. 1996. A single residue exchange within a viral CTL epitope alters proteasome-mediated degradation resulting in lack of antigen presentation. *Immunity* 5:115–24

10. Pircher H, Moskophidis D, Rohrer U, et al. 1990. Viral escape by selection of cytotoxic T cell–resistant virus variants in vivo. *Nature* 346:629–33

11. McMichael A. 1998. T cell responses and viral escape. *Cell* 93:673–76

12. Koenig S, Conley AJ, Brewah YA, et al. 1995. Transfer of HIV-1-specific cytotoxic T lymphocytes to an AIDS patient leads to selection for mutant HIV variants and subsequent disease progression. *Nat. Med.* 1:330–36

13. Borrow P, Lewicki H, Wei X, et al. 1997. Antiviral pressure exerted by HIV-1-specific cytotoxic T lymphocytes (CTLs) during primary infection demonstrated by rapid selection of CTL escape virus. *Nat. Med.* 3:205–11

14. Price DA, Goulder PJ, Klenerman P, et al. 1997. Positive selection of HIV-1 cytotoxic T lymphocyte escape variants during primary infection. *Proc. Natl. Acad. Sci. USA* 94:1890–95

15. Goulder PJ, Phillips RE, Colbert RA, et al. 1997. Late escape from an immunodominant cytotoxic T-lymphocyte response associated with progression to AIDS. *Nat. Med.* 3:212–17

16. Mortara L, Letourneur F, Gras-Masse H, et al. 1998. Selection of virus variants and emergence of virus escape mutants after immunization with an epitope vaccine. *J. Virol.* 72:1403–10

17. Evans DT, O'Connor DH, Jing P, et al. 1999. Virus-specific cytotoxic T-lymphocyte responses select for amino-acid variation in simian immunodeficiency virus Env and Nef. *Nat. Med.* 5:1270–6

18. Evans DT, Jing P, Allen TM, et al. 2000. Definition of five new simian immunodeficiency virus cytotoxic T-lymphocyte epitopes and their restricting major histocompatibility complex class I molecules: evidence for an influence on disease progression. *J. Virol.* 74:7400–10

19. Allen TM, O'Connor DH, Jing P, et al. 2000. Tat-specific cytotoxic T lymphocytes select for SIV escape variants during resolution of primary viraemia. *Nature* 407:386–90

20. McMichael AJ, Phillips RE. 1997. Escape of human immunodeficiency virus from immune control. *Annu. Rev. Immunol.* 15:271–96

21. Walker BD, Goulder PJ. 2000. AIDS. Escape from the immune system. *Nature* 407:313–14

22. Baba TW, Liska V, Hofmann-Lehmann R, et al. 2000. Human neutralizing monoclonal antibodies of the IgG1 subtype protect against mucosal simian-human immunodeficiency virus infection. *Nat. Med.* 6:200–6

23. Gauduin MC, Parren PW, Weir R, et al. 1997. Passive immunization with a human

monoclonal antibody protects hu-PBL-SCID mice against challenge by primary isolates of HIV-1. *Nat. Med* 3:1389–93

24. Mascola JR, Stiegler G, VanCott TC, et al. 2000. Protection of macaques against vaginal transmission of a pathogenic HIV-1/SIV chimeric virus by passive infusion of neutralizing antibodies. *Nat. Med.* 6:207–10

25. Parren PW, Ditzel HJ, Gulizia RJ, et al. 1995. Protection against HIV-1 infection in hu-PBL-SCID mice by passive immunization with a neutralizing human monoclonal antibody against the gp120 CD4-binding site. *AIDS* 9:F1–6

26. Shibata R, Igarashi T, Haigwood N, et al. 1999. Neutralizing antibody directed against the HIV-1 envelope glycoprotein can completely block HIV-1/SIV chimeric virus infections of macaque monkeys. *Nat. Med.* 5:204–10

27. McKeating JA, Gow J, Goudsmit J, et al. 1989. Characterization of HIV-1 neutralization escape mutants. *AIDS* 3:777–84

28. McKnight A, Weiss RA, Shotton C, et al. 1995. Change in tropism upon immune escape by human immunodeficiency virus. *J. Virol.* 69:3167–70

29. Mo H, Stamatatos L, Ip JE, et al. 1997. Human immunodeficiency virus type 1 mutants that escape neutralization by human monoclonal antibody IgG1b12. off. *J. Virol.* 71:6869–74

30. Reitz MS Jr., Wilson C, Naugle C, et al. 1988. Generation of a neutralization-resistant variant of HIV-1 is due to selection for a point mutation in the envelope gene. *Cell* 54:57–63

31. Schonning K, Jansson B, Olofsson S, Hansen JE. 1996. Rapid selection for an N-linked oligosaccharide by monoclonal antibodies directed against the V3 loop of human immunodeficiency virus type 1. *J. Gen. Virol.* 77:753–58

32. Watkins BA, Buge S, Aldrich K, et al. 1996. Resistance of human immunodeficiency virus type 1 to neutralization by natural antisera occurs through single amino acid substitutions that cause changes in antibody binding at multiple sites. *J. Virol.* 70:8431–37

33. Yoshiyama H, Mo H, Moore JP, Ho DD. 1994. Characterization of mutants of human immunodeficiency virus type 1 that have escaped neutralization by a monoclonal antibody to the gp120 V2 loop. *J. Virol.* 68:974–78

34. Thali M, Charles M, Furman C, et al. 1994. Resistance to neutralization by broadly reactive antibodies to the human immunodeficiency virus type 1 gp120 glycoprotein conferred by a gp41 amino acid change. *J. Virol.* 68:674–80

35. Park EJ, Vujcic LK, Anand R, et al. 1998. Mutations in both gp120 and gp41 are responsible for the broad neutralization resistance of variant human immunodeficiency virus type 1 MN to antibodies directed at V3 and non-V3 epitopes. *J. Virol.* 72:7099–107

36. Montelaro RC, Parekh B, Orrego A, Issel CJ. 1984. Antigenic variation during persistent infection by equine infectious anemia virus, a retrovirus. *J. Biol. Chem.* 259:10539–44

37. Salinovich O, Payne SL, Montelaro RC, et al. 1986. Rapid emergence of novel antigenic and genetic variants of equine infectious anemia virus during persistent infection. *J. Virol.* 57:71–80

38. Scott JV, Stowring L, Haase AT, et al. 1979. Antigenic variation in visna virus. *Cell* 18:321–27

39. Pancino G, Chappey C, Saurin W, Sonigo P. 1993. B epitopes and selection pressures in feline immunodeficiency virus envelope glycoproteins. *J. Virol.* 67:664–72

40. Siebelink KH, Rimmelzwaan GF, Bosch ML, et al. 1993. A single amino acid substitution in hypervariable region 5 of the envelope protein of feline immunodeficiency virus allows escape from virus neutralization. *J. Virol.* 67:2202–8

41. Siebelink KH, Huisman W, Karlas JA,

et al. 1995. Neutralization of feline immunodeficiency virus by polyclonal feline antibody: simultaneous involvement of hypervariable regions 4 and 5 of the surface glycoprotein. *J. Virol.* 69:5124–27

42. Andrus L, Prince AM, Bernal I, et al. 1998. Passive immunization with a human immunodeficiency virus type 1–neutralizing monoclonal antibody in Hu-PBL-SCID mice: isolation of a neutralization escape variant. *J. Infect. Dis.* 177:889–97

43. Nara PL, Smit L, Dunlop N, et al. 1990. Emergence of viruses resistant to neutralization by V3-specific antibodies in experimental human immunodeficiency virus type 1 IIIB infection of chimpanzees. *J. Virol.* 64:3779–91

44. Beaumont T, van Nuenen A, Broersen S, et al. 2001. Reversal of human immunodeficiency virus type 1 IIIB to a neutralization-resistant phenotype in an accidentally infected laboratory worker with a progressive clinical course. *J. Virol.* 75:2246–52

45. di Marzo Veronese F, Reitz MS Jr., Gupta G, et al. 1993. Loss of a neutralizing epitope by a spontaneous point mutation in the V3 loop of HIV-1 isolated from an infected laboratory worker. *J. Biol. Chem.* 268:25894–901

46. Weiss SH, Goedert JJ, Gartner S, et al. 1988. Risk of human immunodeficiency virus (HIV-1) infection among laboratory workers. *Science* 239:68–71

47. Albert J, Abrahamsson B, Nagy K, et al. 1990. Rapid development of isolate-specific neutralizing antibodies after primary HIV-1 infection and consequent emergence of virus variants which resist neutralization by autologous sera. *AIDS* 4:107–12

48. Arendrup M, Nielsen C, Hansen JE, et al. 1992. Autologous HIV-1 neutralizing antibodies: emergence of neutralization-resistant escape virus and subsequent development of escape virus neutralizing antibodies. *J. Acquir. Immune Defic. Syndr.* 5:303–7

49. Bradney AP, Scheer S, Crawford JM, et al. 1999. Neutralization escape in human immunodeficiency virus type 1-infected long-term nonprogressors. *J. Infect. Dis.* 179:1264–67

50. Tremblay M, Wainberg MA. 1990. Neutralization of multiple HIV-1 isolates from a single subject by autologous sequential sera. *J. Infect. Dis.* 162:735–37

51. Zhang PF, Chen X, Fu DW, et al. 1999. Primary virus envelope cross-reactivity of the broadening neutralizing antibody response during early chronic human immunodeficiency virus type 1 infection. *J. Virol.* 73:5225–30

52. Burns DP, Collignon C, Desrosiers RC. 1993. Simian immunodeficiency virus mutants resistant to serum neutralization arise during persistent infection of rhesus monkeys. *J. Virol.* 67:4104–13

53. Regier DA, Desrosiers RC. 1990. The complete nucleotide sequence of a pathogenic molecular clone of simian immunodeficiency virus. *AIDS Res. Hum. Retroviruses* 6:1221–31

54. Burns DP, Desrosiers RC. 1991. Selection of genetic variants of simian immunodeficiency virus in persistently infected rhesus monkeys. *J. Virol.* 65:1843–54

55. Burns DP, Desrosiers RC. 1994. Envelope sequence variation, neutralizing antibodies, and primate lentivirus persistence. *Curr. Top. Microbiol. Immunol.* 188:185–219

56. Chan DC, Kim PS. 1998. HIV entry and its inhibition. *Cell* 93:681–84

57. Weissenhorn W, Dessen A, Calder LJ, et al. 1999. Structural basis for membrane fusion by enveloped viruses. *Mol. Membr. Biol.* 16:3–9

58. Burton DR. 1997. A vaccine for HIV type 1: the antibody perspective. *Proc. Natl. Acad. Sci. USA* 94:10018–23

59. Moore JP, Cao Y, Qing L, et al. 1995. Primary isolates of human immunodeficiency virus type 1 are relatively resistant to neutralization by monoclonal antibodies to gp120, and their neutralization is

not predicted by studies with monomeric gp120. *J. Virol.* 69:101–9

60. Parren PW, Burton DR, Sattentau QJ. 1997. HIV-1 antibody—debris or virion? *Nat. Med.* 3:366–67

61. Berger EA, Murphy PM, Farber JM. 1999. Chemokine receptors as HIV-1 coreceptors: roles in viral entry, tropism, and disease. *Annu. Rev. Immunol.* 17:657–700

62. Doms RW, Moore JP. 2000. HIV-1 membrane fusion: targets of opportunity. *J. Cell Biol.* 151:F9–14

63. Bandres JC, Wang QF, O'Leary J, et al. 1998. Human immunodeficiency virus (HIV) envelope binds to CXCR4 independently of CD4, and binding can be enhanced by interaction with soluble CD4 or by HIV envelope deglycosylation. *J. Virol.* 72:2500–4

64. Dumonceaux J, Nisole S, Chanel C, et al. 1998. Spontaneous mutations in the *env* gene of the human immunodeficiency virus type 1 NDK isolate are associated with a CD4-independent entry phenotype. *J. Virol.* 72:512–19

65. Edinger AL, Mankowski JL, Doranz BJ, et al. 1997. CD4-independent, CCR5-dependent infection of brain capillary endothelial cells by a neurovirulent simian immunodeficiency virus strain. *Proc. Natl. Acad. Sci. USA* 94:14742–47

66. Endres MJ, Clapham PR, Marsh M, et al. 1996. CD4-independent infection by HIV-2 is mediated by fusin/CXCR4. *Cell* 87:745–56

67. Hoffman TL, LaBranche CC, Zhang W, et al. 1999. Stable exposure of the co-receptor-binding site in a CD4-independent HIV-1 envelope protein. *Proc. Natl. Acad. Sci. USA* 96:6359–64

68. Kolchinsky P, Mirzabekov T, Farzan M, et al. 1999. Adaptation of a CCR5-using, primary human immunodeficiency virus type 1 isolate for CD4-independent replication. *J. Virol.* 73:8120–26

69. Reeves JD, McKnight A, Potempa S, et al. 1997. CD4-independent infection by HIV-2 (ROD/B): use of the 7-transmembrane receptors CXCR-4, CCR-3, and V28 for entry. *Virology* 231:130–34

70. Sullivan N, Sun Y, Sattentau Q, et al. 1998. CD4-Induced conformational changes in the human immunodeficiency virus type 1 gp120 glycoprotein: consequences for virus entry and neutralization. *J. Virol.* 72:4694–703

71. Wyatt R, Sodroski J. 1998. The HIV-1 envelope glycoproteins: fusogens, antigens, and immunogens. *Science* 280:1884–88

72. Labrosse B, Treboute C, Alizon M. 2000. Sensitivity to a nonpeptidic compound (RPR103611) blocking human immunodeficiency virus type 1 Env-mediated fusion depends on sequence and accessibility of the gp41 loop region. *J. Virol.* 74:2142–50

73. Sattentau QJ, Zolla-Pazner S, Poignard P. 1995. Epitope exposure on functional, oligomeric HIV-1 gp41 molecules. *Virology* 206:713–17

74. Edwards TG, Hoffman TL, Baribaud F, et al. 2001. Relationships between CD4 independence, neutralization sensitivity, and exposure of a CD4-induced epitope in a human immunodeficiency virus type 1 envelope protein. *J. Virol.* 75:5230–39

75. Kolchinsky P, Kiprilov E, Sodroski J. 2001. Increased neutralization sensitivity of CD4-independent human immunodeficiency virus variants. *J. Virol.* 75:2041–50

76. Means RE, Matthews T, Hoxie JA, et al. 2001. Ability of the V3 loop of simian immunodeficiency virus to serve as a target for antibody-mediated neutralization: correlation of neutralization sensitivity, growth in macrophages, and decreased dependence on CD4. *J. Virol.* 75:3903–15

77. Moore JP, Sodroski J. 1996. Antibody cross-competition analysis of the human immunodeficiency virus type 1 gp120 exterior envelope glycoprotein. *J. Virol.* 70:1863–72

78. Parren PW, Burton DR. 2001. The antiviral activity of antibodies in vitro and in vivo. *Adv. Immunol.* 77:195–262

79. Starcich BR, Hahn BH, Shaw GM, et al. 1986. Identification and characterization of conserved and variable regions in the envelope gene of HTLV-III/LAV, the retrovirus of AIDS. *Cell* 45:637–48

80. Gregory T, Hoxie J, Watanabe C, Spellman M. 1991. Structure and function in recombinant HIV-1 gp120 and speculation about the disulfide bonding in the gp120 homologs of HIV-2 and SIV. *Adv. Exp. Med. Biol.* 303:1–14

81. Hoxie JA. 1991. Hypothetical assignment of intrachain disulfide bonds for HIV-2 and SIV envelope glycoproteins. *AIDS Res. Hum. Retroviruses* 7:495–99

82. Leonard CK, Spellman MW, Riddle L, et al. 1990. Assignment of intrachain disulfide bonds and characterization of potential glycosylation sites of the type 1 recombinant human immunodeficiency virus envelope glycoprotein (gp120) expressed in Chinese hamster ovary cells. *J. Biol. Chem.* 265:10373–82

83. Wyatt R, Kwong PD, Desjardins E, et al. 1998. The antigenic structure of the HIV gp120 envelope glycoprotein. *Nature* 393:705–11

84. Kwong PD, Wyatt R, Robinson J, et al. 1998. Structure of an HIV gp120 envelope glycoprotein in complex with the CD4 receptor and a neutralizing human antibody. *Nature* 393:648–59

85. Cao J, Sullivan N, Desjardin E, et al. 1997. Replication and neutralization of human immunodeficiency virus type 1 lacking the V1 and V2 variable loops of the gp120 envelope glycoprotein. *J. Virol.* 71:9808–12

86. Stamatatos L, Cheng-Mayer C. 1998. An envelope modification that renders a primary, neutralization-resistant clade B human immunodeficiency virus type 1 isolate highly susceptible to neutralization by sera from other clades. *J. Virol.* 72:7840–45

87. Overbaugh J, Rudensey LM. 1992. Alterations in potential sites for glycosylation predominate during evolution of the simian immunodeficiency virus envelope gene in macaques. *J. Virol.* 66:5937–48

88. Back NK, Smit L, De Jong JJ, et al. 1994. An N-glycan within the human immunodeficiency virus type 1 gp120 V3 loop affects virus neutralization. *Virology* 199:431–38

89. Schonning K, Jansson B, Olofsson S, et al. 1996. Resistance to V3-directed neutralization caused by an N-linked oligosaccharide depends on the quaternary structure of the HIV-1 envelope oligomer. *Virology* 218:134–40

90. Chackerian B, Rudensey LM, Overbaugh J. 1997. Specific N-linked and O-linked glycosylation modifications in the envelope V1 domain of simian immunodeficiency virus variants that evolve in the host alter recognition by neutralizing antibodies. *J. Virol.* 71:7719–27

91. Cheng-Mayer C, Brown A, Harouse J, et al. 1999. Selection for neutralization resistance of the simian/human immunodeficiency virus SHIVSF33A variant in vivo by virtue of sequence changes in the extracellular envelope glycoprotein that modify N-linked glycosylation. *J. Virol.* 73:5294–300

92. Reiter JN, Means RE, Desrosiers RC. 1998. A role for carbohydrates in immune evasion in AIDS. *Nat. Med.* 4:679–84

93. Frankel AD, Young JA. 1998. HIV-1: fifteen proteins and an RNA. *Annu. Rev. Biochem.* 67:1–25

94. Desrosiers RC, Lifson JD, Gibbs JS, et al. 1998. Identification of highly attenuated mutants of simian immunodeficiency virus. *J. Virol.* 72:1431–37

95. Deacon NJ, Tsykin A, Solomon A, et al. 1995. Genomic structure of an attenuated quasi species of HIV-1 from a blood transfusion donor and recipients. *Science* 270:988–91

96. Ringler DJ, Mori K, Panicali PK, et al. 1991. Importance of the nef gene for maintenance of high virus loads and for development of AIDS. *Cell* 65:651–62

97. Kirchhoff F, Greenough TC, Brettler DB,

et al. 1995. Brief report: absence of intact nef sequences in a long-term survivor with nonprogressive HIV-1 infection. *N. Engl. J. Med.* 332:228–32

98. Mariani R, Kirchhoff F, Greenough TC, et al. 1996. High frequency of defective nef alleles in a long-term survivor with nonprogressive human immunodeficiency virus type 1 infection. *J. Virol.* 70:7752–64

99. Herna Remkema G, Saksela K. 2000. Interactions of HIV-1 NEF with cellular signal transducing proteins. *Front. Biosci.* 5:D268–83

100. Saksela K. 1997. HIV-1 Nef and host cell protein kinases. *Front. Biosci.* 2:d606–18

101. Greenberg ME, Bronson S, Lock M, et al. 1997. Co-localization of HIV-1 Nef with the AP-2 adaptor protein complex correlates with Nef-induced CD4 down-regulation. *EMBO J.* 16:6964–76

102. Le Gall S, Erdtmann L, Benichou S, et al. 1998. Nef interacts with the mu subunit of clathrin adaptor complexes and reveals a cryptic sorting signal in MHC I molecules. *Immunity* 8:483–95

103. Lock M, Greenberg ME, Iafrate AJ, et al. 1999. Two elements target SIV Nef to the AP-2 clathrin adaptor complex, but only one is required for the induction of CD4 endocytosis. *EMBO J.* 18:2722–33

104. Piguet V, Chen YL, Mangasarian A, et al. 1998. Mechanism of Nef-induced CD4 endocytosis: Nef connects CD4 with the mu chain of adaptor complexes. *EMBO J.* 17:2472–81

105. Ploegh HL. 1998. Viral strategies of immune evasion. *Science* 280:248–53

106. Andersson M, Paabo S, Nilsson T, Peterson PA. 1985. Impaired intracellular transport of class I MHC antigens as a possible means for adenoviruses to evade immune surveillance. *Cell* 43:215–22

107. Burgert HG, Kvist S. 1985. An adenovirus type 2 glycoprotein blocks cell surface expression of human histocompatibility class I antigens. *Cell* 41:987–97

108. York IA, Roop C, Andrews DW, et al. 1994. A cytosolic herpes simplex virus protein inhibits antigen presentation to CD8+ T lymphocytes. *Cell* 77:525–35

109. Ishido S, Wang C, Lee BS, et al. 2000. Downregulation of major histocompatibility complex class I molecules by Kaposi's sarcoma-associated herpesvirus K3 and K5 proteins. *J. Virol.* 74:5300–9

110. Coscoy L, Ganem D. 2000. Kaposi's sarcoma-associated herpesvirus encodes two proteins that block cell surface display of MHC class I chains by enhancing their endocytosis. *Proc. Natl. Acad. Sci. USA* 97:8051–56

111. Collins KL, Chen BK, Kalams SA, et al. 1998. HIV-1 Nef protein protects infected primary cells against killing by cytotoxic T lymphocytes. *Nature* 391:397–401

112. Collins KL, Baltimore D. 1999. HIV's evasion of the cellular immune response. *Immunol. Rev.* 168:65–74

113. Schwartz O, Marechal V, Le Gall S, et al. 1996. Endocytosis of major histocompatibility complex class I molecules is induced by the HIV-1 Nef protein. *Nat. Med.* 2:338–42

114. Cohen GB, Gandhi RT, Davis DM, et al. 1999. The selective downregulation of class I major histocompatibility complex proteins by HIV-1 protects HIV-infected cells from NK cells. *Immunity* 10:661–71

115. Greenberg ME, Iafrate AJ, Skowronski J. 1998. The SH3 domain-binding surface and an acidic motif in HIV-1 Nef regulate trafficking of class I MHC complexes. *EMBO J.* 17:2777–89

116. Mangasarian A, Piguet V, Wang JK, et al. 1999. Nef-induced CD4 and major histocompatibility complex class I (MHC-I) down-regulation are governed by distinct determinants: N-terminal alpha helix and proline repeat of Nef selectively regulate MHC-I trafficking. *J. Virol.* 73:1964–73

117. Swigut T, Iafrate AJ, Muench J, et al. 2000. Simian and human immunodeficiency virus Nef proteins use different

surfaces to downregulate class I major histocompatibility complex antigen expression. *J. Virol.* 74:5691–701

118. Haase AT. 1999. Population biology of HIV-1 infection: viral and CD4+ T cell demographics and dynamics in lymphatic tissues. *Annu. Rev. Immunol.* 17:625–56

119. Ho DD, Neumann AU, Perelson AS, et al. 1995. Rapid turnover of plasma virions and CD4 lymphocytes in HIV-1 infection. *Nature* 373:123–26

120. Wei X, Ghosh SK, Taylor ME, et al. 1995. Viral dynamics in human immunodeficiency virus type 1 infection. *Nature* 373:117–22

121. Finkel TH, Tudor-Williams G, Banda NK, et al. 1995. Apoptosis occurs predominantly in bystander cells and not in productively infected cells of HIV- and SIV-infected lymph nodes. *Nat. Med.* 1:129–34

122. Lane HC, Depper JM, Greene WC, et al. 1985. Qualitative analysis of immune function in patients with the acquired immunodeficiency syndrome. Evidence for a selective defect in soluble antigen recognition. *N. Engl. J. Med.* 313:79–84

123. Rosenberg ES, Walker BD. 1998. HIV type 1-specific helper T cells: a critical host defense. *AIDS Res. Hum. Retroviruses* 14(Suppl. 2):S143–47

124. Pitcher CJ, Quittner C, Peterson DM, et al. 1999. HIV-1-specific CD4+ T cells are detectable in most individuals with active HIV-1 infection, but decline with prolonged viral suppression. *Nat. Med.* :518–25

125. Clerici M, Stocks NI, Zajac RA, et al. 1989. Interleukin-2 production used to detect antigenic peptide recognition by T-helper lymphocytes from asymptomatic HIV-seropositive individuals. *Nature* 339:383–85

126. Rosenberg ES, Altfeld M, Poon SH, et al. 2000. Immune control of HIV-1 after early treatment of acute infection. *Nature* 407:523–26

127. Chun TW, Stuyver L, Mizell SB, et al. 1997. Presence of an inducible HIV-1 latent reservoir during highly active antiretroviral therapy. *Proc. Natl. Acad. Sci. USA* 94:13193–97

128. Finzi D, Hermankova M, Pierson T, et al. 1997. Identification of a reservoir for HIV-1 in patients on highly active antiretroviral therapy. *Science* 278:1295–300

129. Pierson T, McArthur J, Siliciano RF. 2000. Reservoirs for HIV-1: mechanisms for viral persistence in the presence of antiviral immune responses and antiretroviral therapy. *Annu. Rev. Immunol.* 18:665–708

130. Wong JK, Hezareh M, Gunthard HF, et al. 1997. Recovery of replication-competent HIV despite prolonged suppression of plasma viremia. *Science* 278:1291–95

131. Finzi D, Siliciano RF. 1998. Viral dynamics in HIV-1 infection. *Cell* 93:665–71

132. Blankson JN, Siliciano RF. 2002. The challenge of viral reservoirs in HIV-1 infection. *Annu. Rev. Med.* 53:557–93

133. Ada G. 1999. The immunology of vaccination. In *Vaccines*, ed. SA Plotkin, WA Orenstein, pp. 28–39. Philadelphia: Saunders

Annu. Rev. Med. 2002. 53:519–40

BREAST CANCER RISK REDUCTION:
Strategies for Women at Increased Risk

Rowan T. Chlebowski
*Harbor-UCLA Research and Education Institute, 1124 W. Carson Street, Torrance,
California 90502-2064; e-mail: rchlebow@whi.org*

Key Words   selective estrogen receptor modulators (SERMs), prophylactic
mastectomy, prophylactic oophorectomy, tamoxifen, raloxifene

■ **Abstract**   Breast cancer risk reduction now represents an achievable medical objective. Current interventions include selective estrogen receptor modulators (SERMs),
prophylactic surgery, and lifestyle change. For SERMs, current evidence supports
tamoxifen use for breast cancer risk reduction whereas raloxifene requires further
study. Prophylactic mastectomy and prophylactic oophorectomy, effective in retrospective clinical experiences, should be considered only for women at substantial
risk willing to accept the irreversible consequences of these procedures. Although dietary fat intake is under clinical trial evaluation, lifestyle change, including weight
loss, dietary change, and increased physical activity, can be recommended based
on other health considerations. Use of any intervention requires careful breast cancer risk assessment, risk-benefit calculations, and informed decision making with
full patient participation. Future breast cancer risk assessment may incorporate additional biologic measures of estrogen exposure and/or analyses of collected breast
cells. Under active evaluation are novel SERMs, aromatase inhibitors/inactivators,
gonadotrophin-releasing hormone agonists, retinoids, statins, and tyrosine kinase and
cyclooxygenase-2 inhibitors.

INTRODUCTION

Breast cancer is the second leading cause of cancer death in the United States.
It is the most common cancer in U.S. women, with about 193,000 invasive plus
30,000 noninvasive cancers anticipated for the year 2001 (1). The decrease in
breast cancer mortality during the past decade is largely attributed to screening mammography and adjuvant therapy for early-stage disease (2). In addition,
breast cancer risk can now be more readily estimated and risk-reducing interventions have been identified (3). The body of evidence relating breast cancer risk
reduction to the current management of otherwise healthy women is reviewed
below.

0066-4219/02/0218-0519$14.00   **519**

BREAST CANCER RISK ASSESSMENT

Before considering interventions to reduce the occurence of breast cancer, a thorough assessment of breast cancer risk is critical (4, 5). Factors consistently associated with breast cancer risk include age, family history, age at menarche and menopause, age at first live birth, breast biopsy number, atypical hyperplasia on breast biopsy, and exogenous estrogen use (6, 7).

Several models have been proposed to facilitate breast cancer risk assessment. The most useful model, which has received the most attention for validation, was developed by Gail and colleagues based on initial observations in the Breast Cancer Detection Demonstration Project population of women having serial screening mammograms (8). This model was slightly modified for use in the National Surgical Adjuvant Breast Project (NSABP) Prevention Trial and further modified to adjust for the lower breast cancer risk of Hispanic women (9). The model incorporates the number of first-degree relatives with breast cancer (0, 1, or $\geq$2), age at menarche (<12, 12 to 13, or $\geq$14 years), and age at first live birth (<20 to 24, 25 to 29 or nulliparous, or $\geq$30 years), the number of breast biopsies (0, 1, or $\geq$2), as well as race (white, black, Hispanic, Asian/Pacific Islander, American Indian/Alaskan native, unknown) and presence of atypical hyperplasia on breast biopsy. A software program available from the National Cancer Institute facilitates calculation of five-year and lifetime risk of breast cancer (9).

The relative risk of populations undergoing Gail Model assessment has resulted in consistent replication of projected and actual breast cancer risk for the entire group (10). However, the model has been shown to have only modest discriminatory accuracy in predicting which individual women will develop breast cancer. In a recent analysis, women classified in the highest risk decile had only 2.8 times the risk of those in the lowest decile (10). Nonetheless, this model is the best available tool for general clinical use (11).

Because the Gail Model does not incorporate age at breast cancer diagnosis, family history of ovarian cancer, family history of breast or ovarian cancer in other than first-degree relatives, or ethnic background more likely to be associated with germline mutation carrier status (i.e., Ashkenazi Jewish background), such information must be collected to determine if use of the Gail Model is appropriate in an individual circumstance.

The full range of issues related to genetic-susceptibility testing and, in particular, evaluation for BRCA1 and BRCA2 are reviewed in detail elsewhere (4, 5). Women whose history suggests germline mutation associated with breast cancer risk should be referred for genetic counseling. Such factors include known BRCA1 and BRCA2 mutation in the family, breast and ovarian cancer in the same family member, two or more family members <50 years old with breast cancer, male breast cancer, one or more family members <50 years of age with breast cancer plus Ashkenazi ancestry, and ovarian cancer plus Ashkenazi ancestry. Although estimates vary, each of these categories carries ~10% or greater risk of having a germline mutation associated with breast cancer. For women outside these categories, use of the Gail Model is appropriate as long as there are no family members with breast cancer diagnosed under age 50. In those circumstances, the Claus Model tables, which incorporate more detailed family history but exclude other risk factors, should be used (12). Although the process appears complicated, the information that determines whether the Gail Model is appropriate can be collected in a few minutes.

Germline mutations that increase breast cancer risk include BRCA1 and BRCA2. Such mutations are estimated to account for <5% of all breast cancers. Women with such mutations have an increased lifetime risk of breast and ovarian cancer, with breast cancer risk estimated at 60%–85% (5). The issues related to identification of individuals with BRCA1 and BRCA2 mutations are complex (5). Although published decision aids compare predicted outcomes of various interventions (13–15), these projections are based on inferences of intervention effectiveness drawn from observational reports.

For women without germline mutations that greatly increase their breast cancer risk, current attempts to improve risk assessment incorporate anthropometrics (16), mammographic density (17), bone mineral density (18), sensitive plasma estrogen determinations (19), and cytology or genetic and molecular markers from breast sampling (20). These factors, discussed below, are not yet appropriate for general use in the clinic.

Effective communication about cancer risk to otherwise healthy women represents a major new challenge, and several strategies are under evaluation (21–23). Updated information on breast cancer risks directed toward a nonmedical audience is available from the Internet at the National Cancer Institutes PDQ[R] breast cancer prevention site, http://cnetdb.nci.nih.gov/index.html, and proprietary sites such as www.realage.com.

CHEMOPREVENTION

Because breast cancer is associated with endogenous (19) and exogenous (24, 25) estrogens, breast cancer therapy commonly incorporates hormone-based interventions. Tamoxifen (Nolvadex[®], Astra-Zeneca), a selective estrogen receptor modulator with both estrogen agonist and antagonist properties, is widely used for breast cancer therapy (26). When studies in early-stage breast cancer using tamoxifen adjuvant therapy demonstrated substantial, statistically significant reduction in contralateral breast cancer risk (27–29), several groups initiated clinical trials of tamoxifen for breast cancer risk reduction.

The NSABP Tamoxifen Prevention Trial evaluated whether tamoxifen (20 mg/day) could reduce breast cancer risk in women whose five-year risk was similar to that of a 60-year-old woman ($\geq$1.66%). In this trial, which randomized 13,388 women to tamoxifen or placebo, tamoxifen reduced the risk of invasive breast cancer by 49% ($p < 0.00001$), an effect almost exclusively seen against receptor-positive tumors (30). Consequently, cancers developing in patients on tamoxifen were more likely to be receptor-negative (30, 31). Risk was also substantially reduced in women with a history of lobular carcinoma in situ (LCIS) (by 56%) or atypical ductal hyperplasia (by 86%).

Two other trials, the Royal Marsden Tamoxifen Prevention Trial (32) and the Italian Randomized Trial of Tamoxifen in Hysterectomized Women (33, 34), did not find tamoxifen to be associated with breast cancer risk reduction. The apparent contradiction in the results of these three trials has been extensively discussed (3, 35, 36); the U.S. and European trials differ in size, characteristics of study populations, adherence, and use of hormone replacement therapy (HRT) (allowed in the British and Italian studies). Although the question is not entirely resolved, a meta-analysis indicates that the results of the three trials are compatible with a 40% reduction in breast cancer incidence (37). The International Breast Intervention Study (IBIS), a British/Australian multicenter placebo-controlled trial, is attempting to determine whether overall health gain is associated with tamoxifen use in otherwise healthy women (36). Because the NSABP Prevention Trial was stopped when a difference in breast cancer incidence emerged, based on the recommendation of the Data Safety Monitoring Board, none of the existing tamoxifen trials provides evidence that tamoxifen influences mortality or overall health when used to reduce the risk of breast cancer.

Taking into account the entire experience with tamoxifen in a variety of breast cancer settings, including its effects on contralateral breast cancer in adjuvant trials (38), the U.S. Food and Drug Administration (FDA) approved tamoxifen for the "reduction of breast cancer risk in women at increased risk for this disease" (3). A Technology Assessment by the American Society of Clinical Oncology recommended that women at increased breast cancer risk (defined as a risk of at least 1.7% over five years) "may be offered tamoxifen to reduce their risk after an informed decision-making process with careful consideration of risks and benefits" (39). The Candian Task Force on Preventive Health Care has published a guideline with similar recommendations (40). Tamoxifen at 20 mg/day for a five-year period is the recommended dose, since adjuvant trials do not support longer periods of therapy (41).

After >20 years of clinical experience in breast cancer therapy, tamoxifen's side effects are well defined. It is generally well-tolerated but is rarely associated with life-threatening instances of endometrial cancer and vascular events reflecting estrogen agonist effects on these systems (26, 30, 42). Such side effects are of special significance when considering use of tamoxifen for risk reduction.

The most frequent side effects of tamoxifen are symptoms of estrogen deficiency (such as hot flashes), which increase in ~20% of women. The risk of thromboembolic events increases by approximately threefold and the risk of stroke by somewhat less, with absolute risk of both increasing with age. The excess mortality from vascular events is about 1 per 1000 among older women using tamoxifen.

Uterine abnormalities are associated with tamoxifen use and may persist after tamoxifen is discontinued (43, 44). Endometrial cancer is increased three- to fourfold in postmenopausal women taking tamoxifen (excluding hysterectomized women). This risk is increased by prior estrogen use and by obesity (45). Endometrial cancer risk associated with estrogen use in HRT has largely been successfully mitigated by systemic progestins (46). However, since progestins may act as breast mitogens (25), their use with tamoxifen is not recommended. Although progesterone/progestogen-releasing intrauterine systems are under evaluation to determine whether they mitigate tamoxifen effects on the uterus (47), they are not available for routine use. It is not established whether tamoxifen affects endometrial cancer prognosis (30, 48).The excess mortality from endometrial cancer is about 1 per 1000 among older women using tamoxifen, excluding hysterectomized women. Although no screening test for endometrial cancer has proven to improve outcome, women given tamoxifen should have annual pelvic examinations, a detailed gynecological history, and evaluation for abnormal vaginal discharge or bleeding (49).

Tamoxifen maintains bone density in postmenopausal women (50), but effects on bone in premenopausal women are mixed (51, 52). Tamoxifen use was associated with a moderate reduction in fracture risk in the NSABP Prevention Trial (30).

Despite a favorable effect on lipid profile (53), tamoxifen does not influence coronary heart disease events. Tamoxifen did not decrease coronary heart disease in the NSABP Prevention Trial (30, 54). In addition, the Early Breast Cancer Trialist Cooperative Group Overview of adjuvant tamoxifen trials reported no effect on mortality from causes other than breast cancer (38, 55). The same overview suggested that some of the favorable (contralateral breast cancer risk reduction) and unfavorable (increased endometrial cancer risk) effects of tamoxifen "carry over" for at least five years after tamoxifen use is terminated (55).

Recent studies indicate no evidence that tamoxifen adversely influences psychosocial or sexual functions (56, 57). Tamoxifen does not increase depression or decrease mental function as measured by screening questionnaires (30, 56, 58). Based on the purported favorable effects of estrogen on cognition (59), tamoxifen's effects on mental function have received increasing attention to establish whether the drug's function is largely agonist or antagonist toward the central nervous system. In a recent report, proton magnetic resonance spectroscopy (^{1}HMRS) was used to determine levels of myo-inositol, a marker of glial activity reflecting brain injury, in a cross-sectional observational study of women ≥ 65 years old who were using tamoxifen, conjugated estrogen, or no hormones. Both estrogen and especially tamoxifen significantly ($p < 0.01$) reduced myo-inositol levels consistent with agonist action on brain estrogen receptors, predicting that tamoxifen use will be associated with neuroprotection (60). In a large cross-sectional study of nursing home residents, women who received tamoxifen were less likely to have diagnosed Alzheimer's disease, were significantly ($p < 0.01$) more independent in activities of daily living, and had better cognitive skills for decision making (61). In a study utilizing a mail-in questionnaire to assess cognition in 1163 women with breast cancer, cognitive function was similar in tamoxifen users and nonusers, although current tamoxifen users had registered more complaints about memory problems (62). Taken together, these results reduce concern that tamoxifen may adversely influence cognition and indicate that centrally mediated symptoms of estrogen deficiency such as hot flashes may not predict adverse effects on cognition.

Although women with ductal carcinoma in situ (DCIS) were not eligible for the NSABP Prevention Trial, their risk for subsequent contralateral cancer exceeds that for women with atypical ductal hyperplasia or LCIS. Because tamoxifen reduced risk of subsequent breast cancers in women with DCIS when given at the time of diagnosis (63), tamoxifen could be considered for breast cancer risk reduction in women with a history of DCIS. Women with a history of diagnosed breast cancer also have increased risk (~0.6% per year) of contralateral breast cancer (38). Women in this category with receptor-positive breast cancer should receive tamoxifen for five years as part of their cancer therapy. However, the risk of contralateral breast cancer is not reduced in women with receptor-negative breast cancers when given tamoxifen, as reported in the most recent Early Breast Cancer Trialist update (55), and tamoxifen should not be used in this setting.

Despite ongoing experience with combined tamoxifen and estrogen in European risk reduction trials (32, 33, 64), currently there is insufficient information to judge whether estrogen addition to tamoxifen modulates tamoxifen's influence on breast cancer or its toxicity profile. Thus, use of combined tamoxifen and estrogen for breast cancer risk reduction is not recommended.

The use of tamoxifen to reduce breast cancer risk in women with BRCA1 or BRCA2 germline mutations, which greatly increased breast cancer risk, is based on observational study results. A case control study found that breast cancer patients with germline mutations who received tamoxifen were half as likely to develop contralateral breast cancer as were women whose therapy did not include tamoxifen (65). A larger effect was seen in women who also had an oophorectomy. In the NSABP and Royal Marsden risk reduction trials, analysis for BRCA1 and BRCA2 in participants is under way. However, it is unclear whether sufficient germline mutation carriers will be identified to allow tamoxifen efficacy in the randomized trials to be determined with statistical power. Tamoxifen's effects on breast cancer risk reduction in African-American women are inferred from the fact that tamoxifen reduced contralateral breast cancer risk in African-American women in studies of early-stage breast cancer (66).

When tamoxifen is being considered for breast cancer risk reduction, determination of breast cancer risk by the process outlined above is the first step. Subsequently, the risks and benefits of tamoxifen use are determined. To facilitate this process, Gail et al. (67), using information from a variety of sources in addition to the NSABP Prevention Trial, generated tabular estimates of net benefit and risk of tamoxifen use in groups of woman based on the variables of five-year breast cancer risk, age, presence or absence of uterus, and race. These tables estimate the net number of clinical events per 10,000 women given tamoxifen for five years. The events of invasive breast cancer, fracture, stroke, pulmonary emboli, and endometrial cancer are each assigned a weight of one, whereas noninvasive breast cancer and deep venous thrombosis are assigned one half. The process does not provide mortality projections and does not incorporate emerging information suggesting that tamoxifen has significant "carry-over" effects on some of these endpoints. Nonetheless, the tables provide a useful framework for clinical decision making and suggest that tamoxifen is most beneficial in younger women at higher breast cancer risk and in hysterectomized women.

In all categories, tamoxifen is associated with fewer benefits in African-American than in white women, largely because of a higher baseline risk of vascular disease and lower risk of osteoporosis and fracture anticipated in the African-American population. Efforts are under way to develop methods to estimate tamoxifen effects on overall survival when given for breast cancer risk reduction (68), but such models are not yet available for clinical use.

RALOXIFENE

Raloxifene (Evista®, Lilly) is a selective estrogen receptor modulator. Its FDA-approved indication is for prevention and therapy of osteoporosis (69, 70). Raloxifene has only modest activity against established breast cancer in the clinic (71) but inhibits mammary cancer development in preclinical systems (72).

Raloxifene influence on breast cancer risk has been reported from several trials where other diseases were primary study endpoints. The Multiple Outcomes of Raloxifene Evaluation (MORE) trial randomized 7705 women with osteoporosis to receive either 60 or 120 mg of raloxifene or placebo daily. In recently updated results (73, 74), 61 invasive breast cancers were confirmed and, in the pooled raloxifene arms, a substantially reduced risk of breast cancer was seen (RR 0.28; 0.17–0.46 CI).

In a post-hoc analysis, the estrogen exposure of participants was estimated using composite laboratory and clinical parameters, which included estradiol determinations with sensitive assays (75). Breast cancers were more frequent in the higher estrogen exposure groups, and raloxifene use was significantly associated with lower breast cancer risk in both the low and high estrogen subgroups. However, women with highest bone density (suggestive of higher lifetime estrogen exposure) and those with a family history of breast cancer experienced a significantly greater benefit than women with lower bone density or without a family history. The authors suggest that estrogen exposure may be prognostic of cancer development and predictive of risk-reduction intervention effectiveness. This provocative hypothesis will require prospective confirmation.

A meta-analysis of nine randomized trials comparing raloxifene to placebo (including the MORE trial) have reported a somewhat smaller (54%) reduction in breast cancer risk (76). Two ongoing studies with breast cancer as primary or coprimary endpoint, the Study of Tamoxifen And Raloxifene (STAR) (35) and Raloxifene for Use in The Heart (RUTH) (77), will provide additional information on the effects of raloxifene on breast cancer risk. Because studies of raloxifene with breast cancer as primary study endpoint have yet to be reported, the use of raloxifene for breast cancer risk reduction remains investigational, but ongoing studies could alter this assessment (39, 40).

Raloxifene at the 60-mg/day dose used for osteoporosis is relatively well-tolerated (78). Information on raloxifene's toxicity and therefore its therapeutic utility is currently limited to postmenopausal women. In this population, raloxifene does not treat hot flashes but causes a slight increase in their frequency (79). Raloxifene is associated with approximately a threefold increase in vascular events, similar in magnitude to those associated with tamoxifen or estrogen (70). Raloxifene has not caused endometrial poliferation in initial clinical studies, nor has endometrial cancer risk been associated with raloxifene use in ongoing studies (80). Raloxifene favorably influences lipid profile (81, 82). The effect of raloxifene on coronary heart disease events is a major focus of the aforementioned RUTH trial.

The influence of raloxifene on cognitive function is also receiving attention (83). The MORE study serially evaluated postmenopausal women with six tests of cognitive function and found no overall difference in cognitive score between women taking raloxifene and those on placebo. However, there was a trend toward less decline in the combined raloxifene groups on tests of verbal memory and attention (84).

In preclinical studies, raloxifene stimulated ovarian cancers in vitro (85) and tamoxifen-resistant breast cancers in athymic mice (86). The clinical relevance of these observations is unknown, but they suggest that routine raloxifene use should be for its approved indications of osteoporosis prevention and therapy.

AROMATASE INHIBITORS/INACTIVATORS

Aromatase inhibitors, which act by reducing estrogen levels through inhibition of the enzyme aromatase, are receiving increasing attention in breast cancer management. Anastrozole (Arimedex®, Astra-Zeneca) and letrozole (Femara®, Novartis) are currently approved for initial therapy of metastatic breast cancer in postmenopausal women (87). These agents, along with the aromatase inactivator exemestane (Aromasin®, Pharmacia & Upjohn), are potential candidates for breast cancer risk reduction as well. They are at least as active as and possibly superior to tamoxifen as first-line hormonal therapy in metastatic breast cancer; furthermore, they have a more favorable toxicity profile and are expected to have less influence on the endometrium and vascular events.

All the above-mentioned compounds are components of ongoing adjuvant breast cancer trials, one of which will also evaluate the effect on contralateral breast cancer with implications for breast cancer risk reduction use. The Anastrozole, Tamoxifen, Alone or in Combination (ATAC) trial is a randomized double-blind study comparing tamoxifen to anastrozole and the combination in over 9000 postmenopausal women with early-stage resected breast cancer (88). Results are anticipated in late 2001. At present, no clinical trial data support use of aromatase inhibitors/inactivators for breast cancer risk reduction.

RETINOIDS

Fenretinide is a synthetic derivative of all-trans retinoic acid. This vitamin A analog has been evaluated in a randomized trial of nearly 3000 women with early breast cancer; contralateral breast cancer was the study endpoint. Although no overall effect was seen, a post-hoc analysis suggested reduced contralateral breast cancer risk in premenopausal women receiving fenretinide (89). The agent was well-tolerated, and a fenretinide and tamoxifen combination is being evaluated in young high-risk women (90).

PROPHYLACTIC SURGERY

Although prophylactic mastectomy has been used for many years, a recent prospective study of 139 women with BRCA mutations strongly supports a role for this intervention in breast cancer risk reduction (91). In this report, prophylactic bilateral mastectomy reduced the incidence of breast cancer compared to regular surveillance. Previously, a retrospective analysis from the Mayo Clinic of a cohort of 639 women at increased breast cancer risk reported bilateral mastectomy reduced breast cancer risk and mortality by about 90% (92), although concerns have been raised that the analytic methodology used may overestimate the survival benefit (93). Using a similar observational study design, Mayo Clinic investigators also observed comparable reduction in breast cancer risk with prophylactic mastectomy in women with BRCA1 or BRCA2 germline mutations (94). Supporting the concept that removal of breast mass can reduce breast cancer risk are reports of reduced risk following breast reduction surgery (95, 96). One report estimated the amount of breast tissue removed in breast reduction surgery and collected information on other breast cancer risk factors (96). Women who had more breast tissue removed ($\geq$1800 versus <600 g removed) had lower breast cancer risk (RR 0.24, 0.1–0.5 CI) after adjustment for other breast cancer risk factors.

Although most reports of bilateral mastectomies involve subcutaneous mastectomy with nipple preservation, substantial breast tissue is left behind in such procedures, and the currently recommended procedure is total mastectomy with nipple removal with or without reconstruction. Because some patients who have prophylactic mastectomies later express regret (97), this procedure should be considered only by premenopausal women at very high risk for breast cancer who are willing to accept an irreversible procedure after careful risk-benefit discussion.

Observational study results suggest that bilateral oophorectomy performed before menopause substantially reduces breast cancer risk (93, 98, 99). However, the overview of all randomized clinical trials of oophorectomy performed for early-stage breast cancer in patients <50 years old did not demonstrate reduction in contralateral breast cancer (100). In a cohort study of known BRCA1 mutation carriers, bilateral oophorectomy was associated with a nearly 50% reduction in the calculated risk of breast cancer (98). Such results are supported by other retrospective reports of prophylactic oophorectomy in inherited breast/ovarian cancer families (99). Consideration of this surgery is of special significance in BRCA1 and BRCA2 carriers, given the potential role of bilateral oophorectomy in modulating, though not eliminating, ovarian cancer risk (93). The surgical complications of oophorectomy, along with the potential medical consequences of early menopause, are discussed in detail elsewhere (93). Bilateral oophorectomy can be considered for breast cancer risk reduction in premenopausal women at extremely high risk.

Although clinical trials have not been reported, the use of gonadotropin-releasing hormone (GNRH) analogs to reduce estrogens in premenopausal women is likely to have effects similar to those of oophorectomy on breast cancer risk. Combinations of GNRH analogs with low-dose estrogen (101) and selective estrogen receptor modulators (87) are under way, but no clinical outcome results are available.

In both advanced and adjuvant breast cancer therapy, tamoxifen plus ovarian suppression with GNRH analogs was more effective than ovarian suppression alone (102, 103). In this context, an observational study has suggested that the effect of tamoxifen on contralateral breast cancer risk reduction in women with BRCA1 mutations was increased by prophylactic oophorectomy (65). Taken together, these reports suggest that an additional consideration in women with germline mutations who have had prophylactic oophorectomy is whether tamoxifen should also be given.

LIFESTYLE AND RISK REDUCTION

Observational study results have linked several lifestye factors with increased breast cancer risk, including increased dietary fat intake (104), increased body weight (105), increased alcohol intake (106), decreased intake of several micronutrients in fruits and vegetables (107, 108), and decreased physical activity (109).

Despite controversy regarding dietary fat and breast cancer risk (104, 110, 111), the weight of evidence has supported several ongoing full-scale randomized trials exploring this connection. In addition, several of these trials incorporate fruit and vegetable intake to variable degrees (112, 113). The feasibility of maintaining a nearly 50% reduction in dietary fat intake has been demonstrated (112, 114, 115), and ongoing full-scale trials have completed accrual in both primary and secondary settings (112, 113, 116). In the largest such study, the dietary-modification component of the Women's Health Initiative, over 47,000 postmenopausal women have been randomized to a reduced-fat dietary program or to a control group. Study outcomes of the Women's Health Initiative include all-cause mortality, breast and colon cancer, and coronary heart disease, with results anticipated by 2005.

None of the current full-scale dietary studies incorporating fat intake reduction were designed to reduce energy intake or achieve weight loss. Consequently, these studies have reported only moderate weight loss of about two to four pounds (116, 117). Thus, the association of obesity with breast cancer risk will require separate investigation.

In observational studies of postmenopausal women, obesity is associated with higher estrogen levels and substantially increased breast cancer risk (6, 16, 19). Such association may be mediated by increased estrogen produced from body fat through androgen-to-estrogen conversion (19). The situation in premenopausal women is more complex, since estrogens from adipose tissue may suppress ovarian estrogen production, somewhat decreasing breast cancer risk (6). These data suggest that obesity, especially weight gain in postmenopausal women, should be avoided to modulate breast cancer risk.

Any current recommendations regarding lifestye change and breast cancer risk must be based on observational and preclinical studies. However, for an obese, sedentary, postmenopausal woman with a high dietary fat intake, weight loss can be recommended based on other health considerations. The National Institute of Health (NIH) recently has endorsed guidelines regarding the evaluation, identification, and treatment of obesity, with target intervention objectives and proven strategies for chronic weight loss including dietary change, exercise, behavior modification, and ongoing medical supervision (118). The definitive role of weight loss and maintenance on breast cancer risk awaits prospective clinical trials. However, given the documented influence of weight loss on other conditions affecting women's health, the nature of the intervention as a return to the "evolutionary norm" (119), and the availability of proven weight reduction strategies (118), a program of weight loss in obese women could reasonably be recommended to improve health.

Table 1 summarizes the current status of potential breast cancer risk reduction interventions.

EXOGENOUS ESTROGEN AND BREAST CANCER RISK

Although HRT is in wide use for estrogen-deficiency symptom management and osteoporosis prevention and therapy, there are no randomized trial results to provide reliable estimates of its effects on breast cancer risk or overall health (120). The Women's Health Initiative has randomized over 27,000 women to HRT or placebo (113), but results are not anticipated until 2005. Observational reports suggest that HRT with estrogen alone or in combination with progestins is associated with increased breast cancer risk, and that longer duration and combination use are associated with greater risk (121, 122). A composite analysis reported ~6 excess breast cancers per 1000 women for 10 years of estrogen use (24).

The widespread concept of a very favorable risk-benefit ratio for HRT, as incorporated in decision aids (123), is largely based on HRT's reputed effects on

TABLE 1   Status of potential breast cancer risk reduction interventions

Intervention	Summary of current status
Chemoprevention:	
Tamoxifen	The only FDA approved intervention for breast cancer risk reduction; placebo controlled trials still ongoing in Europe
Raloxifene (in postmenopausal women)	Support from analysis as secondary endpoint in a randomized trial; definite prospective trials ongoing
Fenretinide	Negative randomized trial (contralateral breast cancer); post-hoc analysis suggested benefit in premenopausal women
Anastrozole (in postmenopausal women)	FDA approved for breast cancer therapy; adjuvant trial powered to assess affect on contralateral breast cancer completed accrual and results pending
Prophylactic surgery:	
Bilateral mastectomy	Support from one prospective and several observational studies; no randomized trials
Bilateral oophorectomy (in premenopausal women)	Support from several observational studies; analysis in randomized adjuvant trials on contralateral breast cancer negative
*Lifestyle changes:**	
Reduction in fat intake	Observational reports mixed; ongoing randomized trial has completed accrual and results pending
Increase in exercise	Support from observational reports only
Weight maintenance/loss (in postmenopausal women)	Support from observational reports only
Reduction in alcohol intake	Support from observational reports only

*These lifestyle changes could be recommended based on return to "evolutionary norm" and influence on other medical events.

coronary heart disease. However, recent results (124), including reports from randomized clinical trials (125, 126), raise questions as to whether estimates of coronary heart disease effects based on lipid profile change and observational studies accurately predict clinical results in postmenopausal women with or without prior heart disease.

Like tamoxifen, HRT can result in life-threatening vascular events (and endometrial cancer for users of estrogen alone). The commonly accepted 30%–40% reduction in coronary heart disease events attributed to HRT is coming under increasing skepticism, and alternatives to estrogen are available for osteoporosis and estrogen deficiency symptoms (127). Therefore, long-term HRT use should be subject to the same rigorous risk-benefit analysis outlined for tamoxifen use (120).

Most observational studies also associate oral contraceptive use, especially recent use, with moderate increase in breast cancer risk in younger women (128). More recently, breast feeding has been associated with reduced breast cancer risk

(129). The association between induced abortion and breast cancer is controversial, with mixed results and methodologic concerns (130, 131).

Phytoestrogens are plant-derived compounds with estrogen agonist and antagonist effects that are available as nutritional supplements. Although they are associated with reduced breast cancer in some observational studies, the epidemiologic results are complex and mixed (132, 133). Phytoestrogens have no established role in breast cancer risk reduction.

BREAST CANCER RISK ASSESSMENT IN THE FUTURE

In the future, breast cancer risk assessment may incorporate additional biologic measures of ongoing and/or lifetime estrogen exposure, including bone density, mammographic breast density, and, in postmenopausal women, circulatory estradiol levels.

Increased bone mineral density, believed to reflect lifetime estrogen exposure, has been consistently related to increased breast cancer risk in cohort reports (74, 134). In one prospective study, 8905 women at least 65 years were followed for a mean of 6.5 years after a single bone-mineral density determination of the wrist, forearm, and heel. The risk of breast cancer for women in the highest quartile of cumulative bone density was 2.7 times greater than the risk for women in the lowest quartile (134).

Mammographic breast density is increased with estrogen exposure and has also been associated with increased breast cancer risk (17). Because breast density reduction has been associated with tamoxifen (135) and dietary fat intake reduction (17), it may represent a surrogate for breast cancer risk reduction. This intriguing possibility will require confirmation in outcome studies that provide a breast cancer risk reduction intervention coupled with breast density determinations. Such a trial is ongoing as a substudy of the aforementioned Women's Health Initiative (113).

Information from observational cohorts indicates that recently available estradiol assays may allow a two- to sixfold discrimination of breast cancer risk among postmenopausal women, comparing risks in lowest versus highest estradiol quintiles (19, 136, 137). Such results are based on new assays with greatly increased sensitivity, which can make determinations on samples that are undetectable with conventional clinical assays. Although these assays are not widely available at present, confirmation of the relationships between estrogen level and risk could greatly facilitate identification of women at sufficient risk to benefit from risk reduction interventions.

A further refinement of risk assessment currently under active evaluation is the collection of breast cells by a variety of techniques including periareolar fine-needle aspiration, routine operative breast endoscopy (ROBE), and ductal lavage through microcatheters (ProDuct Health, CA) (138, 139). The recovered cells are then examined by a range of histological, biochemical, and molecular techniques potentially associated with breast cancer risk. Initial results are promising and provide a means of identifying potentially active agents for full-scale interventions (140). For example, Fabian and coworkers (138) found that hyperplasia with atypical atypia seen in periareolar fine-needle aspiration cytology samples from otherwise healthy women, in conjunction with Gail Model risk, identified a group of women ($n = 66$) with an extremely high five-year breast cancer risk of over 25% compared with no breast cancer development in women without atypia whose Gail risk was below the median for the group ($n = 179$, $p < 0.001$). The potential of molecular biology to refine future risk assessment is suggested by the preliminary studies of Everon and colleagues (139). They tested cells collected from breast ducts by methylation-specific PCR for three specific genes that were hypermethylated in >30% of breast cancer patients. Using this approach, pathologically confirmed breast cancer was subsequently diagnosed in two women who had methylated markers in their ductal-lavage fluid at a time when their mammogram and physical examination were negative.

OTHER STRATEGIES UNDER EVALUATION FOR BREAST CANCER RISK REDUCTION

The increasing array of agents under clinical evaluation for breast cancer risk reduction includes novel selective estrogen-receptor modulators, aromatase inhibitors/inactivators, GNRH agonists, retinoids, vitamin D derivatives, and inhibitors of tyrosine kinase and cyclooxygenase-2 (141). The status of several of these agents is reviewed below.

Novel estrogen-receptor modulators, including EM-652 (142) and LY- 353381 (143), continue under development with potential for a more favorable risk-benefit profile.

Several classes of drugs currently in wide clinical use for seemingly unrelated clinical problems are receiving attention for breast cancer risk reduction as well. Information from the Study of Osteoporotic Fractures, involving postmenopausal women, suggests that statins (used for cholesterol reduction) are associated with a substantially lower rate of breast cancer (2.1 cases per 1000 woman-years among statin users versus 4.7 cases per 1000 woman-years among nonusers; $p < 0.001$) (144). This follows the observation that use of simvastatin, one of the statins, resulted in a 27% reduction in cancer deaths for men and women randomized to the statin compared with placebo ($p = 0.09$) (145). Also receiving attention are cyclooxygenase-2 inhibitors (141). Despite ongoing controversy (146), some observational reports indicate substantial breast cancer risk reduction associated with these compounds (147). Attempts to confirm such observations are ongoing in large, established cohorts of women, since statins and cyclooxygenase-2 inhibitors are widely used in the general population for other indications.

A growing array of agents are directed at new molecular targets for breast cacner prevention (20). One example, ZD 1839 (Iressa), is an oral epidermal growth factor receptor tyrosine kinase inhibitor with low toxicity, which is in phase III clinical evaluation in advanced cancer. In preclinical studies, this agent has demonstrated growth inhibition against human DCIS in a nude mouse system (148). The development of all these interventions should be accelerated by use of previously discussed models incorporating serial evaluation of molecular and cytologic markers of breast cancer risk.

ACKNOWLEDGMENT

Some of the work reported here was supported by grants from the National Institutes of Health (GCRC MO1-RR-00-425, RO1-CA-45504, and NO1-WH-4-2120).

Visit the Annual Reviews home page at www.AnnualReviews.org

LITERATURE CITED

1. Greenlee RT, Hill-Harmon MB, Murray T, Thun M. 2001. Cancer statistics, 2001. *CA Cancer J. Clin.* 51:15–36
2. Peto R, Boreham J, Clarke M, et al. 2000. UK and USA breast cancer deaths down 25% in year 2000 at ages 20–69 years. *Lancet* 355(9217):1822
3. Chlebowski RT. 2000. Primary care. Reducing the risk of breast cancer. *N. Engl. J. Med.* 343(3):191–98
4. Armstrong K, Eisen A, Weber B. 2000. Assessing the risk of breast cancer. *N. Engl. J. Med.* 342(8):564–71
5. Nathanson KN, Wooster R, Weber BL. 2001. Breast cancer genetics: What we know and what we need to know. *Nat. Med.* 7(5):552–56
6. Key TJ, Verkasalo PK, Banks E. 2001. Epidemiology of breast cancer. *Lancet* 2:133–40
7. McPherson K, Steel CM, Dixon JM. 2000. ABC of breast diseases. Breast cancer—epidemiology, risk factors, and genetics. *BMJ* 321(7261):624–28
8. Gail MH, Brinton LA, Byar DP, et al. 1989. Projecting individualized probabilities of developing breast cancer for white females who are being examined annually. *J. Natl. Cancer Inst.* 81:1879–86
9. National Cancer Institute. 2001. Breast Cancer Risk Assessment Tool v.2 for Health Care Providers. www.nci.nih.gov/
10. Rockhill B, Spiegelman D, Byrne C, et al. 2001. Validation of the Gail et al. model of breast cancer risk prediction and implications for chemoprevention. *J. Natl. Cancer Inst.* 93(5):358–66
11. Gail MH, Costantino JP. 2001. Validating and improving models for projecting the absolute risk of breast cancer. *J. Natl. Cancer Inst.* 93(5):334–35
12. Claus EB, Risch N, Thompson WD. 1994. Autosomal dominant inheritance of early-onset breast cancer. Implications for risk prediction. *Cancer* 73(3):643–51
13. Schrag D, Kuntz KM, Garber JE, Weeks JC. 1997. Decision analysis—effects of prophylactic mastectomy and oophorectomy on life expectancy among women with BRCA1 or BRCA2 mutations. *N. Engl. J. Med.* 336:1465–71
14. Grann VR, Jacobson JS, Whang W, et al. 2000. Prevention with tamoxifen or other hormones versus prophylactic surgery in BRCA1/2-positive women: a decision analysis. *Cancer J. Sci. Am.* 6:13–20
15. Eisinger F, Charafe-Jauffret E, Jacquemier J, et al. 2001. Tamoxifen and breast cancer risk in women harboring a BRCA1

germline mutation: computed efficacy, effectiveness and impact. *Int. J. Oncol.* 18(1):5–10

16. Morimoto LM, White E, McTiernan A, et al. 2001. Anthropometrics and risk of breast cancer in postmenopausal women: the Women's Health Initiative. *Proc. Am. Assoc. Cancer Res.* 42:4768 (Abstr.)

17. Boyd NF, Martin LJ, Stone J, et al. 2001. Mammographic densities as a marker of human breast cancer risk and their use in chemoprevention. *Curr. Oncol. Rep.* 3(4):314–21

18. Cauley JA, Lucas FL, Kuller LH, et al. 1996. Bone mineral density and risk of breast cancer in older women: the study of osteoporotic fractures. *JAMA* 276:1404–8

19. Clemons M, Goss P. 2001. Estrogen and the risk of breast cancer. *N. Engl. J. Med.* 344:276–85

20. Bange J, Zwick E, Ullrich A. 2001. Molecular targets for breast cancer therapy and prevention. *Nat. Med.* 7(5):548–52

21. Arkin EB. 1999. Cancer risk communication—what we know. *J. Natl. Cancer Inst. Monogr.* 25:182–85

22. Lipkus IM, Kuchibhatla M, McBride CM, et al. 2000. Relationships among breast cancer perceived absolute risk, comparative risk, and worries. *Cancer Epidemiol. Biomarkers Prev.* 9(9):973–75

23. Smedira HJ. 2000. Practical issues in counseling healthy women about their breast cancer risk and use of tamoxifen citrate. *Arch. Intern. Med.* 160:3034–42

24. Collaborative Group on Hormonal Factors in Breast Cancer. 1997. Breast cancer and hormone replacement therapy: collaborative reanalysis of data from 51 epidemiological studies of 52,705 women with breast cancer and 108,411 women without breast cancer. *Lancet* 350(9084):1047–59

25. Schairer C, Lubin J, Troisi R, et al. 2000. Menopausal estrogen and estrogen—progestin replacement therapy and breast cancer risk. *JAMA* 283:485–91

26. Osborne CK. 1998. Tamoxifen in the treatment of breast cancer. *N. Engl. J. Med.* 339:1609–18

27. Cuzick J, Baum M. 1985. Tamoxifen and contralateral breast cancer. *Lancet* ii:282

28. Fisher B, Constantino J, Redmond C, et al. 1989. A randomized clinical trial evaluating tamoxifen in the treatment of patients with node-negative breast cancer who have estrogen-receptor positive tumors. *N. Engl. J. Med.* 320:479–84

29. Powles TJ, Hardy JR, Ashley SE, et al. 1989. Chemoprevention of breast cancer. *Breast Cancer Res. Treat.* 14:23–31

30. Fisher B, Costantino JP, Wickerham DL, et al. 1998. Tamoxifen for prevention of breast cancer: report of the National Surgical Adjuvant Breast and Bowel Project P-1 Study. *J. Natl. Cancer Inst.* 90:1371–88

31. Li CI, Malone KE, Weiss NS, Daling JR. 2001. Tamoxifen therapy for primary breast cancer and risk of contralateral breast cancer. *J. Natl. Cancer Inst.* 93:1008–13

32. Powles T, Eeles R, Ashley S, et al. 1998. Interim analysis of the incidence of breast cancer in the Royal Marsden Hospital tamoxifen randomised chemoprevention trial. *Lancet* 352:98–101

33. Veronesi U, Maisonneuve P, Costa A, et al. 1998. Prevention of breast cancer with tamoxifen: preliminary findings from the Italian randomized trial among hysterectomized women. *Lancet* 352:93–97

34. Decensi A, Rotmensz N, Maisonneuve P, et al. 2001. Prevention of breast cancer with tamoxifen. Update of the Italian trial in hysterectomized women. *Proc. Am. Assoc. Cancer Res.* 42:4441 (Abstr.)

35. Vogel V. 2000. Breast cancer prevention: a review of current evidence. *CA Cancer J. Clin.* 50(3):157–70

36. Eeles RA, Powles TJ. 2000. Chemoprevention options for BRCA1 and BRCA2 mutation carriers. *J. Clin. Oncol.* 18(Suppl. 21):93S–99S

37. Cuzick J. 2000. Future possibilities in the prevention of breast cancer: breast cancer prevention trials. *Breast Cancer Res.* 2(4):258–63

38. Early Breast Cancer Trialists' Collaborative Group. 1998. Tamoxifen for early breast cancer: an overview of the randomized trials. *Lancet* 351:1451–67

39. Chlebowski RT, Collyar DE, Somerfield M, Pfister DG for the American Society of Clinical Oncology Working Group. 1999. American Society of Clinical Oncology technology assessment of breast cancer risk reduction strategies. Tamoxifen and raloxifene. *J. Clin. Oncol.* 17(6):1939–55

40. Levine M, Moutquin JM, Walton R, Feightner J. 2001. Chemoprevention of breast cancer. *Can. Med. Assoc. J.* 164(12):1681–90

41. Fisher B, Dignam J, Bryant J, Wolmark N. 2001. Five versus more than five years of tamoxifen for lymph node–negative breast cancer: updated findings from the National Surgical Adjuvant Breast and Bowel Project B-14 randomized trial. *J. Natl. Cancer Inst.* 93(9):684–90

42. Braithwaite RS, Lau J, Chlebowski RT, et al. 2000. A meta-analysis of vascular and neoplastic outcomes associated with tamoxifen. *Med. Decis. Making* 20:485 (Abstr.)

43. Barakat RR, Gilewski TA, Almadrones L, et al. 2000. Effect of adjuvant tamoxifen on the endometrium in women with breast cancer: a prospective study using office endometrial biopsy. *J. Clin. Oncol.* 18:3459–63

44. Bertelli G, Valenzano M, Del Mastro L, et al. 2001. Endometrial abnormalities in breast cancer patients receiving adjuvant tamoxifen persist after treatment completion. *Proc. Am. Soc. Clin. Oncol.* 20:36a, Abstr. 142

45. Bernstein L, Deapen D, Cerhan JR, et al. 1999. Tamoxifen therapy for breast cancer and endometrial cancer risk. *J. Natl. Cancer Inst.* 91:1654–62

46. The Writing Group for the PEPI Trial. 1995. Effects of estrogen or estrogen/progestin regimens on heart disease risk factors in postmenopausal women. The Postmenopausal Estrogen/Progestin Interventions (PEPI) Trial. *JAMA* 273(3):199–208

47. Gardner FJ, Konje JC, Abrams KR, et al. 2000. Endometrial protection from tamoxifen-stimulated changes by a levonorgestrel-releasing intrauterine system: a randomised controlled trial. *Lancet* 356:1711–17

48. Beelen BL, Gallee MLR, Hollema MPW, et al. 2000. Risk and prognosis of endometrial cancer after tamoxifen for breast cancer. *Lancet* 356(9233):881–87

49. Suh-Burgmann EJ, Goodman A. 1999. Surveillance for endometrial cancer in women receiving tamoxifen. *Ann. Intern. Med.* 131:127–35

50. Love RR, Mazess RB, Tormey DC, et al. 1988. Bone mineral density in women with breast cancer treated with adjuvant tamoxifen for at least two years. *Breast Cancer Res. Treat.* 12:297–302

51. Powles TJ, Hickish T, Kanis JA, et al. 1996. Effect of tamoxifen on bone mineral density measured by dual-energy x-ray absorptiometry in healthy premenopausal and postmenopausal women. *J. Clin. Oncol.* 14:78–84

52. Sverrisdottir A, Fornander T, Rutqvist LE. 2001. Bone mineral density in premenopausal patients in a randomized trial of adjuvant endocrine therapy (ZIPP-TRIAL). *Proc. Am. Soc. Clin. Oncol.* 20:25a, Abstr. 96

53. Bilimoria MM, Jordan VC, Morrow M. 1996. Additional benefit of tamoxifen for postmenopausal patients. In *Tamoxifen: A Guide for Clinicians and Patients*, ed. VC Jordan, pp. 75–89. Huntington, NY: PRR

54. Reis SE, Costantino JP, Wickerham DL, et al. 2001. Cardiovascular effects of tamoxifen in women with and without heart disease: breast cancer prevention trial. National Surgical Adjuvant Breast and Bowel Project Breast Cancer Prevention

Trial Investigators. *J. Natl. Cancer Inst.* 93(1):16–21

55. Peto R. 2000. *Tamoxifen as adjuvant breast cancer therapy.* Presented at NIH Consens. Dev. Conf. Adjuvant Therapy for Breast Cancer, Nov. 21, Bethesda, MD. http://videocast.nih.gov

56. Fallowfield L, Fleissig A, Edwards R, et al. 2001. Tamoxifen for the prevention of breast cancer: psychosocial impact on women participating in two randomized controlled trials. *J. Clin. Oncol.* 19(7):1885–92

57. Berglund G, Nystedt M, Bolund C, et al. 2001. Effect of endocrine treatment on sexuality in premenopausal breast cancer patients: a prospective randomized study. *J. Clin. Oncol.* 9(11):2788–96

58. Day R, Gary PA, Costantino JP, et al. 1999. Health-related quality of life and tamoxifen in breast cancer prevention: a report for the National Surgical Adjuvant Breast and Bowel Project P-1 Study. *J. Clin. Oncol.* 17:2659–69

59. McEwen BS, Alves SE. 1999. Estrogen actions in the central nervous system. *Endocr. Rev.* 20(3):279–307

60. Chlebowski RT, Ernst T, Chang L, et al. 2001. Tamoxifen and estrogen effects on brain chemistry determined by MRI spectroscopy. *Proc. Am. Soc. Clin. Oncol.* 20:28a, Abstr. 108

61. Breuer B, Anderson R. 2000. The relationship of tamoxifen with dementia, depression, and dependence in activities of daily living in elderly nursing home residents. *Women Health* 31:71–85

62. Paganini-Hill A, Clark LJ. 2001. Preliminary assessment of cognitive function in breast cancer patients treated with tamoxifen. *Breast Cancer Res. Treat.* 64(2):165–76

63. Fisher B, Digman J, Wolmark N, et al. 1999. Tamoxifen in treatment of intraductal breast cancer. National Surgical Adjuvant Breast and Bowel Project B-24 randomized controlled trial. *Lancet* 353:1993–2000

64. Bonanni B, Guerrieri-Gonzaga A, Rotmensz N, et al. 2000. Hormonal therapy and chemoprevention. *Breast J.* 6(5):317–23

65. Narod SA, Brunet JS, Ghadirian P, et al. 2000. Tamoxifen and risk of contralateral breast cancer in BRCA1 and BRCA2 mutation carriers: a case-control study. Hereditary Breast Cancer Clinical Study Group. *Lancet* 356(9245):1876–81

66. McCaskill-Stevens W, Bryant J, Costantino J, et al. 2000. Incidence of contralateral breast cancer (CBC), endometrial cancer (EC) and thromobembolic events (TE) in African American (AA) women receiving tamoxifen for treatment of primary breast cancer. *Proc. Am. Soc. Clin. Oncol.* 19:70a, Abstr. 269

67. Gail MH, Costantino JP, Bryant J, et al. 1999. Weighing the risks and benefits of tamoxifen treatment for preventing breast cancer. *J. Natl. Cancer Inst.* 9(21):1829–46

68. Col NF, Hirota LK, Pauker SG, et al. 1999. Tamoxifen for the primary prevention of breast cancer: Which women benefit from treatment? *Med. Decis. Making* 19:526, Abstr.

69. Delmas PD, Bjarnasan NG, Mitlak BH, et al. 1997. Effects of raloxifene on bone mineral density, serum cholesterol concentrations, and uterine endometrium in postmenopausal women. *N. Engl. J. Med.* 337:1641–47

70. Khovidhunkit W, Shoback DM. 1999. Clinical effects of raloxifene in women. *Ann. Intern. Med.* 130(5):431–39

71. Gradishar W, Glusman J, Lu Y, et al. 2000. Effects of high dose raloxifene in selected patients with advanced breast carcinoma. *Cancer* 88(9):2047–53

72. Jordan VC, Morrow M. 1999. Tamoxifen, raloxifene, and the prevention of breast cancer. *Endocr. Rev.* 20(3):253–78

73. Cummings RS, Eckert S, Krueger KA, et al. 1999. The effect of raloxifene on risk of breast cancer in postmenopausal women. *JAMA* 281:2189–97

74. Cauley JA, Norton L, Lippman ME, et al. 2001. Continued breast cancer risk reduction in postmenopausal women treated with raloxifene: 4-year results from the MORE trial. Multiple outcomes of raloxifene evaluation. *Breast Cancer Res. Treat.* 65(2):125–34

75. Lippman ME, Krueger KA, Eckert S, et al. 2000. *Indicators of lifetime estrogen exposure: effect on breast cancer incidence and interaction with raloxifene therapy in MORE Trial participants.* Annu. San Antonio Breast Cancer Symp., 23rd, Dec. 6–9, Abstr. 5

76. Jordan VC, Glusman JE, Eckert S, et al. 1998. Raloxifene reduces incident primary breast cancer: integrated data from multicenter, double-blind, placebo-controlled, randomized trials in post-menopausal women. *Breast Cancer Res. Treat. Proc.* 21:227 (Abstr.)

77. Saitta A, Morabito N, Frisina N, et al. 2001. Cardiovascular effects of raloxifene hydrochloride. *Cardiovasc. Drug Rev.* 19(1):57–74

78. Strickler R, Stovall DW, Merritt D, et al. 2000. Raloxifene and estrogen effects on quality of life in healthy postmenopausal women: a placebo-controlled randomized trial. *Obstet. Gynecol.* 96(3):359–65

79. Cohen FJ, Lu Y. 2000. Characterization of hot flashes reported by healthy postmenopausal women receiving raloxifene or placebo during osteoporosis prevention trials. *Maturitas* 34(1):65–73

80. Fugere P, Scheele WH, Shah A, et al. 2000. Uterine effects of raloxifene in comparison with continuous-combined hormone replacement therapy in postmenopausal women. *Am. J. Obstet. Gynecol.* 182(3):568–74

81. Walsh BW, Kuller LH, Wild RA, et al. 1998. Effects of raloxifene on serum lipids and coagulation factors in healthy postmenopausal women. *JAMA* 279:1445–85

82. De Leo V, La Marca A, Morgante G, Lanzetta D, Setacci C, Petraglia F. 2001. Randomized control study of the effects of raloxifene on serum lipids and homocysteine in older women. *Am. J. Obstet. Gynecol.* 184(3):350–53

83. Nickelsen T, Lufkin EG, Riggs BL, et al. 1999. Raloxifene hydrochloride, a selective estrogen receptor modulator: safety assessment of effects on cognitive function and mood in postmenopausal women. *Psychoneuroendocrinology* 24(1):115–28

84. Yaffe K, Krueger K, Sarkar S, et al. 2001. Cognitive function in postmenopausal women treated with raloxifene. *N. Engl. J. Med.* 344(16):1207–13

85. Paulson LM. 2001. Raloxifene stimulates ovarian cancer growth in culture. *Eur. Soc. Hum. Reprod.* 42:138–42

86. O'Regan RM, Gajdos C, Dardes R, et al. 2001. Effect of raloxifene after tamoxifen on breast and endometrial cancer growth. *Proc. Am. Soc. Clin. Oncol.* 20:25a, Abstr. 95

87. Goss PE, Strasser K. 2001. Aromatase inhibitors in the treatment and prevention of breast cancer. *J. Clin. Oncol.* 19(3):881–94

88. Jackson TL, Duffy SRG. 2000. The ATAC (Arimidex, Tamoxifen, Alone or in Combination) Trial: transvaginal ultrasound scan findings overestimate observed pathological findings in postmenopausal gynaecologically asymptomatic women before treatment. *Breast Cancer Res. Treat.* 64:64, Abstr. 233

89. Veronesi U, De Palo G, Marubini E, et al., for the fenretinide investigators. 1999. Randomized trial of fenretinide to prevent second breast malignancy in women with early breast cancer. *J. Natl. Cancer Inst.* 91(21):1847–56

90. Camerini T, Mariani L, De Palo G, et al. 2001. Safety of the synthetic retinoid fenretinide: long-term results from a controlled clinical trial for the prevention of contralateral breast cancer. *J. Clin. Oncol.* 19(6):1664–70

91. Meijers-Heijboer H, van Geel B, van Putten WL, et al. 2001. Breast cancer after

prophylactic bilateral mastectomy in women with a BRCA1 or BRCA2 mutation. *N. Engl. J. Med.* 345(3):159–64

92. Hartman LC, Schaid DJ, Woods JE, et al. 1999. Efficacy of bilateral prophylactic mastectomy in women with a family history of breast cancer. *N. Engl. J. Med.* 340(2):77–84

93. Eisen A, Rebbeck TR, Wood WC, Weber BL. 2000. Prophylactic surgery in women with a hereditary predisposition to breast and ovarian cancer. *J. Clin. Oncol.* 18(9): 1980–95

94. Hartman LC, Schaid D, Sellers T, et al. 2000. Bilateral prophylactic mastectomy (PM) in BRCA1/2 mutation carriers. *Proc. Am. Assoc. Cancer Res.* 41:222 (Abstr.)

95. Boice JD Jr, Friis S, McLaughlin JK, et al. 1997. Cancer following breast reduction surgery in Denmark. *Cancer Causes Control* 8(2):253–58

96. Brinton LA, Persson I, Boice JD Jr, et al. 2001. Breast cancer risk in relation to amount of tissue removed during breast reduction operations in Sweden. *Cancer* 91(3):478–83

97. Borgen PI, Hill AD, Tran KW, et al. 1998. Patient regrets after bilateral prophylactic mastectomy. *Surg. Oncol.* 5(7):603–6

98. Rebbeck TR, Levin AM, Eisen A, et al. 1999. Breast cancer risk after bilateral prophylactic oophorectomy in BRCA1 mutation carriers. *J. Natl. Cancer Inst.* 91(17):1475–77

99. Struewing JP, Watson P, Easton DF, et al. 1995. Prophylactic oophorectomy in inherited breast/ovarian cancer families. *Monogr. J. Natl.Cancer Inst.* 17:33–35

100. Early Breast Cancer Trialists' Collaborative Group. 1996. Ovarian ablation in early breast cancer: an overview of the randomized trials. *Lancet* 348:1189–96

101. Spicer DV, Ursin G, Parisby V, et al. 1994. Changes in mammographic densities induced by a hormonal contraceptive designed to reduce breast cancer risk. *J. Natl. Cancer Inst.* 86:431–36

102. Klijn JG, Blamey RW, Boccardo F, Tominaga T, Duchateau L, Sylvester R. 2001. Combined tamoxifen and luteinizing hormone-releasing hormone (LHRH) agonist versus LHRH agonist alone in premenopausal advanced breast cancer: a meta-analysis of four randomized trials. *J. Clin. Oncol.* 19:343–53

103. Davidson N, O'Neill A, Vukov A, et al. 1999. Effect of chemohormonal therapy in premenopausal, node (+), receptor (+) breast cancer: an Eastern Cooperative Oncology Group Phase III Intergroup Trial (E5188, INT-0101). *Proc. Am. Soc. Clin. Oncol.* 18:67a, Abstr. 249

104. Prentice RL. 2000. Future possibilities in the prevention of breast cancer: fat and fiber and breast cancer research. *Breast Cancer Res.* 2(4):268–76

105. Willet WC, Dietz WH, Colditz GA. 1999. Guidelines for a healthy weight. *N. Engl. J. Med.* 341(6):427–31

106. Willett WC, Stampfer MJ, Colditz GA, et al. 1987. Moderate alcohol consumption and the risk of breast cancer. *N. Engl. J. Med.* 316(19):1174–88

107. Zhang S, Hunter DJ, Forman MR, et al. 1999. Dietary carotenoids and vitamins A, C, and E and risk of breast cancer. *J. Natl. Cancer Inst.* I91(6):547–56

108. Zhang S, Hunter DJ, Hankinson SE, et al. 1999. A prospective study of folate intake and the risk of breast cancer. *JAMA* 281(17):1632–37

109. Thune I, Brenn T, Lund E, et al. 1997. Physical activity and the risk of breast cancer. *N. Engl. J. Med.* 336(18):1269–75

110. Hunter DJ, Spiegelman D, Adami HO, et al. 1996. Cohort studies of fat intake and the risk of breast cancer: a pooled analysis. *N. Engl. J. Med.* 334(6):356–61

111. Lee MM, Lin SS. 2000. Dietary fat and breast cancer. *Annu. Rev. Nutr.* 20:221–48

112. Pierce JP, Faerber S, Wright FA, et al. 1997. Feasibility of a randomized trial of a high-vegetable diet to prevent breast cancer recurrence. *Nutr. Cancer* 28:282–88

113. The Women's Health Initiative Study

Group. 1998. Design of the Women's Health Initiative Clinical Trial and Observational Study. *Controlled Clin. Trials* 19:61–82

114. Boyd NF, Cousins M, Lockwood G, Tritchler D. 1992. Dietary fat and breast cancer risk: the feasibility of a clinical trial of breast cancer prevention. *Lipids* 27(10):821–26

115. Chlebowski RT, Blackburn GL, Buzzard IM, et al. 1993. Adherence to a dietary fat intake reduction program in postmenopausal women receiving therapy for early breast cancer. The Women's Intervention Nutrition Study. *J. Clin. Oncol.* 11:2072–80

116. Chlebowski RT, Blackburn G, Winters B, et al. 2000. Long term adherence to dietary fat reduction in the Women's Intervention Nutrition Study. *Proc. Am. Soc. Clin. Oncol.* 19:78a, Abstr. 300

117. Rock CL, Thomson C, Cann BJ, et al. 2001. Reduction in fat intake is not associated with weight loss in most women after breast cancer diagnosis. *Cancer* 91(1):25–34

118. National Institutes of Health/National Heart, Lung and Blood Institute. 1998. Clinical guideline on the identification, evaluation, and treatment of overweight and obesity in adults. *Obes. Res.* 6:51S–210S

119. Barrett-Connor E. 1999. A pill for all by the year 2000? *Prev. Med.* 28:600–7

120. Manson JE, Martin KA. 2001. Postmenopausal hormone replacement therapy. *N. Engl. J. Med.* 345(1):34–40

121. Schairer C, Persson I, Falkeborn M, et al. 1997. Breast cancer risk associated with gynecologic surgery and indications for such surgery. *Int. J. Cancer* 70:150–54

122. Ross RK, Paganini-Hill A, Wan PC, Pike MC. 2000. Effect of hormone replacement therapy on breast cancer risk: estrogen versus estrogen plus progestin. *J. Natl. Cancer Inst.* 92(4):328–32

123. O'Connor AM, Tugwell P, Wells GA, et al. 1998. A decision aid for women considering hormone therapy after menopause: decision support framework and evaluation. *Patient Educ. Couns.* 33:267–79

124. Grodstein F, Manson JE, Stampfer MJ. 2001. Postmenopausal hormone use and secondary prevention of coronary events in the Nurses' Health Study. A prospective, observational study. *Ann. Intern. Med.* 135(1):1–8

125. Hulley S, Grady D, Bush T, et al. 1998. Randomized trial of estrogen plus progestin for secondary prevention of coronary heart disease in postmenopausal women. Heart and Estrogen/progestin Replacement Study (HERS) Research Group. *JAMA* 280(7):605–13

126. Lenfant C. 2000. *Preliminary trends in the Women's Health Initiative*, Apr. 3. Bethesda, MD: Natl. Heart Lung Blood Inst. Commun. Off.

127. Loprinzi CL, Barton DL, Rhodes D. 2001. Management of hot flashes in breast-cancer survivors. *Lancet Oncol.* 2:199–204

128. Ursin G, Ross RK, Sullivan-Halley J, et al. 1998. Use of oral contraceptives and risk of breast cancer in young women. *Breast Cancer Res. Treat.* 50(2):175–84

129. Tryggvadottir L, Tulinius H, Eyfjord JE, et al. 2001. Breastfeeding and reduced risk of breast cancer in an Icelandic cohort study. *Am. J. Epidemiol.* 154(1):37–42

130. Melbye M, Wohlfahrt J, Olsen JH, et al. 1997. Induced abortion and the risk of breast cancer. *N. Engl. J. Med.* 336(2):81–85

131. Rookus MA, van Leeuwen FE. 1996. Induced abortion and risk for breast cancer: reporting (recall) bias in a Dutch case-control study. *J. Natl. Cancer Inst.* 88(23):1759–64

132. Ingram D, Sanders K, Kolybaba M, Lopez D. 1997. Case-control study of phyto-oestrogens and breast cancer. *Lancet* 350:990–94

133. Den Tonkelaar I, Keinan-Bokar L, Veer PV, et al. 2001. Urinary phytoestrogens

and postmenopausal breast cancer risk. *Cancer Epidemiol. Biomarkers Prev.* 10(3):223–28

134. Zmuda JM, Cauley JA, Ljung BM, et al. 2001. Bone mass and breast cancer risk in older women: differences by stage at diagnosis. *J. Natl. Cancer Inst.* 93(12):930–36

135. Chow CK, Venzon D, Jones EC, et al. 2000. Effect of tamoxifen on mammographic density. *Cancer Epidemiol. Biomarkers Prev.* 9(9):917–21

136. Cauley JA, Lucas FL, Kuller LH, et al. 1999. Elevated serum estradiol and testosterone concentrations are associated with a high risk of breast cancer. *Ann. Intern. Med.* 130:270–77

137. Hankinson SE, Willett WC, Manson JE, et al. 1998. Plasma sex steroid hormone levels and risk of breast cancer in postmenopausal women. *J. Natl. Cancer Inst.* 90(17):1292–99

138. Fabian CJ, Kimler BF, Zalles CM, et al. 2000. Short-term breast cancer prediction by random periareolar fine-needle aspiration cytology and the Gail risk model. *J. Natl. Cancer Inst.* 92(15):1217–27

139. Evron E, Dooley WC, Umbricht CB, et al. 2001. Detection of breast cancer cells in ductal lavage fluid by methylation-specific PCR. *Lancet* 357(9265):1335–36

140. Kimler BF, Fabian CJ, Wallace DD. 2000. Breast cancer chemoprevention trials using the fine-needle aspiration model. *J. Cell. Biochem. Suppl.* 34:7–12

141. Fabian CJ. 2001. Breast cancer chemoprevention: beyond tamoxifen. *Breast Cancer Res.* 3(2):99–103

142. Labrie F, Labrie C, Belanger A, et al. 1999. EEM-652 (SCH 57068), A third generation SERM acting as pure antiestrogen in the mammary gland and endometrium. *J. Steroid Biochem. Mol. Biol.* 69(1–6):51–84

143. Munster PN, Buzdar A, Dhingra K, et al. 2001. Phase I study of a third-generation selective estrogen receptor modulator, LY353381. HCL, in metastatic breast cancer. *J. Clin. Oncol.* 19(7):2002–9

144. Cauley JA, Zmuda JM, Bauer DC, et al. 2001. Does statin use reduce the risk of breast cancer in older women? A prospective study. *Proc. Am. Soc. Clin. Oncol.* 20:413a, Abstr. 1647

145. Pedersen TR, Wilhelmsen L, Faergeman O, et al. 2000. Follow-up study of patients randomized in the Scandinavian simvastatin survival study (4S) of cholesterol lowering. *Am. J. Cardiol.* 86(3):257–62

146. Egan KM, Stampfer MJ, Giovannucci E, et al. 1996. Prospective study of regular aspirin use and the risk of breast cancer. *J. Natl. Cancer Inst.* 88(14):941–42

147. Harris RE, Kasbari S, Farrar WB. 1999. Prospective study of nonsteroidal antiinflammatory drugs and breast cancer. *Oncol. Rep.* 6(1):71–73

148. Chan KC, Knox WF, Gandhi A, et al. 2001. Blockade of growth factor receptors in ductal carcinoma in situ inhibits epithelial proliferation. *Br. J. Surg.* 88(3):412–18

Annu. Rev. Med. 2002. 53:541–55

POTENTIAL NEW THERAPIES FOR THE TREATMENT OF HIV-1 INFECTION

Jon H. Condra, Michael D. Miller, Daria J. Hazuda, and Emilio A. Emini
Merck Research Laboratories, West Point, Pennsylvania 19486;
e-mail: emilio_emini@merck.com

Key Words   protease, reverse transcriptase, integrase, entry inhibitors, assembly inhibitors

■ **Abstract**   The development and clinical use of chemotherapeutic agents for the treatment of persistent HIV-1 infection over the past decade has profoundly and favorably affected the course of HIV-1 disease for many infected individuals. Unfortunately, the long-term use of these therapies is complicated by unwanted metabolic side effects, by issues of adherence, and by the selection of viral variants with reduced susceptibility. These complications have spurred the search for new anti-HIV-1 agents having improved pharmacological properties and expressing activity against viral variants resistant to the currently available agents. This brief review describes the current state of this search as well as potentially novel viral targets for chemotherapeutic intervention.

INTRODUCTION

Following the identification of the human immunodeficiency virus type 1 (HIV-1) as the causative agent of the acquired immunodeficiency syndrome (AIDS), an intensive effort was mounted to identify and develop drugs to inhibit the virus' replication and prevent AIDS-related disease. Initial work focused on inhibitors of two well-characterized, essential viral enzymes: the reverse transcriptase (RT) and the protease (PR). All antiretroviral drugs currently approved for clinical use are directed against one of these targets.

With the advent of highly potent drugs and with their widespread use in increasingly effective combinations, it has become possible to suppress viral replication for extended periods of time in many patients and to halt, and often reverse, the immunosuppression that is the hallmark of AIDS. This has been reflected by dramatic reductions in the incidence of AIDS-related opportunistic infections and deaths.

Because all available antiretroviral drugs are targeted against the viral replicative machinery, they are effective only against actively replicating viruses and only as long as they continue to be taken regularly. In the absence of adequate immunological control (generally compromised in AIDS patients), interruption of therapy, even after prolonged viral suppression, is often accompanied by a rapid resurgence of viral replication and immunological decline. Unless a mechanism can be found to clear viral reservoirs and/or mount a suppressive anti-HIV-1 immune response (e.g., by immunization), it is likely that lifelong control of viral replication will require lifelong therapy.

Accordingly, the long-term clinical effectiveness of these potent drugs is limited by the ability of patients to adhere to their complex dosing regimens and to tolerate their side effects. Over time, inadequate drug exposures due to limitations of drug efficacy or to inadequate adherence may permit viral replication in the presence of drug, leading to the emergence of drug-resistant viruses.

The 15 drugs that are currently approved for the treatment of HIV-1 infection fall into three therapeutic classes: the nucleoside (and nucleotide) analog RT inhibitors (NRTIs), the nonnucleoside RT inhibitors (NNRTIs), and the protease inhibitors (PIs). Because of their similar chemical structures and mechanisms of action, the emergence of viral resistance to one drug frequently results in cross-resistance to other, often all, members of the same therapeutic class. Thus, in practice, the development of viral resistance narrows the future therapeutic options much more than the existence of these 15 drugs would imply, and there remains an urgent need for new and effective drugs that will be convenient, well-tolerated, and capable of suppressing viruses that are resistant to existing drugs.

The aggressive search for new effective antiretroviral drugs therefore continues, and as additional viral targets have been identified, they have provided new opportunities for drug discovery. In addition, many new drugs directed against the RT and protease, designed to address many existing deficiencies, are in development. This review highlights some of the most promising drug candidates in new and existing drug classes that may enter the AIDS treatment armamentarium over the next few years. The reader is also referred to the article by Wlodawer in this volume (1).

NEW DRUGS AGAINST EXISTING VIRAL TARGETS

Nucleoside and Nucleotide Analogs

The greatest challenges in the development of new, effective NRTIs relate to safety, tolerability, and drug resistance. Because these are analogs of the natural substrates for DNA synthesis, potent activity against viral polymerases may be accompanied by inhibition of cellular enzymes, and the permissible doses of many existing NRTIs become limited by toxicity. The many host enzymes, both known and unknown, involved in nucleotide metabolism make it difficult to anticipate these toxicities before large-scale animal or human safety studies, which are generally done late in the drug development process. Accordingly, most efforts to identify new NRTIs address drug potency, pharmacokinetics, and activity against viral isolates resistant to existing NRTIs.

One of the most promising drugs in the newest generation of investigational compounds is tenofovir (PMPA), under development by Gilead Sciences. As a nucleotide analog, it is metabolized intracellularly to the active drug, tenofovir diphosphate (PMPApp), which acts as a DNA chain terminator. Although resistance to many existing NRTIs is mediated by the removal of inhibitor from the terminated chain, tenofovir is thought to bind to the enzyme at a site from which removal is inefficient (1a). Consistent with this interpretation, tenofovir retains activity against many viral isolates that are highly resistant to existing NRTIs, although resistance is conferred by the K65R RT substitution and by insertions at codon T69 (2). Both of these mutations are selected by multiple NRTIs and mediate broad loss of viral susceptibility to the NRTIs (3). The tenofovir prodrug, tenofovir disoproxil fumarate, has demonstrated antiviral activity in two phase III clinical trials and is currently under consideration for marketing approval for HIV-1 therapy.

Other NRTIs currently in development include emtricitabine [2′,3′-dideoxy-5-fluoro-3′-thiacytidine (FTC)] and diaminopurine dioxolane/dioxolane guanosine (DAPD/DXG), both by Triangle Pharmaceuticals. FTC is a close analog of 3TC (4), an approved and widely used NRTI, but has somewhat greater potency and the potential for once-daily dosing (5). DAPD/DXG has demonstrated good tolerability and antiviral efficacy in phase I/II studies (6) and activity in vitro against some NRTI-resistant viruses (7).

Nonnucleoside Reverse Transcriptase Inhibitors

Although current NNRTIs have demonstrated potent antiviral activity in vitro and in HIV-1-infected patients, they are highly vulnerable to the emergence of drug-resistant viral variants. Accordingly, efforts to develop new NNRTIs have focused on agents that will retain activity against viruses resistant to existing members of this drug class.

TMC-120 (R147681) and TMC-125 (R165335), both under development by Tibotec, are intended to retain activity against wild-type and common NNRTI-resistant viruses. When selected in culture, resistant variants arose more slowly in the presence of TMC-120 or TMC-125 than in the presence of the approved NNRTIs nevirapine or efavirenz (8), although the selected RT amino acid substitutions, L100I, Y181C; Y188L, and G190E, are characteristically selected by the existing NNRTIs. In phase I/II clinical studies, TMC-120 demonstrated potent antiretroviral activity over a seven-day period (9), but its potential to select resistant viruses in vivo is currently unknown.

Several investigational NNRTIs from DuPont Pharmaceuticals, DPC 082, DPC 083, DPC 961, and DPC 963, have demonstrated potent (low-nanomolar) inhibition of wild-type virus and various NNRTI-resistant mutant viruses in vitro, and reduced human serum protein binding compared with currently used NNRTIs (10). However, no data on human pharmacokinetics of these compounds are yet available, and their potential clinical utility remains to be determined.

Protease Inhibitors

Although the HIV-1 protease inhibitors (PIs) have exhibited potent suppression of viral replication in infected patients, their long-term clinical utility is limited by side effects and viral drug resistance. New-generation PI development efforts have focused on compounds that retain activity against existing PI-resistant variants, either owing to differences in resistance specificity, or with sufficient in vivo drug exposure and potency to overcome drug-resistant viruses.

Tipranavir (TPV), discovered by researchers at Pharmacia-Upjohn and now being developed by Boehringer-Ingelheim, has a nonpeptidyl structure whose interaction with the protease depends less on the amino acid side-chains of the protease than those of earlier PIs (11, 12). Accordingly, the inhibition of the protease by TPV is less affected by many amino acid substitutions that confer significant resistance to other PIs (13). Codosing of TPV with ritonavir, which inhibits TPV's metabolism, is necessary to achieve efficacious drug exposures. Although reported virological responses to TPV in early clinical studies were moderate (14), further improvements in formulation may permit sufficient drug exposures for greater therapeutic utility.

BMS-232632, in phase III clinical trials by Bristol Myers-Squibb, is being developed to be the first HIV PI intended for once-daily dosing. In a phase II clinical study of therapy-naive patients receiving BMS-232632, in addition to the NRTIs d4T and ddI, about 68% of patients receiving 400 mg BMS doses of the PI experienced sustained HIV-1 suppression (15). At this dose, however, about 30% of patients also experienced dose-related grade 3 or 4 hyperbilirubinemia. Although blood levels of BMS-232632 can be increased by ritonavir coadministration (16), the tolerability of this increased exposure remains to be determined.

Other investigational PIs designed to retain activity against resistant viral variants are in preclinical development. These include DPC 681 and DPC 684 (17), from DuPont Pharmaceuticals, and TMC126 (18), from Tibotec. These compounds have low-picomolar inhibitory activity against wild-type HIV-1, with minimal losses of potency against several PI-resistant viral variants. However, owing to the great diversity of mutational patterns found in natural viral populations and the early developmental stages of these compounds, their clinical potential against PI-resistant viruses awaits further testing.

NEW DRUGS AGAINST NOVEL VIRAL TARGETS

Integrase Inhibitors

Integrase is the third of the enzymatic proteins encoded by HIV-1. Integrase catalyzes the insertion of the HIV-1 DNA into the genome of the host cell. Integration is required for stable maintenance of the viral genome and HIV-1 gene expression. Many compounds have been shown to inhibit integrase activity in biochemical assays (reviewed in 19, 20), but it is only recently that the 1,3 diketo acid analogs have been shown to inhibit HIV-1 replication by preventing integration (21).

Integrase is required for the three specific steps in integration: (*a*) assembly of a specific complex (viral preintegration complex) on the HIV-1 DNA, (*b*) 3′ endonucleolytic processing of the viral DNA 3′ termini, and finally (*c*) strand transfer, or joining of the viral and cellular DNAs (reviewed in 22, 23). Each of these steps can be performed in vitro using recombinantly expressed integrase protein and short oligonucleotide substrates to represent the viral ends (24, 25). Diketo acid analogs are highly selective, potent inhibitors of strand transfer. Specific inhibition of strand transfer has been documented both in vitro and in HIV-1–infected cells (21, 26). Inhibition of strand transfer during HIV-1 infection allows the viral DNA to become accessible to metabolism by cellular recombination and repair enzymes. The products of cellular metabolism are integration incompetent and unstable; thus, these inhibitors effectively produce an irreversible block of viral replication.

Integration is a complex process and it is not easy to assign an inhibitor mechanism of action in the infected cell. A variety of small molecules have been shown to inhibit the activity of integrase in biochemical assays, but the biological activity of many of these compounds was, upon later analysis, shown to be the result of their effects on viral fusion and entry (19, 20). The biological activity of the diketo acids, as inhibitors of integrase, has been validated by a careful analysis of their mechanism in infected cells, as well as by the selection and characterization of resistant viral variants (21, 27). Viruses selected for lessened susceptibility to the diketo acids harbor specific amino acid substitutions in the integrase active site (T66I, S153Y, and M154I). When two or more of these mutations are introduced into either the virus or the recombinantly expressed enzyme, diketo acid resistance is engendered in both virological and biochemical assays (21). Interestingly, these mutations mediate substantially decreased integrase enzymatic function in biochemical assays. Resistant viral variants also exhibit impaired replicative capacity in cell culture, possibly accounting for the observation that viral resistance selection in culture typically requires months of continual passage in the presence of inhibitor.

The diketo acids were identified in assays specifically biased to identify inhibitors of strand transfer using recombinant integrase assembled onto immobilized oligonucleotides as a surrogate for authentic HIV-1 preintegration complexes. The relative potencies of these analogs in strand transfer assays are comparable to assays using viral preintegration complexes isolated from HIV-1–infected cells (21). These compounds therefore provide the first validation of an assay using recombinantly expressed integrase to identify biologically relevant integrase inhibitors. Modifications of the originally identified compounds have led to the derivation of integrase inhibitors that exhibit antiviral activities in vitro that are comparable to many of the clinically effective antiretroviral agents currently available (28). The observation that compounds with the necessary potency and specificity can be derived thus bodes well for the future development of integrase inhibitors as chemotherapeutic agents for the treatment of HIV-1. The identification of 1,3 diketo acid analogs as bona fide inhibitors of integration and the elucidation of their distinct mechanism of action as specific inhibitors of the strand transfer activity of integrase validate a new approach for exploiting this important chemotherapeutic target.

Viral Entry Inhibitors

THE MOLECULAR BASIS OF HIV-1 ENTRY   An infectious HIV-1 virion consists of a nucleoprotein core surrounded by a lipid bilayer membrane derived from the cell that produced the virion. Infection of a new cell requires that the core, which contains the viral genome and proteins required for subsequent steps in the viral life cycle, be delivered into the cytoplasm of the host cell. The virus membrane and the plasma membrane of the host cell represent physical barriers between the core and its obligate destination. To breach these topological barriers, enveloped viruses have evolved genes encoding proteins that catalyze the fusion of viral and cellular membranes and thereby place the core in the host cell cytoplasm. In the case of HIV-1, the viral membrane fusion machinery is thought to be wholly contained in the virally encoded envelope glycoproteins, gp120 and gp41. A brief description of the structure and function of the envelope glycoproteins in HIV-1 entry follows (for more extensive reviews, see 29–31).

The gp120/gp41 glycoproteins are proteolytic products of a 160-kDa precursor, gp160. The gp120, or SU (surface), subunit remains noncovalently associated with the gp41, or TM (transmembrane), subunit following proteolysis, probably in trimeric form. These proteins are found on the surfaces of infectious virions, where they function together to bind appropriate receptors on target cells (see below) and subsequently to catalyze the fusion of virus and cell membranes. Receptor binding is a function of the gp120 subunit. The correct engagement of cell surface receptors by gp120 is thought to activate the membrane fusion function of gp41, thus coupling specific target cell recognition to viral entry.

Early studies indicated that gp120 binds with high affinity to the human CD4 molecule found notably on helper T cells but also on other cell types. This finding provided an attractive explanation for one of the major clinical features of HIV-1 infection, the profound depletion of CD4+ T cells. However, CD4 alone is insufficient to trigger gp120/gp41-driven membrane fusion. Activation of the membrane fusion function requires gp120 to engage a second receptor, or coreceptor, after first binding to CD4. The coreceptor can be one of any number of seven-transmembrane domain, G-protein-coupled receptors for chemokines, but the chemokine receptors CCR5 and CXCR4 are generally thought to serve as the major coreceptors for HIV-1 strains in vivo (31). Diverse HIV-1 isolates display various patterns of coreceptor usage owing to differences in the amino acid sequence of highly variable regions of the gp120 subunit.

The gp41 subunit displays structural features, implicated in membrane fusion activity, that are highly similar to those found in the corresponding envelope glycoproteins of other enveloped viruses (32–36). Although the triggering mechanism differs among different virus envelope proteins, the conserved structural features support the idea that these proteins use a common strategy to catalyze virus-cell membrane fusion. These structural features include two heptad repeat regions [designated HR1 (or "N") and HR2 (or "C")] in the ectodomain and two stretches of hydrophobic amino acids that are described below. The proteins trimerize primarily because of the formation of a three-stranded parallel coiled coil consisting of one HR1 heptad repeat from each of three protomers. Structural studies indicate that in their most stable state, each of these trimeric proteins contains a characteristic "trimer-of-hairpins" motif, in which the three HR2 (or C) regions pack in antiparallel fashion into grooves along the three-stranded coiled coil. The trimer-of-hairpins arrangement thus forms a rigid protein rod that, because of its antiparallel packing, brings the two ends of the ectodomain together at one end.

There are two conserved hydrophobic stretches in gp41, namely the "fusion peptide," located at the amino terminus of the glycoprotein, and the transmembrane domain, which anchors the protein in the viral membrane. The fusion peptide is believed to insert into the target cell membrane in response to the appropriate triggering stimulus, yielding a single polypeptide chain that is simultaneously anchored in two different membranes. Notably, the two heptad repeat regions that form the trimer of hairpins lie between the fusion peptide and the transmembrane domain. Therefore the trimer of hairpins, regardless of the pathway by which it is formed, brings both the fusion peptide and the transmembrane domains together at one end of the protein rod. By extension, this arrangement should bring the viral and cellular membranes quite near each other, too. However, it is not yet clear whether this close apposition is sufficient to drive membrane fusion or whether other undefined steps are required subsequently.

In principle, antiviral drugs could block HIV-1 entry by inhibiting gp120-CD4 binding, gp120-coreceptor binding, or gp41 function, and in fact each of these potential targets has been exploited by multiple inhibitors in cell culture systems. Indeed, there is now at least one inhibitor in each mechanistic class being tested in clinical trials. The remainder of this section describes each of the inhibitors in current clinical trials.

INHIBITION OF GP120 BINDING TO CD4: PRO542   Over the years, numerous attempts have been made to use various forms of soluble CD4 to inhibit the interaction between gp120 and its receptor. All have failed to yield a successful chemotherapeutic agent. The most recent form of CD4 in development consists of a fusion of the first two domains of CD4 to human IgG2. This molecule, first described by Maddon and colleagues (37) and dubbed PRO542 by Progenics, Inc., is tetravalent, i.e., it contains four gp120 binding sites. PRO542 blocks replication of numerous HIV-1 isolates in cell culture with typical IC_{90} values of 25 μg/ml or less, although some isolates are resistant (38, 39). PRO542's in vitro properties are compatible with possible clinical use if therapeutically relevant levels can be reached and maintained in vivo.

Two clinical trials designed to measure pharmacokinetic properties and initial antiviral efficacy of PRO542 have been reported (40, 41). Both demonstrated that it is possible to achieve sustained levels of PRO542 in people and that such sustained levels can exert an antiviral effect. The drawbacks to this therapy are the required dose and mode of delivery. The clinical studies suggest that doses of 5–10 mg/kg will be needed to obtain therapeutic plasma levels of PRO542. Patients will need to receive intravenous infusions, probably weekly, of relatively large amounts of protein. The studies performed to date have been short-term, so it is difficult to assess how efficacious and tolerable PRO542 will be over a period of months to years and how readily viral variants resistant to PRO542 will emerge.

INHIBITION OF GP120 BINDING TO CORECEPTOR   The discovery of HIV-1 coreceptors brought new potential therapeutic targets to light (42; see 31 for review). The principle that blocking coreceptor access could inhibit HIV-1 replication was proven by two observations: (*a*) Natural ligands of CXCR4 and CCR5 block replication of certain virus strains, and (*b*) CD4+ lymphocytes from humans lacking cell-surface CCR5, owing to CCR5 gene mutations, are resistant to infection by CCR5-dependent HIV-1 strains. Remarkably, only five years after the first reports describing the HIV-1 coreceptors, inhibitors of viral interaction with CXCR4 and CCR5 were identified and tested in early clinical trials.

CXCR4 INHIBITOR AMD3100   The bicyclam AMD3100 (referred to as JM3100 in earlier literature) was first identified as an anti-HIV-1 agent in1994, prior to the discovery of the viral coreceptors (43). Originally thought to be an inhibitor of a postentry step, AMD3100 was subsequently found to bind specifically to CXCR4 (44, 45). The compound blocks replication of CXCR4-dependent HIV-1 strains but not of CCR5-dependent strains. An isolate of HIV-1 selected in vitro for resistance to AMD3100 and displaying cross-resistance to heparin, dextran sulfate, and other polyanionic compounds was found to have mutations in gp120 (44). AMD3100 also showed some antiviral activity in the scid-hu thy/liv mouse model, suggesting the possibility that AMD3100 might work as an antiviral agent in humans (46). Results of a phase I safety and pharmacokinetic study of AMD3100 in healthy volunteers were recently reported (47). The compound had no oral bioavailability; however, single doses administered by subcutaneous injection (40 or 80 μg/kg) or intravenous infusion (10, 20, 40, or 80 μg/kg) yielded detectable plasma concentrations of AMD3100. At the highest dose, plasma concentrations of AMD3100 were above 30 ng/ml for 8 h and above 10 ng/ml for 12 h. Because AMD3100 is reported to block replication of HIV-1 strains with typical IC_{50}s of 10 ng/ml in vitro and $\sim$40 ng/ml in scid-hu mice, the authors cite this as evidence that AMD3100 can remain in plasma at therapeutically meaningful levels for some time. Nonetheless, the company pursuing development of the compound, Anormed, recently announced discontinuation of the development effort for AMD 3100, apparently because of poor clinical tolerability.

Additional inhibitors of viral-CXCR4 interaction in preclinical studies include the peptidic inhibitors ALX40-4C (48), T22 (49), T134, and T140 (50). A serious concern for the development of any CXCR4 antagonist, however, is the possibility of mechanism-based toxicity suggested by the results of studies in mice lethally irradiated and then reconstituted with hematopoietic cells from mice lacking CXCR4. These studies showed that continued presence of CXCR4 is required for normal hematopoiesis in adult mice (51–53), raising the possibility that long-term antagonism of CXCR4 could result in impairment of hematopoiesis.

CCR5 INHIBITOR SCH-C   Although many small-molecule CCR5 inhibitors have been described, early clinical data have been reported for only one, compound SCH-C from Schering-Plough. No data have appeared in the literature, but results of a phase I trial were reported at the eighth Conference on Retroviruses and Opportunistic Infection (54). The compound was generated by a medicinal chemistry effort to optimize a lead identified in a high-throughput screen for CCR5 antagonists. SCH-C blocks the activities of the natural ligands of CCR5 and was reported to be highly specific for the CCR5 receptor when tested against a panel of 50 G-protein–coupled receptors. SCH-C was also shown to be a potent inhibitor of infection by CCR5-dependent HIV-1 strains, including numerous primary HIV-1 isolates with a mean IC_{90} of ~20 nM. A phase I dose-ranging study in uninfected volunteers showed SCH-C to have acceptable pharmacokinetics. At an oral dose of 200 mg, plasma levels exceeded 20 nM for 72 h. These results suggest the possibility that SCH-C could be administered once daily. However, one potentially serious problem with the compound was observed in that some subjects receiving the highest dose displayed cardiac QT wave prolongations, a potentially serious adverse event. It remains to be seen whether development of SCH-C will be stopped because of this side effect. Other CCR5-directed agents in preclinical or early clinical development include TAK779, a small-molecule CCR5 inhibitor (55, 56); PRO440, an anti-CCR5 monoclonal antibody (57, 58); several structural classes of small molecules reported by Merck (59–61); and the small-molecule compound SCH-D. This latter compound was reported by Schering-Plough to be more potent than SCH-C, with a mean IC_{90} of 4 nM, and to have oral bioavailability and pharmacokinetic properties in rats and monkeys similar to those of SCH-C (54).

gp41 INHIBITOR T-20 (PENTAFUSIDE)   Long before the existence of any structural information about gp41, synthetic peptides overlapping the two heptad repeat regions HRI [e.g., DP-107 (62)] and HRII [e.g., DP-178 (63)] were found to block HIV-1 replication in cell culture. In particular, DP-178 had remarkable potency, with an IC_{90} of about 0.3 nM (63). The eventual understanding that these two regions of gp41 play an important role in viral fusion and entry provided an attractive model to explain the antiviral activity of the synthetic peptides (30). The discovery of an extremely potent inhibitor that blocks HIV-1 replication by a novel mechanism raised the possibility that DP-178 itself might be clinically useful. As a relatively large (36 amino acids) synthetic peptide, however, DP-178 raised formidable obstacles for development, particularly regarding manufacturing and dosing. Despite these challenges, Trimeris and its partner, F. Hoffmann-La Roche, have developed this agent, now called T-20, into a viable therapeutic agent for HIV-1 infection. The first clinical trial of T-20, reported in 1998, was performed in HIV-1-infected subjects (64). Patients received one of four dose levels (3, 10, 30, or 100 mg) of intravenous infusions twice daily for 14 days. A significant reduction in plasma virus levels was seen in individuals receiving 30 mg or 100 mg doses. Numerous subsequent phase I and II clinical trials have confirmed the overall safety and antiviral efficacy of T-20 and have helped work out issues of formulation, dosing, and route of administration (65). Phase III trials are in progress.

gp41 INHIBITOR T1249   One problem likely to arise as T-20 is administered to greater numbers of patients is the emergence of resistant virus strains. Indeed, resistant viruses have been selected in cell culture, and as expected such viruses have mutations in the gp41 coding sequence (66). How the development of resistance will affect T-20's clinical utility is unknown, but to circumvent this potential problem, Trimeris and Roche have developed a second-generation gp41 peptide inhibitor. This peptide, T-1249, is a 39-mer representing a hybrid of sequences from HIV-1 and HIV type 2 that overlaps the T-20 region and contains a pharmacokinetic-enhancing domain present in T-20. The peptide is reportedly more potent than T-20 in vitro and is active against T-20-resistant HIV-1 strains. Results of a phase I/II trial of T-1249, conducted in HIV-1-infected subjects, showed that T-1249 can mediate a decrease of virus levels in patients following twice-daily subcutaneous administration (67). Expanded clinical trials are ongoing.

Viral Assembly Inhibitors

Assembly and release of HIV-1 are primarily governed by the viral gag (68) and vpu (69) proteins. It might be possible to discover and develop drugs that block assembly or release by binding to one of these components. Indeed, there is one known example of a small molecule that has antiviral efficacy in vivo and is thought to inhibit assembly by binding to a gag protein (70). This compound, a tripeptide with the sequence Gly-Pro-Gly-NH_2 (GPG), is being developed by Tripep AB, who have presented unpublished results from a two-week clinical trial (70). Plasma virus levels declined modestly in three of nine patients receiving the highest oral dose of GPG (4 g three times daily). Nonetheless, the observed antiviral efficacy is remarkable in light of GPG's relatively low potency against HIV-1 in cell culture (reported IC50s of 2.7–37 μM) (71). GPG was originally thought to inhibit HIV-1 replication by blocking viral entry, because the peptide corresponds to a conserved sequence in the gp120 V3 domain involved in coreceptor interaction (72). Subsequently, it was shown that this compound works against a wide variety of clinical isolates irrespective of coreceptor usage (71) and does not inhibit any step of the virus life cycle from entry through translation (73). Data from

Tripep indicate that GPG binds to the capsid (p24) protein, possibly interfering with gag oligomerization and hence disrupting the assembly pathway (70). Once the mechanism is better understood, it may be possible to discover more potent compounds that work by the same mechanism and that may be more effective clinically.

CONCLUSION

One approach to the search for new anti-HIV-1 therapeutic agents is to concentrate on discovering and developing novel versions of inhibitors whose modes of action are identical to those of inhibitors currently in clinical use. A critical characteristic of such agents is the potential for in vivo antiviral activity directed against viral variants resistant to the available drugs. The second approach, perhaps more promising, is the development of antiviral agents directed against novel HIV-1 targets. These targets are likely to include the HIV-1 integrase enzyme, various steps in the viral entry process into host cells, and various steps in the viral assembly process. Agents directed against a series of diverse targets may also exhibit noted synergistic antiviral activity when used together in patients. Unfortunately, the scientific uncertainties of the drug development process are such that many of the compounds described in this review may not be successfully developed into clinically usable drugs; nonetheless, each has at least proved the utility and value of the approach used to discover it. The extensive ongoing research efforts will undoubtedly result within a few years in a notable expansion of the number and quality of chemotherapeutic agents available to treat persistent HIV-1 infection and mitigate its clinical consequences.

Visit the Annual Reviews home page at www.AnnualReviews.org

LITERATURE CITED

1. Wlodawer A. 2002. Rational approach to drug design through structural biology. *Annu. Rev. Med.* 53:595–614
1a. Tuske S, Sarafianos SG, Clark AD, et al. 2001. Crystal structure of HIV-1 reverse transcriptase with template-primer terminated with the acyclic nucleotide reverse transcriptase inhibitor tenofovir. *Antiviral Ther.* 6(Suppl. 1):35–6 (Abstr.)
2. Miller MD, Margot NA, Hertogs K, et al. 2000. Anti-HIV activity profile of tenofovir (PMPA) against a panel of nucleoside-resistant clinical samples. *Antiviral Ther.* 5(Suppl. 3):4–5
3. Schinazi RF, Larder BA, Mellors JW. 2000. Mutations in retroviral genes associated with drug resistance: 2000–2001 update. *Int. Antiviral News* 8:65–91
4. Schinazi RF, McMillan A, Cannon D, et al. 1992. Selective inhibition of human immunodeficiency viruses by racemates and enantiomers of cis-5-fluoro-1-[2-(hydroxymethyl)-1,3-oxathiolan-5-yl]cytosine. *Antimicrob. Agents Chemother.* 36:2423–31
5. Van Der Horst C, Sanne I, Wakeford C, et al. 2001. Two randomized, controlled equivalence trials of emtricitibine (FTC)

to lamivudine (3TC). See Ref. 74, p. 48 (Abstr.)

6. Richman DD, Kessler H, Eron J, et al. 2000. Anti-HIV activity and tolerability of DAPD, a novel dioxolane guanosine RT inhibitor: initial results of a phase I/II 14-day monotherapy clinical trial. See Ref. 75, p. 200

7. Borroto-Esoda K, Mewshaw J, Wakefield D, et al. 1999. DAPD: a novel nucleoside inhibitor of HIV-1 replication, is active against drug-resistant isolates of HIV-1 from patients failing standard nucleoside therapy. *Abstr. 39th Intersci. Conf. Antimicrobial Agents and Chemother.*, *Sept. 26–29, San Francisco*, p. 316 (Abstr.)

8. de Bethune M-P, Azijn H, Andries K, et al. 2001. In vitro selection experiments demonstrate reduced development of resistance with TMC 120 and TMC 125 compared with first generation non-nucleoside reverse transcriptase inhibitors. *Antiviral Ther.* 6(Supp. 1):6 (Abstr.)

9. Gruzdev B, Horban A, Boron-Kaczmarska A, et al. 2001. TMC120, a new non-nucleoside reverse transcriptase inhibitor, is a potent antiretroviral in treatment naive, HIV-1 infected subjects. See Ref. 74, p. 46

10. Corbett JW, Ko SS, Rodgers JD, et al. 2000. Inhibition of clinically relevant mutant variants of HIV-1 by quinazolinone non-nucleoside reverse transcriptase inhibitors. *J. Med. Chem.* 43:2019–30

11. Poppe SM, Slade DE, Chong KT, et al. 1997. Antiviral activity of the dihydropyrone PNU-140690, a new nonpeptidic human-immunodeficiency-virus protease inhibitor. *Antimicrob. Agents Chemother.* 41:1058–63

12. Turner SR, Strohbach JW, Tommasi RA, et al. 1998. Tipranavir (PNU-140690): a potent, orally bioavailable nonpeptidic HIV protease inhibitor of the 5,6-dihydro-4-hydroxy-2-pyrone sulfonamide class. *J. Med. Chem.* 41:3467–76

13. Back NKT, van Wijk A, Remmerswaal D, et al. 2000. In vitro tipranavir susceptibility of HIV-1 isolates with reduced susceptibility to other protease inhibitors. *AIDS* 14:101–2

14. Wang Y, Daenzer C, Wood R, et al. 2000. The safety, efficacy and viral dynamics analysis of tipranavir, a new-generation protease inhibitor, in a phase II study in antiretroviral-naive HIV-1-infected patients. See Ref. 75, p. 201

15. Squires K, Gatell J, Piliero P, et al. 2001. AI424-007: 48-week safety and efficacy results from a Phase II study of a once-daily HIV-1 protease inhibitor (PI), BMS-232632. See Ref. 74, p. 47

16. O'Mara E, Mummaneni V, Bifano M, et al. 2001. Pilot study of the interaction between BMS-232632 and ritonavir. See Ref. 74, p. 268

17. Erickson-Viitanen SK, Kaltenbach R, Getman D, et al. 2001. DPC 681 and DPC 684: Resistance and cross-resistance profiles of second-generation HIV protease inhibitors. See Ref. 74, p. 46

18. Erickson JW, Gulnik S, Suvorov L, et al. 2001. A femtomolar HIV-1 protease inhibitor with subnanomolar activity against multidrug resistant HIV-1 strains. See. Ref. 74, p. 46

19. Pommier Y, Neamati N. 1999. Inhibitors of human immunodeficiency virus integrase. In *Advances in Virus Research*, ed. K Maramorosch, F Murphy, A Shatkin, 52:427. New York: Academic

20. Pommier Y, Marchand C, Neamati N. 2000. Retroviral integrase inhibitors year 2000: update and perspectives. *Antiviral Res.* 47:139–48

21. Hazuda DJ, Felock P, Witmer M, et al. 2000. Inhibitors of strand transfer that prevent integration and inhibit HIV-1 replication in cells. *Science* 287:646–50

22. Brown PO. 1998. Retroviruses. In *Retroviruses*, ed. JM Coffin, SH Hughes, HE Varmus, pp. 161–203. Cold Spring Harbor, NY: Cold Spring Harbor Lab. Press

23. Esposito D, Craigie R. 1999. HIV integrase structure and function. *Adv. Virus Res.* 52:319–33

24. Hazuda D, Felock PJ, Hastings JC, et al. 1997. Discovery and analysis of inhibitors of the human immunodeficiency integrase. *Drug Des. Discov.* 15:17–24

25. Jones KS, Coleman J, Merkel GW, et al. 1992. Retroviral integrase functions as a multimer and can turn over catalytically. *J. Biol. Chem.* 267:16037–40

26. Espeseth AS, Felock P, Wolfe A, et al. 2000. HIV-1 integrase inhibitors that compete with the target DNA substrate define a unique strand transfer conformation for integrase. *Proc. Natl. Acad. Sci. USA* 97:11244–49

27. Butler SL, Hansen MS, Bushman FD. 2001. A quantitative assay for HIV DNA integration in vivo. *Nat. Med.* 7:631–34

28. Wai JS, Egbertson MS, Payne LS, et al. 2000. 4-Aryl-2,4-dioxobutanoic acid inhibitors of HIV-1 integrase and viral replication in cells. *J. Med. Chem.* 43:4923–26

29. Wyatt R, Sodroski J. 1998. The HIV-1 envelope glycoproteins: fusogens, antigens, and immunogens. *Science* 280:1884–88

30. Chan DC, Kim PS. 1998. HIV entry and its inhibition. *Cell* 93:681–84

31. Berger EA, Murphy PM, Farber JM. 1999. Chemokine receptors as HIV-1 coreceptors: roles in viral entry, tropism, and disease. *Annu. Rev. Immunol.* 17:657–700

32. Bullough PA, Hughson FM, Skehel JJ, et al. 1994. Structure of influenza haemagglutinin at the pH of membrane fusion. *Nature* 371:37–43

33. Carr CM, Kim PS. 1993. A spring-loaded mechanism for the conformational change of influenza hemagglutinin. *Cell* 73:823–32

34. Carr CM, Chaudhry C, Kim PS. 1997. Influenza hemagglutinin is spring-loaded by a metastable native conformation. *Proc. Natl. Acad. Sci. USA* 94:14306–13

35. Chan DC, Fass D, Berger JM, et al. 1997. Core structure of gp41 from the HIV envelope glycoprotein. *Cell* 89:263–73

36. Caffrey M, Cai M, Kaufman J, et al. 1998. Three-dimensional solution structure of the 44 kDa ectodomain of SIV gp41. *EMBO J.* 17:4572–84

37. Allaway GP, Davis-Bruno KL, Beaudry GA, et al. 1995. Expression and characterization of CD4-IgG2, a novel heterotetramer that neutralizes primary HIV type 1 isolates. *AIDS Res. Hum. Retroviruses* 11:533–39

38. Trkola A, Pomales AB, Yuan H, et al. 1995. Cross-clade neutralization of primary isolates of human immunodeficiency virus type 1 by human monoclonal antibodies and tetrameric CD4-IgG. *J. Virol.* 69:6609–17

39. Gauduin MC, Allaway GP, Maddon PJ, et al. 1996. Effective ex vivo neutralization of human immunodeficiency virus type 1 in plasma by recombinant immunoglobulin molecules. *J. Virol.* 70:2586–92

40. Jacobson JM, Lowy I, Fletcher CV, et al. 2000. Single-dose safety, pharmacology, and antiviral activity of the human immunodeficiency virus (HIV) type 1 entry inhibitor PRO 542 in HIV-infected adults. *J. Infect. Dis.* 182:326–29

41. Shearer WT, Israel RJ, Starr S, et al. 2000. Recombinant CD4-IgG2 in human immunodeficiency virus type 1-infected children: phase 1/2 study. The Pediatric AIDS Clinical Trials Group Protocol 351 Study Team. *J. Infect. Dis.* 182:1774–79

42. Feng Y, Broder CC, Kennedy PE, et al. 1996. HIV-1 entry cofactor: functional cDNA cloning of a seven-transmembrane, G protein-coupled receptor [see comments]. *Science* 272:872–77

43. De Clercq E, Yamamoto N, Pauwels R, et al. 1994. Highly potent and selective inhibition of human immunodeficiency virus by the bicyclam derivative JM3100. *Antimicrob. Agents Chemother.* 38:668–74

44. Schols D, Este JA, Henson G, et al. 1997. Bicyclams, a class of potent anti-HIV agents, are targeted at the HIV coreceptor fusin/CXCR-4. *Antiviral Res.* 35:147–56

45. Donzella GA, Schols D, Lin SW, et al.

1998. AMD3100, a small molecule inhibitor of HIV-1 entry via the CXCR4 coreceptor. *Nat. Med.* 4:72–77

46. Datema R, Rabin L, Hincenbergs M, et al. 1996. Antiviral efficacy in vivo of the anti-human immunodeficiency virus bicyclam SDZ SID 791 (JM 3100), an inhibitor of infectious cell entry. *Antimicrob. Agents Chemother.* 40:750–54

47. Hendrix CW, Flexner C, MacFarland RT, et al. 2000. Pharmacokinetics and safety of AMD-3100, a novel antagonist of the CXCR-4 chemokine receptor, in human volunteers. *Antimicrob. Agents Chemother.* 44:1667–73

48. Doranz BJ, Grovit-Ferbas K, Sharron MP, et al. 1997. A small-molecule inhibitor directed against the chemokine receptor CXCR4 prevents its use as an HIV-1 coreceptor. *J. Exp. Med.* 186:1395–400

49. Murakami T, Nakajima T, Koyanagi Y, et al. 1997. A small molecule CXCR4 inhibitor that blocks T cell line-tropic HIV-1 infection. *J. Exp. Med.* 186:1389–93

50. Tamamura H, Xu Y, Hattori T, et al. 1998. A low-molecular-weight inhibitor against the chemokine receptor CXCR4: a strong anti-HIV peptide T140. *Biochem. Biophys. Res. Commun.* 253:877–82

51. Ma Q, Jones D, Springer TA. 1999. The chemokine receptor CXCR4 is required for the retention of B lineage and granulocytic precursors within the bone marrow microenvironment. *Immunity* 10:463–71

52. Ma Q, Jones D, Borghesani PR, et al. 1998. Impaired B-lymphopoiesis, myelopoiesis, and derailed cerebellar neuron migration in CXCR4- and SDF-1-deficient mice. *Proc. Natl. Acad. Sci. USA* 95:9448–53

53. Kawabata K, Ujikawa M, Egawa T, et al. 1999. A cell-autonomous requirement for CXCR4 in long-term lymphoid and myeloid reconstitution. *Proc. Natl. Acad. Sci. USA* 96:5663–67

54. Reyes G. 2001. Development of CCR5 antagonists as a new class of anti-HIV therapeutic. See Ref. 74, p. 285

55. Baba M, Nishimura O, Kanzaki N, et al. 1999. A small-molecule, nonpeptide CCR5 antagonist with highly potent and selective anti-HIV-1 activity. *Proc. Natl. Acad. Sci. USA* 96:5698–703

56. Shiraishi M, Aramaki Y, Seto M, et al. 2000. Discovery of novel, potent, and selective small-molecule CCR5 antagonists as anti-HIV-1 agents: synthesis and biological evaluation of anilide derivatives with a quaternary ammonium moiety. *J. Med. Chem.* 43:2049–63

57. Olson WC, Rabut GE, Nagashima KA, et al. 1999. Differential inhibition of human immunodeficiency virus type 1 fusion, gp120 binding, and CC-chemokine activity by monoclonal antibodies to CCR5. *J. Virol.* 73:4145–55

58. Trkola A, Ketas TJ, Nagashima KA, et al. 2001. Potent, broad-spectrum inhibition of human immunodeficiency virus type 1 by the CCR5 monoclonal antibody PRO 140. *J. Virol.* 75:579–88

59. Dorn CP, Finke PE, Oates B, et al. 2001. Antagonists of the human CCR5 receptor as anti-HIV-1 agents. 1. Discovery and initial structure-activity relationships for 1-amino-2-phenyl-4-(piperidin-1-yl)butanes. *Bioorg. Med. Chem. Lett.* 11:259–64

60. Finke PE, Meurer LC, Oates B, et al. 2001. Antagonists of the human CCR5 receptor as anti-HIV-1 agents. 2. Structure-activity relationships for substituted 2-Aryl-1-[N-(methyl)-N-(phenylsulfonyl)amino]-4-(piperidin-1-yl)butanes. *Bioorg. Med. Chem. Lett.* 11:265–70

61. Hale JJ, Budhu RJ, Mills SG, et al. 2001. 1,3,4-trisubstituted pyrrolidine CCR5 receptor antagonists. 1. Discovery of the pyrrolidine scaffold and determination of its stereochemical requirements. *Bioorg. Med. Chem. Lett.* 11:1437–40

62. Wild C, Oas T, McDanal C, et al. 1992. A synthetic peptide inhibitor of human immunodeficiency virus replication: correlation between solution structure and viral inhibition. *Proc. Natl. Acad. Sci. USA* 89:10537–41

63. Wild CT, Shugars DC, Greenwell TK, et al. 1994. Peptides corresponding to a predictive alpha-helical domain of human immunodeficiency virus type 1 gp41 are potent inhibitors of virus infection. *Proc. Natl. Acad. Sci. USA* 91:9770–74

64. Kilby JM, Hopkins S, Venetta TM, et al. 1998. Potent suppression of HIV-1 replication in humans by T-20, a peptide inhibitor of gp41-mediated virus entry [see comments]. *Nat. Med.* 4:1302–7

65. Lalezari J, Drucker J, Demasi R, et al. 2001. A controlled phase II trial assessing three doses of T-20 in combination with abacavir, amprenavir, low dose ritonavir and efavirenz in non-nucleoside naïve protease inhibitor experienced HIV-1 infected adults. See Ref. 74, p. 277

66. Rimsky LT, Shugars DC, Matthews TJ. 1998. Determinants of human immunodeficiency virus type 1 resistance to gp41-derived inhibitory peptides. *J. Virol.* 72:986–93

67. Eron J, Merigan T, Kilby M, et al. 2001. A 14-day assessment of the safety, pharmacokinetics, and antiviral activity of T-1249, a peptide inhibitor of membrane fusion. See Ref. 74, p. 67

68. Freed EO. 1998. HIV-1 gag proteins: diverse functions in the virus life cycle. *Virology* 251:1–15

69. Klimkait T, Strebel K, Hoggan MD, et al. 1990. The human immunodeficiency virus type 1-specific protein vpu is required for efficient virus maturation and release. *J. Virol.* 64:621–29

70. Vahlne A. 2001. Tripeptides that inhibit HIV-1: discovery and mode of action. *Abstr. Meet., HIV Therapeutics: Searching for the Next Generation, Feb 28–Mar 1*. London: SMI Group

71. Su J, Andersson E, Horal P, et al. 2001. The nontoxic tripeptide glycyl-prolyl-glycine amide inhibits the replication of human immunodeficiency virus type 1. *J. Hum. Virol.* 4:1–7

72. Su J, Palm A, Wu Y, et al. 2000. Deletion of the GPG motif in the HIV type 1 V3 loop does not abrogate infection in all cells. *AIDS Res. Hum. Retroviruses* 16:37–48

73. Su J, Naghavi MH, Jejcic A, et al. 2001. The tripeptide glycyl-prolyl-glycine amide does not affect the early steps of the human immunodeficiency virus type 1 replication. *J. Hum. Virol.* 4:8–15

74. 2001. *Abstracts of 8th Conference on Retroviruses and Opportunistic Infections, Feb. 4–8, Chicago*

75. 2000. *Abstracts of 7th Conference on Retroviruses and Opportunistic Infections, Jan. 30–Feb. 2, San Francisco*

Annu. Rev. Med. 2002. 53:557–93

THE CHALLENGE OF VIRAL RESERVOIRS IN HIV-1 INFECTION

Joel N. Blankson, Deborah Persaud, and Robert F. Siliciano
*Departments of Medicine and Pediatrics, Johns Hopkins University School of Medicine,
Baltimore, Maryland 21205; e-mail: rsilicia@welch.jhu.edu*

Key Words   AIDS, latency, HAART, sanctuary, persistence

■ **Abstract**   A viral reservoir is a cell type or anatomical site in association with
which a replication-competent form of the virus accumulates and persists with more
stable kinetic properties than the main pool of actively replicating virus. This article reviews several cell types and anatomical sites proposed as potential reservoirs for HIV-1.
It is now clear that HIV-1 persists in a small reservoir of latently infected resting memory
$CD4^+$ T cells, which shows minimal decay even in patients on highly active antiretroviral therapy (HAART). The persistence of virus in this reservoir is consistent with the
biology of these cells and the long-term persistence of immunologic memory. The viral
replication that continues in patients on suppressive HAART may also contribute to
the stability of this reservoir. There may be other reservoirs, but the latent reservoir in
resting $CD4^+$ T cells appears to be sufficient to guarantee lifetime persistence of HIV-1
in the majority of patients on current HAART regimens, and unless new approaches
are developed, eradication will not be possible. The clinical implications of this and
other HIV-1 reservoirs are discussed.

INTRODUCTION

Advances in the treatment of HIV-1 infection have dramatically reduced the death
rate from AIDS in the United States since 1996, when protease inhibitor–based
combination therapy regimens came into widespread use (1). In 1997, several
groups reported that combinations of a protease inhibitor with two nucleoside
analogue inhibitors of HIV-1 reverse transcriptase could reduce plasma virus to
undetectable levels in many patients (2–4). The success of protease inhibitors
exemplifies the power of rational drug design (see review by Wlodawer in this
volume, 4a). Potent new nonnucleoside reverse transcriptase inhibitors (NNRTIs)
have also been developed (5), and it is now clear that many different combinations
of three or more antiretroviral drugs will produce durable suppression of HIV-1
replication (6). This approach for the treatment of HIV-1 infection has become
known as highly active antiretroviral therapy (HAART). Patients who responded
well to HAART show a significant degree of immune reconstitution (see review
by Sempowski & Haynes in this volume, 6a). The excellent suppression of viral

replication achieved by many patients on HAART initially raised hopes for virus eradication (4).

In light of these remarkable therapeutic advances, it is interesting that the recently revised Department of Health and Human Services guidelines for the treatment of HIV-1 infection take a more conservative position on when antiretroviral therapy should be started (6). Clinical immunodeficiency does not develop until the CD4 count has declined from a normal level of 1000 cells/μl to <200 cells/μl, a process that takes an average of 10 years. Whereas previous guidelines recommended treating asymptomatic, chronically infected patients whose CD4 counts had fallen to <500 cells/μl, the revised guidelines state that it may be advisable to wait until the CD4 count has fallen to 350 cells/μl. The change in treatment strategy reflects growing awareness of the long-term toxicity of the drug regimens (7, 8; reviewed in 9) and a new pessimism about the possibility of virus eradication.

This pessimism has been occasioned by two findings. First, HIV-1 persists in reservoirs, the best-defined of which is a small pool of latently infected resting memory CD4$^+$ T cells carrying an integrated form of the viral genome (10, 11). This population of latently infected cells persists in adults (12–15) and children (16) receiving HAART. Second, there is evidence of ongoing virus production even in patients on HAART in whom viremia is suppressed to undetectable levels (17–21). This review considers the underlying basic science and the clinical implications of viral reservoirs and of the low level of virus production that continues in patients on HAART.

VIRAL DYNAMICS

Any discussion of HIV-1 persistence should begin with a review of the dynamics of viral replication in vivo. The quantitative analysis of HIV-1 replication in vivo has greatly advanced understanding of AIDS pathogenesis and antiretroviral therapy, and it will probably be useful in the study of many other viral infections. Progress was made possible by the development in 1993 of a quantitative assay for virus particles in the blood and the discovery that viremia is measurable throughout the course of the infection, even during the prolonged asymptomatic period between primary HIV-1 infection and the development of AIDS (22). Viremia was quantitated by an RT-PCR assay that detects genomic viral RNA in virus particles. The next fundamental advance was the realization by Ho and Shaw that, over the short term (days to weeks), viremia is relatively constant in individual patients and that perturbations in this quasi-steady state might provide insights into the dynamics of the virus production in vivo (23, 24). In 1995, they demonstrated that following the initiation of treatment with potent inhibitors of HIV-1 protease or reverse transcriptase, there was a rapid, exponential drop in viremia—a decline of 100-fold in a matter of days. They proposed that because both classes of drugs block new infection of susceptible cells, the normal equilibrium between virus production and virus clearance was disrupted, thereby revealing the decay characteristics of virus-producing compartments. The rapid drop in viremia immediately suggested that the half-life of plasma virus is very short (minutes to hours) (25), a conclusion confirmed by recent particle infusion studies (26). An even more important conclusion was that the half-life of the cells that produce almost all of the plasma virus is also very short, probably <1 day (23–25). In situ hybidization studies have shown that most virus-producing cells are CD4$^+$ T cells (27), mainly activated CD4$^+$ T cells. These cells die very quickly after infection, either from viral cytopathic effects or from attack by cytolytic T lymphocytes (CTL). It was this discovery that raised hopes that HAART might eradicate the infection.

An important corollary of rapid death of productively infected cells is that the steady-state level of viremia in an untreated individual must reflect a continuous process of new infection of susceptible cells at a rate that balances this rapid death. In an untreated patient, large numbers of CD4$^+$ T cells become infected daily. The reverse transcription process that occurs in each of those cells has a sufficiently high error rate (28, 29) that viral genomes with every possible single point mutation arise daily (30). Perelson and colleagues have estimated that if 10^8 new cells are infected per day, then not only are all possible single point mutations in the 10-kb HIV-1 genome generated daily, but almost 1% of all possible double mutations are generated each day (31). This finding has enormous implications for the evolution of drug resistance mutations and viral escape from immune effector mechanisms. Treatment failure is almost inevitable when drugs are given individually, particularly drugs for which a single point mutation confers resistance (24).

The next major development was the realization that simultaneous treatment with multiple drugs could overcome the striking propensity of the virus to evolve resistance to any single agent. Combinations of three potent antiretroviral drugs started at the same time reduced plasma HIV-1 RNA to undetectable levels in many patients (2–4). The limit of detection of current "ultrasensitive" RT-PCR assays for HIV-1 is 50 copies/ml of plasma. In the majority of patients with no preexisting drug resistance mutations, initiation of HAART can reduce the level of viremia from typical values of 10,000–100,000 copies/ml to <50 copies/ml. Because viral replication is directly linked to CD4 depletion and disease progression (32), this drop in viral replication has profound clinical significance.

Careful analysis of the kinetics of viral decay following the initiation of HAART showed that the decay is biphasic (4). After the rapid initial two-log drop, plasma virus levels fall more slowly (Figure 1). This probably reflects the decay of a different population of infected cells, cells that are not as readily killed when productively infected by HIV-1. It is necessary to postulate that in an untreated patient, these cells contribute only a small proportion of the plasma virus. The contribution of this compartment becomes apparent only when replication is suppressed by antiretroviral drugs. The half-life of the compartment responsible for this second phase of decay was estimated to be 1–4 weeks (4). A biphasic decay process was also observed directly in in situ hybidization studies of productively infected mononuclear cells in the lymphoid tissues (33). Children with perinatally acquired HIV-1 infection have the same biphasic decay process (34).

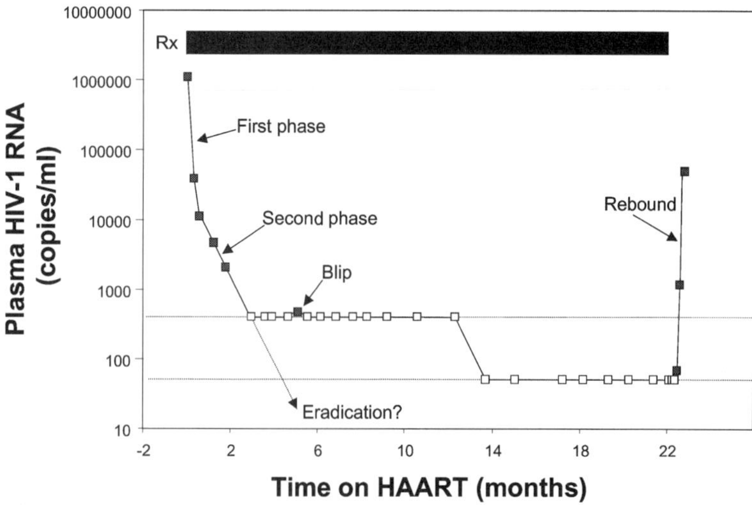

Figure 1   Plasma virus levels in a patient treated with HAART during primary HIV-1 infection. The first and second phases of decay are indicated. The second phase of decay reduces viremia below the limit of detection of the standard assay for plasma HIV-1 RNA (400 copies/ml). When a more sensitive assay for plasma HIV-1 RNA (50 copies/ml) became available, viremia was still below the limit of detection (indicated by the open symbols). Dotted lines indicate the limits of detection of the standard and ultrasensitive assays for plasma HIV-1 RNA. If HAART stopped all new infection of susceptible cells and if there were no viral reservoirs, then the second-phase decay would result in eradication in 2–3 years. However, even in patients with undetectable levels of viremia, the virus persists, as indicated by the presence of a stable reservoir of latently infected resting memory CD4$^+$ T cells, occasional low-level positive plasma HIV-1 RNA determinations (blips), continued production of low levels of virus detectable by special methods, and the rapid rebound of viremia observed if therapy is stopped.

The nature of the cellular or anatomical reservoir that is responsible for the second phase in the classic viral decay curve is still unclear. One possibility is that the relevant cells may be infected macrophages, which at least in vitro are less susceptible to the cytopathic effects of the virus than are CD4$^+$ lymphoblasts (35, 36). In principle, macrophages can continue to release virus for their normal lifespan. In uninfected individuals, macrophage turnover is balanced by the continuous production of new monocytes in the bone marrow. Monocytes circulate for less than a day and enter the tissues, where they differentiate into macrophages. The half-life of tissue macrophages has been estimated at about two weeks (37), consistent with the kinetics of the second phase of decay of plasma virus following initiation of HAART. The frequency of infected macrophages in the tissues is also consistent with the idea that macrophages are the source of virus during the second phase of decay. In most published studies, only a small fraction of the total macrophage population is infected (10, 38, 39), but among all cells that are productively infected, macrophages may comprise on the order of 10%, at least in early stages of the infection (27). Careful studies of simian immunodeficiency virus (SIV) infection in the rhesus monkey have shown that most of the productively infected cells ($>80\%$) are $CD4^+$ T cells, even immediately following inoculation by mucosal routes. Productively infected macrophages are present at lower levels. Interestingly, the proportion of infected cells that are macrophages increases dramatically in patients with end-stage disease who have opportunistic infections (40). In the primate model, most of the plasma virus is produced by macrophages at late stages of the infection, when most of the $CD4^+$ T cells have been depleted by a highly pathogenic recombinant simian/human immunodeficiency virus (SHIV) (41). In summary, the level of infection of macrophages in vivo is consistent with the idea that the second phase of decay reflects the turnover of infected macrophages.

Two other cell populations may also contribute to the second phase of decay. Haase and colleagues have shown that some virus-producing cells in vivo are $CD4^+$ T cells that are not fully activated (27). As is discussed below, the virus does not replicate in T cells that are in a resting state. However, there may be partially activated states that permit lower levels of replication, levels that do not cause rapid destruction of the cells. These infected $CD4^+$ T cells in a lower state of activation may turn over with a longer half-life than the fully activated $CD4^+$ lymphoblasts that are responsible for the first phase of decay. It has also been suggested that the virus that appears during the second phase of decay may be mobilized from follicular dendritic cells (FDCs) in the germinal centers of the peripheral lymphoid tissue (42–46). FDCs do not appear susceptible to productive infection (47) but can trap virus particles on their surfaces. In situ hybridization studies suggest that this pool of trapped extracellular virions declines with a half-life on the order of two weeks in patients on HAART (33), although a longer half-life (9.5 weeks) has been observed in a model system in which HIV-1 is injected into mice and then rescued from FDCs. Although there is evidence that some virions bound to FDCs can retain infectivity in this mouse model (48, 49), the virus recovered may represent a tiny fraction of the virus initially bound. It is not yet clear how rapidly the infectivity of the bound virus is lost. FDC-bound virus is likely to attach to the cells via Fc and complement receptors, and although elegant mathematical models of virus dissociation from FDCs suggest that this compartment could contribute to the second phase of decay (50, 51), the extent to which FDCs serve as a repository for infectious virus in vivo in humans remains unclear.

THE ERADICATION HYPOTHESIS

In 1997, Perelson and colleagues published an elegant mathematical analysis suggesting that the second phase of decay might be rapid enough to allow complete elimination of the virus in 2–3 years of treatment provided there were no additional reservoirs (4). This prediction was based on the assumption that the most stable form of the virus in vivo was the compartment responsible for the second-phase decay, a compartment with a half-life of two weeks. Although the starting number of infected cells in this compartment was unknown, even a reservoir of 10^{12} cells (equivalent to the estimated total body number of lymphocytes) would decay to <1 cell in about three years. This hypothesis challenged defeatist notions about the impossibility of curing retroviral infections. Underlying the hypothesis was the striking observation that most of the virus in the plasma is produced by populations of cells that turn over rapidly. Thus, if HAART regimens could completely stop all new infection of susceptible cells and if there were no additional long-lived viral reservoirs, then eradication would be possible. However, in the past few years, it has become clear that current HAART regimens may not completely stop viral replication and that stable viral reservoirs do exist, making eradication extremely difficult.

DEFINITION OF A VIRAL RESERVOIR

Before considering several potential reservoirs that could allow persistence of HIV-1, it is important to define the term reservoir. In the context of virus eradication within a given infected individual, we define a viral reservoir as a cell type or anatomical site in association with which a replication-competent form of the virus accumulates and persists with more stable kinetic properties than in the main pool of actively replicating virus.

This definition has two critical elements. First, in order to be biologically significant, a reservoir must preserve some replication-competent form of the virus that can replenish the population of infected cells in the future. Thus, defective proviral sequences or decayed virus particles do not represent a reservoir. The second critical element of the definition is stability. Viruses can persist either as virions or in infected cells. Virions are subject to inactivating biochemical decay processes, such as the dissociation of the gp120 and gp41 subunits of the env protein (52–55). Infected host cells are subject to lysis by host CTL (56–63). Therefore, a viral reservoir must have a biologically plausible mechanism that allows the virus to escape from biochemical decay processes or, in the case of a cellular reservoir, from immune effector mechanisms. In addition, for a cellular reservoir, the turnover of the relevant host cell type must be slower that the turnover of the main pool of infected cells that sustains the infection. Thus, it is possible to view infected macrophages and FDC-bound virus particles as reservoirs for HIV-1 because they turn over more slowly than the infected CD4$^+$ lymphoblasts that produce most of the plasma virus. However, as discussed below, these reservoirs lack the stability needed to account for the long-term persistence of HIV-1 in patients on HAART.

As a consequence of the stability of viral reservoirs, viral species arising at different times in the infection should be present in the reservoir (64). In the case of a virus such as HIV-1 that shows continuous evolutionary change (65), there should be recent as well as archival sequences in the reservoir, and both forms should be capable of being released. The presence of archival sequences thus represents an important test for the stability that is part of the definition of a biologically significant viral reservoir.

Table 1 lists cell types that have been proposed as viral reservoirs in HIV-1 infection. Only some of the proposed reservoirs for HIV-1 meet the definition outlined above.

Another concept important to the discussion of viral persistence is latency. Latency is a reversibly nonproductive state of infection—in other words, the term describes an infected cell that is not producing virus but retains the capacity to do so under appropriate conditions. A reservoir need not be latent. A slowly turning over population of productively infected cells could in principle serve a reservoir function. However, in HIV-1 infection, the reservoir for which there is now the best evidence is a small but extremely stable pool of latently infected resting memory CD4$^+$ T cells (10, 11).

THE LATENT RESERVOIR FOR HIV-1 IN RESTING MEMORY CD4$^+$ T CELLS

Current hypotheses regarding the formation of the latent reservoir in resting memory CD4$^+$ T cells are based on normal T cell physiology (Figure 2) (reviewed in 66). Naive T cells emerge from the thymus and circulate in a resting state until they are activated by an appropriate antigen. They then undergo blast transformation, proliferate, and carry out their functions. Some of these activated cells survive and go back to a resting state as memory cells, the biological function of which is to persist for long periods, allowing future responses to the same antigen (67, 68). Activated CD4$^+$ T cells are preferentially infected by HIV-1 (69). These cells progress quickly through the steps of reverse transcription, integration of the viral genome into host cell DNA, virus gene expression, and virus production. As discussed above, most of these cells die quickly after infection, with a half-life of one day.

The sequence of events is different when HIV-1 interacts with resting CD4$^+$ T cells. The frequently transmitted forms of HIV-1 that utilize the chemokine receptor CCR5 can enter a subset of resting memory cells that express sufficient levels of CCR5 to support infection (70). R5 viruses do not enter naive CD4$^+$ T cells, since these cells do not express CCR5 (70–72). X4 viruses can enter resting CD4$^+$ T cells whether they belong to the naive or memory subsets because of the broad expression of this coreceptor (71, 73). Following viral entry into resting CD4$^+$ T cells, the genomic viral RNA is reverse transcribed into DNA. Initial studies suggested that this process was not completed in resting cells, possibly because of low levels of nucleotides (74–77). Other studies (78; T. Pierson, R. F. Siliciano, manuscript in preparation) suggest that reverse transcription can be completed in resting CD4$^+$ T cells, albeit slowly, and that viral replication is blocked at a subsequent step such as import of the preintegration complex containing the reverse-transcribed HIV-1 DNA into the nucleus (79). In any event,

TABLE 1 Reservoirs for HIV-1 (see text for references)

Cell type	Anatomic location	Form of virus	Half-life (months)	Viral genes expressed	Mechanism of virus release	Affected by immune response?	Affected by antiretroviral drugs?	Replication-competent?	Long-term persistence in patients on HAART	Presence of archival vius	Comments
Resting memory CD4+ T cells	Blood, lymph node, other peripheral lymphoid organs, tissues	Integrated HIV-1 DNA	6–44	No	Activation by antigen	No	No	Yes	>5 yrs	Yes	Allows life-time persistence of HIV-1 in most patients on HAART. May also be widely distributed in nonlymphoid tissues
Resting naive CD4+ T cells	Blood, lymph nodes, other peripheral lymphoid organs	Integrated HIV-1 DNA	No data	No	Activation by antigen	No	No	Yes	>5 yrs	Yes	Present at lower frequency than latently infected resting memory cells
Recently infected resting CD4+ T cells	Blood, lymph node, other peripheral lymphoid organs, tissues	Reverse-transcribed, unintegrated HIV-1 DNA	<0.25	No	Activation by antigen	No	Yes, if reverse transcription is not complete	Yes	No	No	Not a reservoir due to short half-life
Macrophages	Many tissues	Integrated HIV-1 DNA	0.5?	Yes	Active virus production	Yes	No	Yes	No data	No data	May be responsible for second phase of decay
Follicular dendritic cells	Germinal centers in lymph node and spleen	Virions opsonized by antibody and complement	0.5, 2.4	No	No data	Already bound by antibody	No	Yes?	Demonstrated in 1 pt	No data	Most work done in mouse model
B cells	Blood, lymph nodes, other peripheral lymphoid organs	Complement opsonized virions	No data	No	No data	No data	No	Yes	No data	No data	Replication competent virus found on surface of B cells in patients with viral load >10,000 copies/ml
Monocytes	Blood	Integrated?	Days	Yes	Constitutive	Yes	No	Yes	Yes	No data	Not a reservoir, may reflect ongoing replication
CD4+ subset of NK cells	Blood	No data	No data	No data	No data	No data	No data	Yes	Yes	No data	Virus can be isolated from CD4+ NK cells of patients on HAART

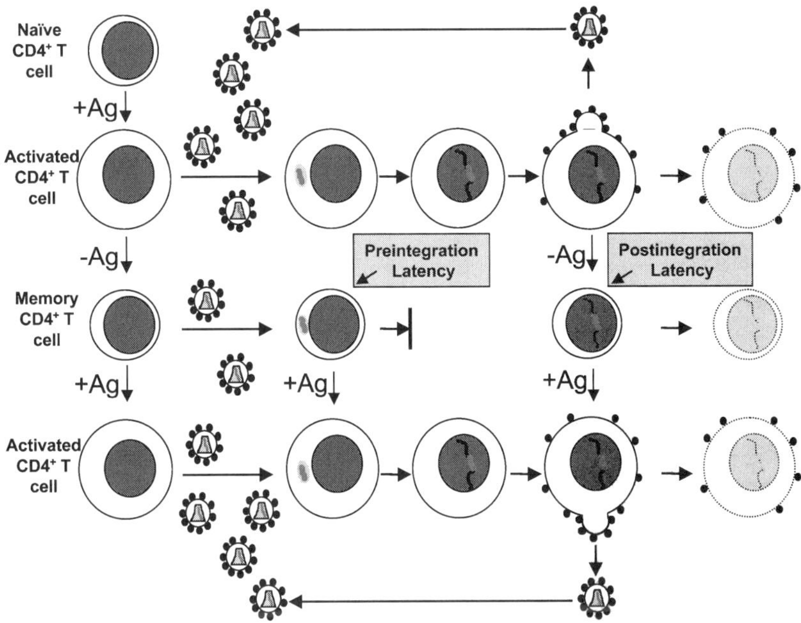

Figure 2 Establishment of the latent reservoir in resting memory CD4$^+$ T cells. Transitions between resting (small) and activated (large) CD4$^+$ T cells are illustrated by vertical arrows. The normal generation of memory CD4$^+$ T cells is illustrated on the left. These cells are derived from antigen (Ag)-activated CD4$^+$ T cells that revert back to a resting memory state. These memory cells survive for long periods, allowing responses to the same Ag in the future. The memory cell compartment may be maintained by a process of proliferative renewal. Successive steps in the life cycle of the virus are indicated by horizontal arrows. R5 isolates can infect activated CD4$^+$ T cells but may also infect a subset of resting memory CD4$^+$ T cells that express sufficient amounts of CCR5. Following infection of resting memory CD4$^+$ T cells, there is a block in the virus life cycle, probably at the level of nuclear import of the preintegration complex containing the viral genome. Resting cells with unintegrated HIV-1 DNA probably represent a relatively labile reservoir for the virus (preintegration latency). Productive infection requires Ag-driven activation of recently infected resting CD4$^+$ cells or, more commonly, direct infection of Ag-activated CD4$^+$ T cells. Productively infected cells generally die within a few days from cytopathic effects of the infection or host cytolytic effector mechanisms, but some infected lymphoblasts survive long enough to go back to a resting state, thereby establishing a stable latent reservoir of resting memory CD4$^+$ T cells with integrated HIV-1 DNA (postintegration latency).

recently infected resting CD4$^+$ T cells provide for a form of latency in the sense that if the cells are activated by antigen before the preintegration complex becomes nonfunctional, then they can go on to produce virus (74, 78, 80). In vitro studies suggest that in the absence of activation this preintegration form of latency decays with a half-life of ∼1–6 days (T. Pierson, R. F. Siliciano, manuscript in preparation). Although labile, this preintegration form of latency is the most prevalent form in untreated HIV-1 infection (10, 16, 81) and is readily detected in all DNA PCR and virus culture methods that do not include special procedures to distinguish integrated and unintegrated forms of viral DNA.

A much more stable form of latent infection arises when activated CD4$^+$ T cells that have integrated HIV-1 DNA survive long enough to revert back to a resting memory state, like their uninfected counterparts (10, 11). This results in a stably integrated form of HIV-1 DNA in a memory T cell, whose biological function is to survive for long periods. Interestingly, HIV-1 gene expression is linked to T cell activation because the HIV-1 long terminal repeat (LTR), which regulates the expression of viral genes, is activated by host transcription factors such as NFκB that are turned on in activated cells and turned off in resting cells (82, 83). Thus, resting CD4$^+$ T cells in this postintegration state of latent infection may have little or no expression of HIV-1 genes. Resting T cells are among the most quiescent cells in the body, as is obvious from their morphology. The cells have only a tiny rim of cytoplasm surrounding the nucleus. They carry out few active functions; they are designed to wait. Thus, resting CD4$^+$ T cells with integrated HIV-1 are an ideal long-term viral reservoir.

The first evidence of resting CD4$^+$ T cells with integrated HIV-1 DNA in vivo was published in 1995 (11). Proving that these cells were present in infected individuals required the isolation of very pure populations of resting CD4$^+$ T cells. It was then necessary to show that purified populations of resting CD4$^+$ T cells contained cells with integrated HIV-1 DNA. This was accomplished using an inverse PCR assay that selectively detects integrated forms of HIV-1 DNA (10, 11). Finally, it was necessary to show that replication-competent virus could be rescued from these cells by the addition of activating stimuli (10, 11). The assay used most extensively to detect latently infected cells involves culturing limiting dilutions of purified resting CD4$^+$ T cells under conditions in which they become efficiently activated, allowing latently infected cells to begin to produce virus that can then be amplified by the addition of CD4$^+$ lymphoblasts from normal donors. The activation step is critical to the definition of latency; without an activating stimulus, virus is not recovered from these resting cells. Thus, any virus obtained following activation can be considered to have come from the latent reservoir. Another important point about this assay is that because of the limiting dilution format, the assay detects viruses grown up from individual latently infected cells. Thus, any virus detected in this assay is capable of enormous in vitro expansion and is therefore likely to be pathogenic.

In the pre-HAART era, this assay and other molecular methods were used to characterize the latent reservoir in resting CD4$^+$ T cells, and the following conclusions were drawn (10):

- Latently infected resting CD4$^+$ T cells with integrated HIV-1 DNA are present in all infected individuals but only at low frequency. Less than 0.01% of resting CD4$^+$ T cells carry integrated HIV-1 DNA.

- Latently infected cells express high levels of CD4 but do not express markers of T cell activation, including the early activation marker CD69, the α chain of the IL-2 receptor, and the late activation marker HLA-DR.

- The frequencies of latently infected cells are similar in blood and lymph node.

- The yield of virus increases with degree of purification of resting CD4$^+$ T cells, suggesting that these cells represent the major reservoir for HIV-1 in blood and lymph node.

- Most latently infected cells belong to the memory subset of resting CD4$^+$ T cells, as expected based on the model presented in Figure 2.

With the advent of HAART, the critical question became whether these cells would persist after HAART had suppressed viremia to undetectable levels. This issue was studied in highly compliant patients who had maintained suppression of viremia on HAART for long periods. Three groups simultaneously found latently infected cells in every patient (12–14). Moreover, initial cross-sectional studies suggested that the frequency of these cells did not appear to decline with increasing time on HAART (12).

This conclusion was verified by longitudinal studies in a larger series of patients at the Johns Hopkins Hospital. These studies confirmed the absence of significant decay in the latent reservoir (15). Statistical analysis of the data suggested a half-life of 44 months for this compartment (Figure 3). In fact, the slope of the decay curve was not statistically different from zero. This decay is much slower that the second phase viral decay curve (half-life of two weeks) and is even slower than the turnover rate of memory T cells in uninfected humans, for which a half-life of about six months has been reported (84, 85). Other investigators have identified rare cases in which the decay rate appears to approach this six-month half-life (18, 86). These have typically been patients treated during primary infection or patients with unusually good suppression of viral replication on HAART. Patients in the Hopkins cohort who were treated during primary HIV-1 infection did not show a more rapid decay of latently infected cells. Most importantly, recent studies of the Hopkins cohort have shown that in patients with stable suppression of viral replication on HAART for >5 years, the number of latently infected cells is essentially the same as when HAART was started, confirming the extremely long half-life of the latent reservoir in most patients on HAART (J. D. Siliciano, R. F. Siliciano, unpublished results). Eradication of the latent reservoir is likely to require at least five or six logs of decay (10). With a half-life of 44 months, this would require over 60 years of suppressive HAART (15). In summary, most of the current data confirm the original prediction (15) that the latent reservoir for HIV-1 in resting memory CD4$^+$ T cells will allow lifetime

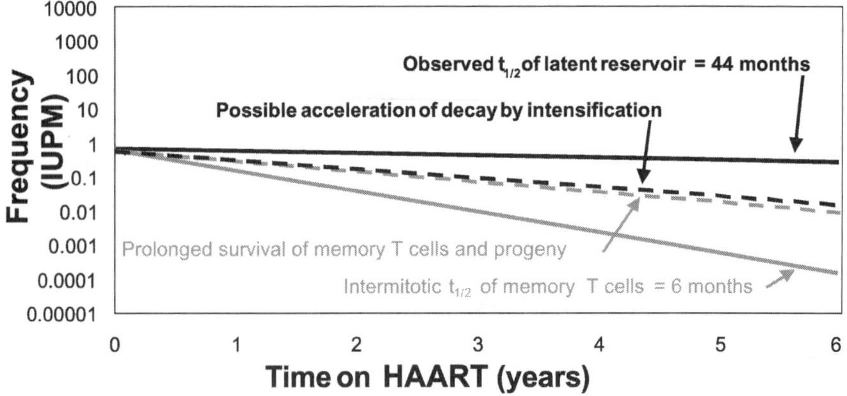

Figure 3 Factors influencing the decay of the latent reservoir in resting memory CD4[+] T cells in patients on HAART. The frequency of latently infected cells in the resting CD4[+] T cell population is plotted versus time on HAART. IUPM = infectious units per million resting CD4[+] T cells. In most patients with suppression of viremia to <50 copies/ml, the reservoir decays only very slowly (solid black line, half-life = 44 months). In some patients, a decay rate approaching six months has been observed. This is close to the reported intermitotic half-life of memory T cells in uninfected humans (half-life = 6 months, solid grey line). If immunologic memory is maintained by occasional homeostatic proliferation of memory T cells, the actual half-life of an infected memory cell and its clonal progeny may be much longer than six months (dotted grey line). If memory cells with integrated HIV-1 DNA can go through this proliferative process without succumbing to viral cytopathic effects or host CTLs, then the half-life of the latent reservoir will also be much longer than six months. The proliferative renewal process may determine the theoretical minimum half-life of the latent reservoir. If ongoing viral replication is reseeding the reservoir, then intensification of the HAART regimen may shorten the half-life of the latent reservoir (dotted black line), but not beyond the theoretical minimum half-life determined by the intrinsic stability of memory T cells.

persistence of the virus at least in the vast majority of patients on current HAART regimens.

Several hypotheses have been put forward to explain the mechanism of HIV-1 latency at the molecular level (see 66 for a review). Some early studies suggested a post-transcriptional mechanism in which HIV-1 mRNA's encoding structural proteins were spliced, preventing production of virus particles (87, 88). However, the absence in resting CD4[+] T cells of active forms of transcription factors required for efficient HIV-1 gene expression suggested that latency might operate at the transcriptional level (82, 83). Recent studies in patients with stable suppression of viral replication on HAART suggest that latently infected cells contain no detectable HIV-1 RNA, consistent with the idea that HIV-1 gene expression is completely shut off in latently infected cells (M. Hermankova, R. F. Siliciano, unpublished results). This would mean that targeting latently infected cells would be virtually impossible because they differ from uninfected cells only by the presence of 10 Kb of integrated but transcriptionally silent HIV-1 DNA.

The latent reservoir is established early in the course of HIV-1 infection. A stable reservoir is established even in patients who are treated with HAART during primary HIV-1 infection (12, 89–91).

Of further concern is the finding that this reservoir is present in perinatally infected children (16, 92). In a cohort of children with suppression of viremia to undetectable levels on HAART, the reservoir was shown to persist with the same stable kinetics observed in adults (16).

A corollary of the stable persistence of HIV-1 in memory T cells is that a rebound in viremia will occur if therapy is interrupted. With only extremely rare exceptions (93), plasma virus levels rebound after cessation of therapy, typically in about two weeks (94–98). To determine whether this latent reservoir is a source of the rebound virus, Zhang et al. examined variable regions of the HIV-1 *env* genes of rebounding viruses in eight patients who went off effective HAART regimens (95). *Env* sequences were compared to *env* sequences of viruses isolated from resting CD4$^+$ T cells during treatment. Comparisons were made using a PCR assay for length polymorphisms in variable regions of *env*. In five patients, *env* sequences from rebound viruses were identical in length to latent reservoir sequences. The authors concluded that in this subset of patients, the rebound virus was probably derived from latently infected CD4$^+$ T cells. Using a different electrophoretic approach, Chun et al. have also observed similarities between the rebound virus and viruses in the latent reservoir in some but not all patients (96). Another study found that rebounding viruses were similar to viruses present when therapy was started (98). The simplest interpretation of these studies is that, in many cases, viruses in the latent reservoir resemble the rebound virus, and that differences may reflect sampling problems, the presence of additional long-term reservoirs for HIV-1, or the failure of HAART to completely halt viral replication (99).

MECHANISMS FOR PERSISTENCE OF THE LATENT RESERVOIR

Two distinct but not mutually exclusive hypotheses attempt to account for the extraordinary stability of the latent reservoir. The first hypothesis is that the stability reflects the basic biology of memory T cells; the stability of the latent reservoir is then no more surprising than the fact that immunity to measles is lifelong. HIV-1 has simply taken advantage of a fundamental characteristic of the immune system, the immunologic memory that resides in long-lived resting lymphocytes. Recent studies in mice have provided a much better understanding of immunologic memory. After the initial expansion of antigen-specific T cells in response to an infection, there is a loss of some of the activated cells and then the stable persistence, in the absence of antigen, of a relatively constant number of specific memory T cells for the lifespan of the animal (100, 101). The memory T cell population also appears to be stable in humans. For example, hepatitis C–specific memory CD4$^+$ T cells can be readily detected in patients who appear to have cleared the infection 20 years previously (102).

The only available estimates of the half-life of memory T cells in uninfected humans come from studies of the survival of T cells with chromosomal abnormalities induced by therapeutic irradiation (84, 85). Because these forms of DNA damage kill cells that go through the cell cycle, the studies measure only the intermitotic half-life of the cells, i.e., the average time required for the cells to either die or divide. For memory T cells, the intermitotic half-life is approximately six months. The cells do not necessarily die after this time; some divide in a homeostatic process that ensures long-term persistence of the appropriate antigenic specificities. The mechanism involved in this homeostatic proliferative process is unclear but does not depend on antigen. It is possible that the relevant proliferative signals drive the cells through the cell cycle without fully activating expression of latent HIV-1. If this is the case, then the reservoir may be maintained by cell division rather than viral replication, making elimination by antiretroviral therapy essentially impossible (Figure 3).

The alternative hypothesis to explain the stability of the latent reservoir is that although HAART reduces viremia below the limit of detection, it fails to stop all viral replication; new cells are entering the reservoir, constantly "topping it off." If HAART stopped all new infection of susceptible cells and the only viruses entering the plasma were derived from the activation of latently infected cells, then viremia would fall to even lower levels. These two mechanisms of persistence may be related in that the latent reservoir may release virus that fuels this ongoing replication while ongoing replication may replenish the latent reservoir.

What is the evidence of ongoing virus replication in patients on HAART who have undetectable viral loads? The most direct evidence is that free virus can be measured in the plasma by extremely sensitive assays. Patients whose plasma virus levels are undetectable by conventional ultrasensitive assays (<50 copies/ml) often have positive determinations when even more sensitive assays for viral RNA are used (limit of detection = 5–50 copies/ml) (17, 21). Many patients have isolated low-level positive plasma HIV-1 RNA determinations by standard clinical assays ("blips") (86). In addition, when patients are switched from three-drug regimens to simpler two-drug "maintenance" regimens, breakthrough viremia is observed in a significant fraction of patients, suggesting that current three-drug regimens barely contain viral replication (103, 104). Productively infected cells expressing HIV-1 RNA can be detected by in situ hybridization or RT-PCR in individuals who are aviremic on HAART (105). Molecular assays for unintegrated forms of HIV-1 DNA also suggest the presence of recently infected cells, consistent with ongoing replication (19, 20). Finally, in some aviremic patients, viruses with altered *env* sequences arise, consistent with ongoing replication (18, 106). However, some patients on HAART show no *env* evolution. Interestingly, there is only limited evidence for evolution in the *pol* gene despite the stringent selection enforced by antiretroviral drug regimens.

In considering these studies, it is very important to distinguish between virus released by previously infected cells and virus release resulting from continual cycles of infection. Virus particles can be released into the plasma by cells infected long ago, such as cells in the latent reservoir that become activated. However, the critical question in patients on HAART is whether there are continuous new cycles of infection of susceptible cells. This distinction is important because the evolution of drug resistance depends on mutation introduced in the error-prone reverse transcription step in each new cycle of infection. Unfortunately, most of the assays used to document ongoing virus replication do not make this critical distinction. Thus, in principle, low-level viremia could result from the release of virus from chronically infected cells or latently infected cells that become activated. The same is true for blips and RNA+ cells. Detection of recently infected cells would provide evidence for new cycles of infection.

To look for recent infection, most investigators have focused on 2LTR circles (19, 20). These circular forms of the HIV-1 genome are generated when reverse-transcribed HIV-1 DNA enters the nucleus and undergoes an aberrant end-to-end ligation reaction instead of integrating into the host cell genome. These circles represent a dead end for replication. It has been suggested that 2LTR circles are unstable, and they have been used as a marker of recent infection (19, 20). However, other studies indicate that the circles are very stable and thus should not be used as a marker of very recent infection (T. Kieffer et al., manuscript submitted; F. Bushman, personal communication). Therefore, at present, sequence evolution remains the best indication of the degree of ongoing virus replication in patients on HAART who have undetectable viremia.

EVOLUTION OF DRUG RESISTANCE IN PATIENTS ON HAART

The evolution of HIV-1 in patients on HAART is a subject of great interest, not only because it provides evidence of new cycles of replication that may replenish viral reservoirs but also because it is a critical factor in determining whether HAART can suppress viral replication without the eventual development of drug resistance. Pioneering studies by Richman and colleagues have shown that resistance can develop when viremia is consistently in the low but detectable range (20–400 copies/ml) (107), but it remains unclear whether evolution continues in fully compliant patients with suppression of viremia to <50 copies/ml, the limit of detection of the current "ultrasensitive" assay. This is a difficult question because there is very little virus in the plasma to analyze.

Viruses in the latent reservoir have been analyzed for drug resistance mutations. In one study, new, HAART-selected drug resistance mutations were detected in the latent reservoir of patients with suboptimal suppression of viral replication

(108). However, in most studies, new resistance mutations have not been readily apparent (12, 13, 16). What is clear is that in patients who have had prior therapy with one- or two-drug regimens that failed to control viremia, resistant viruses selected by this nonsuppressive therapy enter the latent reservoir and then persist there even after the patients go on suppressive HAART regimens (16, 108). Thus, viruses with drug resistance mutations can enter the latent reservoir when patients are viremic. Once suppression to <50 copies/ml has been achieved, there appears to be little additional turnover in the latent reservoir (16). In essence, this reservoir behaves like an archive of all the viral species that were previously circulating at high levels in the patient. The archival character of the latent viruses isolated from resting CD4$^+$ T cells clearly demonstrates that these cells function as a viral reservoir as defined above. The clinical significance of this finding is that drug-resistant viruses can enter the reservoir during conditions of high-level viremia and persist there for life. In this context, the idea of "recycling" drugs that were part of failing regimens is highly problematic.

Interestingly, even in patients who have developed high levels of drug resistance after years of nonsuppressive drug regimens, it is still possible to find wild-type, drug-sensitive virus persisting in the latent reservoir along with the resistant virus (16, 108). This finding is significant in light of recent studies showing that wild-type virus reappears after treatment interruption in patients who are failing HAART with multidrug-resistant virus (109). Studies of the latent reservoir by Persaud and colleagues (manuscript in preparation) indicate that this wild-type virus does not result from classic genetic reversion of multidrug-resistant virus back to wild-type, drug-sensitive virus. Rather, it simply reflects reemergence of wild-type virus that entered the latent reservoir before any treatment occurred. Of course, the reemergence of wild-type virus does not mean the resistant virus is gone. The resistant virus is also stored in the latent reservoir and can reemerge under appropriate selective conditions.

Recently, Persaud and colleagues have shown that it is possible to directly analyze the low-level plasma virus present in patients with suppression of viral replication to <50 copies/ml on HAART (110). The plasma sequences obtained were phylogenetically intermingled with latent reservoir sequences obtained from the same patient, consistent with the idea that the latent reservoir is the source of at least some of the plasma virus. Analysis of drug resistance mutations in viruses obtained from patients with <50 copies/ml revealed a very consistent pattern in which the only drug resistance mutations found were those selected by prior nonsuppressive therapy. For example, in patients who had no prior therapy and who had undetectable plasma HIV-1 RNA for 3–4 years on HAART, no mutations were found. This was true even in patients whose HAART regimen included 3TC, a drug for which a single point mutation—which frequently appears as the first mutation in patients failing HAART (111)—gives high-level resistance (112, 113). Thus, in these patients, drug-sensitive virus continues to be released into the plasma at low levels for 3–4 years without accumulation of even the earliest of resistance mutations. These results indicate that the low-level viremia observed in patients who have

<50 copies/ml of HIV-1 RNA does not require the evolution of partial resistance. The simplest explanation for the continuous production of low levels of drug-sensitive virus over the course of several years without accumulation of resistance mutations is that these viruses come from the latent reservoir. Of course, if prior nonsuppressive therapy has led to the generation of resistant viruses, these will continue to be released into the plasma as well.

APPROACHES FOR ELIMINATING THE LATENT RESERVOIR

Given the long half-life of the latent reservoir, it is unlikely that eradication of HIV-1 will be possible with the current HAART regimens. Several strategies for dealing with this difficult problem have been proposed.

Intensification of HAART

The strategy of intensifying HAART is based on the assumptions that ongoing HIV-1 replication occurs even in patients on current HAART regimens who have undetectable levels of viremia and that this ongoing replication replenishes the latent reservoir. It would follow that the measured or apparent decay rate of the latent reservoir may actually be slower than the intrinsic decay rate of latently infected cells, which is the decay rate that would be observed if new cycles of infection could be completely suppressed (Figure 3). In support of this concept, Ramratnam and colleagues demonstrated that in patients who have no history of blips, the latent reservoir decays with a half-life of approximately six months, which is close to the intermitotic half-life of memory T cells (86). However, the majority of patients studied had one or more blips on monthly follow-up over the course of 1–3 years and had no significant decay in the latent reservoir, consistent with results from other cohorts (15). These results are important because they point to one potential benefit of more potent drug regimens. Unfortunately, the patients studied appear to represent a very select group, and it remains unclear how frequently decay of the latent reservoir occurs in the average group of patients who have responded well to current HAART regimens. In a recent follow-up study, Ho and colleagues intensified the regimens of patients who had intermittent blips (114). The reverse transcriptase inhibitor abacavir with or without efavirenz was added to the standard HAART regimens of five patients, and the frequency of blips, as well as the decay rate of the latent reservoir, was compared to that of five control patients on standard HAART who had similar episodes of intermittent viremia. After intensification, the median half-life of the latent reservoir decreased from 31 months to 10 months ($p = 0.016$). This group has also proposed that novel, highly potent regimens may control viremia better. Antiretroviral therapy–naive patients were treated with a regimen containing lamivudine, tenofovir, efavirenz, and ritonavir/lopinavir (115). This regimen is unusual for patients with drug-sensitive virus in that, in addition to the nucleoside and nucleotide analogs, it includes a nonnucleoside reverse transcriptase inhibitor (NNRTI) as well as a protease inhibitor. These patients had a significantly faster first-phase decay of plasma HIV-1 RNA than patients who had received standard HAART. Based on the decay rate of plasma virus in the two sets of patients, these investigators suggested that the efficacy of standard HAART was only 79% of the new regimen. However, by week 4, the difference between the two groups in the mean change in viral loads was no longer significant. It was suggested that with the more efficacious new regimen, the likelihood of ongoing replication is much lower, and this may translate into a quicker decay rate of the latent reservoir. However, this regimen will probably be more toxic, and no salvage therapy exists for patients who fail it.

In summary, intensification of HAART may produce some increase in the decay rate of the latent reservoir by stopping residual viral replication. However, even with completely suppressive regimens, the intrinsic stability of latent reservoir in resting memory T cells may render eradication unachievable (Figure 3).

T Cell Activation

Other investigators have attempted to "flush out" latent virus by nonspecifically activating T cells in patients on HAART. The rationale is that the activation of quiescent cells will cause latent virus to be released. The presence of antiretroviral drugs should prevent the subsequent productive infection of susceptible cells by the released virus. Prins and colleagues used a combination of OKT3, a monoclonal antibody (mAb) specific for the CD3 complex on T cells, and interleukin-2 (IL-2) in three patients on HAART with plasma virus levels below 5 copies/ml (116). This OKT3/IL-2 regimen effectively activated T cells in these patients, as the vast majority of the cells expressed the activation molecule CD38. As expected with this degree of T cell activation, severe toxicity was seen in each patient, and one patient developed transient renal failure and severe hypotension. Interestingly, during therapy, all three patients had increased HIV-1 RNA levels in lymph nodes and one patient had a transient peak of viremia (1500 copies/ml). Despite the massive T cell activation achieved with this regimen, the frequency of latently infected cells remained unchanged in one patient. Low frequencies prior to OKT3/IL-2 in the other two patients prevented statistical analysis. Clearly, given the severe toxicity seen, as well as the development of host antibodies to the OKT3 mAb, this regimen does not represent a feasible or effective approach for targeting the latent reservoir.

Other investigators have examined the use of IL-2 alone or in combination with other cytokines. It should be noted that resting CD4$^+$ T cells do not express CD25, the α chain of the high-affinity IL-2 receptor, and therefore should not be efficiently activated by this cytokine. Nonetheless, Chun and colleagues studied patients on HAART who had received multiple cycles of intermediate doses of IL-2 and compared the frequency of latently infected CD4$^+$ T cells in these patients to the frequencies in another group of patients who had been treated with HAART alone (117). In 3 of the 14 patients on HAART and IL-2, no latently infected cells were detected in peripheral blood even after analysis of a very large number of resting CD4$^+$ cells (100–330 $\times$ 10^6). However, when HAART was discontinued in these patients, a rebound in plasma viremia was universally seen, and the rate of rebound was identical to that of patients who had not been treated with IL-2 (94). Several more recent studies have failed to confirm an effect of IL-2 on the latent reservoir (118–120).

Immunologic Approaches

Because eradication of the latent reservoir with prolonged HAART is unlikely, some investigators are focusing on stimulating the immune system to contain viral replication. One approach for doing so was based on the well-publicized "Berlin patient," who was treated with HAART shortly after seroconversion but interrupted therapy twice during the first six months (93). After six months, he declined further treatment, and surprisingly, no viremia was detected during 18 months of follow-up after drug cessation. Latently infected cells were found in this patient, ruling out HIV-1 eradication. Rather, it appeared that the patient's immune system was capable of controlling viral replication. Indeed, subsequent studies showed that he had a strong $CD4^+$ T cell response to the HIV-1 gag protein (90), a response normally only seen in long-term nonprogressors who are also able to contain viral replication (121). There is no clear evidence that either early intervention with HAART or the drug interruptions were responsible for this patient's later ability to spontaneously control viremia. Nonetheless, his success led to trials of structured treatment interruptions (STIs) in an attempt to enhance HIV-1-specific immunity in patients on HAART.

STIs are appealing for two reasons. First, HIV-1-specific immunity decreases with time on HAART. The limited viral replication caused by the interruption of therapy may boost the HIV-1-specific immune response. In addition, STIs provide a break from the demands and toxicities of HAART regimens. Most STI studies in chronically infected patients have shown only modest improvements in HIV-1-specific immunity (122, 123), and patients were generally not able to control viremia for prolonged periods (122–125). In contrast, for some patients treated with HAART during primary HIV-1 infection, repeated STIs have shown striking effects, with some patients maintaining low viral loads off therapy for >1 year (97). This may reflect the fact that early treatment allows development of a strong HIV-1-specific $CD4^+$ T cell response (97, 121), a crucial element of HIV-1-specific immunity that is missing in most chronically infected patients. This would suggest that therapeutic vaccination with HIV-1 antigens may restore the $CD4^+$ T cell response in chronically infected patients on HAART and thus lead to immune control of viruses emerging from the latent reservoir when therapy is discontinued.

Hege and colleagues have employed a novel approach to target infected cells released from the latent reservoir (126). The approach utilizes autologous T cells engineered to express the extracellular CD4 domain linked to the ζ chain of the CD3 complex (CD4-ζ). The CD4 domain binds gp120 on the surface of infected cells, initiating signals through the ζ chain that result in the death of the target cells (127). When transduced with CD4-ζ, both $CD4^+$ and $CD8^+$ T cells kill gp120-expressing target cells in a non–MHC-restricted manner (126). Although it is not clear that latently infected cells express gp120 on the cell surface, CD4-ζ–expressing T cells may kill these cells when they became activated and thus prevent other cells from becoming infected. To address this possibility, patients on HAART were infused with 3×10^{10} CD4-ζ–modified or unmodified autologous T cells and followed for 24 weeks. Patients receiving the CD4-ζ–modified cells had a modest but statistically significant decrease in the frequency of latently infected cells. Although this suggests that gene therapy may help control ongoing viral replication, the time and expense involved in this technology may make it unpractical.

OTHER RESERVOIRS FOR HIV-1 IN INFECTED INDIVIDUALS

HIV-1 infection of many different cell types has been analyzed in vitro. However, the significance of these studies is unclear given that productive infection in vivo is seen almost exclusively in cells expressing CD4, namely CD4[+] T cells and macrophages (128). Therefore, this review focuses on infection of cells for which a plausible mechanism of HIV-1 entry has been defined and for which the potential for reservoir function exists. The potential reservoir function of macrophages and FDCs is considered above. In the following section, other potential cellular and anatomical reservoirs for HIV-1 are briefly considered. Table 1 summarizes the characteristics of these reservoirs.

Naive CD4[+] T Cells

Resting CD4[+] T cells that have previously encountered antigen are the principal reservoir for HIV-1. Most of the HIV-1 detected in CD4[+] T cells is in cells that express the memory marker CD45RO, a splice variant of the transmembrane phosphatase CD45 (129, 130). It is now clear that expression of RA or RO isoforms of CD45 alone is insufficient to identify naive T cells and memory T cells. Some activated cells express CD45RA, which is found on naive cells, and most express CD45RO. For these reasons, caution must be used in interpreting studies that rely solely on CD45 isoform expression. Several studies using multiple parameters to distinguish naive and memory T cells also suggest that most of the latent HIV-1 resides in memory cells (10, 70, 131). Nevertheless, a minor proportion of the latent virus in resting CD4[+] T cells is found in naive cells (70, 131). Given that R5 viruses do not enter resting naive CD4[+] T cells (70, 72), it is unclear how these cells become infected. Possibly infection occurs during differentiation in the thymus, when the cells assume a more activated phenotype (132). Alternatively, memory cells with integrated HIV-1 DNA may revert to a naive phenotype.

CD8[+] T Cells

There have been occasional reports of HIV-1 infection of CD8[+] T cells (reviewed in 133), especially in patients with late-stage disease (134). Recently, a mechanism for infection of these cells has been proposed. CD8$^+$ T cells express CD4 upon in vitro activation (135–137). It remains to be determined whether or at what frequency CD8$^+$ T cells harbor replication-competent HIV-1 in vivo and whether the kinetic characteristics of infected CD8$^+$ T cells are consistent with a reservoir function.

Monocytes

Monocytes, the circulating precursors of tissue macrophages, express low levels of CD4. Three recent studies have examined whether monocytes function as a reservoir for HIV-1 in patients on HAART (138–140). In two studies, replication-competent virus was isolated from monocytes (138, 140). Sonza et al. suggest that infected monocytes are actively expressing HIV-1 genes (140).

Although macrophages can clearly serve a reservoir function, the idea that monocytes can function as a long-term reservoir for HIV-1 is clearly inconsistent with the normal turnover of these cells. Labeling studies demonstrate that monocytes are derived from bone marrow precursors in a differentiation process that lasts <2 weeks. Monocytes circulate for a few days at most before leaving the circulation to become tissue macrophages. Thus, monocytes per se lack the requisite longevity to be a reservoir for HIV-1. The detection of HIV-1 in monocytes may reflect relatively recent infection of these cells by the low level of virus that continues to be released in patients on HAART.

B Cells

There is minimal evidence that B cells are infected in vivo. However, a recent study suggests that virions can bind to the surfaces of B cells in a manner similar to that described above for FDCs (141). Replication-competent virus can be rescued from the cells but only in patients with high levels of viremia.

Dendritic Cells

Blood-derived dendritic cells (DCs), which are distinct from FDCs and are important in the presentation of antigens to T cells, can bind virus and transmit it to the CD4$^+$ T cells with which they interact during the course of an immune response (142–144). A recently discovered lectin-like receptor expressed by DCs, called DS-SIGN, can interact with carbohydrate ligands on gp120, facilitating attachment of virions to DCs (145). Following stimulation with inflammatory cytokines, immature tissue DCs migrate to the lymph nodes, where they present antigens taken up in the tissues to T cells in the lymph nodes. It has been proposed that in this way DCs may carry virions to the nodes, where they mediate infection of CD4$^+$ T cells (145). Whether DCs themselves are infectable is controversial, and as yet there is no evidence that these cells serve a reservoir function as defined above.

NK cells

A recent study suggests that a small fraction of NK cells express both CD4 and HIV-1 coreceptors (A. Valentin, et al., manuscript submitted). Interestingly, this population can be increased in some patients with HIV-1 infection. The cells support HIV-1 replication in vitro. Viral DNA can be detected in purified CD4$^+$ NK cells from patients on HAART, and replication-competent virus can be isolated. These results suggest that this subpopulation of NK cells might also function as an HIV-1 reservoir.

ANATOMICAL RESERVOIRS

Lymphoid Organs

At any given time, only 2% of lymphocytes are in the circulation, the remainder being distributed throughout the peripheral lymphoid organs and the tissues. Most investigators believe that viral replication occurs predominantly in the peripheral lymphoid organs, especially the spleen, lymph nodes, and gut-associated lymphoid tissue (GALT) (146–148). The GALT appears to be an important site of active viral replication, possibly reflecting high levels of T cell activation (147). The extent of infection is greater in the lymph nodes than in the peripheral blood (146). In patients on suppressive HAART regimens, cells expressing HIV-1 RNA are found in the lymph nodes even when RT-PCR assays for free virus in the plasma, cerebrospinal fluid (CSF), and genitourinary secretions are negative (148). The cells that constitute the best-defined HIV-1 reservoir, latently infected resting memory CD4$^+$ T cells, are found in blood and lymph node at similar frequencies (10). Recent studies in mice suggest that memory T cells are also widely distributed in nonlymphoid tissues (149). If this proves to be true in humans, then the total size of the latent reservoir could be much greater than the original estimate of 10^6 cells (10).

Lymphocytes develop in the primary lymphoid organs, thymus and bone marrow, and these sites are also possible reservoirs. The extent of infection of thymocytes in vivo is unknown. HIV-1 infection appears to accelerate the thymic involution that normally occurs with age. Thymocyte depletion is seen in a model in which human fetal liver and thymus are implanted into SCID mice (150). The decline in naive CD4$^+$ and CD8$^+$ T cells in the peripheral blood of infected individuals has been interpreted as indicating a defect in thymopoeisis in HIV-1 infection (151, 152), a conclusion that is supported by the finding that naive T cell levels increase upon control of viral replication with HAART (153). Thymic size can be measured radiologically, but direct measurement of function requires other approaches (154), such as the quantitation of T cell receptor excision circles (TRECs) produced as a by-product of the VDJ recombination reactions that occur in the thymus as new T cells are generated (155, 156). These DNA circles are stable in cells after the gene rearrangements that produce functional T cell receptors. Low TREC levels in peripheral blood CD4$^+$ and CD8$^+$ T cells have been observed in some HIV-1-infected adults, with partial reversal upon treatment. Interpretation of TREC measurements is complicated by the fact that TRECs can be diluted out by proliferation of mature T cells (157). Nevertheless, available evidence supports the idea that HIV-1 infection may interfere with T cell production to some extent. Whether the thymus functions as a reservoir as defined above remains to be determined.

Central Nervous System

In the pre-HAART era, neurological problems were common among HIV-1-infected individuals. HIV-associated dementia (HAD), unique dementia syndrome resulting from the direct effects of HIV-1 on the central nervous system (CNS), developed in 15%–20% of patients (158). The capacity of HIV-1 to cause CNS disease raises important questions about whether the virus can persist there (see 159 for a review).

HIV-1 gains access to the CNS from the bloodstream, probably by ingress of infected monocytes/macrophages. Heightened trafficking may occur with peripheral activation of monocytes in late-stage HIV-1 infection, which is generally when HAD occurs. In an extensive study in the SIV system, SIV-infected cells were not detected in the CNS of monkeys during the asymptomatic stage of the infection (160). Following progression to AIDS, SIV infection in the CNS was detected by in situ hybridization (160, 161). The current consensus is that the principal cellular target for HIV-1 in the CNS is the macrophage or microglial cell. A large study in clinically well-characterized adults found no convincing evidence for HIV-1 DNA in neurons, endothelial cells, or oligodendrocytes (162). Certain strains of HIV-1 might have an increased propensity to invade (neurotropism) and cause damage in the nervous system (neurovirulence). Brain isolates tend to be more macrophage-tropic with specifically conserved regions in a portion of the envelope, the V3 domain (163, 164). Studies of genotype (165) and phenotype (166) of virus isolated from CSF versus plasma in HIV-1 disease have suggested compartmentalization of HIV-1 replication in the CNS.

Several short-term studies have reported a markedly slower decay rate of HIV-1 RNA in the CSF than in the plasma, especially in patients with HAD (167–169). It follows that the CNS may serve as a reservoir, especially in patients with HAD. Patients who have been on HAART for extended periods generally have undetectable CSF viral loads (94, 125, 148), although CSF viral loads do not correlate perfectly with the viral burden present in brain parenchyma (170). If HIV-1 replication does occur in the CNS, then achieving adequate levels of antiretroviral drugs in this compartment is clearly important. Levels of NRTIs (171) and protease inhibitors (172, 173) are generally lower in the CSF than in the plasma. The protease inhibitors are substrates of the P-glycoprotein transporter (174, 175). Much higher levels of these drugs are achieved in the brains of P-glycoprotein knockout mice (176, 177). Animal models have shown that the NRTIs AZT and ddI are also pumped out of the CNS by a distinct transport system (178). Thus, subtherapeutic levels of these drugs may be present in the CNS. The presence of different drug resistance patterns in paired plasma and CSF HIV-1 isolates in patients on non-suppressive antiretroviral regimens supports this hypothesis (179–181).

The poor penetrations of some antiretroviral drugs into the CNS raised concerns that HAART might produce undetectable or low plasma HIV-1 RNA levels while allowing significantly higher replication in the CNS (182). However, despite these concerns, there have been relatively few clinical examples of "CNS escape." In fact, significant reductions in the incidence rates of HAD have been noted since 1996 (183–185). HAART actually improves neuropsychological performance and radiological abnormalities in HAD (186–188). It is therefore still unclear whether the CNS can serve as a long-term reservoir for HIV-1 in patients with good suppression of viral replication.

The Genitourinary Tract

The genitourinary tract is a potential reservoir for HIV-1 partly because of its unique vascular adaptations, such as the blood-testes barrier, and the poor penetration of some antiretroviral drugs. T cells and macrophages isolated from semen of HIV-1-infected men harbor provirus (189). Similar studies in HIV-1-infected females have implicated cervical macrophages (190, 191) and lymphocytes (192) as targets of HIV-1 infection. Several studies looking at the genotype and phenotype of virus isolated from plasma versus genital secretions in HIV-1-infected patients have suggested possible compartmentalization of HIV-1 replication in the genitourinary tract (193, 194). Thus, it is possible that the cells responsible for the local production of virus in this compartment also act as reservoirs. This would be particularly important if antiretroviral drugs had limited penetration into genitourinary secretions. The NRTIs AZT, d4T, 3TC, and ddI, as well as the NNRTIs nevirapine and efavirenz, achieve high concentrations in seminal fluids (reviewed in 195). Although the protease inhibitor indinavir achieves high levels in semen, preliminary studies have suggested poor penetration by saquinavir and ritonavir and variable penetration by amprenavir (195). A recent study measuring paired drug concentrations in plasma and cervical fluids suggested surprisingly poor penetration of most NRTIs and protease inhibitors in cervical secretions (196). Consistent with these data are reports that show different patterns of drug resistance in plasma and genital secretions in patients failing therapy (196–199). Nevertheless, despite suboptimal concentrations of some antiretrovirals, HAART regimens that suppress viremia to <50 copies/ml can also suppress HIV-1 replication in the genitourinary tract such that free virus in the seminal fluid is difficult to detect (17, 148, 200).

Latently infected seminal cells were found in two of seven patients on HAART with undetectable levels of plasma virus (200). These cells produced replication-competent virus when they were activated and cultured in vitro. The exact nature of these cells could not be determined, and proviral HIV-1 sequences were found in both CD3-positive and CD3-negative fractions (200). The reservoir probably has a long half-life, since one of the patients had been on therapy for 39 months. Genotypic analysis revealed no drug resistance mutations. Thus, this reservoir appears to be archival. Resistance mutations were seen in virus obtained from seminal cells of a patient on a suppressive HAART regimen who had prostatitis (201). A possible explanation is that in cases of local inflammation, latently infected cells become activated, and viral replication then occurs in an environment where nonsuppressive drug concentrations exist. This could potentially lead to drug resistance mutations in the genitourinary tract but not necessarily in peripheral blood. It may thus be very important to prevent inflammatory conditions such as prostatitis and pelvic inflammatory disease in patients on HAART.

A recent study of patients with HIV-1 nephropathy suggests that the kidney can be a reservoir of HIV-1 infection (202). In situ hybridization was performed in tissue obtained from renal biopsies in HIV-1-infected patients with renal disease. Nef and/or gag mRNA transcripts were found in renal parenchymal cells in samples from 14 of 20 patients, including all 4 patients with undetectable plasma viral loads. The mechanism of the HIV-1 infection of renal epithelial cells in vivo is unclear. A small percentage of the cells may express CD4 and CXCR4 (203), but CCR5, the other major coreceptor for HIV-1, is not present (204). It remains to be determined whether these cells release infectious virus, how rapidly they turn over, and how often infection of these cells occurs in patients without renal disease.

CONCLUSIONS

A viral reservoir is a cell type or anatomical site in association with which a replication-competent form of the virus accumulates and persists with more stable kinetic properties than in the main pool of actively replicating virus. It is now clear that HIV-1 persists in a small reservoir of resting memory CD4$^+$ T cells. The virus in this reservoir appears to be latent, since no virus is produced by these cells unless they are activated by antigen. In fact, these cells do not appear to be making any HIV-1 RNA or protein. Therefore, the only difference between a latently infected cell and its uninfected counterpart is a small amount of extra DNA representing the HIV-1 genome. It will be very difficult to eliminate this reservoir with any available form of treatment. This reservoir shows minimal decay in the vast majority of patients on current HAART regimens. The persistence of virus in this reservoir is totally consistent with the biology of these cells and the long-term persistence of immunologic memory. A low level of ongoing viral replication that continues in patients on suppressive HAART regimens may also contribute to the stability of this reservoir.

The best evidence that resting CD4$^+$ T cells serve as a reservoir in HIV-1 infection comes from studies demonstrating the archival character of viruses in this reservoir. The reservoir does turn over when patients are viremic, and drug-resistant viruses can be deposited in this reservoir. However, the degree of turnover depends on the level of viremia. In patients with suppression of viral replication to <50 copies/ml, there is little further turnover of the reservoir. Thus, the latent reservoir serves as a permanent archive for all wild-type and drug-resistant viruses generated previously.

Even in patients with suppression of viral replication to <50 copies/ml, a low level of viremia persists. The viruses in the plasma resemble and may be derived from viruses in the latent reservoir with perhaps some limited additional amplification at a level that does not allow detectable evolution of drug resistance. The presence of this low-level viremia detectable by special methods does not mean that the virus has begun on the mutational pathway leading to drug resistance. Wild-type viruses can be released into the plasma for several years without new resistance mutations. These results suggest that long-term suppression of viral replication is possible. However, resistant viruses selected by prior nonsuppressive therapy continue to enter the plasma whether or not the relevant drug is still being used, and evolution does occur at slightly higher levels of viremia.

There may be other reservoirs, but the latent reservoir in resting CD4$^+$ T cells appears sufficient to guarantee lifetime persistence of HIV-1 in the majority of patients on current HAART regimens, and unless new approaches are developed, eradication will not be possible.

CLINICAL IMPLICATIONS

The clinical implications of new research on viral reservoirs are still not completely clear. However, there is reasonable consensus on the following points:

1. With current regimens, eradication of the infection is not a reasonable goal because of the persistence of latent HIV-1 in resting memory CD4$^+$ T cells.

2. In compliant patients, current HAART regimens come close to stopping virus evolution.

3. The latent reservoir stores all forms of the virus that circulate at high levels. This means that wild-type viruses are likely to reemerge in patients who are failing therapy with resistant virus and are taken off treatment. However, the reappearance of wild-type virus does not mean that resistant virus is gone; it will have also been stored in the reservoir.

ACKNOWLEDGMENTS

This work was supported by NIH grant AI43222 to R.F.S., by an NRSA fellowship to J.N.B., and by grants from the Doris Duke Charitable Foundation and the Elizabeth Glaser Pediatric AIDS Foundation to D. P.. We thank other members of the lab for helpful discussions.

Visit the Annual Reviews home page at www.AnnualReviews.org

LITERATURE CITED

1. Palella FJ, Delaney KM, Moorman AC, et al. 1998. Declining morbidity and mortality among patients with advanced human immunodeficiency virus infection. *N. Engl. J. Med.* 338:853–60

2. Hammer SM, Squires KE, Hughes MD, et al. 1997. A controlled trial of two nucleoside analogues plus indinavir in persons with human immunodeficiency virus infection and CD4 cell counts of 200 per cubic millimeter or less. AIDS Clinical Trials Group 320 Study Team. *N. Engl. J. Med.* 337:725–33

3. Gulick RM, Mellors JW, Havlir D, et al.

1997. Treatment with indinavir, zidovudine, and lamivudine in adults with human immunodeficiency virus infection and prior antiretroviral therapy. *N. Engl. J. Med.* 337:734–39

4. Perelson AS, Essunger P, Cao Y, et al. 1997. Decay characteristics of HIV-1-infected compartments during combination therapy. *Nature* 387:188–91

4a. Wlodawer A. 2002. Rational approach to AIDS drug design through structural biology. *Annu. Rev. Med.* 53:595–614

5. Staszewski S, Morales-Ramirez J, Tashima KT, et al. 1999. Efavirenz plus zidovudine and lamivudine, efavirenz plus indinavir, and indinavir plus zidovudine and lamivudine in the treatment of HIV-1 infection in adults. Study 006 Team. *N. Engl. J. Med.* 341:1865–73

6. Panel on Clinical Practices for Treatment of HIV Infection. Department of Health and Human Services. 2001. Guidelines for the use of antiretroviral agents in HIV-infected adults and adolescents. http://www.hivatis.org

6a. Sempowski GD, Haynes BF. 2002. Immune reconstitution in patients with HIV infection. *Annu. Rev. Med.* 53:269–84

7. Carr A, Samaras K, Chisholm DJ, Cooper DA. 1998. Pathogenesis of HIV-1-protease inhibitor-associated peripheral lipodystrophy, hyperlipidaemia, and insulin resistance. *Lancet* 351:1881–83

8. Brinkman K, Smeitink JA, Romijn JA, Reiss P. 1999. Mitochondrial toxicity induced by nucleoside-analogue reverse-transcriptase inhibitors is a key factor in the pathogenesis of antiretroviral-therapy-related lipodystrophy. *Lancet* 354:1112–15

9. Richman DD. 2001. HIV chemotherapy. *Nature* 410:995–1001

10. Chun T-W, Carruth L, Finzi D, et al. 1997. Quantitation of latent tissue reservoirs and total body load in HIV-1 infection. *Nature* 387:183–88

11. Chun T-W, Finzi D, Margolick J, et al. 1995. Fate of HIV-1-infected T cells *in vivo*: rates of transition to stable latency. *Nat. Med.* 1:1284–90

12. Finzi D, Hermankova M, Pierson T, et al. 1997. Identification of a reservoir for HIV-1 in patients on highly active antiretroviral therapy. *Science* 278:1295–300

13. Wong JK, Hezareh M, Gunthard HF, et al. 1997. Recovery of replication-competent HIV despite prolonged suppression of plasma viremia. *Science* 278:1291–95

14. Chun TW, Stuyver L, Mizell SB, et al. 1997. Presence of an inducible HIV-1 latent reservoir during highly active antiretroviral therapy. *Proc. Natl. Acad. Sci. USA* 94:13193–97

15. Finzi D, Blankson J, Siliciano JD, et al. 1999. Latent infection of CD4+ T cells provides a mechanism for lifelong persistence of HIV-1, even in patients on effective combination therapy. *Nat. Med.* 5:512–17

16. Persaud D, Pierson T, Ruff C, et al. 2000. A stable latent reservoir for HIV-1 in resting CD4+ T lymphocytes in infected children. *J. Clin. Invest* 105:995–1003

17. Dornadula G, Zhang H, VanUitert B, et al. 1999. Residual HIV-1 RNA in blood plasma of patients taking suppressive highly active antiretroviral therapy. *JAMA* 282:1627–32

18. Zhang L, Ramratnam B, Tenner-Racz K, et al. 1999. Quantifying residual HIV-1 replication in patients receiving combination antiretroviral therapy. *N. Engl. J. Med.* 340:1605–13

19. Furtaldo MR, Callaway DS, Phair JP, et al. 1999. Persistence of HIV-1 transcription in peripheral blood mononuclear cells in patients receiving potent antiretroviral therapy. *N. Engl. J. Med.* 340:1614–22

20. Sharkey ME, Teo I, Greenough T, et al. 2000. Persistence of episomal HIV-1 infection intermediates in patients on highly active anti-retroviral therapy. *Nat. Med.* 6:76–81

21. Yerly S, Kaiser L, Perneger TV, et al. 2000. Time of initiation of antiretroviral therapy: impact on HIV-1 viraemia. The Swiss HIV Cohort Study. *AIDS* 14:243–49

22. Piatak M Jr, Saag MS, Yang LC, et al. 1993. High levels of HIV-1 in plasma during all stages of infection determined by competitive PCR. *Science* 259:1749–54

23. Ho DD, Neumann AU, Perelson AS, et al. 1995. Rapid turnover of plasma virions and CD4 lymphocytes in HIV-1 infection. *Nature* 373:123–26

24. Wei X, Ghosh SK, Taylor ME, et al. 1995. Viral dynamics in human immunodeficiency virus type 1 infection. *Nature* 373:117–22

25. Perelson AS, Neumann AU, Markowitz M, et al. 1996. HIV-1 dynamics in vivo: virion clearance rate, infected cell lifespan, viral generation time. *Science* 271:1582–86

26. Zhang LQ, Dailey PJ, He T, et al. 1999. Rapid clearance of simian immunodeficiency virus particles from plasma of rhesus macaques. *J. Virol.* 73:855–60

27. Zhang Z, Schuler T, Zupancic M, et al. 1999. Sexual transmission and propagation of SIV and HIV in resting and activated CD4+ T cells. *Science* 286:1353–57. Erratum. 286(5448):2273

28. Preston BD, Poiesz BJ, Loeb LA. 1988. Fidelity of HIV-1 reverse transcriptase. *Science* 242:1168–71

29. Roberts JD, Bebenek K, Kunkel TA. 1988. The accuracy of reverse transcriptase from HIV-1. *Science* 242:1171–73

30. Coffin JM. 1995. HIV population dynamics in vivo: implications for genetic variation, pathogenesis, and therapy. *Science* 267:483–89

31. Perelson AS, Essunger P, Ho DD. 1998. Dynamics of HIV-1 and CD4+ lymphocytes in vivo. *AIDS* 11 (Suppl. A):S17–S34

32. Mellors JW, Rinaldo CW Jr, Gupta P, et al. 1996. Prognosis in HIV-1 infection predicted by the quantity of virus in plasma. *Science* 272:1167–70

33. Cavert W, Notermans DW, Staskus K, et al. 1997. Kinetics of response in lymphoid tissue to antiretroviral therapy of HIV-1 infection. *Science* 276:960–64

34. Luzuriaga K, Wu H, McManus M, et al. 1999. Dynamics of human immunodeficiency virus type 1 replication in vertically infected infants. *J. Virol.* 73:362–67

35. Ho DD, Rota TR, Hirsh MS. 1986. Infection of monocyte/macrophages by human T lymphotropic virus type III. *J. Clin. Invest.* 77:1712–20

36. Nicolson JKA, Gross GD, Callaway CS, McDougal JS. 1986. In vitro infection of human monocytes with T lymphotrophic virus type III/lymphadenopathy–associated virus (HTLV-III/LAV). *J. Immunol.* 137:323–29

37. Van Furth R. 1989. Origin and turnover of monocytes and macrophages. *Curr. Top. Pathol.* 79:125–50

38. Sierra-Madero JC, Toossi Z, Hom DL, et al. 1994. Relationship between load of virus in alveolar macrophages from human immunodeficiency virus type 1–infected persons, production of cytokines, and clinical status. *J. Infect. Dis.* 169:18–27

39. McIlroy D, Autran B, Cheynier R, et al. 1996. Low infection frequency of macrophages in the spleens of HIV+ patients. *Res. Virol.* 147:115–21

40. Orenstein JM, Fox C, Wahl SM. 1997. Macrophages as a source of HIV during opportunistic infections. *Science* 276:1857–61

41. Igarashi T, Brown CR, Endo Y, et al. 2001. Macrophages are the principal reservoir and sustain high virus loads in rhesus macaques after the depletion of CD4+ T cells by a highly pathogenic simian immunodeficiency virus/HIV type 1 chimera (SHIV): implications for HIV-1 infections of humans. *Proc. Natl. Acad. Sci. USA* 98:658–63

42. Fox CH, Tenner-Racz K, Racz P, et al. 1991. Lymphoid germinal centers are reservoirs of human immunodeficiency virus type 1 RNA. *J. Infect. Dis.* 164:1051–57

43. Yasutomi Y, Reimann KA, Lord CI, et al.

1993. Simian immunodeficiency virus–specific CD8+ lymphocyte response in acutely infected rhesus monkeys. *J. Virol.* 67:1707–11

44. Embretson J, Zupancic M, Ribas JL, et al. 1993. Massive covert infection of helper T lymphocytes and macrophages by HIV during the incubation period of AIDS. *Nature* 362:359–62

45. Burton GF, Masuda A, Heath SL, et al. 1997. Follicular dendritic cells (FDC) in retroviral infection: host/pathogen perspectives. *Immunol. Rev.* 156:185–97

46. Grouard G, Clark EA. 1997. Role of dendritic and follicular dendritic cells in HIV infection and pathogenesis. *Curr. Opin. Immunol.* 9:563–67

47. Reinhart TA, Rogan MJ, Viglianti GA, et al. 1997. A new approach to investigating the relationship between productive infection and cytopathicity in vivo. *Nat. Med.* 3:218–21

48. Heath SL, Tew JG, Szakal AK, Burton GF. 1995. Follicular dendritic cells and human immunodeficiency virus infectivity. *Nature* 377:7440–44

49. Smith BA, Gartner S, Liu Y, et al. 2001. Persistence of infectious HIV on follicular dendritic cells. *J. Immunol.* 166:690–96

50. Hlavacek WS, Wofsy C, Perelson AS. 1999. Dissociation of HIV-1 from follicular dendritic cells during HAART: mathematical analysis. *Proc. Natl. Acad. Sci. USA* 96:14681–86

51. Hlavacek WS, Stilianakis NI, Notermans DW, et al. 2000. Influence of follicular dendritic cells on decay of HIV during antiretroviral therapy. *Proc. Natl. Acad. Sci. USA* 97:10966–71

52. Gelderblom HR, Reupke H, Pauli G. 1985. Loss of envelope antigens of HTLV-III/LAV, a factor in AIDS pathogenesis. *Lancet* 2:1016–17

53. Schneider J, Kaaden O, Copeland TD, et al. 1986. Shedding and interspecies type sero-reactivity of the envelope glycopolypeptide gp120 of the human immunodeficiency virus. *J. Gen. Virol.* 67:2533–38

54. Moore JP, McKeating JA, Weiss RA, Sattentau QJ. 1990. Dissociation of gp120 from HIV-1 virions induced by soluble CD4. *Science* 250:1139–42

55. McKeating JA, McKnight A, Moore JP. 1991. Differential loss of envelope glycoprotein gp120 from virions of human immunodeficiency virus type 1 isolates: effects on infectivity and neutralization. *J. Virol.* 65:852–60

56. Plata F, Autran B, Martins LP, et al. 1987. AIDS virus-specific cytotoxic T lymphocytes in lung disorders. *Nature* 328:348–51

57. Walker BD, Chakrabarti S, Moss B, et al. 1987. HIV-specific cytotoxic T lymphocytes in seropositive individuals. *Nature* 328:345–48

58. Johnson RP, Walker BD. 1994. Cytotoxic T lymphocytes in human immunodeficiency virus infection: responses to structural proteins. *Curr. Top. Microbiol. Immunol.* 189:35–63

59. Koup RA, Safrit JA, Cao Y, et al. 1994. Temporal association of cellular immune responses with the initial control of viremia in primary human immunodeficiency virus type 1 syndrome. *J. Virol.* 68:4650–55

60. Rinaldo C, Xiao-Li H, Fan Z, et al. 1995. High levels of anti–human immunodeficiency virus type 1 (HIV-1) memory cytotoxic T-lymphocyte activity and low viral load are associated with lack of disease in HIV-1-infected long-term nonprogressors. *J. Virol.* 69:5838–42

61. Jin X, Bauer DE, Tuttleton SE, et al. 1999. Dramatic rise in plasma viremia after CD8+ T cell depletion in simian immunodeficiency virus–infected macaques. *J. Exp. Med.* 189:991–98

62. Schmitz JE, Kuroda MJ, Santra S, et al. 1999. Control of viremia in simian immunodeficiency virus infection by CD8+ lymphocytes. *Science* 283:857–60

63. Allen TM, O'Connor DH, Jing P, et al.

2000. Tat-specific cytotoxic T lymphocytes select for SIV escape variants during resolution of primary viraemia. *Nature* 407:386–90

64. Mullins JI. 2001. *Compartments and reservoirs of HIV infection in vivo.* Presented at Keystone Symp. AIDS Pathogenesis, Keystone, CO, March 2001

65. Shankarappa R, Margolick JB, Gange SJ, et al. 1999. Consistent viral evolutionary changes associated with the progression of human immunodeficiency virus type 1 infection. *J. Virol.* 73:10489–502

66. Pierson T, McArthur J, Siliciano RF. 2000. Reservoirs for HIV-1: mechanisms for viral persistence in the presence of antiviral immune responses and antiretroviral therapy. *Annu. Rev. Immunol.* 18:665–708

67. Ahmed R, Gray D. 1996. Immunological memory and protective immunity: understanding their relation. *Science* 272:54–60

68. Murali-Krishna K, Altman JD, Suresh M, et al. 1998. Counting antigen-specific CD8 T cells: a reevaluation of bystander activation during viral infection. *Immunity* 8:177–87

69. Margolick JB, Volkman DJ, Folks TM, Fauci AS. 1987. Amplification of HTLV-III/LAV infection by antigen-induced activation of T cells and direct suppression by virus of lymphocyte blastogenic responses. *J. Immunol.* 138:1719–23

70. Pierson T, Hoffman TL, Blankson J, et al. 2000. Characterization of chemokine receptor utilization of viruses in the latent reservoir for HIV-1. *J. Virol.* 74:7824–33

71. Mo H, Monard S, Pollack H, et al. 1998. Expression patterns of the HIV type 1 coreceptors CCR5 and CXCR4 on CD4+ T cells and monocytes from cord and adult blood. *AIDS Res. Hum. Retroviruses* 14:607–17

72. Blaak H, van't Wout AB, Brouwer M, et al. 2000. In vivo HIV-1 infection of CD45RA$^+$CD4$^+$ T cells is established primarily by syncytium-inducing variants and correlates with the rate of CD4(+) T cell decline. *Proc. Natl. Acad. Sci. USA* 97:1269–74

73. Chun T-W, Chadwick K, Margolick J, Siliciano RF. 1997. Differential susceptibility of naive and memory CD4+ T cells to the cytopathic effects of infection with HIV-1$_{LAI}$. *J. Virol.* 71:4436–44

74. Zack JA, Arrigo SJ, Weitsman SR, et al. 1990. HIV-1 entry into quiescent primary lymphocytes: molecular analysis reveals a labile, latent viral structure. *Cell* 61:213–22

75. Zack JA, Haislip AM, Krogstand P, Chen ISY. 1992. Incompletely reverse-transcribed human immunodeficiency virus type I genomes function as intermediates in the retroviral life cycle. *J. Virol.* 66:1717–25

76. Korin YD, Zack JA. 1998. Progression to the G1b phase of the cell cycle is required for completion of human immunodeficiency virus type 1 reverse transcription in T cells. *J. Virol.* 72:3161–68

77. Korin YD, Zack JA. 1999. Nonproductive human immunodeficiency virus type 1 infection in nucleoside-treated G0 lymphocytes. *J. Virol.* 73:6526–32

78. Bukrinsky MI, Stanwick TL, Dempsey MP, Stevenson M. 1991. Quiescent T lymphocytes as an inducible virus reservoir in HIV-1 infection. *Science* 254:423–27

79. Bukrinsky MI, Sharova N, Dempsey MP, et al. 1992. Active nuclear import of human immunodeficiency virus type 1 preintegration complexes. *Proc. Natl. Acad. Sci. USA* 89:6580–84

80. Spina CA, Guatelli JC, Richman DD. 1995. Establishment of a stable, inducible form of human immunodeficiency virus type 1 DNA in quiescent CD4 lymphocytes in vitro. *J. Virol.* 69:2977–88

81. Blankson JN, Finzi D, Pierson TC, et al. 2000. Biphasic decay of latently infected CD4+ T cells in acute HIV-1 infection. *J. Infect. Dis.* 182:1636–42

82. Nabel G, Baltimore D. 1987. An inducible transcription factor activates expression of human immunodeficiency virus in T cells. *Nature* 326:711–13

83. Duh EJ, Maury WJ, Folks TM, et al. 1989. Tumor necrosis factor alpha activates human immunodeficiency virus type 1 through induction of nuclear factor binding to the NF-kappa B sites in the long terminal repeat. *Proc. Natl. Acad. Sci. USA* 86:5974 78

84. Michie CA, McLean A, Alcock C, Beverley PC. 1992. Lifespan of human lymphocyte subsets defined by CD45 isoforms. *Nature* 360:264–65

85. McLean AR, Michie CA. 1995. In vivo estimates of division and death rates of human T lymphocytes. *Proc. Natl. Acad. Sci. USA* 92:3707–11

86. Ramratnam B, Mittler JE, Zhang L, et al. 2000. The decay of the latent reservoir of replication competent HIV-1 is inversely correlated with the extent of residual viral replication during prolonged antiretroviral therapy. *Nat. Med.* 6:82–85

87. Pomerantz RJ, Seshamma T, Trono D. 1992. Efficient replication of human immunodeficiency virus type 1 requires a threshold level of Rev: potential implications for latency. *J. Virol.* 66:1809–13

88. Pomerantz RJ, Trono D, Feinberg MB, Baltimore D. 1990. Cells nonproductively infected with HIV-1 exhibit an aberrant pattern of viral RNA expression: a molecular model for latency. *Cell* 61:1271–76

89. Chun T-W, Engel D, Berrey MM, et al. 1998. Early establishment of a pool of latently infected, resting CD4+ T cells during primary HIV-1 infection. *Proc. Natl. Acad. Sci. USA* 95:8869–73

90. Lisziewicz J, Jessen H, Finzi D, et al. 1998. HIV-1 suppression by early treatment with hydroxyurea, didanosine, and a protease inhibitor. *Lancet* 352:199–200

91. Lori F, Jessen H, Lieberman J, et al. 1999. Treatment of human immunodeficiency virus infection with hydroxyurea, didanosine, and a protease inhibitor before seroconversion is associated with normalized immune parameters and limited viral reservoir. *J. Infect. Dis.* 180:1827–32

92. Equils O, Garratty E, Wei LS, et al. 2000. Recovery of replication-competent virus from CD4 T cell reservoirs and change in coreceptor use in human immunodeficiency virus type 1–infected children responding to highly active antiretroviral therapy. *J. Infect. Dis.* 182:751–57

93. Lisziewicz J, Rosenberg E, Lieberman J, et al. 1999. Control of HIV despite the discontinuation of antiretroviral therapy. *N. Engl. J. Med.* 340:1683–84

94. Davey RTJ, Bhat N, Yoder C, et al. 1999. HIV-1 and T cell dynamics after interruption of highly active antiretroviral therapy (HAART) in patients with a history of sustained viral suppression. *Proc. Natl. Acad. Sci. USA* 96:15109–14

95. Zhang L, Chung C, Hu B-S, et al. 2000. Genetic characterization of rebounding HIV-1 after cessation of highly active antiretroviral therapy. *J. Clin. Invest.* 106:839–45

96. Chun TW, Davey RT Jr., Ostrowski M, et al. 2000. Relationship between preexisting viral reservoirs and the re-emergence of plasma viremia after discontinuation of highly active anti-retroviral therapy. *Nat. Med.* 6:757–61

97. Rosenberg ES, Altfeld M, Poon SH, et al. 2000. Immune control of HIV-1 after early treatment of acute infection. *Nature* 407:523–26

98. Imamichi H, Crandall KA, Natarajan V, et al. 2001. Human immunodeficiency virus type 1 quasi species that rebound after discontinuation of highly active antiretroviral therapy are similar to the viral quasi species present before initiation of therapy. *J. Infect. Dis.* 183:36–50

99. Siliciano JD, Siliciano RF. 2000. Latency and viral persistence in HIV-1 infection. *J. Clin. Invest* 106:823–25

100. Murali-Krishna K, Lau LL, Sambhara S, et al. 1999. Persistence of memory CD8

T cells in MHC class I–deficient mice. *Science* 286:1377–81

101. Topham DJ, Doherty PC. 1998. Longitudinal analysis of acute Sendai virus-specific CD4+ T cell response and memory. *J. Immunol.* 161:4530–35

102. Takaki A, Wiese M, Maertens G, et al. 2000. Cellular immune responses persist and humoral responses decrease two decades after recovery from a single-source outbreak of hepatitis C. *Nat. Med.* 6:578–82

103. Havlir DV, Marscher IC, Hirsch MS, et al. 1998. Maintenance antiretroviral therapies in HIV-infected subjects with undetectable plasma HIV RNA after triple drug therapy. *N. Engl. J. Med.* 339:1261–68

104. Pialoux G, Raffi F, Brun-Vezinet R, et al. 1998. Trilege study team: a randomized trial of three maintenance regimens given after three months of induction therapy with zidovudine, lamivudine, and indinavir in previously treated patients. *N. Engl. J. Med.* 338:1269–76

105. Hockett RD, Michael KJ, Derdeyn CA, et al. 1999. Constant mean viral copy number per infected cell in tissues regardless of high, low, or undetectable plasma HIV RNA. *J. Exp. Med.* 189:1545–54

106. Gunthard HF, Frost SDW, Leigh-Brown AJ, et al. 1999. Evolution of envelope sequences of human immunodeficiency virus type 1 in cellular reservoirs in the setting of potent antiviral therapy. *J. Virol.* 73:9404–12

107. Gunthard HF, Wong JK, Ignacio CC, et al. 1998. Human immunodeficiency virus replication and genotypic resistance in blood and lymph nodes after a year of potent antiretroviral therapy. *J. Virol.* 72:2422–28

108. Martinez-Picado J, Kartsonis N, Hanna GJ, et al. 2000. Antiretroviral resistance during successful therapy of human immunodeficiency virus type 1 infection. *Proc. Natl. Acad. Sci. USA* 97:10948–53

109. Deeks SG, Wrin T, Liegler T, et al. 2001. Virologic and immunologic consequences of discontinuing combination antiretroviral-drug therapy in HIV-infected patients with detectable viremia. *N. Engl. J. Med.* 344:472–80

110. Hermankova M, Ray SC, Ruff C, et al. 2001. HIV-1 drug resistance profiles in children and adults with viral load <50 copies/mL receiving combination therapy. *JAMA* 286:196–207

111. Havlir DV, Hellmann NS, Petropoulos CJ, et al. 2000. Drug susceptibility in HIV infection after viral rebound in patients receiving indinavir-containing regimens. *JAMA* 283:229–34

112. Tisdale M, Kemp SD, Parry NR, Larder BA. 1993. Rapid in vitro selection of human immunodeficiency virus type 1 resistant to 3′-thiacytidine inhibitors due to a mutation in the YMDD region of reverse transcriptase. *Proc. Natl. Acad. Sci. USA* 90:5653–56

113. Boucher CA, Cammack N, Schipper P, et al. 1993. High-level resistance to (-) enantiomeric 2′-deoxy-3′-thiacytidine in vitro is due to one amino acid substitution in the catalytic site of human immunodeficiency virus type 1 reverse transcriptase. *Antimicrob. Agents Chemother.* 37:2231–34

114. Ramratnam B, Ribeiro R, He T, et al. 2001. Antiretroviral intensification accelerates the decay of the latent reservoir of HIV-1 and decreases but does not eliminate ongoing virus replication. *Conf. Retroviruses and Opportunistic Infections, 8th, Feb. 4–8, Chicago,* Abstr. 502. Alexandria, VA: IDSA Fdn. Retrovirol. Hum. Health

115. Ho DD, Ramratnam B, Louiie M, Markowitz M. 2001. Latent reservoir and residual HIV-1 replication on antiretroviral therapy. *Conf. Retroviruses and Opportunistic Infections, 8th, Feb. 4–8, Chicago,* Abstr. S17. Alexandria, VA: IDSA Fdn. Retrovirol. Hum. Health

116. Prins JM, Jurriaans S, van Praag RM,

et al. 1999. Immuno-activation with anti-CD3 and recombinant human IL-2 in HIV-1-infected patients on potent antiretroviral therapy. *AIDS* 13:2405–10

117. Chun TW, Engel D, Mizell SB, et al. 1999. Effect of interleukin-2 on the pool of latently infected, resting CD4+ T cells in HIV-1-infected patients receiving highly active anti-retroviral therapy. *Nat. Med.* 5:651–55

118. Dybul M, Chun T-W, Belson M, et al. 2001. A randomized, controlled pilot study of HAART versus HAART plus IL-2 for the treatment of recently acquired HIV infection. *Conf. Retroviruses and Opportunistic Infections, 8th, Feb. 4–8, Chicago*, Abstr. 406. Alexandria, VA: IDSA Fdn. Retrovirol. Hum. Health

119. Stellbrink HJ, Hufert FT, Tenner-Racz K, et al. 1998. Kinetics of productive and latent HIV infection in lymphatic tissue and peripheral blood during triple-drug combination therapy with or without additional interleukin-2. *Antivir. Ther.* 3:209–14

120. Lafeuillade A, Poggi C, Chadapaud S, et al. 2001. Pilot study of a combination of highly active antiretroviral therapy and cytokines to induce HIV-1 remission. *J. Acquired Immune Defic. Syndr.* 26:44–55

121. Rosenberg ES, Billingsley JM, Caliendo AM, et al. 1997. Vigorous HIV-1-specific CD4+ T cell responses associated with the control of viremia. *Science* 278:1447–50

122. Ruiz L, Martinez-Picado J, Romeu J, et al. 2000. Structured treatment interruption in chronically HIV-1 infected patients after long-term viral suppression. *AIDS* 14:397–403

123. Papasavvas E, Ortiz GM, Gross R, et al. 2000. Enhancement of human immunodeficiency virus type 1–specific CD4 and CD8 T cell responses in chronically infected persons after temporary treatment interruption. *J. Infect. Dis.* 182:766–75

124. Lori F, Maserati R, Foli A, et al. 2000.

Structured treatment interruptions to control HIV-1 infection. *Lancet* 355:287–88

125. Garcia F, Plana M, Vidal C, et al. 1999. Dynamics of viral load rebound and immunological changes after stopping effective antiretroviral therapy. *AIDS* 13:F79–F86

126. Mitsuyasu RT, Anton PA, Deeks SG, et al. 2000. Prolonged survival and tissue trafficking following adoptive transfer of CD4zeta gene–modified autologous CD4$^+$ and CD8$^+$ T cells in human immunodeficiency virus–infected subjects. *Blood* 96:785–93

127. Roberts MR, Qin L, Zhang D, et al. 1994. Targeting of human immunodeficiency virus–infected cells by CD8+ T lymphocytes armed with universal T-cell receptors. *Blood* 84:2878–89

128. Zhang Z-Q, Schuler T, Wietgrefe S, et al. 1999. Sexual transmission and propagation of SIV and HIV-1 in activated and quiescent T cells. *Conf. Retroviruses and Opportunistic Infections, 6th, Jan. 31–Feb. 4*, Abstr. 4. Alexandria, VA: IDSA Fdn. Retrovirol. Hum. Health

129. Schnittman SM, Lane HC, Greenhouse J, et al. 1990. Preferential infection of CD4+ memory T cells by human immunodeficiency virus type 1: evidence for a role in the selective T–cell functional defects observed in infected individuals. *Proc. Natl. Acad. Sci. USA* 87:6058–62

130. Sleasman JW, Aleixo LF, Morton A, et al. 1996. CD4+ memory T cells are the predominant population of HIV-1-infected lymphocytes in neonates and children. *AIDS* 10:1477–84

131. Ostrowski MA, Chun TW, Justement SJ, et al. 1999. Both memory and CD45RA+/CD62L+ naive CD4$^+$ T cells are infected in human immunodeficiency virus type 1–infected individuals. *J. Virol.* 73:6430–35

132. Brooks DG, Kitchen SG, Kitchen CM, et al. 2001. Generation of HIV latency during thymopoiesis. *Nat. Med.* 7:459–64

133. Al-Harthi L, Landay A. 2001. Alternative

targets of productive HIV infection: role of CD4 up-regulation on susceptibility of cells to HIV infection. *AIDS Rev.* 3:4–11

134. Livingstone WJ, Moore M, Innes D, et al. 1996. Frequent infection of peripheral blood CD8-positive T lymphocytes. *Lancet* 348:649–54

135. Kitchen SG, Korin YD, Roth MD, et al. 1998. Costimulation of naive CD8$^+$ lymphocytes induces CD4 expression and allows human immunodeficiency virus type 1 infection. *J. Virol.* 72:9054–60

136. Yang LP, Riley JL, Carroll RG, et al. 1998. Productive infection of neonatal CD8+ T lymphocytes by HIV-1. *J. Exp. Med.* 187:1139–44

137. Flamand L, Crowley RW, Lusso P, et al. 1998. Activation of CD8+ T lymphocytes through the T cell receptor turns on CD4 gene expression: implications for HIV pathogenesis. *Proc. Natl. Acad. Sci. USA* 95:3111–16

138. Lambotte O, Taoufik Y, de Goer MG, et al. 2000. Detection of infectious HIV in circulating monocytes from patients on prolonged highly active antiretroviral therapy. *J. Acquired Immune Defic. Syndr.* 23:114–19

139. Zhu T. 2000. HIV-1 genotypes in peripheral blood monocytes. *J. Leukoc. Biol.* 68:338–44

140. Sonza S, Mutimer HP, Oelrichs R, et al. 2001. Monocytes harbour replication-competent, non-latent HIV-1 in patients on highly active antiretroviral therapy. *AIDS* 15:17–22

141. Moir S, Malaspina A, Li Y, et al. 2000. B cells of HIV-1-infected patients bind virions through CD21-complement interactions and transmit infectious virus to activated T cells. *J. Exp. Med.* 192:637–46

142. Pope M, Betles MGH, Romani N, et al. 1994. Conjugates of dendritic cells and memory T lymphocytes from skin facilitate productive infection with HIV-1. *Cell* 78:389–98

143. Cameron PU, Freudenthal PS, Barker JM, et al. 1992. Dendritic cells exposed to human immunodeficiency virus type-1 transmit a vigorous cytopathic infection to CD4$^+$ T cells. *Science* 257:383–87

144. Frankel SS, Wenig BM, Burke AP, et al. 1996. Replication of HIV-1 in dendritic cell–derived syncytia at the mucosal surface of the adenoid. *Science* 272:115–17

145. Geijtenbeek TB, Kwon DS, Torensma R, et al. 2000. DC-SIGN, a dendritic cell–specific HIV-1-binding protein that enhances trans-infection of T cells. *Cell* 587–97

146. Pantaleo G, Graziosi C, Demarest JF, et al. 1993. HIV infection is active and progressive in lymphoid tissue during the clinically latent stage of disease. *Nature* 362:355–58

147. Veazey RS, Demaria MA, Chalifoux LV, et al. 1998. Gastrointestinal tract as a major site of CD4+ T cell depletion and viral replication in SIV infection. *Science* 280:427–31

148. Gunthard HF, Havlir DV, Fiscus S, et al. 2001. Residual human immunodeficiency virus (HIV) type 1 RNA and DNA in lymph nodes and HIV RNA in genital secretions and in cerebrospinal fluid after suppression of viremia for 2 years. *J. Infect. Dis.* 183:1318–27

149. Reinhardt RL, Khoruts A, Merica R, et al. 2001. Visualising the generation of memory T cells in the whole body. *Nature* 410:101–5

150. Su L, Kaneshima H, Bonyhadi M, et al. 1995. HIV-1-induced thymocyte depletion is associated with indirect cytopathicity and infection of progenitor cells in vivo. *Immunity* 2:25–36

151. Roederer M, Dubs JG, Anderson MT, et al. 1995. CD8 naive T cell counts decrease progressively in HIV-infected adults. *J. Clin. Invest.* 95:2061–66

152. Rabin RL, Roederer M, Maldonado Y, et al. 1995. Altered representation of naive and memory CD8 T cell subsets in HIV-infected children. *J. Clin. Invest.* 95:2054–60

153. Autran B, Carcelain G, Li TS, et al. 1997.

Positive effects of combined antiretroviral therapy on CD4$^+$ T cell homeostasis and function in advanced HIV disease. *Science* 277:112–16

154. McCune JM, Loftus R, Schmidt DK, et al. 1998. High prevalence of thymic tissue in adults with human immunodeficiency virus–1 infection. *J. Clin. Invest.* 101:2301–8

155. Douek DC, McFarland RD, Keiser PH, et al. 1998. Changes in thymic function with age and during the treatment of HIV infection. *Nature* 396:690–95

156. Zhang L, Lewin SR, Markowitz M, et al. 1999. Measuring recent thymic emigrants in blood of normal and HIV-1-infected individuals before and after effective therapy. *J. Exp. Med.* 190:725–32

157. Hazenberg MD, Otto SA, Cohen Stuart JW, et al. 2000. Increased cell division but not thymic dysfunction rapidly affects the T-cell receptor excision circle content of the naive T cell population in HIV-1 infection. *Nat. Med.* 6:1036–42

158. Bacellar H, Munoz A, Miller EN, et al. 1994. Temporal trends in the incidence of HIV-1 related neurologic diseases: Multicenter AIDS Cohort Study, 1985–1992. *Neurology* 44:1892–900

159. Glass JD, Johnson RT. 1996. Human immunodeficiency virus and the brain. *Annu. Rev. Neurosci.* 19:1–26

160. Reinhart TA, Rogan MJ, Huddleston D, et al. 1997. Simian immunodeficiency virus burden in tissues and cellular compartments during clinical latency and AIDS. *J. Infect. Dis.* 176:1198–208

161. Zink MC, Spelman JP, Robinson RB, Clements JE. 1998. SIV infection of macaques—modeling the progression to AIDS dementia. *J. Neurovirol.* 4:249–59

162. Takahashi K, Wesselingh SL, Griffin DE, et al. 1996. Localization of HIV-1 in human brain using polymerase chain reaction/in situ hybridization and immunocytochemistry. *Ann. Neurol.* 39:705–11

163. Gartner S, Markovits P, Markovitz DM, et al. 1986. The role of mononuclear phagocytes in HTLV-III/LAV infection. *Science* 233:215–19

164. Chesebro B, Wehrly K, Nishio J, Perryman S. 1992. Macrophage-tropic human immunodeficiency virus isolates from different patients exhibit unusual V3 envelope sequence homogeneity in comparison with T-cell-tropic isolates: definition of critical amino acids involved in cell tropism. *J. Virol.* 66:6547–54

165. Winslow BJ, Pomerantz RJ, Bagasra O, Trono D. 1993. HIV-1 latency due to the site of proviral integration. *Virology* 196:849–54

166. Peeters MF, Colebunders RL, Van den AK, et al. 1995. Comparison of human immunodeficiency virus biological phenotypes isolated from cerebrospinal fluid and peripheral blood. *J. Med. Virol.* 47:92–96

167. Eggers CC, van Lunzen J, Buhk T, Stellbrink HJ. 1999. HIV infection of the central nervous system is characterized by rapid turnover of viral RNA in cerebrospinal fluid. *J. Acquired Immune Defic. Syndr. Hum. Retrovirol.* 20:259–64

168. Cinque P, Presi S, Bestetti A, et al. 2001. Effect of genotypic resistance on the virological response to highly active antiretroviral therapy in cerebrospinal fluid. *AIDS Res. Hum. Retroviruses* 17:377–83

169. Ellis RJ, Gamst AC, Capparelli E, et al. 2000. Cerebrospinal fluid HIV RNA originates from both local CNS and systemic sources. *Neurology* 54:927–36

170. Weinberg JB, Matthews TJ, Cullen BR, Malim MH. 1991. Productive human immunodeficiency virus type 1 (HIV-1) infection of nonproliferating human monocytes. *J. Exp. Med.* 174:1477–82

171. Foudraine NA, Hoetelmans RM, Lange JM, et al. 1998. Cerebrospinal-fluid HIV-1 RNA and drug concentrations after treatment with lamivudine plus zidovudine or stavudine. *Lancet* 351:1547–51

172. Aweeka F, Jayewardene A, Staprans S, et al. 1999. Failure to detect nelfinavir in the cerebrospinal fluid of HIV-1-infected

patients with and without AIDS dementia complex. *J. Acquired Immune Defic. Syndr. Hum. Retrovirol.* 20:39–43

173. Kravcik S, Gallicano K, Roth V, et al. 1999. Cerebrospinal fluid HIV RNA and drug levels with combination ritonavir and saquinavir. *J. Acquired Immune Defic. Syndr.* 21:371–75

174. van Asperen J, Mayer U, van Tellingen O, Beijnen JH. 1997. The functional role of P-glycoprotein in the blood-brain barrier. *J. Pharm. Sci.* 86:881–84

175. Lee CG, Gottesman MM, Cardarelli CO, et al. 1998. HIV-1 protease inhibitors are substrates for the MDR1 multidrug transporter. *Biochemistry* 37:3594–601

176. Kim RB, Fromm MF, Wandel C, et al. 1998. The drug transporter P-glycoprotein limits oral absorption and brain entry of HIV-1 protease inhibitors. *J. Clin. Invest.* 101:289–94

177. Polli JW, Jarrett JL, Studenberg SD, et al. 1999. Role of P-glycoprotein on the CNS disposition of amprenavir (141W94), an HIV protease inhibitor. *Pharm. Res.* 16:1206–12

178. Takasawa K, Terasaki T, Suzuki H, Sugiyama Y. 1997. In vivo evidence for carrier-mediated efflux transport of 3′-azido-3′-deoxythymidine and 2′,3′-dideoxyinosine across the blood-brain barrier via a probenecid-sensitive transport system. *J. Pharmacol. Exp. Ther.* 281:369–75

179. Cunningham PH, Smith DG, Satchell C, et al. 2000. Evidence for independent development of resistance to HIV-1 reverse transcriptase inhibitors in the cerebrospinal fluid. *AIDS* 14:1949–54

180. Stingele K, Haas J, Zimmermann T, et al. 2001. Independent HIV replication in paired CSF and blood viral isolates during antiretroviral therapy. *Neurology* 56:355–61

181. Venturi G, Catucci M, Romano L, et al. 2000. Antiretroviral resistance mutations in human immunodeficiency virus type 1 reverse transcriptase and protease from paired cerebrospinal fluid and plasma samples. *J. Infect. Dis.* 181:740–45

182. Pialoux G, Fournier S, Moulignier A, et al. 1997. Central nervous system (CNS) as sanctuary of HIV-1 in a patient treated with AZT+3TC+indinavir. *Conf. Retroviruses and Opportunistic Infections, 4th,* Abstr. 233. Alexandria, VA: IDSA Fdn. Retrovirol. Hum. Health

183. Brodt HR, Kamps BS, Gute P, et al. 1997. Changing incidence of AIDS-defining illnesses in the era of antiretroviral combination therapy. *AIDS* 11:1731–38

184. Sacktor N, Lyles RH, McFarlane G, et al., The Multicenter AIDS Cohort Study. 1999. HIV-1-related neurological disease incidence changes in the era of highly active antiretroviral therapy. *Neurology* 52 (Suppl. 2):A252–A253 (Abstr. S31.001)

185. Moore RD, Keruly JC, Bartlett JG, Chaisson RE. 1999. Differential effect of HAART on development of opportunistic illness and death in clinical practice. *Conf. Retroviruses and Opportunistic Infections, 6th, Jan. 31–Feb. 4,* Abstr. 691. Alexandria, VA: IDSA Fdn. Retrovirol. Hum. Health

186. Brew BJ, Brown SJ, Catalan J, et al., CNAB 001 Study Team. 1998. Safety and efficacy of abacavir (ABC, 1592) in AIDS dementia complex (Study CNAB 3001). *World AIDS Conf., 12th, Geneva,* Abstr. 32192. Geneva: World AIDS Conf.

187. Filippi CG, Sze G, Farber SJ, et al. 1998. Regression of HIV encephalopathy and basal ganglia signal intensity abnormality at MR imaging in patients with AIDS after the initiation of protease inhibitor therapy. *Radiology* 206:491–98

188. Sacktor NC, Lyles RH, Skolasky RL, et al., for the Multicenter AIDS Cohort Study (MACS). 1999. Combination antiretroviral therapy including protease inhibitors improves HIV-associated cognitive impairment. *Neurology* 52:1640–47

189. Quayle AJ, Xu C, Mayer KH, Anderson

DJ. 1997. T lymphocytes and macrophages, but not motile spermatozoa, are a significant source of human immunodeficiency virus in semen. *J. Infect. Dis.* 176:960–68

190. Nuovo GJ, Forde A, MacConnell P, Fahrenwald R. 1993. In situ detection of PCR-amplified HIV-1 nucleic acids and tumor necrosis factor cDNA in cervical tissues. *Am. J. Pathol.* 143:40–48

191. Pomerantz RJ, de la Monte SM, Donegan SP, et al. 1988. Human immunodeficiency virus (HIV) infection of the uterine cervix. *Ann. Intern. Med.* 108:321–27

192. Van de PP, De Clercq A, Cogniaux-Leclerc J, et al. 1988. Detection of HIV p17 antigen in lymphocytes but not epithelial cells from cervicovaginal secretions of women seropositive for HIV: implications for heterosexual transmission of the virus. *Genitourin. Med.* 64:30–33

193. Kiessling AA, Fitzgerald LM, Zhang D, et al. 1998. Human immunodeficiency virus in semen arises from a genetically distinct virus reservoir. *AIDS Res. Hum. Retroviruses* 14(Suppl. 1):S33–S41

194. Vernazza PL, Eron JJ, Cohen MS, et al. 1994. Detection and biologic characterization of infectious HIV-1 in semen of seropositive men. *AIDS* 8:1325–29

195. Taylor S, Pereira AS. 2001. Antiretroviral drug concentrations in semen of HIV-1 infected men. *Sex Transm. Infect.* 77:4–11

196. Si-Mohamed A, Kazatchkine MD, Heard I, et al. 2000. Selection of drug-resistant variants in the female genital tract of human immunodeficiency virus type 1–infected women receiving antiretroviral therapy. *J. Infect. Dis.* 182:112–22

197. Eron JJ, Vernazza PL, Johnston DM, et al. 1998. Resistance of HIV-1 to antiretroviral agents in blood and seminal plasma: implications for transmission. *AIDS* 12:F181–F189

198. Kroodsma KL, Kozal MJ, Hamed KA, et al. 1994. Detection of drug resistance mutations in the human immunodeficiency virus type 1 (HIV-1) pol gene: differences in semen and blood HIV-1 RNA and proviral DNA. *J. Infect. Dis.* 170:1292–95

199. Byrn RA, Zhang D, Eyre R, et al. 1997. HIV-1 in semen: an isolated virus reservoir. *Lancet* 350:1141

200. Zhang H, Dornadula G, Beumont M, et al. 1998. HIV-1 in the semen of men receiving highly active anti-retroviral therapy. *N. Engl. J. Med.* 339:1803–9

201. Eyre RC, Zheng G, Kiessling AA. 2000. Multiple drug resistance mutations in human immunodeficiency virus in semen but not blood of a man on antiretroviral therapy. *Urology* 55:591

202. Bruggeman LA, Ross MD, Tanji N, et al. 2000. Renal epithelium is a previously unrecognized site of HIV-1 infection. *J. Am. Soc. Nephrol.* 11:2079–87

203. Conaldi PG, Biancone L, Bottelli A, et al. 1998. HIV-1 kills renal tubular epithelial cells in vitro by triggering an apoptotic pathway involving caspase activation and Fas upregulation. *J. Clin. Invest* 102:2041–49

204. Eitner F, Cui Y, Hudkins KL, et al. 1998. Chemokine receptor (CCR5) expression in human kidneys and in the HIV infected macaque. *Kidney Int.* 54:1945–54

Annu. Rev. Med. 2002. 53:595–614

RATIONAL APPROACH TO AIDS DRUG DESIGN THROUGH STRUCTURAL BIOLOGY*

Alexander Wlodawer

Macromolecular Crystallography Laboratory, National Cancer Institute at Frederick, Frederick, Maryland 21702; e-mail: wlodawer@ncifcrf.gov

■ **Abstract** The discovery and development of more than a dozen drugs in the past 15 years for the treatment of AIDS offer an excellent example of progress in the field of rational drug design. At this time, the principal targets are reverse transcriptase and protease, enzymes encoded by the human immunodeficiency virus. The introduction of protease inhibitors, in particular, has drastically decreased the mortality and morbidity associated with AIDS. This review presents the methods used to develop such drugs and discusses the remaining problems, such as the rapid emergence of drug resistance.

INTRODUCTION

The structure-assisted ("rational") drug design and discovery process (1–3) utilizes techniques such as protein crystallography, nuclear magnetic resonance (NMR), and computational biochemistry to guide synthesis of potential drugs. The structural information is used to help explain the basis of effective inhibition and to improve the potency and specificity of new lead compounds. The term "rational drug design" is, however, often misinterpreted. There is nothing irrational about traditional methods, such as screening of compound libraries, and indeed, screening and design are often used together. The complementary methods of computer-aided molecular design (4) and combinatorial chemistry (5) are now routinely employed in both the lead identification and the development phases of drug design. These different approaches have been successfully combined in many cases, although rational drug design is a much more recent phenomenon than screening or serendipity-based techniques.

Many structure-based techniques of drug discovery and development have evolved in the past 20 years during the search for therapeutically useful agents in the treatment of acquired immunodeficiency syndrome (AIDS). This major epidemic is caused by two variants of the human immunodeficiency virus, HIV-1 and HIV-2. The complete nucleotide sequence of HIV-1 (6) shows a relatively simple retrovirus whose genome consists of three open reading frames (ORF), *gag, pol,*

---

*The US Government has the right to retain a nonexclusive, royalty-free license in and to any copyright covering this paper.

595

and *env*. The *gag* ORF contains structural proteins such as capsid, nucleocapsid, and matrix, whereas regulatory proteins are encoded in the multiply spliced *env* ORF. The HIV-1 genome encodes only three unique enzymes, all located within the *pol* ORF. These enzymes, reverse transcriptase (RT), integrase, and protease (PR), have all become targets for drug discovery.

The first AIDS drugs to be identified were nucleoside inhibitors of RT (Figure 1*a*), discovered and developed long before the structure of RT itself was solved (7, 8). However, the development of newer RT-targeted drugs, nonnucleoside inhibitors, is closely coupled to structural investigations of enzyme complexes. Even now, only fragmentary structural data have been described for integrase (9–12); and extensive efforts to discover integrase inhibitors (13) have as yet produced no clinical candidates. Retroviral protease, however, was identified as a potential target early on (14, 15), and the discovery and development of its inhibitors (reviewed in 16–23 and discussed below) exemplify an unqualified success of modern pharmacology and structural biology. Selected aspects of the development of RT-targeted drugs are also mentioned in this review.

DEVELOPMENT OF THE INHIBITORS OF HIV PROTEASE

HIV-1 PR (Figure 1*b*) shares considerable similarity (24) with the much-studied family of aspartic proteases, which includes such mammalian enzymes as pepsin, renin, and chymosin (25). Pepstatin, a signature inhibitor of aspartic proteases (15, 26), inhibits HIV-1 PR and other retroviral proteases; in addition, they are inactivated by mutation of the active-site aspartates (15, 27). Inactivation of HIV-1 PR by either mutation or chemical inhibition leads to the production of immature, noninfectious viral particles (15, 27); thus, the function of this enzyme was shown to be essential for proper virion assembly and maturation. For such reasons, HIV-1 PR became an important target for drug design, and between 1995 and 2001 the U.S. Food and Drug Administration (FDA) has approved six drugs targeting this enzyme, with more certain to come.

Crystallographic and NMR Studies of Retroviral Proteases

The availability of crystal structures of HIV-1 PR was an important reason for the rapid progress in drug development. The structure of the uninhibited enzyme was determined independently in several laboratories (28–30). Crystal structures of HIV-2 PR (31, 32) and simian immunodeficiency virus (SIV) PR (33, 34) also became available. The structures of many complexes of HIV and SIV PRs with inhibitors have been reported in a number of crystal forms at resolutions up to 1.55 Å (35). More than 180 structures of the complexes of HIV-1, HIV-2, and SIV PRs with inhibitors are publicly available in an Internet-accessible database (36). The structures of inhibitor complexes of HIV-1 PR have also been studied using NMR (37–40). NMR combined with computational methods confirmed that a combination of computational models and simulations, along with NMR data,

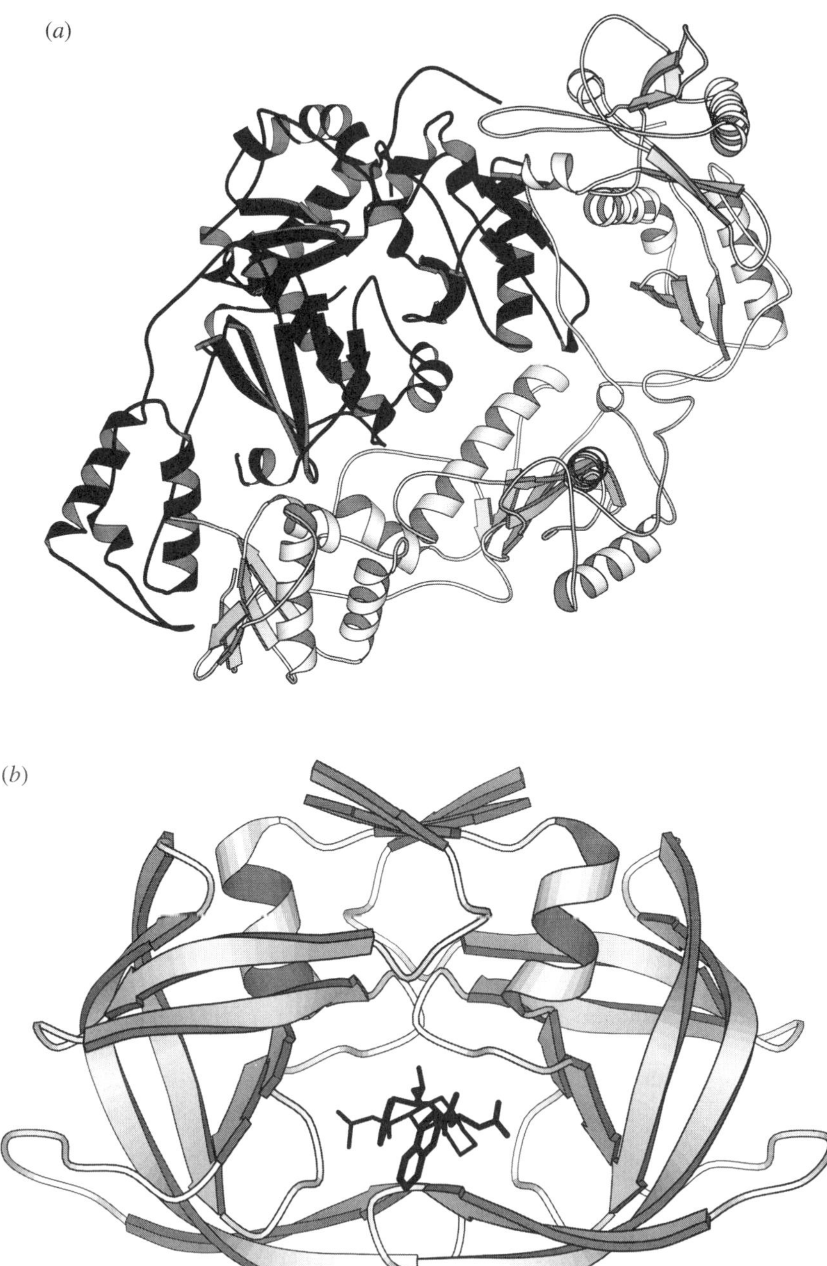

Figure 1 Ribbon diagrams of the enzymes that are targets for the approved AIDS drugs. (*a*) HIV reverse transcriptase (RT), with its active p66 domain shown in grey and the smaller p51 domain in black. (*b*) HIV protease (PR) complexed with the drug saquinavir (in black stick representation). The loops on the right side that cover the inhibitor are the flaps (see text).

can provide a basis for further modification and design (41). The ionization state of the catalytic residues was studied by NMR, using chemically synthesized HIV-1 PR in which the Asp-25 in each monomer was specifically labeled with ^{13}C (42).

The Structure of HIV-1 PR and Enzyme-Inhibitor Interactions

A molecule of HIV-1 PR is composed of two identical protein chains, each containing 99 amino acids (Figure 1b). Each monomer contains nine β strands and a single helix, arranged with internal pseudosymmetry (29). Four antiparallel β strands, two from each molecule, form the principal dimer interface. Another two β strands lead to the active-site triplet (Asp25-Thr26-Gly27). Four of the β strands in the molecular core are organized into a Ψ-shaped sheet characteristic of all aspartic proteases. The active-site triplet is located in a loop whose structure is stabilized by a network of hydrogen bonds. The carboxylate groups of the active-site residues, Asp25 from both chains, are nearly coplanar and in close contact. The active site is covered by two symmetric flaps that change their conformation between the free and inhibited enzymes. This structural feature is different from the single flap present in pepsins. The area adjacent to the active site is the most rigid and most highly conserved in the whole molecule (16, 35), whereas the flaps are the most dynamic. The areas leading to the flaps have been implicated in facilitating motions necessary to allow substrate entry and release (43).

Most of the inhibitors cocrystallized with HIV PR, including all petidomimetic inhibitors, are bound in the protease active site in an extended conformation (16). The hydrogen bonds are made mostly between the main chain atoms of both the enzyme and the inhibitor and follow a similar pattern. The nonhydrolyzable scissile bond analogs of each inhibitor align with the active-site aspartate carboxyl groups Asp25/Asp25'. The hydroxyl group at the nonscissile junction, present in many inhibitors, is positioned between the PR aspartate carboxyl groups, within hydrogen bonding distance of at least one carboxylate oxygen of each aspartate. A feature common to almost all complexes of HIV-1 PR is a buried water molecule that bridges the P2 and P1' CO groups of the inhibitor and the Ile50 and Ile50' NH groups of the flaps. This water is approximately tetrahedrally coordinated and is completely inaccessible to solvent (44). The functional substitution of this water led to the design of a number of inhibitors (see below).

Several distinct subsites (45) that accommodate side chains of the inhibitors can be identified in HIV PR. Owing to the symmetry of the enzyme, subsites on both sides of the peptide bond replacement are practically the same, with only three (S1–S3) well-defined. The protease side chains comprising the pockets S1 and S1', with the exception of the active-site aspartates, are mostly hydrophobic; thus, these subsites are usually occupied by hydrophobic residues, often large. Although the S2 and S2' pockets are hydrophobic, both hydrophilic and hydrophobic residues can occupy these sites. The subsites S3 and S3' can accommodate a variety of residues, with much less specificity, while the parts of the inhibitors extending further are binding, if at all, largely on the surface of the protein.

Computational Studies of the Inhibitor Complexes of HIV-1 PR

Whereas structural studies of HIV-1 PR and its inhibitor complexes have played a very important role in drug design, computational studies were necessary to understand the mode of binding and to optimize inhibitor design. Studies that involved energy minimization using molecular mechanics (46, 47) have shown that the calculated contribution of the main-chain atoms to the total interaction energy ranged from 56% to 68%, providing a substantial contribution to the total binding energy. A study aimed at predicting the activity of HIV-1 PR inhibitors resulted in a high correlation between the interaction energy and the experimentally determined IC_{50} constants for almost 50 inhibitor-enzyme complexes (48). Free energy perturbation calculations coupled with molecular dynamics have been relatively reliable in predicting the free energy of binding by computational methods (49, 50). Such studies were also performed to explain the differences between the binding constants of similar inhibitors (51, 52), to analyze HIV-1 PR mutants and their affinity to different inhibitors (53), or to aid molecular modeling and drug design (54).

A number of docking procedures based on the crystal structures of the inhibitor complexes of HIV-1 PR have been reported. Docking methods and algorithms were tested using the structural data and experimental characteristics by Monte Carlo docking (55) or by comparison with de novo constructed inhibitors using the fragment-based method (56). Other studies examined empirical free energy as a target function in docking and design, showing the advantages of this approach over the calculation of interaction energy (57). These and similar studies have played major roles in the design of a variety of inhibitors, some of which became clinical candidates.

PROTEASE INHIBITORS IN CLINICAL AND PRECLINICAL USE

Several inhibitors of HIV-1 PR (Figure 2) are already in use or in clinical trials as anti-HIV drugs; more are under way (58). Indeed, the availability of these inhibitors has drastically changed the course of the disease and significantly decreased its associated mortality and morbidity (59). Chemical structures of all current clinical inhibitors of HIV-1 PR, and of selected inhibitors that are in advanced clinical trials, are shown in Figure 2.

Saquinavir

Saquinavir (Ro 31-8959, Invirase, Fortavase), from Hoffmann-La Roche, was designed in a rational drug design program initiated with peptide derivatives that were transition-state mimics (60). The basic design criterion relied on the observation that HIV-1 PR cleaves the sequences containing dipeptides Tyr-Pro or Phe-Pro.

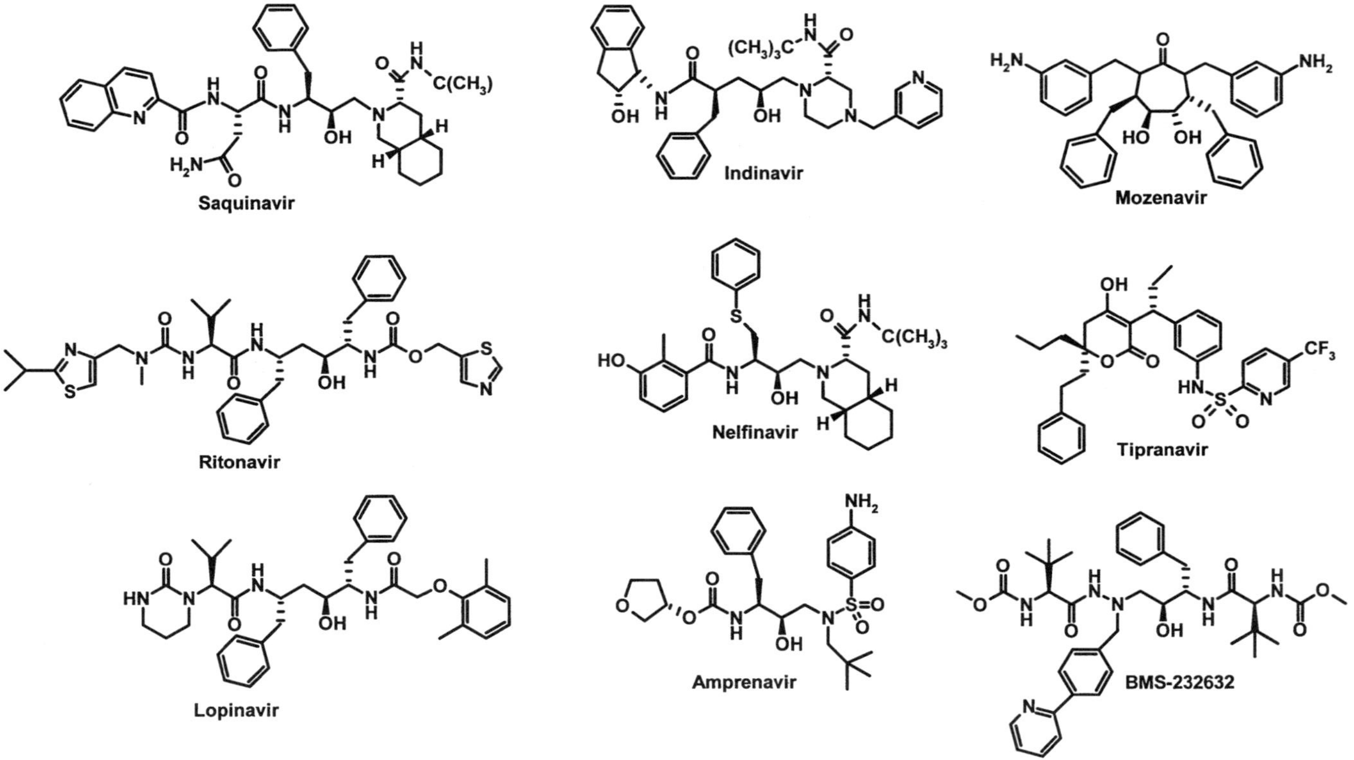

Figure 2 Chemical formulas of the six FDA-approved inhibitors of HIV-1 PR and of other selected inhibitors that are currently in advanced clinical trials.

Mammalian proteases do not cleave peptide bonds followed by a proline; thus, this target promised selectivity. Because reduced amides and hydroxyethylamine isosteres most readily accommodate the imino acid moiety, they were chosen for further studies.

A peptidic inhibitor, Ro 31-8558, was studied crystallographically in complex with HIV-1 PR, showed the expected mode of binding and suggested possible future modifications (61). Replacement of a proline at the P1$'$ subsite by (S,S,S)-decahydro-isoquinoline-3-carbonyl (DIQ) significantly improved the potency of the inhibitors. A compound that included such a modification (Ro 31-8959, saquinavir) (60) exhibited K_i of 0.12 nM at pH 5.5 against HIV-1 PR and was even better against HIV-2 PR ($K_i < 0.1$ nM). It was shown to be highly selective, causing only minor inhibition of human aspartic proteases. Crystallographic study of saquinavir has shown that the carbonyl of the DIQ group is able to maintain the hydrogen bond between the water molecule connecting the inhibitor with the flap regions (Wat301) (62). In 1995, saquinavir became the first protease inhibitor approved by the FDA. It is available in two forms: as Invirase in hard-gel formulation and as Fortovase in soft-gel capsules. The latter formulation considerably increased the bioavailability of the drug.

Ritonavir

The initial basis of the design and development efforts that led to the discovery of Abbott's ritonavir (ABT-538, Norvir) was the symmetry of HIV-1 PR, and the first Abbott inhibitors were also symmetric (63, 64). These inhibitors showed good kinetic profiles but poor bioavailability. In order to enhance the aqueous solubility, the terminal phenyl residues were modified to pyridyl groups (65). A lead compound, A-77003, revealed broad-spectrum activity against both HIV-1 and HIV-2 in a variety of transformed and primary human cell lines. However, crystallographic studies of inhibitor complexes of HIV-1 PR have shown that even symmetric inhibitors may bind to HIV-1 PR in an asymmetric fashion (66). In addition, imposition of symmetry made it difficult to improve bioavailability, which is often influenced by the termini of the inhibitor. For these reasons, a development process that started from symmetric or pseudosymmetric inhibitors led to compounds with significant asymmetry. The knowledge of the superior potency of the deshydroxy diols finally led to creation of a series of compounds, one of which was ABT-538 (ritonavir) (67), ultimately approved by the FDA as Norvir.

It was later shown that ritonavir potentiates the activity of other protease inhibitors, most likely by inhibiting the cytochrome P450 (CYP)-mediated metabolism (68). Because of this property, ritonavir was included in the formulation of a second-generation protease drug, Kaletra (see below).

Indinavir

The development of indinavir (MK-639, L-735,524, Crixivan) by Merck was based on a transition-state mimetic concept (69), previously utilized in design of renin inhibitors (70). A series of peptidomimetic inhibitors of different lengths, containing a hydroxyethylene isostere in an S configuration, was examined, with a number of substitutions of the side chains. Another approach to the design of nanomolar inhibitors of HIV PR led to a series of analogs of L-682,679 in which the carboxyl terminus had been shortened and modified (71). Inclusion of (aminomethyl) benzimidazole provided the most potent compounds in that series, as the imidazole portion appeared to be mimicking a carboxamide, while the phenyl portion was probably contributing additional hydrophobic binding. Some of the inhibitors with excellent IC_{50} values were considerably less potent in cell culture, presumably because of their inability to penetrate the hydrophobic cell membrane. The important conclusion was that as the terminal amide increased in size or polarity, the intrinsic potency improved but not the minimum inhibitory concentration.

The design of indinavir was guided by molecular modeling and X-ray crystal structure of the inhibited enzyme complex (72, 73). This potent inhibitor was highly active against HIV-1 and HIV-2 PRs, both in enzymatic and in tissue culture assays. Indinavir (Crixivan) was orally bioavailable in three animal models and gained FDA approval at the beginning of 1996.

Nelfinavir

Agouron (now part of Pfizer) was one of the first companies established in the 1980s for the explicit purpose of creating drugs through rational design, and nelfinavir (AG-1343, Viracept) is one of the first products of such companies to reach the stage of FDA approval. Nelfinavir was also the first PR drug that was not a peptidomimetic, although peptidomimetics were created along its development pathway. Two early Agouron inhibitors, AG-1002 and AG-1004, had statine isosteres instead of normal peptide bonds in their central parts (74, 75). The best inhibitor in that series had an inhibition constant of about 30 nM.

Iterative protein cocrystal structure analysis of peptidic inhibitors and the replacement of parts of the inhibitors by nonpeptidic substituents (76) were used to design orally bioavailable, nonpeptidic inhibitors. A Monte Carlo program that could generate ligands was used to fill the S1 subsite (77), resulting in the placement of a large cyclopenthylethyl group in this position. Combining the 5-chloro with the dimethylbenzyl and cyclopentyl amides resulted in the best compound in this series, with K_i of about 2 nM, comparable with saquinavir in efficiency.

The final steps in the design of nelfinavir have been described in some detail (78). Nelfinavir contains a novel 2-methyl-3-hydroxybenzamide group, whereas its carboxyl terminus contains the same DIQ group as saquinavir (see above). However, nefinavir is a mesylate salt of a basic amine of DIQ. The P1 subsite is occupied by the S-phenyl group, increasing the potency by an order of magnitude. Nelfinavir's mode of binding to HIV-1 PR was verified by determination of the crystal structure of the complex (78). Nelfinavir (Viracept) was approved by the FDA in 1997 and was the first protease inhibitor to be indicated for pediatric AIDS.

Amprenavir

Amprenavir (VX-478, 141W94, Agenerase), from Vertex Pharmaceuticals and GlaxoSmithKline, shares some structural features with the other successful protease inhibitors described above. Its central core is identical to that of saquinavir, although both ends are quite different. The P2 group consists of tetrahydrofuran carbamate, whereas the P1′–P2′ moieties consist of an isobutylphenyl sulfonamide with an added amide. This design gives amprenavir fewer chiral centers than saquinavir, facilitating synthesis and increasing water solubility to allow oral bioavailability as high as 40%–70% (79). The crystal structure of HIV-1 PR with bound amprenavir has been reported (80). Amprenavir is quite potent against HIV-1 PR ($K_i = 0.6$ nM), whereas its inhibition constant against human aspartic proteases is low. It was also shown to be very potent in vitro against a variety of clinical isolates of HIV-1 (79). Early clinical results indicated that amprenavir was very potent and well-tolerated (81). Amprenavir in a combination with two nucleoside RT inhibitors was more potent than these two inhibitors alone, although less effective than indinavir (82). The necessary dose of amprenavir could be reduced by coadministration with ritonavir (also see below). Prodrug formulations of amprenavir (GW433908) are being developed.

Kaletra

Kaletra, developed at Abbott, was approved by the FDA in the second half of 2000; it is the first second-generation protease inhibitor to reach drug status. It is a mixture of two protease inhibitors: a novel compound, lopinavir (ABT-378), and a smaller amount of ritonavir (a typical pill combination is 133 mg of the former and 33 mg of the latter).

Lopinavir was originally designed to diminish the interactions of the inhibitor with Val82 of HIV-1 PR, a residue that is often mutated in the drug-resistant strains of the virus (83). The core of lopinavir is identical to that of ritonavir. The 5-thiazolyl end group in ritonavir was replaced by the phenoxyacetyl group, and the 2-isopropylthiazolyl group in rotonavir was replaced by a modified valine in which the amino terminus had a six-membered cyclic urea attached. The chemical (84) and therapeutic (85) properties of lopinavir have been reviewed elsewhere. Lopinavir is a very powerful competitive inhibitor of HIV-1 PR ($K_i = 1.3$ pM) against wild-type enzymes, and still excellent against a number of mutants (83). As expected based on the design criteria, lopinavir exhibited much higher potency against a number of drug-resistant mutants of HIV-1 PR than did the competing inhibitors, although new mutants with increased resistance to that compound were observed early on (86). The plasma level of lopinavir decreased very quickly in rats and even faster in humans, but in the presence of subclinical amounts (50 mg) of ritonavir, lopinavir concentration exceeding EC_{50} could be maintained for over 24 h after a single 400 mg dose (84). Kaletra is now considered an important salvage drug, administered after the primary therapy with protease inhibitors has failed.

Other Inhibitors in Clinical Trials

One of the unexpected structural features of complexes between HIV-1 PR and the inhibitors is a conserved water molecule that mediates the contacts between the P2/P1′ carbonyl oxygen atoms of the peptidic inhibitors and the amide groups of Ile50/Ile50′ of the enzyme. Replacement of the tetrahedrally coordinated Wat301 was proposed early on as a possible way of making highly specific protease inhibitors (87), and several groups implemented that suggestion. Scientists from DuPont Merck and from the University of Uppsala designed molecules with a seven-membered cyclic urea ring as the starting pharmacophore (88, 89). Some such inhibitors were symmetric and others were not (90). One of these inhibitors, DMP-450 (mozenavir), with excellent inhibitory properties ($K_i = 0.3$ nM) and high potency against the virus in cell culture, was shown to be orally available in humans (91). As of spring 2001, this inhibitor was in phase I/II clinical trials conducted by Triangle Pharmaceuticals.

A very different inhibitor of HIV-1 PR was created at Pharmacia and is being further developed by Boehringer-Ingelheim. Tipranavir (PNU-140690) is an entirely nonpeptidic compound with $K_i = 5$ pM and $IC_{90} = 100$ nM in antiviral cell culture (92). The discovery of tiprinavir followed a broad screening program that identified a small molecule, phenprocoumon, as a possible template for designing inhibitors of HIV PR. Several potential clinical candidates, each more potent than the last, originated from this combination of screening and rational drug design. Crystal structure analysis of tipranavir has shown that despite its structural differences from the peptidic inhibitors, its mode of interaction with HIV PR is similar in many respects. The lactone oxygen atom of the dihydropyrone ring forms hydrogen bonds with the amide nitrogen atoms of the flap residues, in a manner analogous to Wat301. The 4-hydroxy group is bonded in a pseudosymmetric manner to the two active-site aspartates. This drug is soluble and highly bioavailable (93), and clinical trials are under way. It appears to exhibit significant activity against HIV-1 isolated from patients with multidrug resistance to other protease inhibitors (94).

An azapeptide inhibitor of HIV-1 PR is being developed by Bristol-Myers Squibb under the name of BMS-232632 (95). The principal advantage of this potential drug is its once-daily dosing and lower toxicity. Its most likely future use is in multidrug combination therapy.

DRUGS TARGETING REVERSE TRANSCRIPTASE

Reverse transcriptase is a heterodimer consisting of two chains, p66 and p51 (Figure 1a), encoded by the same gene belonging to the *pol* ORF. The larger chain contains an additional RNase H domain; the rest of the sequence (but not the three-dimensional structure) is the same. The active sites for both primary activities of the enzyme (RNA- or DNA-dependent DNA polymerase, and RNase H) are contained in the p66 domain. The structures of RT have been solved (*a*) in the presence of nonnucleoside inhibitors (see below) (7); (*b*) in a ternary complex with a bound template:primer and Fab (8); (*c*) for the apoenzyme (96); and (*d*) as a covalently trapped catalytic complex with a DNA template:primer and a deoxynucleoside triophosphate (97), among others.

RT inhibitors can be divided into two general classes. The first to be discovered were compounds that act as terminators of chain elongation. These analogs of the nucleoside substrates bind in the substrate-binding site and can inhibit both HIV-1 and HIV-2 RT. Another class of RT inhibitors, nonnucleoside inhibitors (NNIs), are specific to a pocket that is found in the vicinity of the active site in HIV-1 RT but does not exist in HIV-2 RT. These noncompetitive inhibitors were initially identified largely by serendipity, and their practicality as AIDS drugs was initially met with considerable skepticism. However, some NNIs have been found to be excellent drugs when used in combination with other antiretroviral drugs, even though they are largely useless in monotherapy. However, a single dose of NNIs offers considerable protection against mother-to-child transmission of HIV during birth.

Nucleoside Analogs

The inhibitory properties of nucleoside analogs against RT are due either to the lack of 2′ or 3′ hydroxyl groups, or to their replacement by other functional groups. In the case of AZT (azidothymidine, zidovudine), for example, the presence of the 3′-azido group prevents subsequent creation of a 3′-5′ phosphodiester bond and thus terminates the chain. The introduction of nucleoside analogs as potential AIDS drugs was based on the understanding of RT's mechanism of action rather than on the knowledge of its structure, which was unknown when these compounds were introduced. Five nucleoside analogs (NRTIs) have so far been approved by the FDA (Figure 3). Zidovudine (AZT, Retrovir, GlaxoSmithKline) was approved for monotherapy in 1987 as the first generally available AIDS drug, although its efficacy in that mode was shown to be only transitory (98). The drug is delivered orally with very high bioavailability. Another nucleoside analog AIDS drug is didanosine (dideoxyinosine, ddI, Videx), a product of Bristol-Myers Squibb. It is an analog of inosine, lacking both the 2′- and 3′-hydroxyl groups on its ribose moiety. In common with zidovudine, its active form is a triphosphate produced by a cellular enzyme. Its intracellular half-life is 8–24 h, much longer than that of zidovudine, thus allowing once-a-day dosing.

Another drug related to didanosine is zalcitabine (dideoxycytidine; ddC, Hivid), a product of Hoffmann–La Roche. This pyrimidine analog is active against HIV in vitro at very low concentrations, although its plasma half-life is rather short, requiring several daily doses of the drug. The FDA approved Stavudine (d4T, 3′-deoxy-2′-thymidinene, Zerit), a modification of thymidine manufactured by Bristol-Myers Squibb, for the treatment of HIV-infected adults who have received prolonged zidovudine therapy (99). The drug is generally well-tolerated with minimal side effects. Lamivudine (3TC, 3′-thia-2′,3′-dideoxcytidine, Epivir), discovered by BioChem Pharma and developed by GlaxoSmithKline, is also potent against another viral disease, chronic hepatitis B. After it was found that the

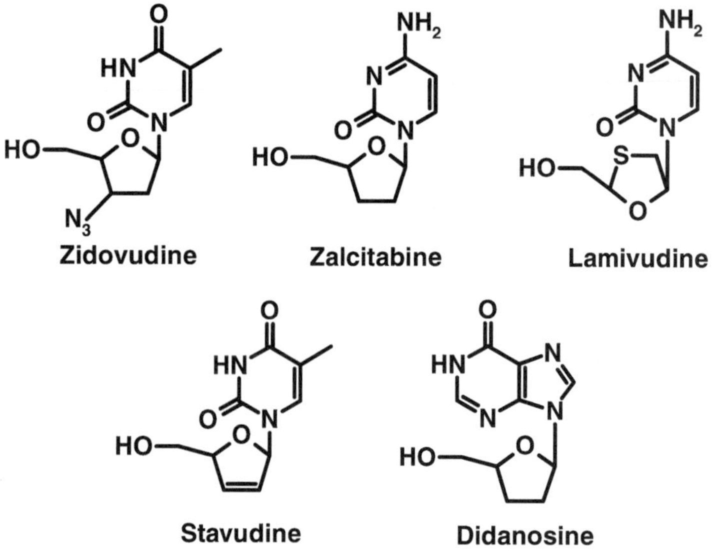

Zidovudine

Zalcitabine

Lamivudine

Stavudine

Didanosine

Figure 3 Chemical formulas of FDA-approved nucleoside inhibitors of HIV-1 RT.

principal mutation in RT that occurs in individuals receiving lamivudine, M184V, prevents resistance to zidovudine, a combination of both drugs (Combivir, which consists of 150 mg of lamivudine combined with 300 mg of zidovudine) was developed. Ziagen (Abacavir) is another nucleoside inhibitor recently developed by GlaxoSmithKline, and Triangle Pharmaceuticals is currently developing emtricitabine (Coviracil). It is clear that the usefulness of the nucleoside AIDS drugs will continue in the foreseeable future.

Nonnucleoside Analogs

Nonnucleoside analogs are potent inhibitors of HIV-1 RT but not of HIV-2 RT. The first such compounds, HEPT (100) and TIBO (101), were discovered to be active in cell culture before their target was identified. Several other members of this heterogeneous class, including nevirapine, were identified in screening programs specifically targeting HIV-1 RT (102). The NNIs bind in a pocket located about 10 Å from the substrate binding site. When bound into that pocket in HIV-1 RT, most NNIs maintain a similar, butterfly-like shape. The mode of action of NNIs is not completely clear, although it has been suggested that their proximity to the active site might alter the conformation of this domain, or that they restrict the motions of the p66 thumb domain (7).

So far, three NNIs have gained FDA approval for use against HIV (103). Their chemical formulas are shown in Figure 4. Nevirapine (Viramune, Boehringer-Ingelheim) was the first to gain approval (in 1996). Nevirapine is highly bioavailable in oral form and induces its own metabolism by activating the hepatic

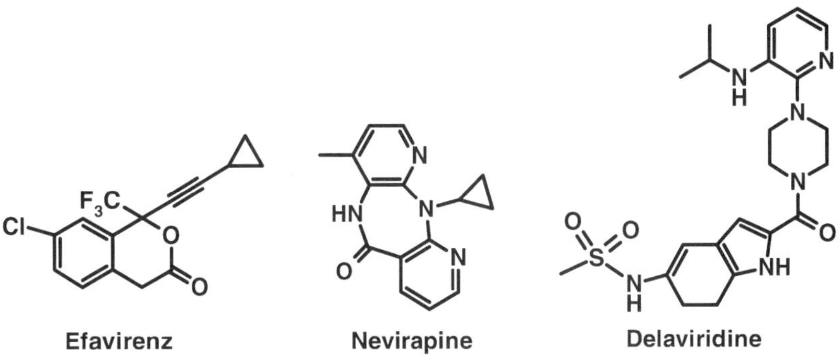

Efavirenz   **Nevirapine**   **Delaviridine**

Figure 4 Chemical formulas of FDA-approved nonnucleoside inhbitors of HIV-1 RT.

cytochrome P450 pathways. Another FDA-approved NNI is delaviridine (Rescriptor), developed by Pharmacia and currently marketed by Pfizer. This compound has a relatively short plasma half-life, requiring several daily doses to maintain its concentration. The third NNI in current clinical use is efavirenz (Sustiva) from DuPont Pharmaceuticals. NNIs are not recommended in monotherapy because of rapid development of resistance, but they are very useful in multidrug combinations.

DEVELOPMENT OF DRUG RESISTANCE

Because retroviral RT has no editing function, transcription errors during nucleic acid replication are very common, and the viral pool contains species with all conceivable mutations. The presence of drugs provides a powerful selection pressure for virus modifications that produce lower susceptibility to such compounds. Development of resistance is often observed only a week or two after initiation of therapy. Rapid appearance of drug-resistant HIV species was considered a major obstacle in the development of newer therapies, such as PR inhibitors or NNIs.

Although nucleoside inhibitors of RT have been in clinical use for almost 15 years, the mechanism of resistance to them has been elucidated only recently (97). The structure of a trapped catalytic complex of RT provided data on the exact location of the incoming deoxynucleoside triphosphate and, by extension, of the nucleoside drugs. Not surprisingly, residues mutated in drug-resistant RT are located in the vicinity of the active site of the enzyme. An analysis of the steric nature of these mutations can also explain why resistance to one class of inhibitors may sensitize the enzyme to another class, forming the basis of sequential therapy. The emergence of resistance to NNIs is particularly rapid, since the binding site for these compounds is not a direct part of the active site of RT (103, 104). As a rule, mutations leading to resistance to NNIs involve residues lining the binding site of these inhibitors. However, it is now clear that resistance can be minimized, both by combining NNIs with other inhibitors and by starting therapy with high concentrations of the drugs. NNIs are generally prescribed in combination with drugs from other classes (105).

A study of mutations resulting from the use of protease inhibitors found that about one third of the residues in HIV-1 PR were mutated in samples obtained after application of 21 drugs (104). Although some of these mutations were in pockets directly adjacent to the inhibitors, other mutations are observed throughout the protein. The appearance of the mutations is usually sequential, and remote mutations usually develop subsequent to the primary ones. The discovery of a pattern of multiple resistance mutations in patients subjected to indinavir monotherapy (106), as well as cross-resistance with six other PR inhibitors, raised serious questions about the efficacy of that category of drugs. However, this initial pessimism was unwarranted, since the use of sufficiently high doses and combination therapies have been quite successful in delaying or overcoming resistance. Drug-resistant mutations of HIV PR are considered so important that resistance studies now precede any attempts to introduce such compounds into clinical practice, as was recently described for lopinavir (86).

Combination therapies (highly active antiretroviral therapy, HAART) using different inhibitors promise the best clinical outcome. However, it is not clear whether it is better to use combinations of different drugs from the same family or drugs belonging to different classes. On one hand, combinations such as ritonavir-saquinavir, nelfinavir-saquinavir, or ritonavir-indinavir combine two similar drugs with distinct resistance patterns and, especially in the case of ritonavir, with different metabolisms. On the other hand, combinations of indinavir or nelfinavir with nevirapine, or indinavir plus efavirenz, assure that the development of resistance will require mutations in two different enzymes, making resistance less likely.

In Western countries, drug treatment is reducing AIDS to a manageable and treatable long-term disease. However, even with all the drugs already on the market, it is clear that the serious nature of the AIDS pandemic and the limitations of the therapies will make it necessary to continue drug development. Until a safe, effective vaccine against HIV has been found, it will be necessary to introduce new therapies and combinations of drugs to counteract the development of resistant variants. The understanding of drug-target interactions on the molecular level, coupled with extensive studies using the techniques of molecular biology, are of great help in achieving rapid success.

Visit the Annual Reviews home page at www.AnnualReviews.org

LITERATURE CITED

1. Appelt K, Bacquet RJ, Bartlett CA, et al. 1991. Design of enzyme inhibitors using iterative protein crystallographic analysis. *J. Med. Chem.* 34:1925–34

2. Gane PJ, Dean PM. 2000. Recent advances in structure-based rational drug design. *Curr. Opin. Struct. Biol.* 10:401–4

3. Klebe G. 2000. Recent developments in structure-based drug design. *J. Mol. Med.* 78:269–81

4. Leach AR. 1996. *Molecular Modelling: Principles and Applications*, pp. 543–85. Singapore: Longman

5. Balkenkohl F, Von Dem Bussche-Hunnefield C, Lansky A, Zechel C. 1996. Combinatorial synthesis of small molecules. *Angew. Chem. Int.* 35:2288–337

6. Ratner L, Haseltine W, Patarca R, et al. 1985. Complete nucleotide sequence of the AIDS virus, HTLV-III. *Nature* 313: 277–84

7. Kohlstaedt LA, Wang J, Friedman JM, et al. 1992. Crystal structure at 3.5 Å resolution of HIV-1 reverse transcriptase complexed with an inhibitor. *Science* 256:1783–90

8. Jacobo-Molina A, Ding J, Nanni RG, et al. 1993. Crystal structure of human immunodeficiency virus type 1 reverse transcriptase complexed with double-stranded DNA at 3.0 Å resolution shows bent DNA. *Proc. Natl. Acad. Sci. USA* 90: 6320–24

9. Dyda F, Hickman AB, Jenkins TM, et al. 1994. Crystal structure of the catalytic domain of HIV-1 integrase: similarity to other polynucleotidyl transferases. *Science* 266:1981–86

10. Bujacz G, Alexandratos J, Zhou-Liu Q, et al. 1996. The catalytic domain of human immunodeficiency virus integrase: ordered active site in the F185H mutant. *FEBS Lett.* 398:175–78

11. Maignan S, Guilloteau JP, Zhou-Liu Q, et al. 1998. Crystal structures of the catalytic domain of HIV-1 integrase free and complexed with its metal cofactor: high level of similarity of the active site with other viral integrases. *J. Mol. Biol.* 282:359–68

12. Chen JC, Krucinski J, Miercke LJ, et al. 2000. Crystal structure of the HIV-1 integrase catalytic core and C-terminal domains: a model for viral DNA binding. *Proc. Natl. Acad. Sci. USA* 97:8233–38

13. Pommier Y, Pilon AA, Bajaj K, et al. 1997. HIV-1 integrase as a target for antiviral drugs. *Antivir. Chem. Chemother.* 8: 463–83

14. Katoh I, Yasunaga T, Ikawa Y, Yoshinaka Y. 1987. Inhibition of retroviral protease activity by an aspartyl proteinase inhibitor. *Nature* 329:654–56

15. Kohl NE, Emini EA, Schleif WA, et al. 1988. Active human immunodeficiency virus protease is required for viral infectivity. *Proc. Natl. Acad. Sci. USA* 85: 4686–90

16. Wlodawer A, Erickson JW. 1993. Structure-based inhibitors of HIV-1 protease. *Annu. Rev. Biochem.* 62:543–85

17. Vacca JP, Condra JH. 1997. Clinically effective HIV-1 protease inhibitors. *Drug Discov. Today* 2:261–72

18. Wlodawer A, Vondrasek J. 1998. Inhibitors of HIV-1 protease: a major success of structure-assisted drug design. *Annu. Rev. Biophys. Biomol. Struct.* 27:249–84

19. Gulnik S, Erickson JW, Xie D. 2000. HIV protease: enzyme function and drug resistance. *Vitam. Horm.* 58:213–56

20. Wlodawer A, Gustchina A. 2000. Structural and biochemical studies of retroviral proteases. *Biochim. Biophys. Acta* 1477:16–34

21. Tomasselli AG, Heinrikson RL. 2000. Targeting the HIV-protease in AIDS therapy: a current clinical perspective. *Biochim. Biophys. Acta* 1477:189–214

22. Sansom C, Wlodawer A. 2000. Drugs targeted at HIV—successes and resistance. In *Computational Analysis of Human Immunodeficiency Virus Molecular Sequences*, ed. A Rodrigo, GH Learn, pp. 269–86. Boston: Kluwer

23. Swanstrom R, Erona J. 2000. Human immunodeficiency virus type-1 protease inhibitors: therapeutic successes and failures, suppression and resistance. *Pharmacol. Ther.* 86:145–70

24. Toh H, Ono M, Saigo K, Miyata T. 1985. Retroviral protease-like sequence in the yeast transposon Ty1. *Nature* 315: 691

25. Davies DR. 1990. The structure and

function of the aspartic proteinases. *Annu. Rev. Biophys. Biomol. Struct.* 19:189–215

26. Katoh I, Yoshinaka Y, Rein A, et al. 1985. Murine leukemia virus maturation: protease region required for conversion from immature to mature form and for virus infectivity. *Virology* 145:280–92

27. Seelmeier S, Schmidt H, Turk V, von der Helm K. 1988. Human immunodeficiency virus has an aspartic-type protease that can be inhibited by pepstatin A. *Proc. Natl. Acad. Sci. USA* 85:6612–16

28. Navia MA, Fitzgerald PM, McKeever BM, et al. 1989. Three-dimensional structure of aspartyl protease from human immunodeficiency virus HIV-1. *Nature* 337:615–20

29. Wlodawer A, Miller M, Jaskólski M, et al. 1989. Conserved folding in retroviral proteases: crystal structure of a synthetic HIV-1 protease. *Science* 245:616–21

30. Lapatto R, Blundell T, Hemmings A, et al. 1989. X-ray analysis of HIV-1 proteinase at 2.7 Å resolution confirms structural homology among retroviral enzymes. *Nature* 342:299–302

31. Tong L, Pav S, Pargellis C, et al. 1993. Crystal structure of human immunodeficiency virus (HIV) type 2 protease in complex with a reduced amide inhibitor and comparison with HIV-1 protease structures. *Proc. Natl. Acad. Sci. USA* 90: 8387–91

32. Mulichak AM, Hui JO, Tomasselli AG, et al. 1993. The crystallographic structure of the protease from human immunodeficiency virus type 2 with two synthetic peptidic transition state analog inhibitors. *J. Biol. Chem.* 268:13103–9

33. Zhao B, Winborne E, Minnich MD, et al. 1993. Three-dimensional structure of a simian immunodeficiency virus protease/inhibitor complex. Implications for the design of human immunodeficiency virus type 1 and 2 protease inhibitors. *Biochemistry* 32:13054–60

34. Rose RB, Rose JR, Salto R, et al. 1993. Structure of the protease from simian immunodeficiency virus: complex with an irreversible nonpeptide inhibitor. *Biochemistry* 32:12498–507

35. Mahalingam B, Louis JM, Reed CC, et al. 1999. Structural and kinetic analysis of drug resistant mutants of HIV-1 protease. *Eur. J. Biochem.* 263:238–45

36. Vondrasek J, van Buskirk CP, Wlodawer A. 1997. Database of three-dimensional structures of HIV proteinases. *Nat. Struct. Biol.* 4:8

37. Wonacott A, Cooke R, Hayes FR, et al. 1993. A series of penicillin-derived C2-symmetric inhibitors of HIV-1 proteinase: structural and modeling studies. *J. Med. Chem.* 36:3113–19

38. Jhoti H, Singh OM, Weir MP, et al. 1994. X-ray crystallographic studies of a series of penicillin-derived asymmetric inhibitors of HIV-1 protease. *Biochemistry* 33:8417–27

39. Yamazaki T, Nicholson LK, Torchia DA, et al. 1994. Secondary structure and signal assignments of human-immunodeficiency-virus-1 protease complexed to a novel, structure-based inhibitor. *Eur. J. Biochem.* 219:707–12

40. Ohno Y, Kiso Y, Kobayashi Y. 1996. Solution conformations of KNI-272, a tripeptide HIV protease inhibitor designed on the basis of substrate transition state: determined by NMR spectroscopy and simulated annealing calculations. *Bioorg. Med. Chem.* 4:1565–72

41. Podlogar BL, Farr RA, Friedrich D, et al. 1994. Design, synthesis, and conformational analysis of a novel macrocyclic HIV-protease inhibitor. *J. Med. Chem.* 37:3684–92

42. Smith R, Brereton IM, Chai RY, Kent SB. 1996. Ionization states of the catalytic residues in HIV-1 protease. *Nat. Struct. Biol.* 3:946–50

43. Rose RB, Craik CS, Stroud RM. 1998. Domain flexibility in retroviral proteases: structural implications for drug resistant mutations. *Biochemistry* 37:2607–21

44. Miller M, Schneider J, Sathyanarayana

BK, et al. 1989. Structure of complex of synthetic HIV-1 protease with a substrate-based inhibitor at 2.3 Å resolution. *Science* 246:1149–52

45. Schechter I, Berger A. 1967. On the size of the active site in proteases. I. Papain. *Biochem. Biophys. Res. Commun.* 27:157–62

46. Sansom CE, Wu J, Weber IT. 1992. Molecular mechanics analysis of inhibitor binding to HIV-1 protease. *Protein Eng.* 5:659–67

47. Gustchina A, Sansom C, Prevost M, et al. 1994. Energy calculations and analysis of HIV-1 protease-inhibitor crystal structure. *Protein Eng.* 7:309–17

48. Holloway MK, Wai JM, Halgren TA, et al. 1995. A priori prediction of activity for HIV-1 protease inhibitors employing energy minimization in the active site. *J. Med. Chem.* 38:305–17

49. Ferguson DM, Radmer RJ, Kollman PA. 1991. Determination of the relative binding free energies of peptide inhibitors to the HIV-1 protease. *J. Med. Chem.* 34:2654–59

50. Tropsha A, Hermans J. 1992. Application of free energy simulations to the binding of a transition-state-analogue inhibitor to HIV protease. *Protein Eng.* 5:29–33

51. Kato R, Takahashi O, Kiso Y, et al. 1994. Solution structure of HIV-1 protease-allophenylnorstatine derivative inhibitor complex obtained from molecular dynamics simulation. *Chem. Pharm. Bull. (Tokyo)* 42:176–78

52. Rao BG, Murcko MA. 1996. Free energy perturbation studies on binding of A-74704 and its diester analog to HIV-1 protease. *Protein Eng.* 9:767–71

53. Schock HB, Garsky VM, Kuo LC. 1996. Mutational anatomy of an HIV-1 protease variant conferring cross-resistance to protease inhibitors in clinical trials. Compensatory modulations of binding and activity. *J. Biol. Chem.* 271:31957–63

54. Wallqvist A, Jernigan RL, Covell DG. 1995. A preference-based free-energy parameterization of enzyme-inhibitor binding. Applications to HIV-1-protease inhibitor design. *Protein Sci.* 4:1881–903

55. Caflisch A, Niederer P, Anliker M. 1992. Monte Carlo docking of oligopeptides to proteins. *Proteins Struct. Funct. Genet.* 13:223–30

56. Rotstein SH, Murcko MA. 1993. GroupBuild: a fragment-based method for de novo drug design. *J. Med. Chem.* 36:1700–10

57. King BL, Vajda S, DeLisi C. 1996. Empirical free energy as a target function in docking and design: application to HIV-1 protease inhibitors. *FEBS Lett.* 384:87–91

58. Tavel JA. 2000. Ongoing trials in HIV protease inhibitors. *Expert Opin. Investig. Drugs* 9:917–28

59. Lavalle C, Aguilar JC, Pena F, et al. 2000. Reduction in hospitalization costs, morbidity, disability, and mortality in patients with AIDS treated with protease inhibitors. *Arch. Med. Res.* 31:515–19

60. Roberts NA, Martin JA, Kinchington D, et al. 1990. Rational design of peptide-based HIV proteinase inhibitors. *Science* 248:358–61

61. Graves BJ, Hatada MH, Miller JK, et al. 1991. The three-dimensional x-ray crystal structure of HIV-1 protease complexed with a hydroxyethylene inhibitor. *Adv. Exp. Med. Biol.* 306:455–60

62. Krohn A, Redshaw S, Ritchie JC, et al. 1991. Novel binding mode of highly potent HIV-proteinase inhibitors incorporating the (R)-hydroxyethylamine isostere. *J. Med. Chem.* 34:3340–42

63. Erickson J, Neidhart DJ, VanDrie J, et al. 1990. Design, activity, and 2.8 Å crystal structure of a C2 symmetric inhibitor complexed to HIV-1 protease. *Science* 249:527–33

64. Erickson JW. 1993. Design and structure of symmetry-based inhibitors of HIV-1 protease. In *Perspectives in Drug Discovery and Design*, ed. PS Anderson, GL Kenyon, GR Marshall, pp. 109–28. Leiden, The Netherlands: ESCOM Sci.

65. Kempf DJ, Marsh KC, Paul DA, et al. 1991. Antiviral and pharmacokinetic properties of C2 symmetric inhibitors of the human immunodeficiency virus type 1 protease. *Antimicrob. Agents Chemother.* 35:2209–14

66. Dreyer GB, Boehm JC, Chenera B, et al. 1993. A symmetric inhibitor binds HIV-1 protease asymmetrically. *Biochemistry* 32:937–47

67. Kempf DJ, Marsh KC, Denissen JF, et al. 1995. ABT-538 is a potent inhibitor of human immunodeficiency virus protease and has high oral bioavailability in humans. *Proc. Natl. Acad. Sci. USA* 92:2484–88

68. Kempf DJ, Marsh KC, Kumar G, et al. 1997. Pharmacokinetic enhancement of inhibitors of the human immunodeficiency virus protease by coadministration with ritonavir. *Antimicrob. Agents Chemother.* 41:654–60

69. Rich DH, Sun CQ, Vara Prasad JV, et al. 1991. Effect of hydroxyl group configuration in hydroxyethylamine dipeptide isosteres on HIV protease inhibition. Evidence for multiple binding modes. *J. Med. Chem.* 34:1222–55

70. Greenlee WJ. 1990. Renin inhibitors. *Med. Res. Rev.* 10:173–236

71. deSolms SJ, Giuliani EA, Guare JP, et al. 1991. Design and synthesis of HIV protease inhibitors. Variations of the carboxy terminus of the HIV protease inhibitor L-682,679. *J. Med. Chem.* 34:2852–57

72. Dorsey BD, Levin RB, McDaniel SL, et al. 1994. L-735,524: the design of a potent and orally bioavailable HIV protease inhibitor. *J. Med. Chem.* 37:3443–51

73. Vacca JP, Dorsey BD, Schleif WA, et al. 1994. L-735,524: an orally bioavailable human immunodeficiency virus type 1 protease inhibitor. *Proc. Natl. Acad. Sci. USA* 91:4096–100

74. Appelt K. 1993. Crystal structures of HIV-1 protease-inhibitor complexes. In *Perspectives in Drug Discovery Design*, ed. PS Anderson, GL Kenyon, GR Marshall, pp. 23–48. Leiden, The Netherlands: ESCOM Sci.

75. Varney MD, Appelt K, Kalish V, et al. 1994. Crystal-structure-based design and synthesis of novel C-terminal inhibitors of HIV protease. *J. Med. Chem.* 37:2274–84

76. Reich SH, Melnick M, Davies JF, et al. 1995. Protein structure-based design of potent orally bioavailable, nonpeptide inhibitors of human immunodeficiency virus protease. *Proc. Natl. Acad. Sci. USA* 92:3298–302

77. Gehlhaar DK, Moerder KE, Zichi D, et al. 1995. De novo design of enzyme inhibitors by Monte Carlo ligand generation. *J. Med. Chem.* 38:466–72

78. Kaldor SW, Kalish VJ, Davies JF, et al. 1997. Viracept (nelfinavir mesylate, AG1343): a potent, orally bioavailable inhibitor of HIV-1 protease. *J. Med. Chem.* 40:3979–85

79. St Clair MH, Millard J, Rooney J, et al. 1996. In vitro antiviral activity of 141W94 (VX-478) in combination with other antiretroviral agents. *Antiviral Res.* 29:53–56

80. Kim EE, Baker CT, Dwyer MD, et al. 1995. Crystal structure of HIV-1 protease in complex with VX-478, a potent and orally bioavailable inhibitor of the enzyme. *J. Am. Chem. Soc.* 117:1181–82

81. Fung HB, Kirschenbaum HL, Hameed R. 2000. Amprenavir: a new human immunodeficiency virus type 1 protease inhibitor. *Clin. Ther.* 22:549–72

82. Noble S, Goa KL. 2000. Amprenavir: a review of its clinical potential in patients with HIV infection. *Drugs* 60:1383–410

83. Sham HL, Kempf DJ, Molla A, et al. 1998. ABT-378, a highly potent inhibitor of the human immunodeficiency virus protease. *Antimicrob. Agents Chemother.* 42:3218–24

84. Wlodawer A. 1999. ABT-378 Abbott Laboratories. *Curr. Opin. Anti-infect. Investig. Drugs* 1:246–50

85. Hurst M, Faulds D. 2000. Lopinavir. *Drugs* 60:1371–79

86. Carrillo A, Stewart KD, Sham HL, et al. 1998. In vitro selection and characterization of human immunodeficiency virus type 1 variants with increased resistance to ABT-378, a novel protease inhibitor. *J. Virol.* 72:7532–41

87. Swain AL, Miller MM, Green J, et al. 1990. X-ray crystallographic structure of a complex between a synthetic protease of human immunodeficiency virus 1 and a substrate-based hydroxyethylamine inhibitor. *Proc. Natl. Acad. Sci. USA* 87:8805–9

88. Lam PY, Jadhav PK, Eyermann CJ, et al. 1994. Rational design of potent, bioavailable, nonpeptide cyclic ureas as HIV protease inhibitors. *Science* 263:380–84

89. Backbro K, Lowgren S, Osterlund K, et al. 1997. Unexpected binding mode of a cyclic sulfamide HIV-1 protease inhibitor. *J. Med. Chem.* 40:898–902

90. Jadhav PK, Ala P, Woerner FJ, et al. 1997. Cyclic urea amides: HIV-1 protease inhibitors with low nanomolar potency against both wild type and protease inhibitor resistant mutants of HIV. *J. Med. Chem.* 40:181–91

91. Hodge CN, Aldrich P, Bacheler LT, et al. 1996. Improved cyclic urea inhibitors of the HIV-1 protease: synthesis, potency, resistance profile, human pharmacokinetics and X-ray crystal structure of DMP 450. *Chem. Biol.* 3:301–14

92. Turner SR, Strohbach JW, Tommasi RA, et al. 1998. Tipranavir (PNU-140690): a potent, orally bioavailable nonpeptidic HIV protease inhibitor of the 5,6-dihydro-4-hydroxy-2-pyrone sulfonamide class. *J. Med. Chem.* 41:3467–76

93. Thaisrivongs S, Strohbach JW. 1999. Structure-based discovery of Tipranavir disodium (PNU-140690E): a potent, orally bioavailable, nonpeptidic HIV protease inhibitor. *Biopolymers* 51:51–58

94. Rusconi S, La Seta CS, Citterio P, et al. 2000. Susceptibility to PNU-140690 (Tipranavir) of human immunodeficiency virus type 1 isolates derived from patients with multidrug resistance to other protease inhibitors. *Antimicrob. Agents Chemother.* 44:1328–32

95. Robinson BS, Riccardi KA, Gong YF, et al. 2000. BMS-232632, a highly potent human immunodeficiency virus protease inhibitor that can be used in combination with other available antiretroviral agents. *Antimicrob. Agents Chemother.* 44:2093–99

96. Jager J, Smerdon SJ, Wang J, et al. 1994. Comparison of three different crystal forms shows HIV-1 reverse transcriptase displays an internal swivel motion. *Structure* 2:869–76

97. Huang H, Chopra R, Verdine GL, Harrison SC. 1998. Structure of a covalently trapped catalytic complex of HIV-1 reverse transcriptase: implications for drug resistance. *Science* 282:1669–75

98. Volberding PA, Lagakos SW, Koch MA, et al. 1990. Zidovudine in asymptomatic human immunodeficiency virus infection. A controlled trial in persons with fewer than 500 CD4-positive cells per cubic millimeter. *N. Engl. J. Med.* 322:941–49

99. Spruance SL, Pavia AT, Mellors JW, et al. 1997. Clinical efficacy of monotherapy with stavudine compared with zidovudine in HIV-infected, zidovudine-experienced patients. A randomized, double-blind, controlled trial. *Ann. Intern. Med.* 126:355–63

100. Baba M, Tanaka H, De Clercq E, et al. 1989. Highly specific inhibition of human immunodeficiency virus type 1 by a novel 6-substituted acyclouridine derivative. *Biochem. Biophys. Res. Commun.* 165:1375–81

101. Pauwels R, Andries K, Desmyter J, et al. 1990. Potent and selective inhibition of HIV-1 replication in vitro by a novel series of TIBO derivatives. *Nature* 343:470–74

102. Merluzzi VJ, Hargrave KD, Labadia M,

et al. 1990. Inhibition of HIV-1 replication by a nonnucleoside reverse transcriptase inhibitor. *Science* 250:1411–13; Erratum. 1991. *Science* 251:362

103. De Clercq E. 1998. The role of non-nucleoside reverse transcriptase inhibitors (NNRTIs) in the therapy of HIV-1 infection. *Antiviral Res.* 38:153–79

104. Schinazi RF, Larder BA, Mellors JW. 1997. Mutations in retroviral genes associated with drug resistance. *Int. Antiviral News* 5:129–42

105. Peiperl L. 2001. HIV InSite knowledge base. Overview of antiretroviral drugs. http://hivinsite.ucsf.edu/InSite.jsp?page = ar-drugs

106. Condra JH, Schleif WA, Blahy OM, et al. 1995. In vivo emergence of HIV-1 variants resistant to multiple protease inhibitors. *Nature* 374:569–71

Annu. Rev. Med. 2002. 53:615–27

MECHANISMS OF CANCER DRUG RESISTANCE

Michael M. Gottesman

Laboratory of Cell Biology, National Cancer Institute, National Institutes of Health, 37 Convent Drive, Bethesda, Maryland 20892-4255; e-mail: mgottesman@nih.gov

Key Words   cancer, multidrug resistance, ABC transporters, drug transport, chemotherapy

■ **Abstract**   The design of cancer chemotherapy has become increasingly sophisticated, yet there is no cancer treatment that is 100% effective against disseminated cancer. Resistance to treatment with anticancer drugs results from a variety of factors including individual variations in patients and somatic cell genetic differences in tumors, even those from the same tissue of origin. Frequently resistance is intrinsic to the cancer, but as therapy becomes more and more effective, acquired resistance has also become common. The most common reason for acquisition of resistance to a broad range of anticancer drugs is expression of one or more energy-dependent transporters that detect and eject anticancer drugs from cells, but other mechanisms of resistance including insensitivity to drug-induced apoptosis and induction of drug-detoxifying mechanisms probably play an important role in acquired anticancer drug resistance. Studies on mechanisms of cancer drug resistance have yielded important information about how to circumvent this resistance to improve cancer chemotherapy and have implications for pharmacokinetics of many commonly used drugs.

INTRODUCTION

The treatment of disseminated cancer has become increasingly aimed at molecular targets derived from studies of the oncogenes and tumor suppressors known to be involved in the development of human cancers (1). This increase in specificity of cancer treatment, from the use of general cytotoxic agents such as nitrogen mustard in the 1940s, to the development of natural-product anticancer drugs in the 1960s such as *Vinca* alkaloids and anthracyclines, which are more cytotoxic to cancer cells than normal cells, to the use of specific monoclonal antibodies (2) and immunotoxins (3) targeted to cell surface receptors and specific agents that inactivate kinases in growth-promoting pathways (4), has improved the response rate in cancer and reduced side effects of anticancer treatment but has not yet resulted in cure of the majority of patients with metastatic disease. A study of the mechanisms by which cancers elude treatment has yielded a wealth of information about why these therapies fail and is beginning to yield valuable information about how to circumvent drug resistance in cancer cells and/or design agents that are not subject to the usual means of resistance.

0066-4219/02/0218-0615$14.00   **615**

HOW DO CANCER CELLS ELUDE CHEMOTHERAPY?

Failure of a patient's cancer to respond to a specific therapy can result from one of two general causes: host factors and specific genetic or epigenetic alterations in the cancer cells. Host factors include poor absorption or rapid metabolism or excretion of a drug, resulting in low serum levels; poor tolerance to effects of a drug, especially in elderly patients, resulting in a need to reduce doses below optimal levels; inability to deliver a drug to the site of a tumor, as could occur with bulky tumors or with biological agents of high molecular weight and low tissue penetration such as monoclonal antibodies and immunotoxins (5); and various alterations in the host-tumor environment that affect response of the tumor including local metabolism of a drug by nontumor cells, unusual features of the tumor blood supply that may affect transit time of drugs within tumors and the way in which cells in a cancer interact with each other and with interstitial cells from the host (6).

To paraphrase Tolstoy in the opening lines of *Anna Karenina*, normal cells are all alike in their response to drugs, but cancer cells each respond in their own way. Each cancer cell from a given patient has a different genetic make-up depending not only on the tissue of origin but also on the pattern of activation of oncogenes and inactivation of tumor suppressors as well as random variations in gene expression resulting from the "mutator" phenotype of most cancers. As a result, every cancer expresses a different array of drug-resistance genes, and cells within a cancer, even though clonally derived, exhibit an enormous amount of heterogeneity with respect to drug resistance. In addition, even if tumors are not intrinsically resistant to a specific anticancer treatment, this genetic and epigenetic heterogeneity in the face of the powerful selection imposed by potent anticancer drugs results in overgrowth of drug-resistant variants and the rapid acquisition of drug resistance by many cancers.

For the past 40 years, researchers have been tabulating the various mechanisms by which cancer cells grown in tissue culture become resistant to anticancer drugs (Figure 1). Some of these mechanisms, such as loss of a cell surface receptor or transporter for a drug, specific metabolism of a drug, or alteration by mutation of the specific target of a drug, all of which occur for antifolates such as methotrexate (7), result in resistance to only a small number of related drugs. In such cases, use of multiple drugs with different mechanisms of entry into cells and different cellular targets allows for effective chemotherapy and high cure rates. All too often, however, cells express mechanisms of resistance that confer simultaneous resistance to many different structurally and functionally unrelated drugs. This phenomenon, known as multidrug resistance (8), can result from changes that limit accumulation of drugs within cells by limiting uptake, enhancing efflux, or affecting membrane lipids such as ceramide (9). These changes block (*a*) the programmed cell death (apoptosis) that is activated by most anticancer drugs (10), (*b*) activation of general response mechanisms that detoxify drugs and repair damage to DNA (11), and (*c*) alterations in the cell cycle and checkpoints that render cells relatively

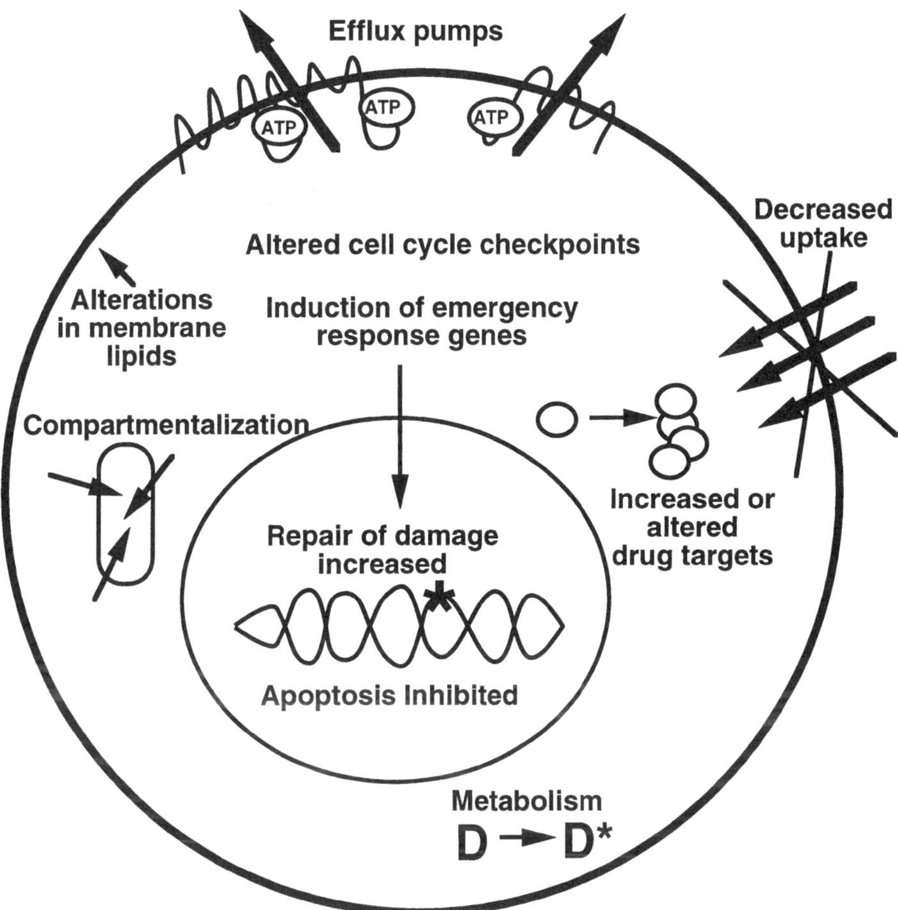

Figure 1 This cartoon summarizes many of the ways in which cultured cancer cells have been shown to become resistant to cytotoxic anticancer drugs. The efflux pumps shown schematically at the plasma membrane include MDR1, MRP family members, and MXR (ABC G2), which is presumed to function as a dimer.

resistant to the cytotoxic effects of drugs on cancer cells. Expression of a major vault protein, termed lung resistance-related protein (LRP), which may regulate nuclear entry of drugs, has also been described in multidrug resistance (11a).

Among these mechanisms, we know the most about those that alter accumulation of drugs within cells (for reviews, see 12, 13). This accumulation results from a balance between drug entry and exit mechanisms. Drugs enter cells in various ways (Figure 2). Each of these mechanisms of entry has been determined to have physiological significance based on detailed uptake studies and on the existence of resistant mutants in which defects in these pathways have been observed.

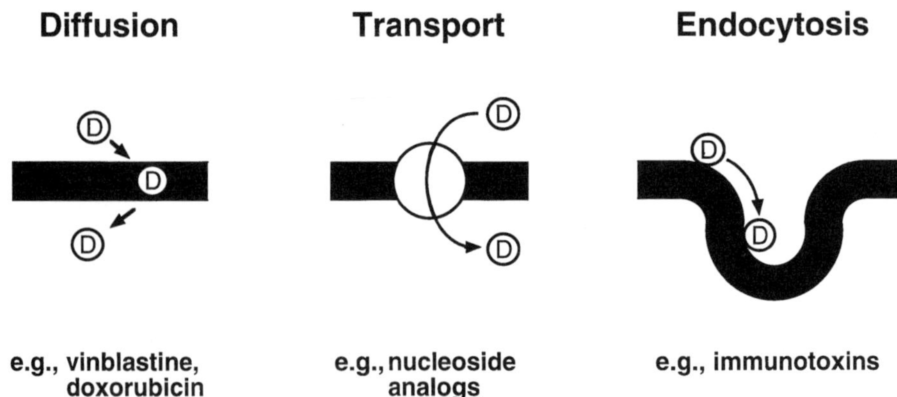

Figure 2   Ways in which drugs can get into cells. Examples are given for the three major routes: diffusion across the plasma membrane, piggy-backing onto a receptor or transporter, and endocytosis.

The remainder of this review focuses on the mechanisms of multidrug resistance resulting from alterations in the pathways of drug uptake or efflux from the cell.

MECHANISMS OF DRUG RESISTANCE THAT INCREASE DRUG EFFLUX FROM CANCER CELLS

It came as something of a surprise that the major mechanism of multidrug resistance in cultured cancer cells was the expression of an energy-dependent drug efflux pump, known alternatively as P-glycoprotein (P-gp) or the multidrug transporter (14, 15). This efflux pump, the product of the *MDR*1 gene in the human (16) and the product of two different related genes, *mdr*1a and *mdr*1b in the mouse (17, 18), was one of the first members described of a large family of ATP-dependent transporters known as the ATP-binding cassette (ABC) family (19). Every living organism has encoded within its genome many members of this family, and they appear to be involved not only in efflux of drugs but in moving nutrients and other biologically important molecules into, out of, and across plasma membranes and intracellular membranes in cells. P-gp is widely expressed in many human cancers, including cancers of the gastrointestinal (GI) tract (small and large intestine, liver cancer, and pancreatic cancer), cancers of the hematopoietic system (myeloma, lymphoma, leukemia), cancers of the genitourinary system (kidney, ovary, testicle), and childhood cancers (neuroblastoma, fibrosarcoma) (20). The human gene most closely related to *MDR*1 is *MDR*2, a phosphatidylcholine transporter expressed in liver whose defect results in inability to form bile and progressive cirrhosis (21).

P-gp, the human *MDR*1 gene product and one of 48 known ABC transporters in the human, is a 170,000-dalton–molecular weight phosphoglycoprotein

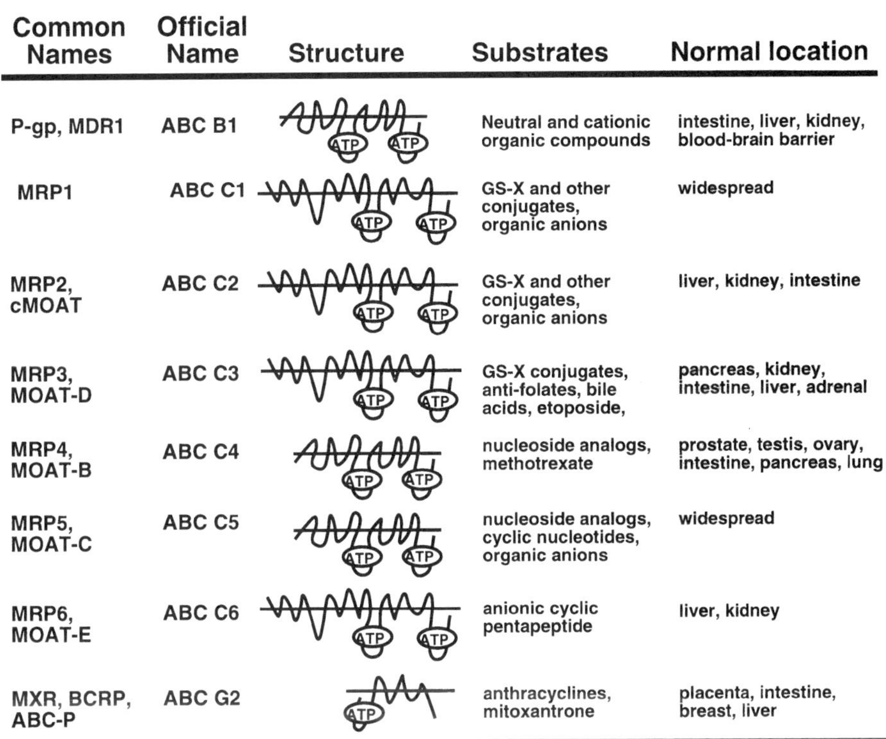

Common Names	Official Name	Structure	Substrates	Normal location
P-gp, MDR1	ABC B1		Neutral and cationic organic compounds	intestine, liver, kidney, blood-brain barrier
MRP1	ABC C1		GS-X and other conjugates, organic anions	widespread
MRP2, cMOAT	ABC C2		GS-X and other conjugates, organic anions	liver, kidney, intestine
MRP3, MOAT-D	ABC C3		GS-X conjugates, anti-folates, bile acids, etoposide,	pancreas, kidney, intestine, liver, adrenal
MRP4, MOAT-B	ABC C4		nucleoside analogs, methotrexate	prostate, testis, ovary, intestine, pancreas, lung
MRP5, MOAT-C	ABC C5		nucleoside analogs, cyclic nucleotides, organic anions	widespread
MRP6, MOAT-E	ABC C6		anionic cyclic pentapeptide	liver, kidney
MXR, BCRP, ABC-P	ABC G2		anthracyclines, mitoxantrone	placenta, intestine, breast, liver

Figure 3   ABC transporters with known drug substrates. Curved lines represent transmembrane domains, and the ATP in the ovals represents the ATP-binding cassettes in these ABC transporters. GS-X represents glutathione conjugates of drugs.

consisting of two ATP binding cassettes and two transmembrane regions, each of which contains six transmembrane domains (16) (Figure 3). P-gp can detect and bind a large variety of hydrophobic natural-product drugs as they enter the plasma membrane. These drugs include many of the commonly used natural-product anticancer drugs such as doxorubicin and daunorubicin, vinblastine and vincristine, and taxol, as well as many commonly used pharmaceuticals ranging from antiarrhythmics and antihistamines to cholesterol-lowering statins (22) and HIV protease inhibitors (23). Binding of these drugs results in activation of one of the ATP-binding domains, and the hydrolysis of ATP causes a major change in the shape of P-gp, which results in release of the drug into the extracellular space (24). Hydrolysis of a second molecule of ATP is needed to restore the transporter to its original state so that it can repeat the cycle of drug binding and release (25, 26). Although the detailed mechanism of action of other ABC transporters is not known, it is presumed that the ATP binding cassette acts as the engine for the transport mediated by members of this large family of transporters.

Because of the promiscuity with which P-gp binds electrically neutral and positively charged hydrophobic drugs within the plasma membrane, many different anticancer drugs and other drugs in common use are substrates for this transport system. Any drug that interacts with the substrate-binding region of P-gp is likely to be a competitive inhibitor of the binding of other drugs. Because of the large size and complex structure of P-gp drug-binding region(s), not all inhibitors have equal potency against all substrates. Active development of potent, specific inhibitors of P-gp is underway as a means to reverse multidrug resistance in cancers, and some have shown activity in sensitizing drug-resistant cancers in patients (see below).

After the discovery of P-gp and the demonstration of its widespread expression in many human cancers, it was found that many multidrug-resistant cancers, such as lung cancers, rarely express P-gp. Using a multidrug-resistant lung cancer cell line as a model system, Deeley and Cole and colleagues cloned another ABC family member, known as *MRP*1 (for multidrug resistance associated protein 1) and showed that it had a broad spectrum of anticancer drug transport activity (27) (Figure 3). MRP1, unlike MDR1, transports negatively charged natural-product drugs and drugs that have been modified by glutathione, conjugation, glucosylation, sulfation, and glucuronylation. In some cases cotransport of glutathione with positively charged drugs such as vinblastine can occur. MRP1 is also widely expressed in many human tissues and cancers (12).

The discovery of MRP1 led to a search for other members of this family, resulting in the discovery of a total of 9 or 10 MRP genes, at least 6 of which have been characterized enough to indicate that they transport anticancer and antiviral compounds (12, 28–32) (Figure 3). Many of these appear to transport drugs potentially important for the treatment of cancer, and their role in conferring drug resistance on cancer cells is under active investigation.

A third ABC transporter for anticancer drugs has been called MXR, BCRP, or ABC-P (33–35) (Figure 3). It was found to be overexpressed in cells selected for resistance to mitoxantrone or anthracyclines. Unlike MDR1 and the MRP family members, it only has one region with six transmembrane domains and a single ATP-binding cassette (see Figure 1) but is presumed to function as a dimer. Recent evidence suggests that the wild-type form of MXR shows a narrower range of substrates for drug transport than a mutant form of the protein in which the amino acid threonine or glycine is substituted for arginine at position 482, which was isolated in the early studies (36). The role of MXR in clinical drug resistance remains to be determined.

Three additional ABC transporters have been implicated in drug transport of potential significance to cancer, including the *MDR*2 gene product (37), a protein named SPGP (sister of P-gp) (38), and ABC A2 (39), but these data are too preliminary to include in our figure. It is also possible that other members of the ABC transporter family in addition to the MDR, MRP, and MXR family members are involved in clinical cancer drug resistance or in drug transport in the human. Based on the known DNA sequences of these genes, efforts to explore their patterns of expression and determine their function are under way. One approach is to examine intrinsically resistant cancers and those that have acquired resistance to anticancer drugs and determine whether expression of other ABC transporters occurs commonly.

DRUG RESISTANCE DUE TO REDUCED UPTAKE OF DRUGS

As illustrated in Figure 2, specific and nonspecific uptake of water-soluble drugs can occur across the plasma membrane based on piggy-backing of these drugs on known transporters involved in uptake of nutrients and other essential low molecular weight molecules and by the process of endocytosis, either receptor-mediated or nonspecific. The latter process has been termed pinocytosis and refers to the general means by which cells "drink" extracellular fluids and internalize the variety of compounds that may be dissolved in the extracellular fluid.

Selection of cells for resistance to drugs that enter cells via receptors or transporters can result in mutations that eliminate or modify these cell surface molecules. For example, resistance to toxic folate analogs such as methotrexate commonly occurs by mutation of one or both of the folate transporters (folate binding protein, and/or the reduced folate transporter) (7). Resistance to nucleoside analogs has been described as a result of mutation of specific nucleoside transporters, etc. In general, these mechanisms of resistance are specific for these nutrient analogs and structurally related compounds.

Very few drugs enter cells by endocytosis. However, some of the newer anticancer agents, such as immunotoxins that bind to cell surface receptors, cannot kill cells unless they are internalized (3). They are generally internalized via receptor-mediated endocytosis. Cancer cell mutants that have defective endocytosis are resistant to both toxins and immunotoxins (40).

Cisplatin is commonly used to treat cancers such as head and neck cancer, testicular cancer, ovarian cancer, and other solid tumors. It is not known with certainty how cisplatin, a water-soluble compound, enters cells (41). Many different cisplatin-resistant cancer cell lines have been isolated in the laboratory. These exhibit a variety of mechanisms of resistance, but reduced accumulation of the drug is commonly seen, as is cross-resistance to methotrexate, heavy metals such as arsenite and arsenate, cadmium and mercury, and resistance to some nucleoside analogs. We have recently shown that cisplatin-resistant cells demonstrating this pattern of cross-resistance and reduced accumulation of the drug have a pleiotropic defect resulting in reduced plasma membrane receptors and transporters and reduced endocytosis (42). In these cells there is no evidence for an energy-dependent efflux pump for cisplatin (43), which has been described by other researchers in different cell lines. These results suggest that cisplatin may enter cells via receptors and/or via endocytosis. Whether clinical resistance to cisplatin by this mechanism also occurs, with attendant cross-resistance to methotrexate and nucleoside analogs, remains to be determined.

CLINICAL RELEVANCE OF LABORATORY STUDIES ON CANCER DRUG RESISTANCE

As noted, it is possible to demonstrate the presence of several different drug efflux pumps in human cancers. Evidence that ABC transporters, especially P-gp, play a significant role in clinical drug resistance has been reviewed extensively and can be summarized as follows: (*a*) Levels of expression of P-gp in many different tumors are high enough to confer significant drug resistance, and the presence of P-gp correlates with drug resistance in several different cancers (20); (*b*) acquisition of drug resistance after chemotherapy is associated with increased P-gp levels (20), and this increased expression occurs via specific molecular mechanisms, such as gene rearrangement and selection of cells showing these rearrangements (44), which argues that the P-gp-expressing cells have a selective advantage; (*c*) acute induction of P-gp has been observed in human tumors following exposure in vivo to doxorubicin (45); (*d*) in early clinical trials testing P-gp modulation in acute leukemia, cells that survived chemotherapy in the presence of modulators, resulting in clinical relapse, had reduced expression of P-gp (46, 47); and (*e*) expression of P-gp in some tumors predicts poor response to chemotherapy with drugs that are transported by P-gp (48).

This evidence has been used to support the introduction of various P-gp inhibitors into the clinic, and many studies using such inhibitors have been reported, with more in progress. The first studies were performed with modulators approved for clinical uses other than inhibition of P-gp. Subsequent studies were performed with "second generation" modulators, compounds with somewhat increased potency but still limited by toxicity. Recently, a new generation of inhibitors has reached clinical testing. These "third generation" inhibitors promise to be nontoxic, more specific, and more potent than the earlier inhibitors used in trials of P-gp modulation. These compounds include XR9576, R101933, Biricodar (VX710), and LY335979.

In studies reported to date, with first generation modulators and with dexverapamil, dexniguldipine, and the cyclosporin D analogue Valspodar (PSC833), there have been no dramatic changes in response rates in a variety of human tumors (49). Cancers such as acute myelocytic leukemia and myeloma, which commonly express P-gp at a low level at presentation and with increasing frequency following chemotherapy, may give higher response rates when a P-gp inhibitor is included in the chemotherapy regimen (49a). Solid tumors, such as renal cell cancer and colon cancer, do not respond significantly despite relatively high levels of expression of P-gp, suggesting that other mechanisms of drug resistance also contribute to the resistance of these solid tumors to many forms of chemotherapy (20). Recent knowledge about other ABC transporters such as MRP transporters and MXR that might contribute to drug resistance has caused clinicians to reconsider what the best inhibitors might be: a nonspecific inhibitor of ABC transporters that might have the broadest spectrum, but a higher likelihood of side effects, or a cocktail of specific inhibitors designed for each individual tumor. Also, there is a strong need to be able to "image" activity of drug transporters in vivo using imaging agents, such as ^{99}mTc-sestamibi, which are substrates for ABC transporters such as P-glycoprotein (50).

One consequence of enumerating the various transporters that handle anticancer drugs was the discovery that these transporters are also involved in pharmacokinetics of many different drugs in common clinical use. For example, P-gp is normally expressed at high levels in the mucosa of the GI tract, in biliary epithelial cells of the liver, in proximal tubule cells of the kidney, in the adrenal cortex, in capillary endothelial cells of the brain, testes and ovary, and in the placenta. These locations argue for a role of P-gp in excretion of drugs from intestine, liver, and kidney into stool, bile and urine; in blocking absorption of drugs from the GI tract; and as a barrier to transport into brain, testes, ovary, and the fetus (23).

The generation of a mouse lacking *mdr*1a and *mdr*1b by insertional mutagenesis demonstrated that loss of P-gp was not lethal to the animals, but they were very susceptible to toxic effects of many different drugs because of increased absorption and neurotoxicity (51). Studies with mice deficient in mdr1a/mdr1b and mrp1 and cell lines derived from these triple knockout [*mdr*1a/1b(−/−), *mrp*1(−/−)] mice indicate that P-gp and MRP1 transporters contribute significantly to the development of resistance to paclitaxel (taxol), anthracyclines, and *Vinca* alkaloids (52). In addition, exposure of these triple knockout mice to therapeutic doses of vincristine resulted in severe damage to bone marrow and gastrointestinal mucosa, indicating that both P-gp and MRP1 are compensatory transporters for *Vinca* alkaloids in these tissues (53). These results suggest that P-gp and MRP1 are important determinants of the pharmacokinetics of many different drugs, and further, that inhibitors of P-gp and possibly MRP1 can be used to enhance uptake of these drugs that are given orally and perhaps to influence their penetration into the central nervous system. Evidence that P-gp serves a normal role in the physiological transport of opioid compounds out of the central nervous system into the bloodstream has also recently been reported (54). Recent data also suggest that a noncoding polymorphism in the P-gp gene is closely linked to levels of expression of P-gp in the GI tract, which results in alterations in absorption of commonly used drugs such as digoxin (55). It is assumed that pharmacogenomic analysis of other ABC transporters, such as the MRP family, will reveal similarly important roles in handling many different drugs.

The knowledge that expression of a drug-resistance gene, such as *MDR*1, can result in clinically significant drug resistance, has led to the idea that drug-resistance genes can be used as selectable markers in gene therapy (56). One of the barriers to successful gene therapy is the inefficiency of transfer of therapeutic genes into target cells. Use of cancer drug–resistance genes as linked markers to allow selection of cells to which therapeutic genes have been transferred has been suggested as a means to improve efficiency of gene therapy. Many different vectors have been developed using *MDR*1 and other drug-resistance genes for gene therapy (57). Clinically, attempts have been made to introduce P-gp into bone marrow cells to protect them from the cytotoxic effects of anticancer drugs. In the mouse this works reasonably well because efficiency of transfer of genes into mouse bone marrow stem cells is relatively high (58). In the human transfer efficiencies are low. Whereas expression of P-gp might have a small selective advantage after taxol treatment of patients undergoing bone marrow transplants in association with breast cancer treatment, the effect is not dramatic or therapeutic (59). In addition, some studies in the mouse suggest that high levels of P-gp in hematopoietic cells may be associated under some circumstances with a myeloproliferative disorder, and more data are needed before additional clinical trials can be attempted (60).

CONCLUSIONS

A great deal is now known about mechanisms of drug resistance in cancer cells. Despite the development of new targeted anticancer therapies, mechanisms that have evolved in mammals to protect cells against cytotoxic compounds in the environment will continue to act as obstacles to successful treatment of cancer. Additional knowledge about these mechanisms of cancer drug resistance may help to design strategies to circumvent resistance and new drugs that are less susceptible to known resistance mechanisms. Some of the knowledge about drug resistance has revealed new mechanisms relevant to normal handling of drugs by the body, and this information will be important in improving drug delivery and distribution in patients.

ACKNOWLEDGMENTS

I am grateful to my many coworkers and colleagues, especially Ira Pastan, who have contributed over the years to the ideas presented in the review, to Susan Bates and Suresh V. Ambudkar for critical reading and comments on the text, and to Gregar D. Odegaarden and Joyce L. Sharrar for help in preparation of the manuscript.

Visit the Annual Reviews home page at www.AnnualReviews.org

LITERATURE CITED

1. Barinaga M. 1997. From bench top to bedside. *Science* 278:1036–39
2. Nabholtz JM, Slamon D. 2001. New adjuvant strategies for breast cancer: meeting the challenge of integrating chemotherapy and trastuzumab (Herceptin). *Semin. Oncol.* 28 (Suppl 3):1–12
3. Pastan I, Kreitman RJ. 1998. Immunotoxins for targeted cancer therapy. *Adv. Drug Deliv. Rev.* 31:53–88
4. Druker BJ, Sawyers CL, Kantarjian H, et al. 2001. Activity of a specific inhibitor of the BCR-ABL tyrosine kinase in the blast crisis of chronic myeloid leukemia and acute lymphoblastic leukemia with the Philadelphia chromosome. *N. Engl. J. Med.* 344:1038–42
5. Pluen A, Boucher Y, Ramanujan S, et al. 2001. Role of tumor-host interactions in interstitial diffusion of macromolecules:

cranial vs. subcutaneous tumors. *Proc. Natl. Acad. Sci. USA* 98:4628–33

6. Green SK, Frankel A, Kerbel RS. 1999. Adhesion-dependent multicellular drug resistance. *Anticancer-Drug Designs* 14: 153–68

7. Longo-Sorbello GS, Bertino JR. 2001. Current understanding of methotrexate pharmacology and efficacy in acute leukemias. Use of newer antifolates in clinical trials. *Haematologica* 86:121–27

8. Gottesman MM, Ambudkar SV, Ni B, et al. 1994. Exploiting multidrug resistance to treat cancer. *Cold Spring Harbor Symp. Quant. Biol.* 59:677–83

9. Liu YY, Han TY, Giuliano AE, et al. 2001. Ceramide glycosylation potentiates cellular multidrug resistance. *FASEB J.* 15: 719–30

10. Lowe SW, Ruley HE, Jacks T, et al. 1993. p53-dependent apoptosis modulates the cytotoxicity of anticancer agents. *Cell* 74: 957–67

11. Synold TW, Dussault I, Forman BM. 2001. The orphan nuclear receptor SXR coordinately regulates drug metabolism and efflux. *Nat. Med.* 7: 584–90

11a. Dalton WS, Scheper RJ. 1999. Lung resistance-related protein: determining its role in multidrug resistance. *J. Natl. Cancer Inst.* 91:1604–5

12. Borst P, Evers R, Kool M, et al. 2000. A family of drug transporters: the multidrug resistance-associated proteins. *J. Natl. Cancer Inst.* 92:1295–301

13. Ambudkar SV, Dey S, Hrycyna CA, et al. 1999. Biochemical, cellular and pharmacological aspects of the multidrug transporter. *Annu. Rev. Pharmacol. Toxicol.* 39:361–98

14. Juliano RL, Ling V. 1976. A surface glycoprotein modulating drug permeability in Chinese hamster ovary cell mutants. *Biochim. Biophys. Acta* 455:152–62

15. Ueda K, Cardarelli C, Gottesman MM, et al. 1987. Expression of a full-length cDNA for the human MDR1 gene confers resistance to colchicine, doxorubicin, and vinblastine. *Proc. Natl. Acad. Sci. USA* 84:3004–8

16. Chen C-J, Chin JE, Ueda K, et al. 1986. Internal duplication and homology with bacterial transport proteins in the *mdr*1 (P-glycoprotein) gene from multidrug-resistant human cells. *Cell* 47:381–89

17. Croop JM, Raymond M, Haber D, et al. 1989. The three mouse multidrug resistance (*mdr*) genes are expressed in a tissue-specific manner in normal mouse tissues. *Mol. Cell. Biol.* 9:1346–50

18. Lothstein L, Hsu SI, Horwitz SB, et al. 1989. Alternate overexpression of two P-glycoprotein genes is associated with changes in multidrug resistance in a J774.2 cell line. *J. Biol. Chem.* 264: 16054–58

19. Higgins CF. 1992. ABC transporters: from microorganisms to man. *Annu. Rev. Cell Biol.* 8:67–13

20. Goldstein LJ, Galski H, Fojo A, et al. 1989. Expression of a multidrug resistance gene in human cancers. *J. Natl. Cancer Inst.* 81:116–24

21. De Vree JML, Jacquemin E, Sturm E, et al. 1998. Mutations in the *MDR3* gene cause progressive familial intrahepatic cholestasis. *Proc. Natl. Acad. Sci. USA* 95: 282–87

22. Bogman K, Peyer AK, Torok M, et al. 2001. HMG-CoA reductase inhibitors and P-glycoprotein modulation. *Br. J. Pharmacol.* 132:1183–92

23. Lee CGL, Gottesman MM. 1998. HIV-1 protease inhibitors and the *MDR*1 multidrug transporter. *J. Clin. Invest.* 101:287–88

24. Ramachandra M, Ambudkar SV, Chen D, et al. 1998. Human P-glycoprotein exhibits reduced affinity for substrates during a catalytic transition state. *Biochemistry* 37:5010–19

25. Sauna ZE, Ambudkar SV. 2000. Evidence for a requirement for ATP hydrolysis at two distinct steps during a single turnover of the catalytic cycle of human

P-glycoprotein. *Proc. Natl. Acad. Sci. USA* 97:2515–20

26. Sauna ZE, Ambudkar SV. 2001. Characterization of the catalytic cycle of ATP hydrolysis by human P-glycoprotein. *J. Biol. Chem.* 276:11653–61

27. Cole SP, Bhardwaj G, Gerlach JH, et al. 1992. Overexpression of a transporter gene in a multidrug-resistant human lung cancer cell line. *Science* 258:1650–54

28. Belinsky MG, Bain LJ, Balsara BB, et al. 1998. Characterization of MOAT-C and MOAT-D new members of the MRP/cMOAT subfamily of transporter proteins. *J. Natl. Cancer Inst.* 90:1735–41

29. Loe DW, Deeley RG, Cole SPC. 1998. Characterization of vincristine transport by the M_r 190,000 multidrug resistance protein (MRP): evidence for cotransport with reduced glutathione. *Cancer Res.* 58:5130–36

30. Borst P, Evers R, Kool M, et al. 1999. The multidrug resistance protein family. *Biochim. Biophys. Acta* 1461:347–57

31. Kool M, Van Der Linden M, de Haas M, et al. MRP3, an organic anion transporter able to transport anti-cancer drugs. *Proc. Natl. Acad. Sci. USA* 96:6914–19

32. Wijnholds J, Mol CAAM, van Deemter L, et al. Multidrug-resistance protein 5 is a multispecific organic anion transporter able to transport nucleotide analogs. *Proc. Natl. Acad. Sci. USA* 97:7476–81

33. Doyle LA, Yang W, Abruzzo LV, et al. 1998. A multidrug resistance transporter from human MCF-7 breast cancer cells. *Proc. Natl. Acad. Sci. USA* 95:15665–70

34. Allikmets R, Schriml LM, Hutchinson A, et al. 1998. A human placenta-specific ATP-binding cassette gene (ABCP) on chromosome 4q22 that is involved in multidrug resistance. *Cancer Res.* 58:5337–39

35. Miyake K, Mickley L, Litman T, et al. 1999. Molecular cloning of cDNAs which is highly overexpressed in mitoxantrone-resistant cells: demonstration of homology to ABC transport genes. *Cancer Res.* 59:8–13

36. Komatani H, Kotani H, Hara Y, et al. 2001. Identification of breast cancer resistant protein/mitoxantrone resistance protein/placenta-specific, ATP-binding cassette transporter as a transporter of NB-506 and J-107088, topoisomerase I inhibitors with an indolocarbazole structure. *Cancer Res.* 61:2827–32

37. Borst P, Zelcer N, van Helvoort A. 2000. ABC transporters in lipid transport. *Biochim. Biophys. Acta* 1486:128–44

38. Childs S, Yeh RL, Hui D, et al. 1998. Taxol resistance mediated by transfection of the liver-specific sister gene of P-glycoprotein. *Cancer Res.* 58:4160–67

39. Laing NM, Belinsky MG, Kruh GD, et al. 1998. Amplification of the ATP-binding cassette 2 transporter gene is functionally linked with enhanced efflux of estramustine in ovarian carcinoma cells. *Cancer Res.* 58:1332–37

40. Lyall RM, Hwang J, Cardarelli C, et al. 1987. *Cancer Res.* 47:2961–66

41. Gately DP, Howell SB. 1993. Cellular accumulation of the anticancer agent cisplatin: a review. *Br. J. Cancer* 67:1171–76

42. Shen D-W, Pastan I, Gottesman MM. 1998. Cross-resistance to methotrexate and metals in human cisplatin-resistant cell lines results from a pleiotropic defect in accumulation of these compounds associated with reduced plasma membrane binding proteins. *Cancer Res.* 58:268–75

43. Shen D-W, Goldenberg S, Pastan I, et al. 2000. Decreased accumulation of [14C]-carboplatin in human cisplatin-resistant cells results from reduced energy-dependent uptake. *J. Cell. Physiol.* 183:108–16

44. Mickley LA, Lee J, Weng Z, et al. 1998. Genetic polymorphism in *MDR*1: a tool for examining allelic expression in normal cells, unselected and drug-selected cell lines, and human tumors. *Blood* 91:1749–56

45. Abolhoda A, Wilson AE, Ross H, et al. 1999. Rapid activation of *MDR*1 gene

expression in human metastatic sarcoma after *in vivo* exposure to doxorubicin. *Clin. Cancer Res.* 5:3352–56

46. List AF, Spier C, Greer J, et al. 1993. Phase I/II trial of cyclosporine as a chemotherapy-resistance modifier in acute leukemia. *J. Clin. Oncol.* 11:1652–60

47. Marie J-P, Bastie J-N, Coloma F, et al. 1993. Cyclosporine A as a modifier agent in the salvage treatment of acute leukemia (AL). *Leukemia* 7:821–24

48. Chan HS, Haddad G, Thorner PS, et al. 1991. P-glycoprotein expression as a predictor of the outcome of therapy for neuroblastoma. *N. Engl. J. Med.* 325:1608–14

49. Bradshaw DM, Arceci R. 1998. Clinical relevance of transmembrane drug efflux as a mechanism of multidrug resistance. *J. Clin. Oncol.* 16:3674–90

49a. Advani R, Saba HI, Tallman MS, et al. 1999. Treatment of refractory and relapsed acute myelogenous leukemia with combination chemotherapy plus the multidrug resistance modulator PSC833 (Valspodar). *Blood* 93:787–95

50. Crankshaw CL, Marmion M, Luker GD, et al. 1998. Novel technetium (III)-Q complexes for functional imaging of multidrug resistance (MDR1) P-glycoprotein. *J. Nucl. Med.* 39:77–86

51. Schinkel AH, Mayer U, Wagenaar E, et al. 1997. Normal viability and altered pharmacokinetics in mice lacking mdr1-type (drug-transporting) P-glycoproteins. *Proc. Natl. Acad. Sci. USA* 94:4028–33

52. Allen JD, Brinkhuis RF, van Deemter L, et al. 2000. Extensive contribution of the multidrug transporter P-glycoprotein and mrp1 to basal drug resistance. *Cancer Res.* 60:5761–66

53. Johnson DR, Finch R, Lin P, et al. 2001. The pharmacological phenotype of combined multidrug-resistance mdr1a/1b- and mrp1-deficient mice. *Cancer Res.* 61:1469–76

54. King M, Su W, Chang A, et al. 2001. Transport of opioids from the brain to the periphery by P-glycoprotein: peripheral actions of central drugs. *Nat. Neurosci.* 4:221–22

55. Hoffmeyer S, Burk O, von Richter O, et al. 2000. Functional polymorphisms of the human multidrug-resistance gene: multiple sequence variations and correlation of one allele with P-glycoprotein expression and activity *in vivo*. *Proc. Natl. Acad. Sci. USA* 97:3473–78

56. Gottesman MM, Hrycyna CA, Schoenlein PV, 1995. Genetic analysis of the multidrug transporter. *Annu. Rev. Genet.* 29:607–49

57. Gottesman MM, Licht T, Zhou Y, et al. 2000. Selectable markers for gene therapy. In *Gene Therapy: Therapeutic Mechanisms and Strategies*, ed. D Lasic, N Templeton, 16:333–52. New York: Marcel Dekker

58. Sorrentino BP, Brandt SJ, Bodine D, et al. 1992. Retroviral transfer of the human *MDR*1 gene permits selection of drug resistant bone marrow cells *in vivo*. *Science* 257:99–103

59. Moscow JA, Huang H, Carter C, et al. 1999. Engraftment of *MDR1* and NeoR gene-transduced hematopoietic cells after breast cancer chemotherapy. *Blood* 94:52–61

60. Bunting KD, Galipeau J, Topham D, et al. 1998. Transduction of murine bone marrow cells with an MDR1 vector enables ex vivo stem cell expansion, but these expanded grafts cause a myeloproliferative syndrome in transplanted mice. *Blood* 92:2269–79

Annu. Rev. Med. 2002. 53:629–57

THALIDOMIDE: Emerging Role in Cancer Medicine

Paul Richardson, Teru Hideshima, and Kenneth Anderson
Jerome Lipper Myeloma Center, Division of Hematologic Oncology, Department of Adult Oncology, Dana-Farber Cancer Institute, Harvard Medical School, Boston, Massachusetts 02115; e-mail: paul_richardson@dfci.harvard.edu

Key Words immunomodulation, antiangiogenesis, myeloma

■ **Abstract** Thalidomide—removed from widespread clinical use by 1962 because of severe teratogenicity—has antiangiogenic and immunomodulatory effects, including the inhibition of tumor necrosis alpha factor. It has now returned to practice as an effective oral agent in the management of various disease states including erythema nodosum leprosum, for which it was approved by the U.S. Food and Drug Administration in 1998, and more recently certain malignancies, including multiple myeloma. Although thalidomide's mechanism of action remains incompletely understood, considerable insight has been generated by extensive preclinical studies in multiple myeloma. Moreover, clinical trials have confirmed benefit in relapsed disease, and the role of thalidomide in treating newly diagnosed patients is currently under study. Its use in other tumors is under evaluation, with promise in renal cell carcinoma, prostate cancer, glioma, and Kaposi's sarcoma. Activity has also been demonstrated in chronic graft-versus-host disease and in symptom relief as part of palliative care.

INTRODUCTION

A tragic event in the history of drug development occurred with the over-the-counter marketing of thalidomide in Europe during the late 1950s for the treatment of pregnancy-associated morning sickness. As early as 1961, reports of teratogenicity and dysmyelia (stunted limb growth) associated with thalidomide use prompted its subsequent withdrawal (1, 2). The return of thalidomide as a therapy in certain conditions stems from its broad array of pharmacoimmunologic effects (3). This rehabilitation was reflected by its approval in 1998 by the U.S. Food and Drug Administration for the short-term treatment of cutaneous manifestations of moderate to severe erythema nodosum leprosum (ENL), along with its use as maintenance therapy to prevent and suppress the cutaneous manifestations of ENL recurrence (3). Thalidomide has since became a treatment of choice for ENL, and its wide spectrum of activity has fostered its application in a variety of disease states (Table 1) (3–5). Because of its teratogenic effects, thalidomide is now used under strict guidelines to prevent fetal exposure to the drug (4).

TABLE 1 Potential therapeutic uses of thalidomide currently under investigation

Cancer and related conditions	Solid tumors (e.g., brain, breast, renal cell carcinoma); hematologic malignancies (e.g., multiple myeloma)
Infectious diseases	HIV/AIDS and related conditions; aphthous ulcerations; wasting syndrome; mycobacterial infections (e.g., tuberculosis)
Autoimmune diseases	Discoid and systemic lupus erythematosus; chronic graft-versus-host disease; inflammatory bowel disease; rheumatoid arthritis; multiple sclerosis
Dermatologic diseases	Behcet's syndrome; prurigo nodularis; pyoderma gangrenosum
Other disorders	Sarcoidosis; diabetic retinopathy; macular degeneration

In the field of medical oncology, the discovery of thalidomide's antiangiogenic properties has coincided with the emerging importance of angiogenesis in tumor growth and progression. Thalidomide has been shown to inhibit angiogenesis induced by basic fibroblast growth factor (β-FGF) in a rabbit cornea micropocket assay and by vascular endothelial growth factor (VEGF) in a murine model of corneal vascularization (6, 7). In human studies, the drug appears to undergo activation to metabolites with antiangiogenic activity (8). Because of these antiangiogenic properties, thalidomide is currently undergoing evaluation in the treatment of various solid tumors, multiple myeloma, and other hematologic malignancies (9–13). Results in multiple myeloma are particularly promising, although thalidomide's antiangiogenic effects are believed to be only part of its antimyeloma activity. Its other potential actions include modulation of adhesion molecules, inhibition of tumor necrosis alpha factor (TNF-α), downregulation of lymphocyte surface molecules, lowering of CD4:CD8 peripheral lymphocyte ratios, and direct effects on myeloma cells themselves (10, 14–18).

This chapter presents a comprehensive review of the pharmacology of thalidomide, a description of preclinical studies in multiple myeloma to illustrate the drug's complex putative mechanisms of action, and a description of clinical studies in multiple myeloma. Studies in other hematologic malignancies are also addressed, as is the status of research in solid tumors and in other cancer-related applications.

PHARMACOLOGY

Thalidomide is a derivative of glutamic acid and is pharmacologically classified as an immunomodulatory agent (19). Structurally, thalidomide contains two amide rings and a single chiral center (Figure 1); its full chemical name is alpha-N{phthalimido}glutarimide [$C13$ $O4$ $N2$ $H9$] and its gram molecular weight is 258.2 (19).

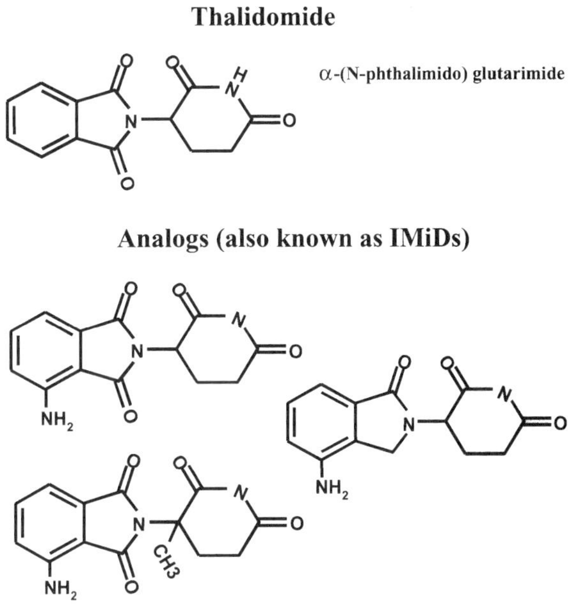

Thalidomide

α-(N-phthalimido) glutarimide

Analogs (also known as IMiDs)

Figure 1 Structures of thalidomide and its potent analogues, immunomodulatory drugs (IMiDs).

The currently available formulation is a nonpolar racemic mixture present as the optically active S and R isomers at physiologic pH, which can effectively cross cell membranes (19, 20). The S isomer has been linked to thalidomide's teratogenic effects, whereas the R isomer appears to be primarily responsible for its sedative properties (7, 20, 21). The isomers rapidly interconvert at physiologic pH in vivo, and thus efforts at formulating only the R isomer have failed to obviate the teratogenic potential of thalidomide (20, 22).

Pharmacokinetics

Pharmacokinetic analysis of thalidomide in humans has been limited by the absence of a suitable intravenous formulation, owing to the drug's instability and poor solubility in water. The pharmacokinetics of thalidomide have therefore been determined only from animal studies and in humans receiving the oral therapy. Single-dose thalidomide trials have been conducted in healthy volunteers, patients with HIV infection, and patients with hormone-refractory prostate cancer (23–27).

As Table 2 shows, the pharmacokinetics appear highly variable. Moreover, in patients with HIV infection, dose adjustments based on both ideal body weight and body surface did not affect this variability (23, 24). As a result of this variability, the pharmacokinetic properties of thalidomide in humans have not been well characterized, and this has confounded the definition of a dose-response effect against human cancer.

TABLE 2   Single dose pharmacokinetic parameters of thalidomide in humans (27)

Population	Dose	Mean apparent pharmacokinetic parameters		
		t_{max}	$t_{1/2}$ (L)	V_d (L)
Elderly patients with hormone-refractory	200 mg	3.3[*]	6.5	66.9
prostate cancer	800 mg	4.4[*]	18.3	165.8
Patients with HIV infection	300 mg	3.4	5.7	78.2
Healthy female volunteers	200 mg	5.8	4.1	53.0
Healthy male volunteers	200 mg	4.4	8.7	120.7

Abbreviations: t_{max}, time to reach maximum concentrations; $t_{1/2}$, elimination half-life; V_d, volume of distribution; HIV, human immunodeficiency virus.

[*]Median value.

Absorption

When oral thalidomide at a dose of 100 mg/kg has been administered in animal studies, maximum serum concentrations were reached within 4 h (28). Absorption was apparently independent of the administered doses and slower than drug elimination. Recent studies in humans show a similar pattern; thalidomide at 200 mg per dose reaches peak concentration (t_{max}) in a mean of ~4 h (23–25, 29).

Distribution

Animal studies have demonstrated a wide distribution of thalidomide throughout most tissues and organs (28). It is present in semen following oral administration in rabbits, but it is not known whether the drug is present in human semen (19, 30). Human pharmacokinetic studies to date also indicate that thalidomide has a large apparent volume of distribution (V_d) (24–26). Further, studies in elderly prostate cancer patients suggest variability in V_d, possibly due to alterations in absorption and plasma protein binding (24).

Metabolism

Thalidomide undergoes rapid and spontaneous nonenzymatic hydrolytic cleavage at physiologic pH to generate up to 50 metabolites, of which five are considered primary metabolites (8, 20, 22, 28, 31). Research efforts to better characterize the biologic properties of the specific metabolites have been complicated by their instability and rapid degradation under physiologic conditions (32). Whereas in vitro studies suggest thalidomide induces cytochrome P-450 isoenzymes in rats, recent evaluation of single- or multiple-dose pharmacokinetic parameters of oral thalidomide at 200 mg daily in healthy human volunteers has indicated that thalidomide does not inhibit or induce its own metabolism over a 21-day period in humans, and thus very little metabolism of thalidomide is thought to occur via the hepatic cytochrome P-450 system (26, 33, 34).

Excretion

Thalidomide appears to be rapidly excreted in urine as its metabolites, with the nonabsorbed portion of the drug excreted unchanged in feces. However, clearance is primarily nonrenal; mean terminal half-lives of the R and S isomers in healthy male human volunteers were measured at 4.6 and 4.8 h, respectively (23, 28, 29). In a study report of urinary excretion data for a single dose (200 mg daily), the elimination half-life was ~8 h, with minimal drug excretion over a 24-h period (23). Both single and multiple dosing of thalidomide in older prostate cancer patients revealed a significantly longer half-life at a higher dose (1200 mg daily) than at a lower dose (200 mg daily) (24). Conversely, no effect of increased age on elimination half-life was identified in the age range of 55–80 years (24). Thus, the effects of renal or hepatic dysfunction on the clearance of thalidomide remain unclear, and additional studies are needed to better characterize age-related or physiologic effects on drug clearance.

Drug Interactions

The only drug that has been systematically evaluated for interaction with thalidomide is oral hormonal contraceptives, which showed no significant interaction. Animal studies suggest that thalidomide enhances the sedative effects of barbituates and alcohol as well as the catatonic effects of chlorpromazine and reserpine. Central nervous system stimulants (including methamphetamine and methylphenidate) appear to counteract the depressant effects of thalidomide (35).

Potential Antitumor Effects

D'Amato et al., while evaluating thalidomide's mechanism of teratogenicity, found that it exhibited antiangiogenic properties (6, 7). They postulated that thalidomide inhibited angiogenesis by interrupting processes induced by β-FGF and/or VEGF (6, 7, 36). Further in vitro studies suggested that the antiangiogenic effect of thalidomide was due to specific metabolites and not the parent compound (37).

Another important property of thalidomide is that it selectively inhibits TNF-α production while leaving the patient's immune system otherwise intact (38). This has led to its application in various disorders characterized by abnormal TNF-α activity, including ENL, mycobacterium tuberculosis infection, graft-versus-host disease, rheumatoid arthritis, systemic lupus erythematosis, multiple sclerosis, Crohn's disease, cancer- and HIV-related cachexia, diabetes mellitus, and endotoxic shock.

The exact mechanism of thalidomide-induced TNF-α inhibition is unclear, but it does appear to differ from other TNF-α inhibitors such as pentoxyfylline and dexamethasone (39, 40). One mechanism postulated is that thalidomide inhibits TNF-α synthesis by accelerating degradation of TNF-α mRNA, resulting in a significant but incomplete suppression of TNF-α protein production (39, 41). Of particular interest is the recent demonstration that thalidomide decreases the binding activity of NF-κB which in turn controls activation of the TNF-α gene (42).

It has also been postulated that thalidomide's effect on angiogenesis may be through TNF-α inhibition, since TNF-α has proangiogenic effects (6). However, the absence of a demonstrable TNF-α effect in experimental models of angiogenesis, coupled with the inability of strong TNF-α inhibitors to directly influence angiogenesis, suggests that thalidomide's antiangiogenic activity is not related to TNF-α inhibition alone (6, 7).

Immunomodulatory Effects

Results of studies evaluating the effects of thalidomide on lymphocytes have been inconsistent (43–45). Emerging evidence suggests that thalidomide does not directly suppress lymphocyte proliferation (14). However, differential effects on T cell stimulation, shifts in T cell responses, and inhibition of proliferation of already stimulated lymphocytes have been shown (17, 44, 46–48). Modification of surface adhesion molecule on leukocytes, inhibition of neutrophil chemotaxis, and effects of cytokines other than TNF-α have been demonstrated, including the inhibition of interleukin (IL)-12 production, enhanced synthesis of IL-2, and inhibition of IL-6 (14, 16, 38, 49–51).

Adverse Effects

Common side effects reported during treatment with thalidomide are summarized in Table 3 (27). Sedation and constipation appear to be the most common adverse effects in cancer patients (9, 13, 36). The most serious adverse effect associated with thalidomide is peripheral neuropathy. There may also be an increased incidence of thromboembolic events, but this appears to be rare when the drug is used as a single agent. However, recent reports have shown thromboembolic complications to be more frequent when the drug is combined with steroids and particularly

TABLE 3   Clinical adverse events reported during thalidomide use (27)

Neurologic	Gastrointestinal	Dermatologic	Miscellaneous
Sedation	Constipation	Exfoliative/erythrodermic	Xerostomia
Dizziness	Nausea	Cutaneous reactions	Weight gain
Mood changes	Increased appetite	Brittle fingernails	Edema of face/limbs
Headaches		Pruritis	Reduction in thyroid hormone secretion
			Hypotension

with anthracycline-based chemotherapy, causing early cessation of one study exploring a combination of thalidomide with doxil and dexamethasone (52, 53). Possible cardiovascular effects of thalidomide include bradycardia and hypotension. The risk of adverse cardiovascular events appears greater in older patients with coronary disease taking multiple blood-pressure-lowering medications along with thalidomide (27).

It is well-known that thalidomide must not be used during pregnancy, and recommended contraceptive methods must be used by both men and women of childbearing potential. The System for Thalidomide Education and Prescribing Safety (STEPS), implemented to ensure the safe distribution of thalidomide, requires a patient's compliance with contraception guidelines and mandatory surveillance procedures. In addition, all healthcare providers who plan to prescribe and/or dispense thalidomide must be registered with the program (4).

Thalidomide-induced peripheral neuropathy commonly presents with numbness of the toes and feet, muscle cramps, weakness, signs of pyramidal tract involvement, and carpal tunnel syndrome (5, 19). Clinical improvement typically occurs upon prompt discontinuation of the drug, but long-standing sensory loss has been documented (54–57). Drug-related neuropathy is characterized as asymmetric, painful, peripheral paresthesia with sensory loss (5, 54–57). The risk of developing peripheral neuropathy during thalidomide treatment increases when high cumulative doses are administered and especially in the elderly (19).

In cancer patients, thalidomide should be used with caution when there is a prior history of neuropathy and when used in combination with other agents known to have neurotoxic effects (27). However, whether the incidence of thalidomide-induced peripheral neuropathy is increased in cancer patients with a history of vinca alkaloid use remains unknown. Safety data from current phase I and II clinical trials of thalidomide in the treatment of solid tumors, multiple myeloma, and hematologic malignancies suggest that peripheral neuropathy occurs in 10%–30% of patients (10, 12, 13, 58).

PRECLINICAL STUDIES OF THALIDOMIDE AND ITS ANALOGS IN MULTIPLE MYELOMA

Although thalidomide was initially used to treat multiple myeloma because of its antiangiogenic effects, the mechanism of its antimyeloma activity appears to be more complex (Figure 2). Preclinical studies of thalidomide and its potent analogs (also known as immunomodulatory drugs, IMiDs) suggest that these drugs act against myeloma in several ways. First, there appears to be a direct effect on the myeloma cell and/or bone marrow stromal cell, which inhibits tumor growth and survival. Second, adhesion of myeloma cells to bone marrow stromal cells (BMSCs) triggers secretion of cytokines, which augment myeloma cell growth and survival (59–61) and confer drug resistance (62); importantly, thalidomide modulates adhesive interactions (14) and thereby may alter tumor cell growth,

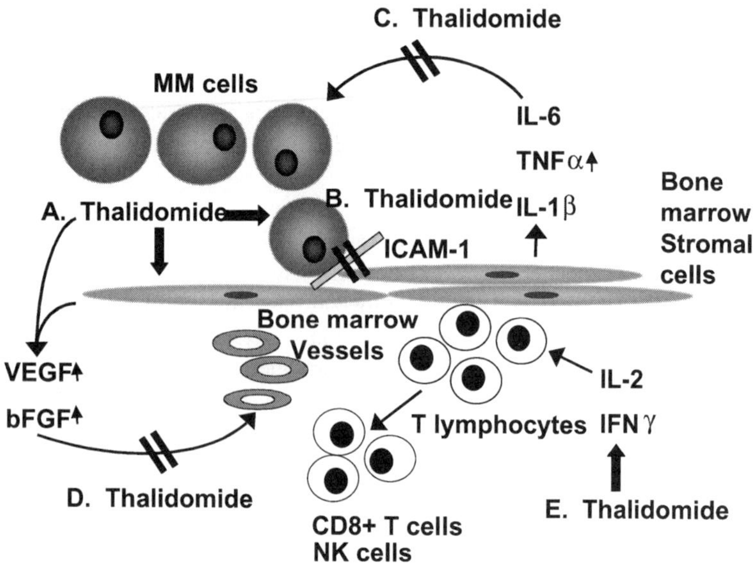

Figure 2 Possible effect of thalidomide on myeloma cells' and bone marrow stromal cells' (BMSCs') microenvironment in vivo. (*A*) Thalidomide directly inhibits myeloma cell growth. (*B*) Thalidomide inhibits myeloma cell adhesion to BMSCs. (*C*) Thalidomide blocks IL-6, TNF-α, and IL-1β secretion from BMSCs. (*D*) Thalidomide blocks the ability of VEGF and β-FGF to stimulate neovascularization of bone marrow. (*E*) Thalidomide induces IL-2 and INF-γ secretion from T cells.

survival, and drug resistance. Third, cytokines secreted into the bone marrow microenvironment by myeloma cells and/or BMSCs, such as IL-6, IL-1β, IL-10, and TNF-α may augment myeloma cell growth and survival (61, 63), and thalidomide may alter their secretion and bioactivity (64). Fourth, thalidomide decreases the secretion of VEGF, IL-6 (65), and βFGF by myeloma and/or BMSCs.

Since IL-6 is known to promote myeloma cell growth and survival, and VEGF has been demonstrated to induce myeloma cell migration (66), thalidomide may directly block tumor cell growth and migration, as well as inhibiting bone marrow angiogenesis (67, 68). Recent studies have demonstrated the direct antitumor activity of thalidomide and IMiDs on myeloma cells (18). IMiDs induce growth inhibition of myeloma cells in a dose-dependent fashion, with an IC$_{50}$ as low as 0.1–1 μM. IMiDs are effective against myeloma cell lines resistant to conventional chemotherapeutic agents such as doxorubicin, melphalan, or mitoxantrone, as well as dexamethasone. Moreover, thalidomide and the IMiDs enhanced the antitumor activity of dexamethasone (Figure 3*a*); conversely, these effects were partially inhibited by IL-6 (Figure 3*b*), a potent myeloma growth and antiapoptotic factor. IMiDs also showed significant activity against drug-resistant patient myeloma cells (Figure 4). The observed clinical activity of thalidomide in patients

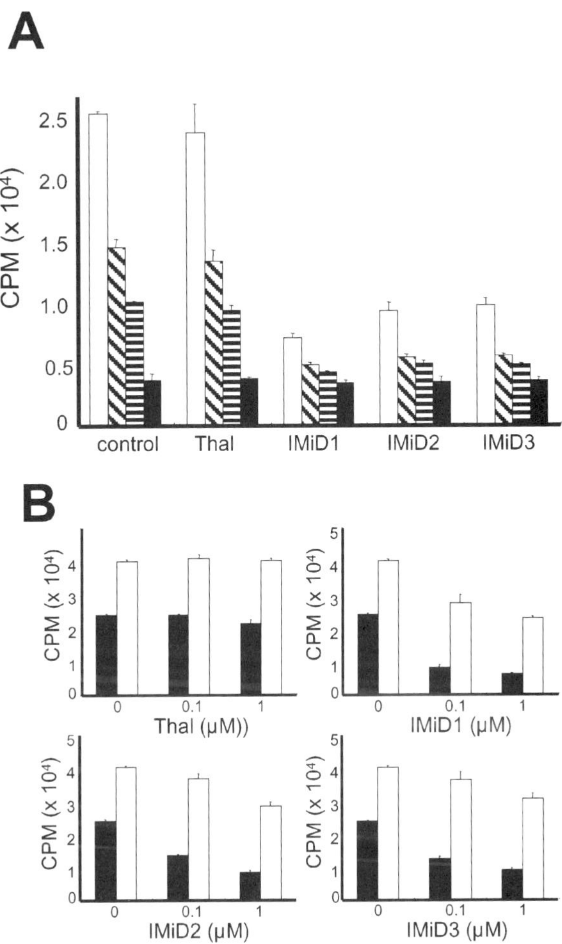

Figure 3   Effect of Dex and IL-6 on response of multiple myeloma cells to thalidomide and the IMiDs. (*a*) MM.1S cells were cultured with 1.0 μM thalidomide, IMiD1, IMiD2, or IMiD3 in control media alone ($\square$) or with 0.001 ($\boxtimes$), 0.01 ($\equiv$), and 0.1 μM ($\blacksquare$) Dex. (*b*) MM.1S cells were cultured in control media alone and with 0.1 and 1.0 μM thalidomide, IMiD1, IMiD2, or IMiD3 either in the presence ($\square$) or absence ($\blacksquare$) of IL-6 (50 ng/ml). In each case, ^{3}H-TdR uptake was measured during the last 8 h of 48-h cultures. Values represent the mean ($\pm$ SD) ^{3}H-TdR (cpm) of triplicate cultures.

with myeloma that is refractory to conventional therapies (69), coupled with our in vivo studies, suggests that thalidomide can overcome resistance to conventional treatments. In addition, our laboratory work suggests that dexamethasone can add to the antiproliferative effect of thalidomide and its analogs in vitro, suggesting potential utility of coupling these agents in novel therapeutics.

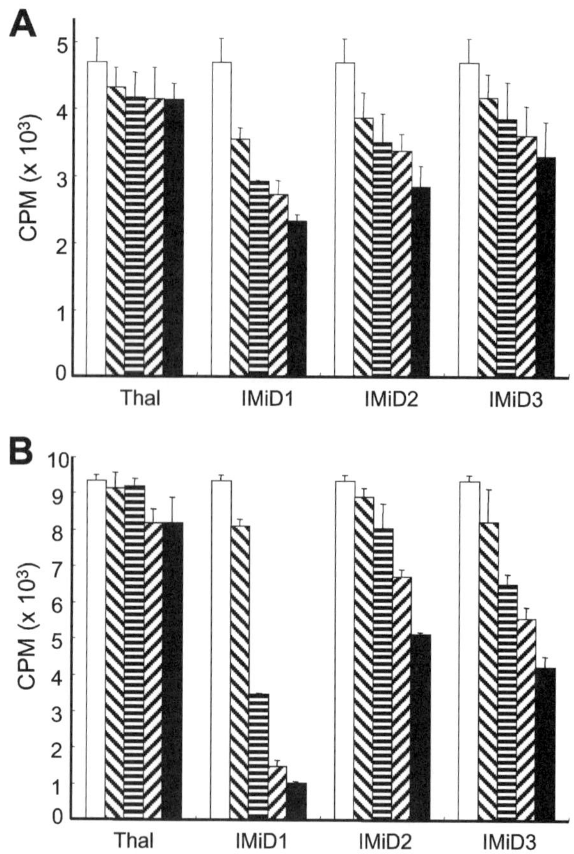

Figure 4   Effect of thalidomide and its analogs on DNA synthesis of patient multiple myeloma cells cultured with control media (□), or with 0.1 μM (▨), 1.0 μM (▤), 10 μM (▧), and 100 μM (■) thalidomide, IMiD1, IMiD2, or IMiD3. In each case, ^{3}H-TdR uptake was measured during the last 8 h of 48-h cultures. Values represent the mean ($\pm$ SD) ^{3}H-TdR (cpm) of triplicate cultures.

The mechanism of growth inhibition induced by thalidomide and its analogs is not totally understood. IMiDs, and to a lesser extent thalidomide, induce apoptosis of myeloma MM.1S cells, as evidenced both by increased sub-G1 cells on PI staining and by increased annexin V–positive cells. In these cells, which characteristically have wild-type p53, exposure to these agents (and dexamethasone) downregulates p21, thereby facilitating G1-to-S transition and enhanced susceptibility to apoptosis. Moreover, p27 is also upregulated by treatment with both thalidomide and IMiDs (T. Hideshima, et al., unpublished data). This profound apoptotic effect may correlate with the fact that complete responses to thalidomide are occasionally observed. The mechanism of thalidomide/IMiDs-induced apoptosis is also not entirely understood. However, our preliminary data indicate the participation of caspase-8 activation in thalidomide/IMiDs-induced apoptosis. IL-6 overcomes the downregulation of p21 induced by these agents, consistent with the increase in DNA synthesis triggered by IL-6 even in the presence of these drugs. In contrast, in Hs Sultan cells and AS cells, derived from a multiple myeloma patient, (which are both wild-type and mutant p53), the IMiDs and thalidomide induce p21 and related G1 growth arrest (Figure 5), thereby conferring protection from apoptosis, as has been observed in other systems (70, 71). Prior studies showed that p21 was constitutively expressed in the majority of myeloma cells and inhibited proliferation in both a p53-dependent and -independent fashion (72).

Previous reports that cells overexpressing p21 protein demonstrate chemoresistance (73) further support the notion that a protective effect of G1 growth arrest is induced by thalidomide and IMiDs in Hs Sultan- and AS-patient-derived myeloma cells. Conversely, the frequent regrowth of progressive myeloma noted

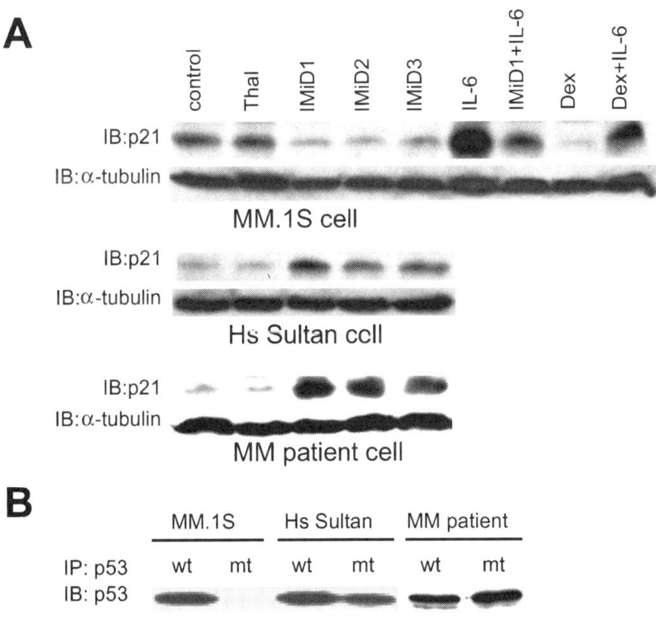

Figure 5 Effect of thalidomide and its analogs on p21 expression in multiple myeloma (MM) cell lines and patient cells. (*a*) MM.1S cells were cultured with 10 μM of thalidomide, IMiD1, IMiD2, and IMiD3 for 48 h. MM.1S cells were also cultured with IL-6 (50 ng/ml) alone and with IMiD1, 10 μM Dex, and Dex plus IL-6. Cells were lysed, subjected to SDS PAGE, transferred to PVDF membrane, and blotted with anti-p21 Ab. The membrane was stripped and reprobed with anti-α-tubulin Ab. (*b*) MM.1S, Hs Sultan, and patient MM cells were lysed and immunoprecipitated with wt-p53 and mt-p53 Ab, transferred to PVDF membrane, and blotted with anti-p53 Ab.

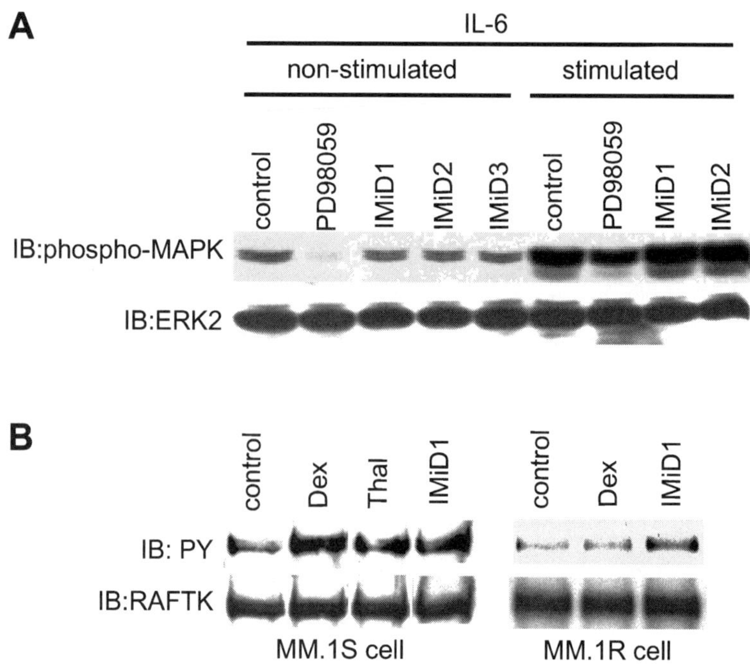

Figure 6 Effect of thalidomide and its analogs on growth and apoptotic signaling in myeloma cell lines, MM.1S and MM.1R cells. (*a*) MM.1S cells were cultured for 48 h in media, with 50 μM of PD98059, and with 10 μM of IMiD1, IMiD2, or IMiD3. Cells were then triggered with 50 ng/ml of IL-6 for 10 min, lysed, transferred to PVDF membrane, and blotted with anti-phospho MAPK Ab. Blots were stripped and reprobed with anti-ERK2 Ab. (*b*) MM.1S and MM.1R cells were treated with thalidomide (100 μM), IMiD 1 (100 μM), or Dex (10 μM) and harvested at 12 h. Total cell lysates were subjected to immunoprecipitation with anti-RAFTK Ab and analyzed by immunoblotting with anti-P-Tyr Ab or anti-RAFTK Ab.

clinically upon discontinuation of thalidomide treatment may correlate with release of drug-related G1 growth arrest. We have previously shown that related adhesion focal tyrosine kinase (RAFTK, Figure 6) mediated dexamethasone-induced myeloma cell apoptosis. Thalidomide and IMiDs, like dexamethasone, induced tyrosine phosphorylation of RAFTK, suggesting a key role of RAFTK in thalidomide- and IMiDs-induced apoptosis. Activation of RAFTK was also found in dexamethasone-resistant, IMiDs-sensitive MM.1R myeloma cells.

Recent studies have also demonstrated that myeloma cell lines and patient myeloma cells produce TNF-α (63). TNF-α in turn triggers IL-6 secretion from BMSCs in a dose-dependent fashion; importantly, TNF-α is a more potent stimulus of IL-6 secretion than TGF-β1 and VEGF (Figure 7). Remarkably, TNF-α also induces NF-κB activation and expression of LFA-1, ICAM-1, VCAM-1, and MUC-1 on myeloma cell lines, as well as ICAM-1 and VCAM-1 on BMSCs.

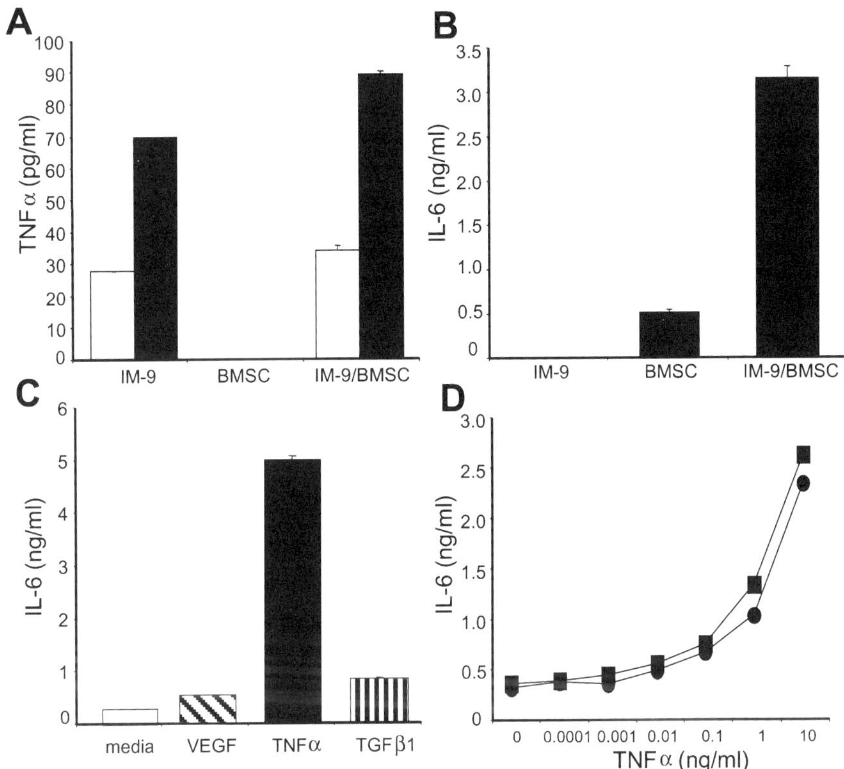

Figure 7 TNF-α secretion from IM-9 multiple myeloma (MM) cells stimulates IL-6 secretion from bone marrow stromal cells (BMSCs). (*a*) IM-9 MM cells, BMSCs, and both together were cultured for 24 h ($\square$) and 48 h ($\blacksquare$). (*b*) IM-9 myeloma cells, BMSCs, and both together were cultured for 48 h. (*c*) BMSCs were cultured for 48 h in the presence of media alone, VEGF (10 ng/ml), TNF-α (10 ng/ml), or TGF-β1 (10 ng/ml). (*d*) Two multiple myeloma patient BMSCs ($\blacksquare$, $\bullet$) were cultured for 24 h with TNF-α (0.0001–10 ng/ml). TNF-α (*a*) or IL-6 (*b*, *c*, *d*) levels were measured in culture supernatants by ELISA. Values represent the mean ($\pm$ SD) of triplicate cultures.

As a result, adherence of myeloma cells to BMSCs is significantly upregulated by TNF-α–related induction of these adhesion molecules. Adherence of myeloma cells to BMSCs induces drug resistance of myeloma cells, induces IL-6 secretion in BMSCs, and activates p44/42 MAPK in myeloma cells, thereby promoting tumor cell growth. Because thalidomide and its analogs are potent inhibitors of TNF-α production, they may not only act directly on myeloma cells but also act indirectly by inhibiting cytokine cross-talk in the myeloma/BMSC microenvironment. In conclusion, TNF-α induces an increase in proliferation, as well as MAPK/ERK activation, in myeloma cells, and it induces IL-6 secretion, as well as NF-κB activation, in BMSCs. TNF-α induces adhesion molecules on myeloma cells and BMSCs, increasing IL-6 secretion and the binding of myeloma cells to BMSCs; conversely, blockade of TNF-α–induced NF-κB activation inhibits these sequelae. These studies confirm a central role for TNF-α in the growth and survival of myeloma cells in the bone marrow milieu and suggest the utility of novel therapeutics targeting TNF-α in multiple myeloma.

Keifer et al. recently reported that thalidomide inhibited NF-κB activation triggered by TNF-α in Jurkat T cells (74). This inhibitory effect of thalidomide on NF-κB activation was mediated by suppression of IκB kinase (IKK) activity. Phosphorylation of IκBα, inhibitory molecule of NF-κB, by IKK is essential for degradation of IκBα. Since adherence of myeloma cells to BMSCs induces IL-6 secretion from BMSCs via NF-κB activation (60), and TNF-α induces adhesion molecules on both myeloma cells and BMSCs also via NF-κB activation, NF-κB may be a novel therapeutic target.

A recent study demonstrated that thalidomide and IMiDs augment natural killer (NK) cell cytotoxicity in multiple myeloma (75). This report showed that thalidomide and IMiDs do not induce T cell proliferation alone but act as co-stimulators to trigger proliferation of anti-CD3-stimulated T cells from multiple myeloma patients, accompanied by an increase in interferon-γ and IL-12 secretion. Treatment of patient peripheral blood mononuclear cells with thalidomide or IMiDs triggered increased lysis of autologous myeloma cells. Furthermore, patients showed an increase in CD3$^-$CD56$^+$ cells in response to thalidomide/IMiDs therapy. Lentzch et al. (76) demonstrated that thalidomide and IMiDs inhibited microvessel density in murine transplanted Hs Sultan cells, resulting in longer survival of IMiD-treated mice than of nontreated mice. These findings strongly support the antiangiogenic effect of thalidomide and IMiDs in vivo.

In summary, extensive preclinical studies in multiple myeloma provide a compelling basis for the development and testing of thalidomide and the IMiDs in a new treatment paradigm to target both the tumor cell and the microenvironment, overcome classical drug resistance, and improve outcome in this presently incurable disease.

CLINICAL STUDIES IN MULTIPLE MYELOMA

Despite recent advances in treatment, including transplantation, myeloma remains incurable and more effective therapies are clearly needed (77, 78). The development of resistance to chemotherapy and radiation, characteristic of myeloma, has spurred research in new biologically derived treatment strategies. The strategy of antiangiogenesis is based on observations that hematologic malignancies, such as multiple myeloma, are associated with intense neovascularization of bone marrow and thus may be angiogenesis-dependent (79, 80). However, although angiogenesis appears well-established as a key component in the growth, progression, and metastatic spread of solid tumors (81), its role in hematologic malignancy remains to be defined, and only relatively recently has clinical investigation suggested its potential in this setting (67, 69, 80, 82–84).

In 1994, Vacca and colleagues reported a high correlation between the extent of bone marrow angiogenesis and the labeling index (LI) of marrow plasma cells and disease activity in patients with multiple myeloma (80). Subsequent studies have confirmed extensive bone marrow vascularization in multiple myeloma (67, 69, 83, 84) and have associated poor prognosis with both elevated levels of angiogenic cytokines, such as β-FGF and VEGF, and increased bone marrow levels of mast cells, which secrete a variety of angiogenic factors (80, 83–85). Moreover, recent reports have shown increased bone marrow angiogenesis in acute lymphoblastic leukemia (ALL) in children (79). Collectively, these findings have provided the rationale for the use of antiangiogenic drugs in the treatment of multiple myeloma and other hematologic malignancies.

Thalidomide therapy for advanced refractory myeloma began after an encouraging initial experience in two patients at the University of Arkansas prompted a large phase II study, which assessed the efficacy and toxicity of single-agent thalidomide in relapsed and refractory multiple myeloma (69). The primary endpoint of this trial was paraprotein response. Additional endpoints included time to response and disease progression, event-free survival, overall survival, and improvement in other laboratory parameters. Of the 84 patients enrolled, 76 had relapsed after receiving high-dose chemotherapy. Oral thalidomide was administered as a single agent for a median of 80 days (range 2–46). The starting dose was 200 mg taken at night, and this was escalated by 200 mg every 2 weeks to a maximum of 800 mg. The median patient age was 58 years (range 38–77); the majority (73%) were men, and most patients (61%) had IgG myeloma. Chromosome 13 deletion, an unfavorable prognostic marker, was identified in 42% of patients. Analysis of baseline bone marrow biopsy showed that 21% of patients had >50% plasma cell infiltration of their marrow, and 15% had a plasma cell LI >1%. In the patients who received high-dose chemotherapy, the median time from therapy to study entry was 14 months.

The median duration of treatment with thalidomide was 80 days (range 2–465). Most patients received daily doses of 400 mg (86%), with fewer attaining 600 mg/day (68%) and 800 mg/day (55%). Response, defined as $\geq$25% reduction in serum or urine levels of paraprotein, was seen in 27 patients (32%). Remarkably, reductions by $\geq$90% in serum or urine levels of paraprotein were documented in 8 patients (2 with complete remission), and reductions in paraprotein levels were typically apparent within 2 months. In 78% of patients with response, decreases in plasma cell infiltration of bone marrow and increased hemoglobin values were seen. However, microvascular density in bone marrow was unchanged even in responders.

Adverse events, generally mild to moderate, increased in incidence with higher doses. Constipation was frequent but manageable with the use of laxatives. Neuropathy, characterized by paresthesia or numbness, was reported by 12% of patients at the 200 mg dose level and by 28% of patients receiving 800 mg daily. In most cases, this was reversible with dose reduction. Other mild to moderate side effects included weakness, fatigue, and somnolence, which occurred in 34% of patients at the 200 mg dose level and in 43% of those at the 800 mg dose level. More severe adverse events were infrequent (occurring in ≤10% of patients), and hematologic effects were rare. However, 9 patients discontinued thalidomide because of drug intolerance. One responding patient died suddenly on day 37, most likely from sepsis, but a possible relationship to thalidomide could not be ruled out. The incidence of myelosuppression was low; significant leukopenia, anemia, and/or thrombocytopenia occurred in <5% of patients. After 12 months of follow-up, Kaplan-Meier estimates of the mean event-free and overall survival for all patients were 22% and 58%, respectively. Additional patients have been enrolled since this landmark report, and evaluation of a total patient population of 169 is currently ongoing.

Alexanian & Weber recently reported a phase II trial of thalidomide in 45 myeloma patients resistant to conventional therapies (86). Forty-three patients were evaluable for response. Partial response or greater, defined by ≥50% reduction of serum myeloma production and/or ≥75% reduction of Bence-Jones protein, was achieved in 11 patients (26%). Side effects were mild, dose-related, and reversible after dose reduction or interruption of therapy. Consistent with other experiences, common side effects included constipation (66%), fatigue (60%), pruritis or rash (35%), unsteadiness (28%), numbness/tingling/tremor (25%), and dry mouth (24%). Less than 20% of patients experienced other problems, including peripheral edema and venous thrombosis in 3 patients. As in other reports, the authors concluded that thalidomide was active in myeloma and should be evaluated further, either in combination with other drugs or as maintenance therapy.

A smaller study reported on 16 patients (median age, 64) who received a similar oral regimen of thalidomide with a dose range of 200 mg/day for 2 weeks, increased by 200 mg/day every 2 weeks to a maximum of 800 mg/day (87). The median time from myeloma diagnosis to initiation of thalidomide therapy was 32 months. Twenty-five percent of patients had failed stem cell transplant and a majority (88%) had received two or more prior chemotherapy regimens before institution of thalidomide. All patients were evaluable for response. Four (25%) achieved partial response to therapy, defined as ≥50% reduction in serum and urine protein level with a response duration of 2–10 months. Adverse effects included constipation (25%), excessive sedation (25%), fatigue (25%), and rash (19%). A few patients experienced grade 3 sedation and constipation, and one patient discontinued treatment because of peripheral neuropathy and cardiac arrythmia (grade 3). The study therefore confirmed activity of thalidomide in patients with advanced myeloma. Future clinical studies will include correlative analysis of bone marrow angiogenesis, as well as the expression of VEGF, β-FGF, and their receptors to further explore in vivo whether the antimyeloma activity of thalidomide is associated with its antiangiogenic effects. Studies from Europe have since confirmed response rates of 36%–51% in both relapsed and refractory settings with thalidomide at dose ranges of 200 to 800 mg/day (88, 89).

Based on the impressive activity of single-agent thalidomide in refractory and relapsed multiple myeloma, the combination of thalidomide with chemotherapy and dexamethasone is being investigated (thalidomide has nonoverlapping toxicity and a different mechanism of action). Initial clinical experience at Arkansas has shown that the incorporation of thalidomide into the dexamethasone, cyclophosphamide, etoposide, and cisplatinum (DCEP) regimen can induce complete responses in patients with plasma cell leukemia and multiple myeloma (90). The same group is piloting the use of thalidomide in newly diagnosed patients who have received at least one prior cycle of induction chemotherapy. In an ambitious treatment program, patients receive induction chemotherapy with four sequential regimens that include DCEP and CAD (cyclophosphamide, adriamycin, and dexamethasone) followed by peripheral blood stem mobilization and an additional course of DCEP therapy. Eligible patients are then randomized to receive or not receive thalidomide and subsequently undergo tandem transplant. A further randomization follows, and patients receive either four courses of DCEP every three months or a more intense consolidation consisting of eight courses of DCEP and CAD for one year as part of so-called total therapy. Patients are maintained on interferon plus dexamethasone, with or without thalidomide. The results of these studies are awaited with great interest, but because of the complexity of the treatment strategy, meaningful interpretation of the role of thalidomide in this setting will be challenging.

Low-dose thalidomide in combination with dexamethasone and also in combination with biaxin has been reported to be active in relapsed disease in a number of studies (91), and the results of larger trials exploring such approaches are anticipated.

The combination of dexamethasone and thalidomide is under evaluation as therapy for previously untreated patients. The importance of prospective, controlled trials was highlighted by recent reports of life-threatening toxic epidermal necrolysis (19). Thalidomide undergoes spontaneous nonenzymatic cleavage to metabolites, and there is evidence that the levels of these metabolites are affected by dexamethasone. Thus, the use of this combination outside of a closely monitored clinical trial cannot be recommended. Similarly, caution should be exercised when combining thalidomide with other drugs that have the potential to interact with it such as sulphonamides and allopurinol. Moreover, a recent report of thrombotic events in patients treated with a novel combination of dexamethasone, thalidomide, and doxil raises further concerns regarding hypercoagulability, although this seems to be enhanced primarily when the drug is used with other potentially prothrombotic agents (53).

A particularly exciting new area of research involves the thalidomide derivatives. Two classes of such derivatives have been reported: the phosphodiesterase type 4 inhibitors that inhibit TNF-α but have little effect on T cell activation (so-called selective cytokine inhibitory drugs or SelCids), and the IMiDs, another group of phosphodiesterase type 4 inhibitors, which not only inhibit TNF-α but also markedly stimulate T cell proliferation and interferon-γ production. As described above, the IMiDs appear to have significantly greater potency than thalidomide, with a potentially more favorable toxicity profile. On this basis, phase I studies of CC-5013, also known as IMiD 3, are now under way in patients with refractory or relapsed multiple myeloma, and preliminary results are encouraging (92).

CLINICAL STUDIES IN ACUTE MYELOGENOUS LEUKEMIA, MYELODYSPLASTIC SYNDROMES, AND MYELOPROLIFERATIVE DISORDERS

In their seminal paper, Perez-Atayde et al. (79) showed that children with ALL had increased bone marrow vascularity and high urine levels of β-FGF at diagnosis compared with a control group of nonleukemic patients without marrow involvement. Microvessel density was noted to be significantly higher in patients with ALL than in controls. Remarkably, a three-dimensional reconstruction of marrow vascularity showed complex bulging of microvessels in ALL, but no such complex bulging was observed in the control group. Urine β-FGF levels were high in ALL patients before induction therapy, variable during induction, and normalized when complete response was achieved (79). After D'Amato et al. (6) demonstrated direct inhibition of β-FGF-stimulated angiogenesis in a rabbit cornea micropocket assay following oral administration of thalidomide, the therapeutic potential of thalidomide in inhibiting pathologic angiogenesis prompted clinical study in leukemia, with the therapeutic rationale further strengthened by inhibition of TNF-α production by thalidomide in stimulated monocytes (41). Clinical efficacy in a variety of inflammatory conditions, including graft-versus-host disease (GVHD) after allogeneic bone marrow transplantation and renal transplantation, further supports thalidomide's immunomodulatory properties (93–96). Of additional interest was the observation in one study of a reduced risk of leukemia relapse in patients who responded to thalidomide given for GVHD (95). Moreover, metabolites of thalidomide have been shown to have cytotoxic effects on leukemic cells through induction of morphologic differentiation in vitro (97). Given these data and other encouraging studies of thalidomide, clinical investigation has been initiated to assess the efficacy and tolerability of thalidomide in refractory and relapsed acute myelogenous leukemia (AML), high-risk myelodysplastic syndrome, chronic myelogenous leukemia (CML), and other myeloproliferative disorders.

Pilot studies in these settings have been reported in preliminary form (98). Table 4 summarizes the diagnoses in the first 28 patients treated, and Table 5 summarizes adverse effects reported during treatment with thalidomide.

In these studies, thalidomide was administered orally at an initial daily dose of 200 mg at bedtime, which was escalated by 200 mg each week if no grade 2 or greater toxicity was encountered. If grade 2 toxicity occurred, doses were maintained and not escalated. If toxicity persisted, doses were reduced. If grade 3 to 4 toxicity was observed by National Cancer Institute common toxicity

TABLE 4   Specific diagnoses of 28 patients with
hematologic malignancy treated with thalidomide

Diagnosis	No. of patients
Refractory or relapsing AML	10
Myelodyplastic syndromes	9
RAEB	6
RAEB-T	2
CMML-T	1
Ph-positive CML	4
Late chronic phase	2
Accelerated phase	1
Myeloid blastic phase	1
Other myeloproliferative disorders	5
Ph-negative CML	3
Myeloproliferative disorder with myelofibrosis	4
Idiopathic myelofibrosis	4
TOTAL	28

Abbreviations: AML, acute myelogenous leukemia; RAEB, refractory
anemia with excess blasts; RAEB-T, RAEB in transformation; CMML-T,
chronic myelomonocytic leukemia in transformation; Ph, Philadelphia
chromosome; CML, chronic myelogenous leukemia.

criteria, thalidomide was withheld until toxicity decreased to less than grade 3
(98).

In addition to routine clinical assessment every week and then at two- and four-
week intervals, assessed outcome measures included the effects of thalidomide on
bone marrow microvessel density and serum levels of VEGF and β-FGF. Patients
who received at least two weeks of thalidomide therapy were considered evaluable
for response, with response criteria dependent on their underlying disease.

Of the 9 evaluable AML patients reported, 1 achieved hematologic improvement. Of the 6 evaluable myelodysplastic patients, 1 achieved complete response.
Of 2 Philadelphia-chromosome–positive CML patients, 1 achieved stable disease. Of 5 patients with myeloproliferative disorders other than Philadelphia-
positive CML, 3 patients achieved hematologic improvement and 1 had stable
disease. On the basis of these results, a randomized phase II trial evaluating
first-line anthracyline-based combination chemotherapy with or without thalidomide in patients with poor-karyotype AML is ongoing at the M. D. Anderson
Cancer Center, and further studies in myeloprofilerative disease and myelodysplastic syndrome are under way (98).

TABLE 5   Adverse events reported during treatment with thalidomide

Adverse effect	No. (%) of patients
Fatigue	16 (57)
Neurotoxicity, reversible	12 (43)
Sedation, grade 1or 2	7
Confusion, grade 2	2
Paresthesias, grade 2	2
Orthostasis, grade 2	1
Gastrointestinal toxicity	12 (43)
Emesis, grade 1 or 2	2
Constipation, grade 1 or 2	10
Rash or skin dryness	9 (32)
Infection	7 (25)
Pneumonia	3
Cytomegalovirus	1
Cellulitis	1
Gastroenteritis	1
Chronic foot ulcer	1

CLINICAL STUDIES IN THE TREATMENT OF SOLID TUMORS AND OTHER CANCER-RELATED INDICATIONS

Given that neovascularization is required for the growth of solid tumors (99, 100), several studies of thalidomide in the treatment of solid tumors have been pursued. Brain tumor treatment is one example. Slow progress in the treatment of adult high-grade glioma in the past 20 years has stimulated a search for novel treatment strategies in these otherwise lethal neoplasms. Given that gliomas are vascular, angiogenesis inhibition has been studied as a logical approach in the treatment of this disease.

Fine et al. completed a phase II trial of thalidomide in the treatment of adult patients with previously radiated, recurrent high-grade glioma (101). Patients with a histologic diagnosis of anaplastic mixed glioma, anaplastic astrocytoma, or glioblastoma multiforme who had radiographic demonstration of tumor progression after standard external beam radiation, with or without chemotherapy, were eligible. Patients were initially treated with a relatively high dose of thalidomide of 800 mg/day, with increases of 200 mg/day every 2 weeks up to a final daily dose of 1200 mg. Patients were evaluated every 8 weeks for response, by both clinical and radiographic criteria. Of 39 patients accrued, 36 patients were evaluable for both toxicity and response. Constipation and sedation were the predominant toxicities. One patient developed grade 2 peripheral neuropathy after nearly a year of treatment. There were 2 objective radiographic partial responses (6%), 2 minor responses (6%), and 12 patients who appeared to have stable disease (33%). The median survival was 28 weeks, and 8 patients were alive >1 year after starting thalidomide, although almost all had tumor progression. Importantly, changes in serum levels of β-FGF were seen and correlated with time to tumor progression and overall survival. The authors concluded that thalidomide was generally well-tolerated and that there may be antitumor activity in a minority of patients with recurrent high-grade glioma. Future studies of thalidomide were recommended in combination with radiation and chemotherapy, along with additional analyses of surrogate markers of response such as β-FGF, which may reflect antiangiogenic activity and glioma growth. One criticism of this report was that neither responders nor survivors were identified by histology and that glioblastoma multiforme and anaplastic astrocytoma, though both high-grade gliomas, are associated with very different prognoses. Furthermore, the study population had relatively favorable prognostic features, including a median age of 49 years, good performance status in the majority, and no prior chemotherapy in nearly half of the patients enrolled. Moreover, other studies of thalidomide at a lower dose (100 mg/day) in relapsed glioma have reported less favorable overall response rates. Nonetheless, additional trials are being done to explore whether thalidomide has additive or synergistic value in recurrent and early-stage disease.

The experience in breast cancer has been less encouraging. In a recent phase II evaluation of thalidomide in patients with progressive metastatic breast cancer, 28 patients were randomized to receive daily doses of thalidomide at 200 mg/day or 800 mg/day for 8 weeks, subsequently escalated to 1200 mg/day for 8 weeks (101a). Pharmacokinetics and serum growth factor levels were evaluated. No patients had a true partial or complete response. On the 800 mg/day arm, 13 patients had progressive disease before 8 weeks of treatment were completed and 1 patient refused to continue. Dose reduction occurred because of somnolence in 7 patients. Successful dose escalation was achieved in only 5 cases. On the 200 mg/day arm, 12 patients had progressive disease by 8 weeks and 2 had stable disease after 8 weeks, one of whom was removed on week 11 because of grade 3 neuropathy, and the other had progressive disease by week 16. Other adverse events included constipation, fatigue, dry mouth, dizziness, nausea, anorexia, arrhythmia, headaches, skin rash, hypotension, and neutropenia, although no dose modifications were required. Evaluation of circulating angiogenic factors and pharmacokinetic studies failed to provide insight for the lack of drug efficacy. The authors concluded that single-agent thalidomide had little or no activity in patients with heavily pretreated breast cancer and recommended that any further studies include different populations and/or combinations with other agents using lower dose levels.

Other authors have also reported that the benefits of oral thalidomide in patients with advanced cancer are disappointing (102). However, in a recent phase II study of continuous low-dose thalidomide in patients with advanced melanoma, as well as renal cell, ovarian, and breast cancer, 3 of 18 patients with renal cell carcinoma showed partial response and an additional 3 patients experienced stabilization of disease after 6 months (81). Serum and urine concentrations of β-FGF, TNF-α, and VEGF were measured during treatment, and higher levels were associated with progressive disease. In this relatively large trial of 66 patients, thalidomide was administered orally at a daily dose of 100 mg at night. The drug was well-tolerated; no patients developed grade 3 or 4 toxicities, and only a small number of patients experienced mild peripheral neuropathy and lethargy. The authors concluded that further studies evaluating the use of thalidomide at higher doses for advanced renal cell cancer were warranted. In National Cancer Institute phase II trials, thalidomide has shown some evidence of clinical benefit in androgen-independent prostate cancer, prompting studies of thalidomide as neo-adjuvant therapy and in combination with paclitaxel and estramustine in a phase I/II study for the treatment of metastatic, androgen-independent disease.

The activity of thalidomide in AIDS-related Kaposi's sarcoma (KS) has attracted considerable research interest. Thalidomide already has established efficacy in the treatment of oral aphthous ulcers, HIV wasting syndrome, and HIV-related diarrhea, which are well-recognized manifestations of immune dysregulation in this setting. Given thalidomide's activity in the reduction of TNF-α by the accelerated degradation of its mRNA, and the drug's putative antiangiogenic effects, KS is an attractive target (94). In a recent phase II dose-escalation study, HIV-positive patients with biopsy-confirmed KS who had progressed over the 2 months prior to enrollment received an initial dose of 200 mg/day of oral thalidomide (95). Doses were increased to a maximum of 1000 mg/day for up to 1 year, and anti-HIV therapy was maintained during the study period. Of the 20 patients enrolled, aged 29–49 years, all were assessable for toxicity and 17 for response. Eight patients achieved partial response (47%; 95% CI, 23%–73%), and 2 patients had stable disease. The overall response rate was 40% (95% CI, 19%, -64%). The median thalidomide dose at the time of response was 500 mg/day (range 400–1000 mg/day). The median duration of drug treatment was 6.3 months and the median time to progression was 7.3 months. The authors concluded that oral thalidomide was well-tolerated in this population at doses up to 1000 mg/day given for as long as 12 months and that treatment induced clinically meaningful anti-KS responses in a sizeable subset of patients. Additional studies of thalidomide in the treatment of KS are ongoing.

The immunomodulatory and antiinflammatory properties of thalidomide have stimulated interest in the field of GVHD, and over the past decade thalidomide has become established as an adjunctive treatment for chronic GVHD (cGVHD) (103). Vogelsang et al. first demonstrated thalidomide to be safe and effective in 23 patients with cGVHD refractory to conventional treatment and in 21 patients with high-risk GVHD. They observed complete responses in 7 (30%) of 23 patients receiving thalidomide as drug salvage treatment and in 7 (33%) of 21 patients receiving this agent as primary therapy (104). The median duration of therapy was 240 days. Sedation and constipation were the major side effects, and 4 patients discontinued medication because of peripheral neuropathy. Subsequent reports confirmed these results in both adults and children, with the best responses seen in patients with predominantly mucocutaneous involvement by cGVHD (105, 106).

In a larger phase II trial, thalidomide was used as salvage therapy in 80 patients with refractory cGVHD who had failed to respond to prednisone or to prednisone and cyclosporin (107). Sixteen patients (20%) had a sustained response, with 9 complete responses and 7 partial responses. Median duration of response was 16 months, and again most responses were seen in patients with isolated mouth, skin, and liver GVHD but without severe sclerodermatous manifestations. It should be noted that patients were maintained on prednisone and cyclosporine during thalidomide therapy, and 36% of patients discontinued thalidomide because of side effects, which included sedation, constipation, or neuropathy. Skin rash and neutropenia, which had not been reported in prior studies of cGVHD, resulted in discontinuation of the drug in a few patients.

In a more recent study, thalidomide achieved a response in 38% of patients with refractory cGVHD and was well-tolerated. However, side effects including neutropenia and neuropathy led to early discontinuation, and a separate randomized placebo-controlled trial found that the duration of thalidomide treatment had been too short to assess its efficacy in controlling cGVHD (108). At this stage, thalidomide appears to have activity against cGVHD, but whether it should be used as a first-line treatment of cGVHD remains to be defined (11).

Clinical trials of thalidomide in patients with cachexia secondary to terminal cancer are under way, based on encouraging preliminary reports (109). A recent report has also described beneficial effects of the combination of thalidomide and irinotecan for the treatment of metastatic colorectal cancer, with abrogation of dose-limiting gastrointestinal toxicity, including diarrhea and nausea (110). Studies in palliative care have found thalidomide beneficial in relieving chronic nausea, insomnia, and profuse sweating, and as an adjunct in pain control (111).

CONCLUSION

New approaches are needed to target the biological processes associated with disease progression in multiple myeloma and other malignancies, including solid tumors. Antiangiogenic therapy is an appealing strategy for targeting resistant disease, and accumulating evidence suggests that the combination of cytotoxic chemotherapy and antiangiogenic therapy has greater antitumor effects than either strategy alone. Current data suggest that thalidomide, which has antiangiogenic as well as immunomodulatory properties, has major activity in patients with multiple myeloma and holds promise in the treatment of other hematologic malignancies. Results in solid tumors are less encouraging, but patients with certain tumors, such as glioma or renal cell prostate cancer, may benefit. The use of thalidomide in the management of certain treatment-related complications, such as cGVHD, or for the relief of symptoms related to advanced malignancy, are also noteworthy. Finally, the emergence of thalidomide derivatives with considerable potential for improved efficacy and less toxicity provide an exciting platform for future therapies in a wide array of cancers.

ACKNOWLEDGMENT

The authors gratefully acknowledge the contribution of Reggie Deocampo in the preparation of the manuscript.

Visit the Annual Reviews home page at www.AnnualReviews.org

LITERATURE CITED

1. Lenz W. 1968. The susceptible period for thalidomide malformations in man and monkey. *Ger. Med. Mon.* 4:197–98
2. Lenz W. 1996. Malformations caused by drugs in pregnancy. *Am. J. Dis. Child.* 2: 99–106
3. Hales BF. 1999. Thalidomide on the comeback trail. *Nat. Med.* 5:489–90
4. Zeldis JB, Williams BA, Thomas SD, El-sayed ME. 1999. S.T.E.P.S™: a comprehensive program for controlling and monitoring access to thalidomide. *Clin. Ther.* 21:319–30
5. Stirling DI. 1998. Thalidomide and its impact in dermatology. *Semin. Cutan. Med. Surg.* 17:231–42
6. D'Amato RJ, Loughnan MS, Flynn E, Folkman J. 1994. Thalidomide is an inhibitor of angiogenesis. *Proc. Natl. Acad. Sci. USA* 91:4082–85
7. Kenyon BM, Browne F, D'Amato RJ. 1997. Effects of thalidomide and related metabolites in a mouse corneal model of neovascularization. *Exp. Eye Res.* 64: 971–78
8. Bauer KS, Dixon SC, Figg WD. 1998. Inhibition of angiogenesis by thalidomide requires metabolic activation, which is species-dependent. *Biochem. Pharmacol.* 55:1827–34
9. Eisen T, Boshoff C, Vaughan M, et al. 1998. Anti-angiogenic treatment of meta-static melanoma, renal cell, ovarian and breast cancers with thalidomide: a phase II study. *Proc. Am. Soc. Clin. Oncol.* 17: 441a (Abstr.)
10. Figg WD, Bergan R, Brawley O, et al. 1997. Randomized, phase II study of thalidomide in androgen-independent prostate cancer (AIPC). *Proc. Am. Soc. Clin. Oncol.* 16:333a (Abstr.)
11. Fine HA, Loeffler JS, Kyritsis A, et al. 1997. A phase II trial of the anti-angiogenic agent, thalidomide, in patients with recurrent high-grade gliomas. *Proc. Am. Soc. Clin. Oncol.* 16:385a (Abstr.)
12. Long G, Vredenburgh J, Rizzieri DA, et al. 1998. Pilot trial of thalidomide post-autologous peripheral blood progenitor cell transplantation (PBPC) in patients with metastatic breast cancer. *Proc. Am. Soc. Clin. Oncol.* 17:181a (Abstr.)
13. Marx GM, Levi JA, Bell DR, et al. 1999. A phase I/II trial of thalidomide as an antiangiogenic agent in the treatment of advanced cancer. *Proc. Am. Soc. Clin. Oncol.* 18:454a (Abstr.)
14. Geitz H, Handt S, Zwingenberger K. 1996. Thalidomide selectively modulates the density of cell surface molecules involved in the adhesion cascade. *Immunopharmacology* 31:213–21
15. Sampaio EP, Kaplan G, Miranda A, et al. 1993. The influence of thalidomide on the

clinical and immunologic manifestation of erythema nodosum leprosum. *J. Infect. Dis.* 168:408–14

16. Nogueira AC, Neubert R, Helge H, Neubert D. 1994. Thalidomide and the immune system. simultaneous up- and down-regulation of different integrin receptors on human white blood cells. *Life Sci.* 55:77–92

17. Shannon EJ, Ejigu M, Haile-Mariam HS, et al. 1992. Thalidomide's effectiveness in erythema nodosum leprosum is associated with a decrease in CD4+ cells in the peripheral blood. *Lepr. Rev.* 63:5–11

18. Hideshima T, Chauhan D, Shima Y, et al. 2000. Thalidomide and its analogs overcome drug resistance of human multiple myeloma cells to conventional therapy. *Blood* 96:2943–50

19. Tseng S, Pak G, Washenik K, et al. 1996. Rediscovering thalidomide: a review of its mechanism of action, side effects, and potential uses. *J. Am. Acad. Dermatol.* 35:969–79

20. Muller GW. 1997. Thalidomide: from tragedy to new drug discovery. *Chemtech* 1997:210–15

21. Reist M, Carrupt PA, Francotte E, Testa B. 1998. Chiral inversion and hydrolysis of thalidomide: mechanisms and catalysis by bases and serum albumin, and chiral stability of teratogenic metabolites. *Chem. Res. Toxicol.* 11:1521–28

22. Eriksson T, Bjorkman S, Roth B, et al. 1995. Stereospecific determination, chiral inversion in vitro and pharmacokinetics in humans of the enantiomers of thalidomide. *Chirality* 7:44–52

23. Chen TL, Vogelsang GB, Petty BG, et al. 1989. Plasma pharmacokinetics and urinary excretion of thalidomide after oral dosing in healthy male volunteers. *Drug Metab. Dispos.* 17:402–5

24. Figg WD, Raje S, Bauer KS, et al. 1999. Pharmacokinetics of thalidomide in an elderly prostate cancer population. *J. Pharmacol. Sci.* 88:121–25

25. Piscitelli SC, Figg WD, Hahn B, et al. 1997. Single-dose pharmacokinetics of thalidomide in human immunodeficiency virus-infected patients. *Antimicrob. Agents Chemother.* 41:2797–99

26. Scheffler MR, Colburn W, Kook KA, Thomas SD. 1999. Thalidomide does not alter estrogen-progesterone hormone single dose pharmacokinetics. *Clin. Pharmacol. Ther.* 65:483–90

27. Stirling DI. 2000. The pharmacology of thalidomide. *Semin. Hematol.* 37:5–14

28. Faigle JW, Keberle H, Friess W, et al. 1962. The metabolic fate of thalidomide. *Experientia* 18:389–97

29. Teo SK, Colburn WA, Thomas SD. 1999. Single-dose oral pharmacokinetics of three formulations of thalidomide in healthy male volunteers. *J. Clin. Pharmacol.* 39:1162–68

30. Ludwak-Mann C, Schmid K, Keberle H. 1967. Thalidomide in rabbit semen. *Nature* 214:1018–20

31. Schumacher H, Smith RL, Williams RT. 1965. The metabolism of thalidomide: the spontaneous hydrolysis of thalidomide in solution. *Br. J. Pharmacol.* 25:324–27

32. Fabro S, Schumacher H, Smith RL, Stagg RB, Williams RT. 1965. The metabolism of thalidomide: some biological effects of thalidomide and its metabolites. *Br. J. Pharmacol.* 25:352–62

33. Tsambaos D, Bolsen K, Georgiou S, et al. 1994. Effects of oral thalidomide on rat liver and skin microsomal P450 isozyme activities and on urinary porphyrin excretion: interaction with oral hexachlorobenzene. *Arch. Dermatol. Res.* 286:347–49

34. Wiener H, Krivanek P, Tuisl E, Kolassa N. 1980. Induction of drug metabolism in the rat by taglutimide, a sedative-hypnotic glutarimide derivative. *Eur. J. Drug Metab. Pharmacokinet.* 5:93–97

35. Somers GF. 1960. Pharmacological properties of thalidomide (α-phthalimido glutarimide), a new sedative hypnotic drug. *Br. J. Pharmacol.* 15:111–16

36. Kotoh T, Dhar DK, Masunaga R, et al. 1999. Anti-angiogenic therapy of human

esophageal cancers with thalidomide in nude mice. *Surgery* 125:536–44

37. Hastings RC, Trautman JR, Enna CD, Jacobson RR. 1970. Thalidomide in the treatment of erythema nodosum leprosum: with a note on selected laboratory abnormalities in erythema nodosum leprosum. *Clin. Pharmacol. Ther.* 11:481–87

38. Dunzendorfer S, Schratzberger P, Reinisch N, et al. 1997. Effects of thalidomide on neutrophil respiratory burst, chemotaxis, and transmigration of cytokine- and endotoxin-activated endothelium. *Naunyn Schmiedebergs Arch. Pharmacol.* 356:529–35

39. Moreira AL, Sampaio EP, Zmuidzinas A, et al. 1993. Thalidomide exerts its inhibitory action on tumor necrosis factor alpha by enhancing mRNA degradation. *J. Exp. Med.* 177:1675–80

40. Calderon P, Anzilotti M, Phelps R. 1997. Thalidomide in dermatology. New indications for an old drug. *Int. J. Dermatol.* 36:881–87

41. Sampaio EP, Sarno EN, Galilly R, et al. 1991. Thalidomide selectively inhibits tumor necrosis factor alpha production by stimulated human monocytes. *J. Exp. Med.* 173:699–703

42. Turk BE, Jiang H, Liu JO. 1996. Binding of thalidomide to 1-acid glycoprotein may be involved in its inhibition of TNF production. *Proc. Natl. Acad. Sci. USA* 93:7552–56

43. Fernandez LP, Schlegel PG, Baker J, et al. 1995. Does thalidomide affect IL-2 response and production? *Exp. Hematol.* 23:978–85; erratum, 1995. *Exp. Hematol.* 23(12):1324

44. Keenan RJ, Eiras G, Burckart GJ, et al. 1991. Immunosuppressive properties of thalidomide. Inhibition of in vitro lymphocyte proliferation alone and in combination with cyclosporine or FK506. *Transplantation* 52:908–10

45. Moncada B, Baranda ML, Gonzalez-Amaro R, et al. 1985. Thalidomide—effect on T cell subsets as a possible mechanism of action. *Int. J. Lepr. Other Mycobact. Dis.* 53:201–5

46. Haslett P, Hempstead M, Seidman C, et al. 1997. The metabolic and immunologic effects of short-term thalidomide treatment of patients infected with the human immunodeficiency virus. *AIDS Res. Hum. Retroviruses* 13:1047–54

47. McHugh SM, Rifkin IR, Deighton J, et al. 1995. The immunosuppressive drug thalidomide induces T helper cell type 2 (Th2) and concomitantly inhibits Th1 cytokine production in mitogen- and antigen-stimulated human peripheral blood mononuclear cell cultures. *Clin. Exp. Immunol.* 99:160–67

48. Haslett PA, Corral LG, Albert M, Kaplan G. 1998. Thalidomide costimulates primary human T lymphocytes, preferentially inducing proliferation, cytokine production, and cytotoxic responses in the CD8+ subset. *J. Exp. Med.* 187:1885–92

49. Rowland TL, McHugh SM, Deighton J, et al. 1998. Differential regulation by thalidomide and dexamethasone of cytokine expression in human peripheral blood mononuclear cells. *Immunopharmacology* 40:11–20

50. Moller DR, Wysocka M, Greenlee BM, et al. 1997. Inhibition of IL-12 production by thalidomide. *J. Immunol.* 159:5157–61

51. Shannon EJ, Sandoval F. 1995. Thalidomide increases the synthesis of IL-2 in cultures of human mononuclear cells stimulated with Concanavalin-A, Staphylococcal enterotoxin A, and purified protein derivative. *Immunopharmacology* 31:109–16

52. Weber DM, Rankin K, Gavino M. 2000. Thalidomide with dexamethasone for resistant multiple myeloma. *Blood* 96:167a (Abstr.)

53. Osman K, Comenzo R, Rajkumar SV. 2001. Deep venous thrombosis and thalidomide therapy for multiple myeloma. *N. Engl. J. Med.* 21:1951–52

54. Mellin GW, Katzenstein M. 1962. The

saga of thalidomide (concluded): Neuropathy to embryopathy, with case reports of congenital anomalies. *N. Engl. J. Med.* 267:1238–44

55. Aronson IK, Yu R, West DP, et al. 1984. Thalidomide-induced peripheral neuropathy. Effect of serum factor on nerve cultures. *Arch. Dermatol.* 120:1466–70

56. Clemmensen OJ, Olsen PZ, Andersen KE. 1984. Thalidomide neurotoxicity. *Arch. Dermatol.* 120:338–41

57. Fullerton PM, O'Sullivan DJ. 1968. Thalidomide neuropathy: a clinical, electrophysiological, and histological follow-up study. *J. Neurol. Neurosurg. Psychiatry* 31:543–51

58. Singhal S, Mehta J, Eddlemon P, et al. 1998. Marked anti-tumor effect from anti-angiogenesis (AA) therapy with thalidomide (T) in high risk refractory multiple myeloma (MM). *Blood* 92:318a (Abstr.)

59. Uchiyama H, Barut BA, Mohrbacher AF, et al. 1993. Adhesion of human myeloma-derived cell lines to bone marrow stromal cells stimulates interleukin-6 secretion. *Blood* 82:3712–20

60. Chauhan D, Uchiyama H, Akbarali Y, et al. 1996. Multiple myeloma cell adhesion-induced interleukin-6 expression in bone marrow stromal cells involves activation of NF-kappa B. *Blood* 87:1104–12

61. Hallek M, Bergsagel PL, Anderson KC. 1998. Multiple myeloma: increasing evidence for a multistep transformation process. *Blood* 91:3–21

62. Damiano JS, Cress AE, Hazlehurst LA, et al. 1999. Cell adhesion mediated drug resistance (CAM-DR): role of integrins and resistance to apoptosis in human myeloma cell lines. *Blood* 93:1658–67

63. Hideshima T, Chauhan D, Schlossman RL, Richardson P, Anderson KC. 2001. The role of tumor necrosis factor α in the pathophysiology of human multiple myeloma: therapeutic applications. *Oncogene* 20:4519–27

64. Corral LG, Haslett PA, Muller GW, et al. 1999. Differential cytokine modulation and T cell activation by two distinct classes of thalidomide analogues that are potent inhibitors of TNF-alpha. *J. Immunol.* 163:380–86

65. Gupta D, Treon SP, Shima Y, et al. 2001. Adherence of multiple myeloma cells to bone marrow stromal cells upregulates vascular endothelial growth factor secretion: therapeutic applications. *Leukemia.* In press

66. Podar K, Tai Y-T, Davies FE, et al. 2001. Vascular endothelial growth factor (VEGF) triggers signaling cascades mediating multiple myeloma cell growth and migration. *Blood* 98:428–35

67. Vacca A, Ribatti D, Presta M, et al. 1999. Bone marrow neovascularization, plasma cell angiogenic potential, and matrix metalloproteinase-2 secretion parallel progression of human multiple myeloma. *Blood* 93:3064–73

68. Bellamy WT, Richter L, Frutiger Y, Grogan TM. 1999. Expression of vascular endothelial growth factor and its receptors in hematopoietic malignancies. *Cancer Res.* 59:728–33

69. Singhal S, Mehta J, Desikan R, et al. 1999. Antitumor activity of thalidomide in refractory multiple myeloma. *N. Engl. J. Med.* 341:1565–71; erratum, 2000. *N. Engl. J. Med.* 342(5):364

70. Jung J-M, Brunet JM, Ruan S, et al. 1998. Increased level of p21[WAF1,CIP1] in human brain tumors. *Oncogene* 11:2021–28

71. Polyak K, Waldman T, He TC, et al. 1996. Genetic determinants of p53-induced apoptosis and growth arrest. *Genes Dev.* 10:1945–52

72. Urashima M, Teoh G, Chauhan D, et al. 1997. Interleukin-6 overcomes p21WAF1 upregulation and G1 growth arrest induced by dexamethasone and interferon-gamma in multiple myeloma cells. *Blood* 90:279–89

73. Chauhan D, Pandey P, Ogata A, et al. 1997. Cytochrome c-dependent and -independent induction of apoptosis in multiple

myeloma cells. *J. Biol. Chem.* 272:29995–97

74. Keifer JA, Guttridge DC, Ashburner BP, Baldwin JAS. 2001. Inhibition of NF-κB activity by thalidomide through suppression of IκB kinase activity. *J. Biol. Chem.* In press

75. Davies FE, Raje N, Hideshima T, et al. 2001. Thalidomide and immunomodulatory derivatives augment natural killer cell cytotoxicity in multiple myeloma. *Blood* 210–16

76. Lentzch S, LeBlank R, Podar K, et al. 2001. Thalidomide and its immunomodulatory drug inhibit multiple myeloma cell growth and angionenesis in vivo. *Blood.* In press

77. Anderson KC, Hamblin TJ, Traynor A. 1999. Management of multiple myeloma today. *Semin. Hematol.* 36:3–8

78. Stevenson F, Anderson KC. 1999. Introduction to immunotherapy for multiple myeloma—insights and advances. *Semin. Hematol.* 36:1–2

79. Perez-Atayde AR, Sallan SE, Tedrow U, et al. 1997. Spectrum of tumor angiogenesis in the bone marrow of children with acute lymphoblastic leukemia. *Am. J. Pathol.* 150:815–21

80. Vacca A, Ribatti D, Roncali L, et al. 1994. Bone marrow angiogenesis and progression in multiple myeloma. *Br. J. Haematol.* 87:503–8

81. Eisen T, Boshoff C, Mak I, et al. 2000. Continuous low dose thalidomide: a phase II study in advanced melanoma, renal cell, ovarian and breast cancer. *Br. J. Cancer* 82:812–17

82. Munshi N, Wilson CS, Penn J, et al. 1998. Angiogenesis in newly diagnosed multiple myeloma: poor prognosis with increased microvessel density (MVD) in bone marrow biopsies. *Blood* 92:92a (Abstr.)

83. Rajkumar SV, Fonseca R, Witzig TE, et al. 1999. Bone marrow angiogenesis in patients achieving complete response after stem cell transplantation for multiple myeloma. *Leukemia* 13:469–72

84. Nguyen M, Tran C, Barsky S, et al. 1997. Thalidomide and chemotherapy combination: preliminary results of preclinical studies. *Int. J. Oncol.* 10:965–69

85. Ribatti D, Vacca A, Nico B, et al. 1999. Bone marrow angiogenesis and mast cell density increase simultaneously with progression of human multiple myeloma. *Br. J. Cancer* 79:451–55

86. Alexanian R, Webes D. 2000. Thalidomide for resistant and relapsing myeloma. *Semin. Hematol.* 37:22–25

87. Rajkumar SV, Fonseca R, Dispenzieri A, et al. 2000. Thalidomide in the treatment of relapsed multiple myeloma. *Mayo Clin. Proc.* 75:897–901

88. Hus M, Dmoszynska A, Soroka-Wojtaszko, et al. 2001. Thalidomide treatment of resistant or relapsed multiple myeloma patients. *Haematologica* 86:404–8

89. Tosi P, Ronconi S, Zamagni E, et al. 2001. Salvage therapy with thalidomide in multiple myeloma patients relapsing after autologous peripheral blood stem cell transplantation. *Haematologica* 86:409–13

90. Barlogie B, Desikan R, Munshi N, et al. 1999. Single course D.T. PACE anti-angiochemotherapy effects CR in plasma cell leukemia and fulminant multiple myeloma (MM). *Blood* 92:273b (Abstr.)

91. Coleman M, Leonard JP, Nahum K, Michaeli J. 2000. Non-myeloppressive therapy with BLT-DC (Biaxin, low-dose thalidomide and dexamethasone) is highly active in Waldenstrom's macroglobunemia and myeloma. *Blood* 96:167a (Abstr.)

92. Richardson P, Schlossman R, Hideshima T, et al. 2001. A phase I study of the safety and efficacy of CC5013 treatment for patients with relapsed multiple myeloma: preliminary results. VIIIth Int. Myeloma Workshop, May 2001 (Abstr.)

93. Ghigliotti G, Repetto T, Farris A, et al. 1993. Thalidomide: treatment of choice

for aphthous ulcers in patients seropositive for human immunodeficiency virus. *J. Am. Acad. Dermatol.* 28:271–72

94. Jacobson JM, Greenspan JS, Spritzler J, et al. 1997. Thalidomide for the treatment of oral aphthous ulcers in patients with human immunodeficiency virus infection. National Institute of Allergy and Infectious Diseases AIDS Clinical Trials Group. *N. Engl. J. Med.* 336:1487–93

95. Kulkarni S, Powles R, Mehta J, et al. 1998. Thalidomide in GVHD—Is anti-GVHD effect separable from anti-angiogenesis? *Blood* 92:344b (Abstr.)

96. Vogelsang GB, Hess AD, Santos GW. 1988. Thalidomide for the treatment of graft-versus-host disease. *Bone Marrow Transplant.* 3:393–98

97. Hatfill SJ, Fester ED, de Beer DP, et al. 1991. Induction of morphological differentiation in the human leukemic cell line K562 by exposure to thalidomide metabolites. *Leukemia Res.* 15:129–36

98. Thomas DA. 2000. Thalidomide in acute myelogenous leukemia, myelodysplastic syndromes and myeloproliferative disorders. *Semin. Hematol.* 37:26–34

99. Folkman J. 1995. Angiogenesis in cancer, vascular, rheumatoid and other disease. *Nat. Med.* 1:27–31

100. Folkman J. 1995. Clinical applications of research on angiogenesis. *N. Engl. J. Med.* 333:1757–63

101. Fine HA, Figg WD, Jaeckle K, et al. 2000. Phase II trial of the antiangiogenic agent thalidomide in patients with recurrent high-grade gliomas. *J. Clin. Oncol.* 18:708–15

101a. Baidas SM, Winer EP, Fleming GF, et al. 2000. Phase II evaluation of thalidomide in patients with metastatic breast cancer. *J. Clin. Oncol.* 18:2710–17

102. Gutheil J, Finucane D. 2000. Thalidomide therapy in refractory solid tumour patients. *Br. J. Haematol.* 110:754

103. Gaziev D, Galimberti M, Lucarelli G, Polchi P. 2000. Chronic graft-versus-host disease: Is there an alternative to the conventional treatment? *Bone Marrow Transplant.* 25:689–96

104. Vogelsang GB, Farmer ER, Hess AD, et al. 1992. Thalidomide for the treatment of chronic graft-versus-host disease. *N. Engl. J. Med.* 326:1055–58

105. Heney D, Norfolk DR, Wheeldon J, et al. 1991. Thalidomide treatment for chronic graft-versus-host disease. *Br. J. Haematol.* 78:23–27

106. Rovelli A, Arrigo C, Nesi F, et al. 1998. The role of thalidomide in the treatment of refractory chronic graft-versus-host disease following bone marrow transplantation in children. *Bone Marrow Transplant* 21:577–81

107. Parker PM, Chao N, Nademanee A, et al. 1995. Thalidomide as salvage therapy for chronic graft-versus-host disease. *Blood* 86:3604–9

108. Browne PV, Weisdorf DJ, DeFor T, et al. 2000. Response to thalidomide therapy in refractory chronic graft-versus-host disease. *Bone Marrow Transplant.* 26:865–69

109. Bruera E, Neumann CM, Pituskin E, et al. 1999. Thalidomide in patients with cachexia due to terminal cancer: preliminary report. *Ann. Oncol.* 10:857–59

110. Govindarajan R, Heaton KM, Broadwater R, et al. 2000. Effect of thalidomide on gastrointestinal toxic effects of irinotecan. *Lancet* 356:566–67

111. Peuckmann V, Fisch M, Bruera E. 2000. Potential novel uses of thalidomide: focus on palliative care. *Drugs* 60:273–92

SUBJECT INDEX

CUMULATIVE INDEXES

CONTRIBUTING AUTHORS, VOLUMES 49–53

CHAPTER TITLES, VOLUMES 49–53

Cardiovascular System

Hematology/Oncology

HIV

Immunology

Infectious Diseases

Kidney and Urinary System

Prefatory

Psychiatry

Respiratory System

Surgery